Uniquest Series
PHYSIOLOGY

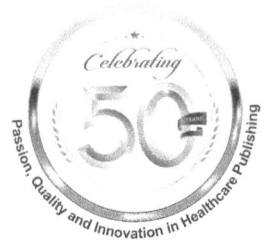

Uniquest Series
PHYSIOLOGY

Editor
V Suganthi MD
Associate Professor
Vinayaka Mission's Kirupananda Variyar Medical College
Salem, Tamil Nadu, India

Associate editor
National Journal of Basic Medical Sciences

Foreword
Milind V Bhutkar

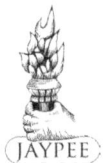

JAYPEE BROTHERS MEDICAL PUBLISHERS
The Health Sciences Publisher
New Delhi | London | Panama

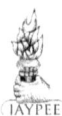
Jaypee Brothers Medical Publishers (P) Ltd

Headquarters

Jaypee Brothers Medical Publishers (P) Ltd
4838/24, Ansari Road, Daryaganj
New Delhi 110 002, India
Phone: +91-11-43574357
Fax: +91-11-43574314
Email: jaypee@jaypeebrothers.com

Overseas Offices

J.P. Medical Ltd
83 Victoria Street, London
SW1H 0HW (UK)
Phone: +44 20 3170 8910
Fax: +44 (0)20 3008 6180
Email: info@jpmedpub.com

Jaypee-Highlights Medical Publishers Inc
City of Knowledge, Bld. 235, 2nd Floor, Clayton
Panama City, Panama
Phone: +1 507-301-0496
Fax: +1 507-301-0499
Email: cservice@jphmedical.com

Jaypee Brothers Medical Publishers (P) Ltd
Bhotahity, Kathmandu
Nepal
Phone: +977-9741283608
Email: kathmandu@jaypeebrothers.com

Website: www.jaypeebrothers.com
Website: www.jaypeedigital.com

© 2019, Jaypee Brothers Medical Publishers

The views and opinions expressed in this book are solely those of the original contributor(s)/author(s) and do not necessarily represent those of editor(s) of the book.

All rights reserved. No part of this publication may be reproduced, stored or transmitted in any form or by any means, electronic, mechanical, photocopying, recording or otherwise, without the prior permission in writing of the publishers.

All brand names and product names used in this book are trade names, service marks, trademarks or registered trademarks of their respective owners. The publisher is not associated with any product or vendor mentioned in this book.

Medical knowledge and practice change constantly. This book is designed to provide accurate, authoritative information about the subject matter in question. However, readers are advised to check the most current information available on procedures included and check information from the manufacturer of each product to be administered, to verify the recommended dose, formula, method and duration of administration, adverse effects and contraindications. It is the responsibility of the practitioner to take all appropriate safety precautions. Neither the publisher nor the author(s)/editor(s) assume any liability for any injury and/or damage to persons or property arising from or related to use of material in this book.

This book is sold on the understanding that the publisher is not engaged in providing professional medical services. If such advice or services are required, the services of a competent medical professional should be sought.

Every effort has been made where necessary to contact holders of copyright to obtain permission to reproduce copyright material. If any have been inadvertently overlooked, the publisher will be pleased to make the necessary arrangements at the first opportunity. The **CD/DVD-ROM** (if any) provided in the sealed envelope with this book is complimentary and free of cost. **Not meant for sale.**

Inquiries for bulk sales may be solicited at: jaypee@jaypeebrothers.com

Uniquest Series: Physiology

First Edition: **2019**

ISBN: 978-93-5270-571-9

Printed at

FOREWORD

It gives me immense pleasure to note that Dr V Suganthi, Associate Professor in Physiology has written a book titled *Uniquest Series: Physiology*.

Today's first MBBS students face a peculiar problem. Officially first MBBS duration is one year but practically students get only about nine months to prepare for the examinations. Combine this with an ever expanding syllabus and falling standards of English language in students fraternity, they really have a tough job at their hands.

Considering this scenario, a book like this one will prove to be invaluable for the students. Dr V Suganthi has more than ten years of teaching experience and she has distilled her experience and expertise in penning this book.

I am sure *Uniquest Series: Physiology* will be of great help for first MBBS students in facing their examination confidently.

Milind V Bhutkar MD MNAMS
Deputy Dean (Administration)
Professor and Head
Department of Physiology
Vinayaka Mission's Kirupananda Variyar Medical College
Salem, Tamil Nadu, India

PREFACE

Physiology, a study of normal functions of the body, is a basic science in medicine. A sound knowledge of Physiology is needed to understand deranged body functions in disease conditions and to learn the Physiological basis of treating diseases.

This book has been written for the benefit of undergraduate students to acquire knowledge and guide them to give appropriate answers to questions in their examinations and to help them clear the exams. Answers are given in three forms: Essays, Short notes and Short answers.

The contents presented in this book are taken from my lecture notes and updates from standard Physiology textbooks.

This question-answer book in Physiology is first of its kind and has been prepared with utmost care and concern for the students.

I would like to welcome suggestions on improving the utility of this book in future.

V Suganthi

ACKNOWLEDGMENTS

I give my sincere thanks to my teachers of Physiology for guiding me in my career, both in academics and research in Physiology.

I wish to thank our Professor and Head of the department Dr Milind V Bhutkar for his support and writing Foreword for this book.

I extend my thanks to all our administrators of Vinayaka Mission's Kirupananda Variyar Medical College, Salem, Tamil Nadu, India, for giving me an opportunity to write this book.

I wish to thank my family members for their constant support and encouragement.

I thank all my students for inspiring me to write this book.

I am very grateful to the whole team of M/s Jaypee Brothers Medical Publishers (P) Ltd, who helped and guided me, Shri Jitendar P Vij (Group Chairman), Mr Ankit Vij (Managing Director), Mr MS Mani (Group President), Ms Pooja Bhandari (Production Head), Ms Chetna Vohra (Associate Director-Content Strategy), Ms Sunita Katla (Executive Assistant to Group Chairman and Publishing Manager), Ms Samina Khan (Executive Assistant Director-Content Strategy), Dr Sneha Kashyap (Development Editor), Ms Seema Dogra (Cover Visualizer), Mr Deepak Saxena (DTP Operator), Mr Narsingh Kumar (Proofreader), Ms Ritika Ahuja (Proofreader), and his team members, for all their support to work in this project and make it a success. Without their cooperation, I could not have completed this project.

CONTENTS

1. MBBS Examination 2003 — 1
2. MBBS Examination 2004 — 27
3. MBBS Examination 2005 — 59
4. MBBS Examination 2006 — 93
5. MBBS Examination 2007 — 133
6. MBBS Examination 2008 — 165
7. MBBS Examination 2009 — 191
8. MBBS Examination 2010 — 222
9. MBBS Examination 2011 — 265
10. MBBS Examination 2012 — 286
11. MBBS Examination 2013 — 311
12. MBBS Examination 2014 — 334
13. MBBS Examination 2015 — 360
14. MBBS Examination 2016 — 372
15. MBBS Examination 2017 — 383
16. MBBS Examination 2018 — 390
    Topic-wise University Questions — 404

MBBS Examination 2003

ANSWER ALL QUESTIONS

I. Essay questions   (15 Marks each)
1. Describe the composition, functions and regulation of salivary secretion.
2. Name the clotting factors. Describe the blood clotting mechanism by intrinsic pathway.
3. Define blood pressure. Give the normal values. Describe the 'Baroreceptor mechanism for regulation of blood pressure'.
4. Explain the role of vestibular apparatus in posture and equilibrium. Add a note on Meniere's syndrome.

II. Short notes   (5 Marks each)
1. Excitation-contraction coupling in skeletal muscle.
2. Erythroblastosis fetalis (EBF).
3. Thyroid function tests.
4. Deglutition.
5. Regulation of gastric juice secretion.
6. Countercurrent exchangers in kidneys.
7. Glomerular filtration.
8. Actions of growth hormone.
9. Testosterone.
10. Milk ejection reflex.
11. Accommodation for near vision.
12. Visceral pain.
13. Sensory cortex.
14. Total peripheral resistance in vascular system.
15. Acclimatization to high altitude.
16. Compliance of lungs.
17. Functions of middle ear.
18. Associative learning.
19. Righting reflexes.
20. Control of food intake.

I. ESSAY QUESTIONS

1. **Describe the composition, functions and regulation of salivary secretion.**

Composition of Saliva

- Rate of secretion—1000–1800 mL/day
- pH—6 to 7.4
- Water—99.95%
- Solids—0.5%
- Solids—organic and inorganic
- Organic—enzymes like ptyalin, lysozyme, lingual lipase, carbonic anhydrase, RNAse, DNAse, others like kallikrein, blood group antigens, IgA, etc. Urea, uric acid, cholesterol and mucin
- Inorganic—Na^+, K^+, Ca^{++}, PO_4, Mg^{++}, Cl^-, HCO_3^-, sulphate, bromide, etc.
- Saliva is Hypotonic. Tonicity depends on the rate of salivary secretion.

Regulation of Salivary Secretion

- Salivary secretion is under neural regulation. It is controlled by the autonomic nerves.

Parasympathetic stimulation: It increases salivary secretion which is watery and low in organic content. Along with acetylcholine released at the nerve terminal, vasoactive intestinal peptide (VIP) is also released by some postganglionic parasympathetic nerves which causes vasodilation and increase blood flow to the gland and thereby increases salivary secretion. Increased secretion through parasympathetic stimulation is by way of reflexes. The reflexes are conditioned and unconditioned reflexes.

Conditioned reflexes: Salivary secretion is increased by thought, sight or smell of food and stimulated by impulses coming from higher centers.

Unconditioned reflex: Secretion is stimulated by placing substances in the mouth thereby stimulating the touch receptors in the oral cavity.

Sympatheic stimulation: It causes vasoconstriction of blood vessels supplying the glands and causes secretion of small amount of thick viscous saliva rich in organic contents.

Functions of Saliva

a. Ptyalin (α-amylase) in saliva splits starches. Action of amylase is maximum at a pH of 6.8. Digestion continues in stomach for some time till the pH becomes less than 4
b. Protective function: Saliva cleans the mouth after a meal and prevents growth of harmful bacteria
c. Saliva contains lysozyme, IgA and lactoferrin for protection. Lysozymes are bacteriocidal and lactoferrin is bacteriostatic in action
d. Saliva facilitates speech
e. It helps in taste of food
f. Mucus in saliva helps in lubrication of food, mastication and swallowing
g. It buffers the gastric juice in stomach
h. Proline rich proteins in the saliva protect the enamel of tooth
i. Saliva dilutes hot and irritant foods and protects buccal mucosa. It also dilutes regurgitated bile and HCl
j. In animals it helps in temperature regulation
k. Helps in excretion of heavy metals, alchohol, morphine, thiocyanate, etc.

2. **Name the clotting factors. Describe the blood clotting mechanism by intrinsic pathway.**

- Blood while flowing in the vessels is fluid in nature, but when the vessel wall is injured or the blood is removed from the body and collected in a test tube it becomes a jelly like mass – the clot
- Clotting or coagulation of blood involves a series of cascade of events in which many clotting factors (proteins in the plasma) are activated in a serial manner. There are many such clotting factors.

They are:
- Factor I—Fibrinogen
- Factor II—Prothrombin
- Factor III—Thromboplastin
- Factor IV—Calcium
- Factor V—Labile factor or proaccelerin
- Factor VI—Non-existant
- Factor VII—Stable factor or proconvertin
- Factor VIII—Antihemophilic factor
- Factor IX—Christmas factor or Plasma thromboplastic component (PTC) or Antihemophilic factor B
- Factor X—Stuart-Prower factor
- Factor XI—Plasma thromboplastin antecedent (PTA) or Antihemophilic factor C
- Factor XII—Hageman factor or Glass factor or Contact factor
- Factor XIII—Laki Lorand factor or fibrin stabilizing factor
- HMW-K—High-molecular-weight kininogen or Fitzgerald factor
- Pre-Ka (Prekallikrein or Fletcher factor)
- Kallikrein—Ka
- Platelet phospholipid—PL.

The coagulation process involves three major steps:
1. Formation of prothrombin activator
2. Conversion of prothrombin to thrombin
3. Conversion of fibrinogen to fibrin.

Formation of Prothrombin Activator is by 2 Mechanisms
1. Extrinsic pathway
2. Intrinsic pathway.

Intrinsic pathway: This pathway is activated when there is injury to vessel wall and exposure of collagen or injury to blood itself.

Steps involved are:
- Injury to vessel wall exposes collagen and activates Factor XII to XIIa
- Factor XIIa activates Factor XI to XIa
- Factor XIa activates Factor IX to IXa
- Factor IXa in the presence of Factor VIII, Ca^{2+} and platelet phospholipids (PPL) activates Factor X to Xa

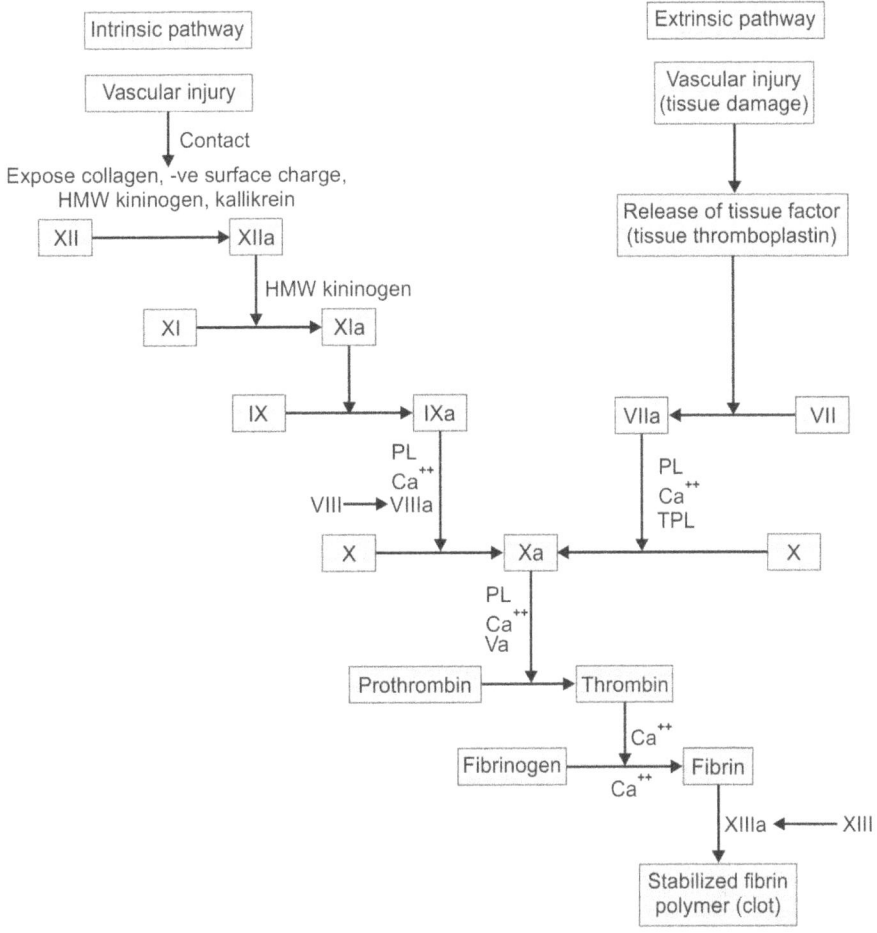

Fig. 1: Mechanism of clotting.
(TPL: Tissue Phospholipid; PL: Platelet phospholipid.)
(*Source:* GK Pal)

- The activated Factor Xa, platelet phospholipids, Factor Va and Ca^{2+} forms the Prothrombin activator (Fig. 1).

Conversion of Prothrombin to Thrombin:

Prothrombin activator in the presence of Ca^{2+} converts prothrombin to thrombin. This happens at the surface of platelets. Thrombin is a proteolytic enzyme.

Conversion of Fibrinogen to Fibrin:

- Thrombin, a proteolytic enzyme removes two pairs of polypeptide chains from each fibrinogen molecule and converts it to fibrin monomer
- The fibrin monomers now polymerize to form long fibrin threads. The fibrin is initially a loose mesh of interlacing strands. This meshwork traps the blood cells
- It is later converted to a dense tight aggregate by formation of covalent cross-linkages. This is catalyzed by Factor XIII and Ca^{2+}. The stabilized fibrin mesh with the trapped blood cells forms the CLOT.

3. **Define blood pressure. Give the normal values. Describe the 'Baroreceptor mechanism for regulation of blood pressure'.**

- Blood pressure (BP) is defined as the lateral pressure exerted by the moving column of blood on the vessel wall. Normal value = 120/80 mm Hg.

Components of BP

- Systolic BP (Normal value; 100-130 mmHg)
- Diastolic BP (Normal value; 60-90 mmHg)
- Pulse pressure (Normal value; 40 mmHg)
- Mean arterial pressure (Calculated as; DBP + 1/3 PP).

I. Neural Regulation of BP

i. Regulation by autonomic nerves
ii. Regulation by Medullary cardiovascular control centers
iii. Regulation by reflexes
   a. Baroreceptor reflex
   b. Chemoreceptor reflex
   c. CNS ischemic response.

i. Regulation by Autonomic Nerves

- Blood vessels are supplied by sympathetic nerves
- They are of two types—sympathetic vasoconstrictor (VC) and vasodilator (VD) fibers
- Sympathetic VC fibers—present in all blood vessels
- Sympathetic VD or cholinergic fibers—present in blood vessels of skeletal muscles, sweat glands and they originate from frontal cortex and reach hypothalamus, midbrain medulla and end in the intermediolateral nucleus (IML) of spinal cord (SC)
- **Sympathetic stimulation results in:** Vaso- and Veno constriction, increase in HR and myocardial contractility and therefore the BP is increased.

ii. Regulation by Medullary Control Centers (Fig. 2)

- There are two areas in the medulla which control the CVS
- They are—vasomotor center (VMC) and cardiac vagal center (CVC)
- VMC—Neuronal cell bodies in the rostral venterolateral medulla (RVLM) constitute the VMC. Axons of these neurons reach the IML of SC. From IML the sympathetic nerves arise and supplies the heart
- CVC—Nucleus tractus solitarius, nucleus ambiguus and dorsal motor nucleus of vagus constitute the CVC
- Stimulation of VMC—↑ HR and contractility, ↑ Vaso- and Veno constriction—↑ BP

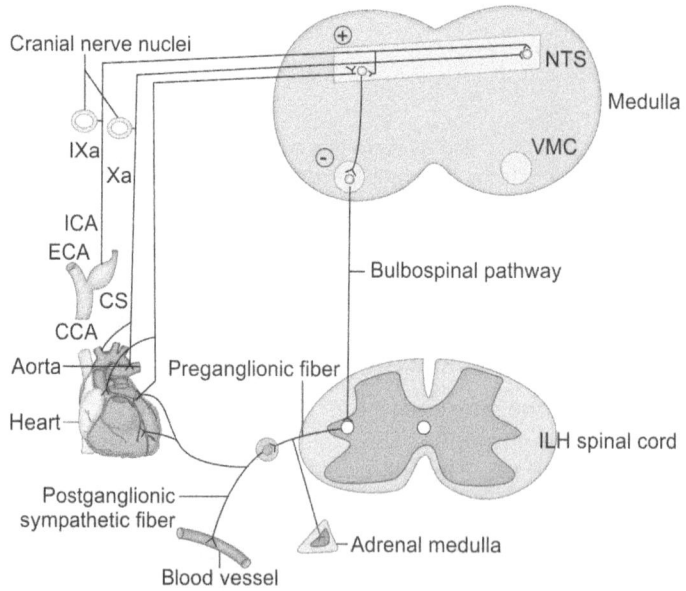

Fig. 2: Medullary cardiovascular centers and Baroreceptor reflex pathway.
(CS: Carotid sinus; CCA: Common carotid artery; ECA: Externa carotid artery; ICA: Internal carotid artery; Xa: Afferents of Vagus nerve; Xe: Efferents of Vagus nerve; IXa: Afferents of Glossopharyngeal nerve; VMC: Vasomotor center; NTS: Nucleus tractus solitarius; ILH: Intermediolateral horn of spinal cord.)
(*Source:* GK Pal)

and on inhibition of VMC the effects are vice versa
- The final pathway from VMC is through sympathetic nerves to the heart
- Stimulation of CVC—↓HR, Decreased vasoconstriction and thereby—↓BP
- Final pathway is through vagus nerve to the heart
- There are inputs coming to VMC, from limbic centers through hypothalamus which are responsible for BP modulation in emotional states like anxiety (Increase in BP and heart rate).

iii. Reflex Regulation of BP
a. **Baroreceptor reflex:**
Baroreceptors:
- There are two types of baroreceptors (BRs) (Fig. 3). High pressure and low pressure baroreceptors
- High pressure BRs are present in the carotid and aortic sinuses
- Low pressure BRs are present in the great veins, right and left atria
- High pressure BRs are there to monitor and correct the day-to-day change in BP as in change of posture from supine to standing position
- They regulate BP maximally when the MAP is between 70-110 mm Hg and stops firing when MAP falls < 40 or rises above 150 mm Hg.

The reflex:
- Most important reflex to regulate BP
- Also called as Sinoaortic reflex (Fig. 4)

- Receptor—carotid and aortic sinuses
- Stimulus—stretch of baroreceptors (as in increased BP)
- Afferents—IXth (supplies carotid sinus) and Xth cranial nerves (aortic sinus)
- Center—Medullary centers NTS, VMC and CVC
- Efferents—sympathetic nerves and vagus nerve
- Effector—heart and blood vessels
- Response—decrease in BP.

When there is increase in MAP above the normal range the baroreceptors are stretched and the stretch receptors present here send impulses through the IX & X cranial nerves to Nucleus tractus solitarius (NTS).

Impulses from NTS will inhibit the VMC and stimulate CVC.

There is decrease in heart rate and myocardial contractility resulting in decrease in cardiac output and decrease in blood pressure.

There is also vasodilatation which results in decrease in diastolic BP.

When there is decrease in MAP there is stimulation of VMC and inhibition of CVC and thereby BP is increased (Fig. 4).

4. Explain the role of vestibular apparatus in posture and equilibrium. Add a note on Meniere's syndrome.

- Vestibular apparatus is present in the inner ear and consists of 3 semicircular canals (SCC) and 2 sac like structures - utricle and saccule
- The receptors for vestibular sensation are the hair cells and they are located in the Cristae in the ampulla of semicircular canals and the macula or Otolithic organ of the utricle and saccule (the receptor organs) as seen in Figure 5
- The hairs of the hair cells are embedded in a thick gelatinous substance called the Cupula
- The receptor organ in utricle and saccule is called the Macula. The macula is an elevation in the sacs. Cupula, here is embedded with calcium carbonate crystals - Otoliths
- The receptor organ of SCC are in Cristae and is located in the ampulla

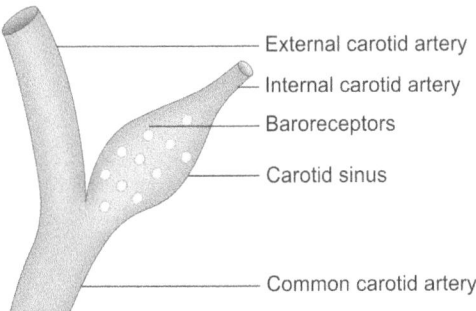

Fig. 3: Barorecptor – carotid sinus.
(*Source:* GK Pal)

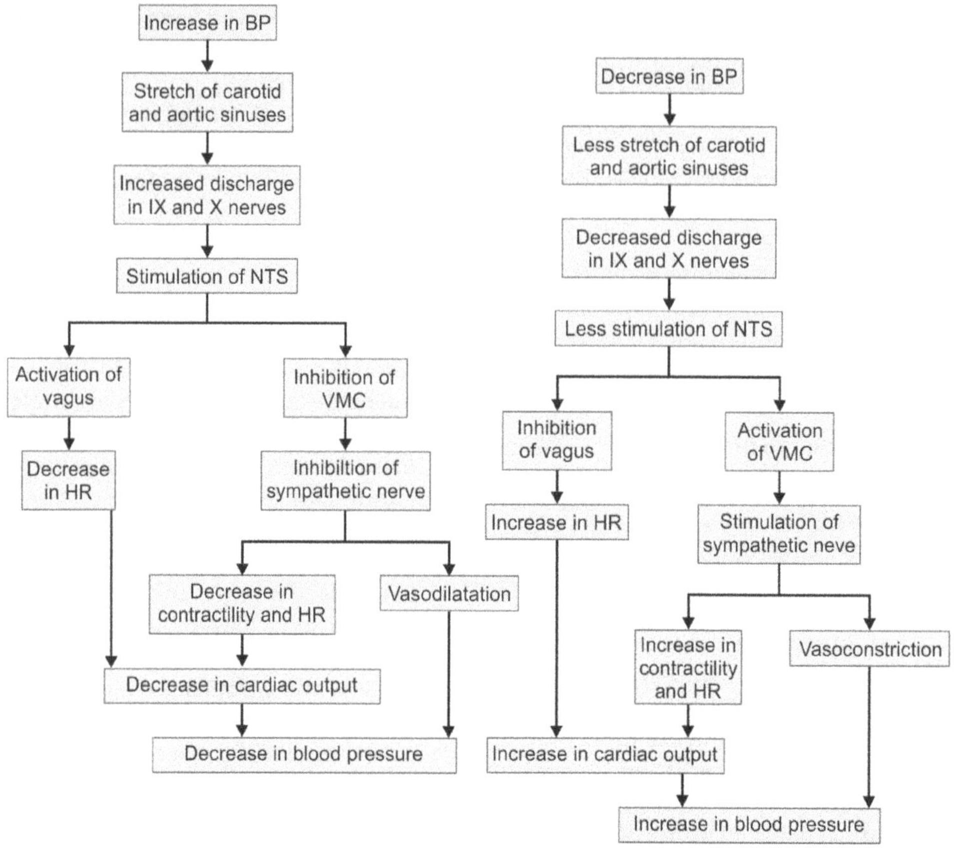

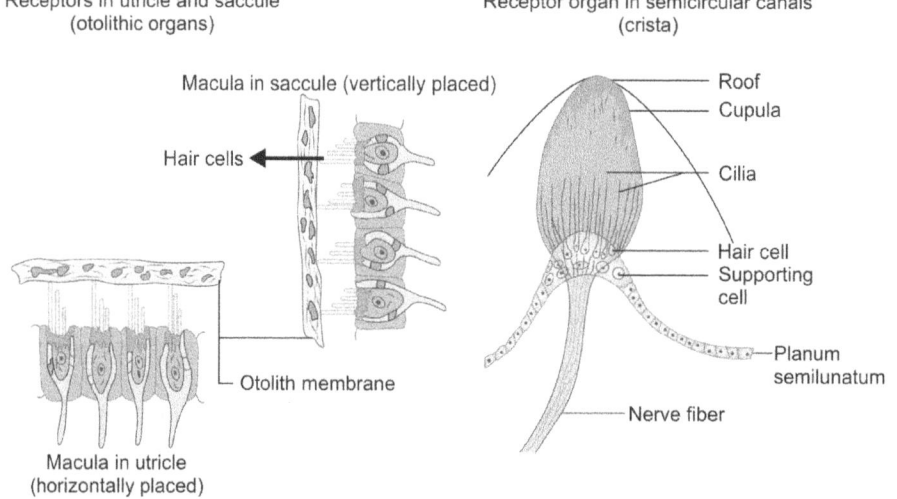

Fig. 4: Regulation of BP by baroreceptors.
(BP: Blood pressure; VMC: Vasomotor center; HR: Heart rate; NTS: Nucleus tractus solitarius)
(*Source:* GK Pal)

Fig. 5: Receptors for vestibular apparatus. Vestibular apparatus has 3 semicircular canals and 2 sac like structures – Utricle and Saccule. The receptor organs are crista in SCC and macula or otolithic organs in utricle and saccule. The receptors are hair cells in these organs.
(*Source:* GK Pal)

- The bases of the hair cells are in contact with the vestibular nerves.

Hair Cells

- The hair cells are the receptors of sensation of equilibrium
- They have hairs arranged in increasing order on the apical surface of the cells
- The largest hair is the Kinocilia and the rest are called as the Stereocilia
- Longest stereocilia is close to kinocilia
- The smaller stereocilia are connected to longer ones by a protein, the TIP LINK proteins which opens cation channels in the hairs
- On stimulation, the hairs can either move towards the largest one or towards the smallest one. When they move towards the largest hair there is depolarization of hair cells and when it moves to opposite side there is hyperpolarization of hair cells
- Depolarization of hair cells will stimulate the vestibular nerves at the bases of hair cells.

Functions of Vestibular Apparatus

- Since these apparatus are present in the inner ear they give information to the brain about the movement of head in relation to space and also body acceleration
- The receptors in utricle and saccule give information about linear acceleration and change in head position in relation to gravity. Saccule responds to vertical accelartion and utricle to horizontal acceleration
- Saccule detects the lateral tilting of the head and utricle detects up and down movement of head and they help in maintaining equilibrium during such movements
- SCC detect angular acceleration as in rotational movements and they send impulses down the vestibulospinal tract to the trunk muscles and help in maintaining posture and equilibrium
- The receptors of SCC have a predictive function and they help the nervous system to make appropriate adjustments to prevent a fall
- Vestibular apparatus have an important role in maintaining posture through various reflexes.

Role of Vestibular Apparatus in Maintaining Posture

- Maintanence of posture is the role of muscle tone especially in the antigravity muscles; the extensors of the back and lower limbs. Regulation of tone is in turn the function of stretch reflex in these muscles
- Vestibular apparatus and the pathways in relation to vestibular apparatus regulate muscle tone and thereby regulate body posture
- Vestibular nucleus in medulla influences muscle tone of antigravity muscles by stimulating α-motor neurons. It is facilitatory to muscle tone
- Impulses from the vestibular apparatus reach vestibular nuclei in medulla, cerebellum and reticular formation
- Vestibular nuclei give rise to vestibulospinal tracts and medial longitudinal bundle and they maintain tone in the antigravity muscles and correlate the adjustments made in the limbs and eyes in response to change in body position
- Vestibular apparatus also provides information of position of head in relation to space and during movements to maintain posture and they also regulate eye movements through postural reflexes.

Postural Reflexes

These reflexes are demonstrated in experimental animals with transections done at various levels of brainstem. These reflexes help in maintaining body posture in various body movements.

1. Tonic Labyrinthine Reflexes

Tonic labyrinthine reflex is demonstrated in a decerebrate animal. The transection of brain is done at the superior border of pons. Following this there is spasticity in all antigravity muscles. This is said to be 'Decerebrate rigidity'. In these animals the rigidity in limbs varies with body position.

- When the animal is in supine position the tone is maximum in antigravity muscles
- When the animal is in prone position the tone is minimum in antigravity muscles
- When the body is in lateral position, the rigidity is less
- These reflexes help to redistribute muscle tone in the limbs to prevent loss of balance when the body is in inclined posture
- *Reflex arc for this reflex:*
  - **Stimulus** is gravity
  - **Receptors** are otolithic organs
  - **Center** is medulla
  - **Response** is contraction of limb extensor muscles.

2. Righting reflexes: These reflexes are demonstrated in a midbrain animal with transection done at the superior border of midbrain.

- They help to keep the head upright and in alignment with the body. They are also called as righting reflexes
- These reflexes are integrated in the nuclei of midbrain.
  Labyrinthine righting reflexes: When the animal is held by its body and tipped from side to side, the animal holds the head erect in response to stimulus (gravity) from the otolithic organ (receptors).

3. Vestibulo-ocular Reflex

Through this reflex, the vestibular apparatus controls eye movements in relation to head movement. This helps to fix the eye in the same point in spite of change in head movement. This is possible due to its connections with the cranial nerve nuclei in midbrain.

4. Vestibular Placing Reaction

- It is integrated in cerebral cortex
- When the snout of a suspended blind-folded animal touches a surface it immediately places both the forepaws on the surface. Exteroceptors are reponsible for the placing reaction
- If a blind-folded animal is suspended in air with one foot touching the surface it can place the foot firmly on the supporting surface. Labyrinthine (Vestibular) and exteroceptors are responsible for the placing reaction
- If an animal is thrown into air it can land firmly with four limbs. It is due to visual, labyrinthine and exteroceptor cues.

Meniere's Disease

- It is a disease affecting the membranous labyrinth of the vestibular apparatus
- There is overdistension of the membranous labyrinth, due to excess secretion of endolymph
- Symptoms are episodic attacks of vertigo, deafness and tinnitus (ringing sensation in the ears)
- Vertigo is due to imbalance of inputs from both ears as one ear may be affected or the disease may be progressive from one ear and may affect the other ear later
- Patient also has nausea, vomiting and sensation of fullness of the affected ear.
- There is no cure for the disease and treatment is symptomatic.
- Drugs are given for reducing the symptoms of vertigo and to control nausea and vomiting.

II. SHORT NOTES

1. **Excitation-contraction coupling in skeletal muscle.**
- The process by which the muscle membrane is excited and is followed by muscle contraction is given as excitation-contraction coupling
- **The steps are given below:**
  - The action potential generated following the End plate potential (EPP) in the motor end plate, moves through the T-tubule and activates the voltage-gated Dihydropyridine receptors (DHPRs) which are present in the T-tubule membrane of the muscle fiber
  - The activated DHPRs open the Ca^{2+} channels named as the ryanodine receptors which are located in the terminal cisterns of the sarcoplasmic reticulum (SR)
  - This releases Ca^{2+} stored in the SR into the cytoplasm and the Ca^{2+}

concentration in cytosol rises by 2,000 times than that of the resting state
- The Ca^{2+} now gets attached to the troponin C subunit
- Troponin C-Ca^{2+} complex now induce a conformational change in the tropomyosin and the tropomyosin is lifted up, exposing the myosin binding sites on actin molecules
- So the myosin heads bind to the actin molecules and cross-bridge cycling starts resulting in muscle contraction.

2. Erythroblastosis fetalis (EBF).

- It is also called as hemolytic disease of the newborn (HDN)
- This is due to Rh incompatability between the mother and fetus
- It happens if the mother is Rh negative and the fetus is Rh positive
- Since Rh system does not follow the 2nd law of Landsteiner's, there are no preformed antibodies in the Rh negative mother's blood
- So in first pregnancy there are no complications
- At the time of parturition, few fetal RBCs enter the mother's circulation
- Mother's immune system recognizes the Rh antigen in the fetal RBCs as foreign antigens and starts producing antibodies for D antigen on fetal RBCs
- These anti-D antibodies belong to IgG type and therefore can cross the placenta
- If the mother conceives for the second time and if that fetus happens to be Rh positive, the anti-D antibodies from mother crosses the placenta and destroys the fetal RBCs resulting in HDN/EBF
- As the number of conceptions increase antibody titre increases and causes more damage to the fetus
- **The symptoms are:**
  a. Anemia—There is agglutination of RBCs following antigen-antibody reaction and the agglutinated RBCs are lysed. This results in severe anemia
  b. Hemolytic jaundice—the released hemoglobin, following hemolysis, is converted to bilirubin and the levels may rise very high resulting in jaundice
  c. Hydrops fetalis— There is generalized edema due to anemia and hypoproteinemia
  d. Erythroblasts start appearing in the circulation due to exaggerated erythropoiesis following severe anemia
  e. Kernicterus—It happens due to hemolysis and formation of excess bilirubin, and the bilirubin crosses the blood-brain barrier (BBB) since the BBB is not fully developed in the fetus. Basal ganglia in the brain, has great affinity for bilirubin and therefore it gets deposited in the basal ganglia. There are motor dysfunctions due to this.

Prevention of EBF: EBF is prevented by administering the mother with anti-D antibodies after delivery of the fetus. Injected antibodies neutralize the antigens which had entered the mother's body and further antibody production is prevented.

Treatment of EBF:
- **Exchange transfusion**—The newborns with the above symptoms are treated with exchange transfusion after birth. This removes sensitized Rh positive RBCs from the blood and is replaced with Rh negative blood. This is continued till the antibodies are removed from the fetal circulation. The transfused blood should be ABO negative and Rh negative
- **Phototherapy** can also be given to reduce bilirubin levels.

3. Thyroid function tests.

- Thyroid function tests help us to identify the status of thyroid gland activity
- It includes estimation of hormone levels, basal metabolic rate, radioactive iodine uptake, thyroid antibody estimation, thyroid scan, serum cholesterol levels and thyroid biopsy.

a. Measurement of thyroid hormones:
- T3 and T4 levels are estimated by ELISA technique
- More importantly free T3 and free T4 levels are estimated

- In primary hyperthyroidism T3 and T4 levels are increased and TSH levels are decreased
- In primary hypothyroidism the opposite is seen.

b. Measurement of plasma TSH levels:
- It is an important test done to identify thyroid status
- In primary hypothyroidism, TSH levels are high and T3 and T4 levels are low, but in secondary hypothyroidism (due to pituitary dysfunction), TSH, T3 and T4 are all low
- In hyperthyroidism TSH levels are low and T3 and T4 levels are high.

c. Radioactive iodine uptake studies:
- Iodine is usually taken up by the thyroid gland for the formation of T3 and T4
- So the uptake of radiactive iodine gives an idea about the function of the gland
- The radioactive forms used are ^{123}I and ^{131}I
- The radioactive iodine (RAI) is given with water and an X-ray counter is placed on the neck and the thyroid uptake is determined
- In hyperthroidism, it is increased and in hypothyroidism, it is decreased.

d. Measurement of basal metabolic rate:
- Normal value is ± 20%, in hyperthyroidism it is increased upto 100% and in hypothyroidism it is decreased upto –30 to –40%.

e. Thyroid antibody detection:
- This test is done to identify antibodies in Grave's disease and Hashimotos thyroiditis
- In Grave's disease antibodies against TSH receptors are detected and in Hashimoto's disease antibodies against thyroglobulin molecule are detected.

f. Thyroid scan:
- Ultrasound scanning of the gland gives a clear idea about the nature of lesions in the gland, either cystic or solid lesions
- CT scan and MRI scan are useful in determining retrosternal and retrotracheal extension of the gland.

g. Fine needle aspiration biopsy:
- It is done in patients with nodular goiter to identify malignancies.

4. Deglutition.

Deglutition is the process of swallowing.
- It is a reflex response integrated in the medulla in nucleus tractus solitarius (NTS) and nucleus ambiguus (NA)
- Afferents pass through the cranial nerves V, IX and X
- Efferents come through cranial nerves V, VII and XII nerves to the tongue and pharynx.

There are 3 phases of deglutition (Figs. 6A to D):
1. Oral or voluntary phase
2. Pharyngeal or involuntary phase
3. Esophageal phase.

Oral phase:
When food enters mouth, tongue forms it into a bolus and pushes it to the oropharynx by pushing up and against the hard palate.

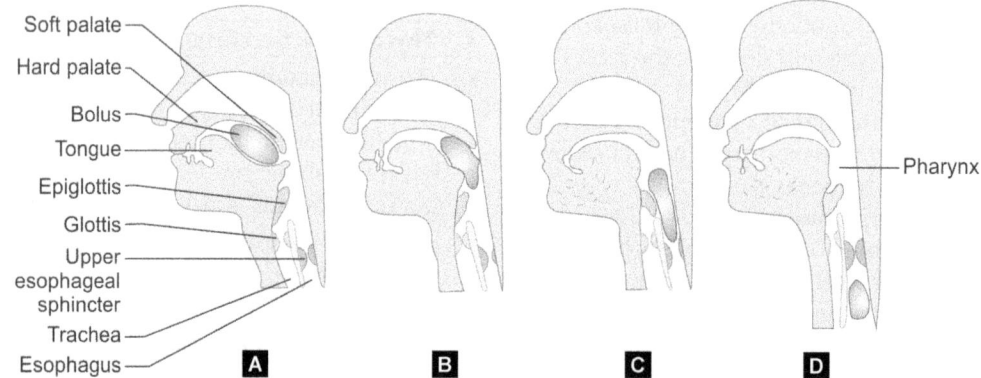

Figs. 6A to D: Phases of deglutition: (A) Oral phase; (B) Bolus enters the pharynx; (C) Pharyngeal phase; (D) Esophageal phase. (*Source:* Sembulingam)

Pharyngeal phase:
- It starts when food enters pharynx
- Soft palate is elevated and closes the nasopharynx and prevents food from entering the nose
- Larynx rises, Vocal cords approximate and Epiglottis closes the laryngeal opening and prevents food from entering the trachea
- Deglutition apnea follows
- Palatopharyngeal folds approximate for selective material to move into the esophagus
- Cricopharyngeus (upper esophageal sphincter) relaxes and bolus enters upper esophagus
- On entering of food into esophagus, the cricopharyngeus closes, vocal cords open and air entry is allowed.

Esophageal phase:
- There are 2 sphincters in the esophagus—upper esophageal sphincter (UES) and lower esophageal sphincter (LES)
- UES is formed by cricopharyngeas muscle which is a skeletal muscle. It opens reflexly at the beginning of swallow
- LES is made of smooth muscle and its actions are regulated by the vagus nerve and other intrinsic nerves. Its main action is to prevent regurgitation of acids from the stomach into esophagus
- Food on reaching esophagus is pushed into the stomach by peristalsis—primary and secondary peristalsis
- Primary peristalsis is initiated by swallowing and is coordinated by vagus nerve
- Secondary peristalsis is initiated by the presence of food in the esophagus and it sweeps the food down towards the stomach, coordinated by the intrinsic nerves.

5. **Regulation of gastric juice secretion.**

Regulation of Gastric Secretion

Neural, humoral and reflex regulation of secretion.

Factors that stimulate:
- Vagus nerve
- Gastrin
- Histamine (refer Fig. 7).

Factors that inhibit:
- Low pH in the stomach
- Somatostatin
- Prostaglandin E2.

Neural regulation:
- Vagus nerve acts on parietal cells by a direct and indirect mechanism to increase HCl secretion
- Direct action is through M3 receptors. Stimulation of vagus releases acetylcholine which acts on the M3 receptors. It results in activation of protein kinases and insertion of proton pumps on the apical membrane of parietal cells
- Indirectly the nerve acts on 'G' cells in the antrum and increases gastrin secretion. The neurotransmitter released here is Gastrin releasing peptide (GRP). Gastrin stimulates HCl secretion.

Humoral regulation:
- Gastrin: Gastrin is a hormone secreted by 'G' cells in the gastric antrum. It is secreted in response to distension of antrum, vagal stimultion and presence of products of digestion in antrum. It acts on parietal cells and inserts H^+-K^+ pumps on the apical membrane of parietal cells. Gastrin also stimulates ECL cells to secrete histamine
- Histamine: Histamine is a potent stimulator of HCl secretion. It acts on H_2 rceptor and increases cAMP levels in the parietal cells and thereby increases HCl secretion
- PGE2: It inhibits secretion of HCl by acting on its receptor and thereby decrease in the cAMP levels (Fig. 7).

Regulation is discussed in terms of:
- Cephalic phase
- Gastric phase
- Intestinal phase.

Cephalic phase:

Nearly 500 mL/hr (45% of total secretion)

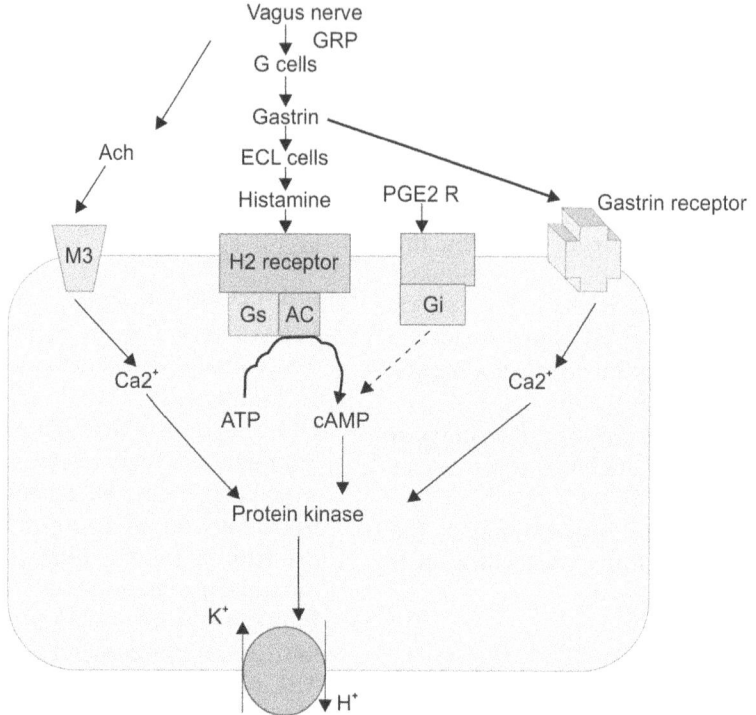

Fig. 7: Parietal cell with the regulating factors for HCl secretion.
(GRP: Gastrin-releasing peptide; ECL cells: Enterochromaffin like cells; ACh: Acetylcholine; M3: Muscarinic receptor 3; Gs; Gi: G proteins; AC: Adenylyl cyclase; PGE2R: Prostaglandin E2 Receptor)

- Initiated by thought, sight, smell, taste of food through vagus nerve
- Emotions also affect secretion through impulses from hypothalamus (refer Fig. 8).

Gastric phase:
- About 50% of total secretion happens in this phase. Food in stomach induces secretion by:
  - Distension of body of stomach (through the reflexes—vagal reflex)
  - Distension of antrum (through the gastrin secretion)
  - By presence of products of partial digestion of protein (through the gastrin secretion).

Intestinal phase:
- It begins when chyme enters the intestine
- Intestinal influence is inhibitory for gastric secretion. It is by:
  - Enterogastric reflex—by distension of intestine, presence of acid and products of digestion in the intestine will inhibit secretion.

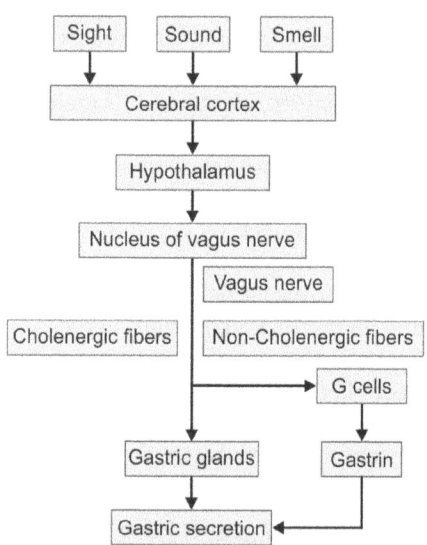

Fig. 8: Cephalic phase of regulation of HCl secretion.
(*Source:* GK Pal)

- Hormonal mechanism (through the hormones)—CCK, secretin, GIP, neurotensin, etc—enterogastrone. All the above hormones inhibit gastric secretion.

6. Countercurrent exchangers in kidneys.

- Countercurrent mechanism in general is a mechanism in which fluids flow in opposite directions in closely placed structures
- In kidneys, the countercurrent mechanism is used to generate and maintain a hyperosmolar gradient from the outer to inner region of the medulla, highest osmolality is at the tip of the renal papillae
- Hyperosmolar medullary interstitium is essential for the process of concentration of urine
- Only in the presence of this hyperosmolar interstitium ADH can reabsorb water from the collecting ducts through aquaporins
- The countercurrent system in the kidneys has two components—the countercurrent multiplier and countercurrent exchanger
- The descending and ascending loops of henle act as the countercurrent multiplier. Flow of fluid in descending loop is towards the deeper parts of medulla and is highly permeable to water and in the ascending limb the flow of fluid is towards the cortex and it is totally impermeable to water and permeable only to solutes. This selective permeability of the loops of henle helps in generating a hyperosmolar gradient in the medulla
- Vasa recta acts as the countercurrent exchanger. The flow of blood in the ascending and descending limbs of the vasa recta helps in maintaining the hyperosmolar environment created by the countercurrent multiplier as shown in Figure 9
- The ascending and descending limbs of vasa recta are also selectively permeable to water and solutes
- Solutes come out of the ascending limb and enters descending limb and water enters the ascending limb and moves out into the general circulation. Solutes get circulated in the deeper parts of the medulla and

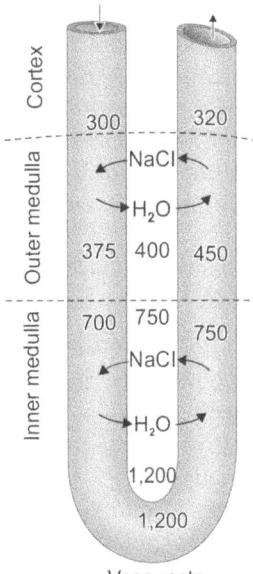

Fig. 9: Vasa recta (Countercurrent exchanger).
(*Source:* Sembulingam).

thereby the vasa recta prevents the dilution of solutes in the medullary interstitium
- This is the mechanism by which the countercurrent exchanger is able to maintain the hyperosmolar medullary gradient generated by the countercurrent multiplier.

7. Glomerular filtration.

Formation of urine involves 3 steps:
1. Glomerular filtration
2. Tubular reabsorption
3. Tubular secretion.

Glomerular filtration is ultrafiltration of plasma across the glomerular membrane.

The glomerular membrane is a 3 layered structure. It includes:
1. The capillary endothelial cell lining
2. Epithelium lining the Bowman's capsule, made of podocytes
3. Between them, the basement membrane.
- The total area of membrane is 0.8 m^2
- The capillary endothelial cells are fenestrated with pores of 70–90 nm diameter
- The podocytes have filtration slits of 25 nm diameter
- So the membrane permits passage of substances upto 4 nm diameter and excludes substances above 8 nm

- The presence of sialoproteins in the capillary wall which are negatively charged substances repel the negatively charged substances in plasma from getting filtered
- **Plasma** is filtered across the glomerular membrane and all constituents of plasma except the proteins are present in the filtrate
- The osmolality of the ULTRAFILTRATE is 300 mosm/L.

Factors regulating glomerular filtration:
- Hydrostatic pressure gradient across the capillary wall
- Osmotic pressure gradient across the capillary wall
- Filtration coefficient:
  - Size of the capillary bed—depends on mesangial cell activity
  - Permeability of the membrane—molecular size and electrostatic charge.

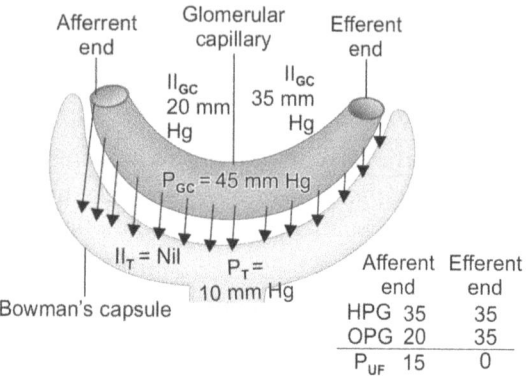

Fig. 10: Mechanism of filtration along the glomerular capillary. In contrast to systemic capillaries filtration happens along the entire capillary.
(P_{GC}: Capillary hydrostatic pressure; P_T: Bowman's space hydrosatic pressure; π_{GC}: Glomerular capillary oncotic pressure; π_T: Osmotic pressure in Bowman's space; HPG: Hydrostatic pressure gradient; OPG: Osmotic pressure gradient)
(*Source:* GK Pal)

Glomerular Filtration Rate (GFR)

- GFR refers to the volume of the glomerular filtrate formed per unit time by all the nephrons in both the kidneys. The normal value is 125 mL/min or 7.5 L/Hr or 180 L/day
- Mechanism of filtration across the glomerular capillary is similar to the mechanism of filtration across any of the systemic capillaries as shown in Figure 10.

GFR is expressed as:

$$GFR = K_f [(P_{GC} - P_T) - (\pi_{GC} - \pi_T)]$$

GFR = Glomerular filtration rate
K_f = Filtration coefficient of the membrane and it is 12.5 m²/min/mm Hg. It is the product of glomerular capillary wall conductivity and effective filtration surface area.
P_{GC} = Glomerular capillary hydrostatic pressure.
P_T = Hydrostatic pressure in Bowman's space.
π_{GC} = Glomerular capillary oncotic pressure.
π_T = Oncotic pressure in Bowman's space.

Factors Regulating GFR
a. **Surface area of filtration membrane:** It is altered by the contraction or relaxation of the mesangial cells. Contraction of mesangial cells decrease the surface area of filtration and relaxation increases it. Contraction is induced by angotensin II, endothelin, antidiuretic hormone (ADH), etc. and relaxation is stimulated by atrial notriuretic pressure (ANP), Dopamine, cAMP and Prostaglandin E2 (PGE2).
b. **Permeability of glomerular membrane** for neutral substances of less than 4 nm molecular diameter is favored and neutral substances above 8 nm are not filtered. Between 4 to 8 nm the filtration is inversely proportional to diameter of substances. There are negatively charged sialoproteins lining the glomerular membrane which prevents negatively charged particles like albumin from getting filtered even though it is 6 nm in diameter. Permeability is increased in hypoxia and presence of toxic substances.
c. **Hydrostatic pressure in glomerulus:** It is higher than in other capillaries in the body as the efferent arterioles (the outlet of glomerulus) is more constricted and offers more resistance than the afferent arterioles (the inlet for glomerulus) which are short and staright branches. So factors which increase efferent arteriolar constriction will increase the hydrostatic

pressure in the glomerulus. Changes in the systemic blood pressure will affect renal perfusion and thereby the filtration. The hydrostatic pressure in the glomerulus at the afferent and efferent end is 45 mm Hg.

d. **Hydrostatic pressure in Bowman's space:** This is the pressure exerted by the filtered fluid in the Bowman's space and it opposes filtration. Normally it is 10 mm Hg. It increases in conditions of obstruction of urinary tract as in ureteric calculi blocking the flow of fluid in the tubule.

e. **Oncotic pressure in the glomerulus:** GFR is inversely proportional to oncotic pressure. It is exerted by the plasma proteins. The capillary oncotic pressure at afferent end is 25 mm Hg and at efferent end it is 35 mm Hg. This is because as the fluid leaves the capillary from afferent to efferent ends, the concentration of plasma proteins increases and thereby oncotic pressure increases. So in conditions of hyperproteinemia or hemoconcentration oncotic pressure rises and GFR decreases. In hypoprotenemia GFR is increased.

f. **Oncotic pressure in Bowman's space:** It is very negligible because no protein is filtered into the Bowman's space.

g. **Effective filtration pressure:** It is the net outward pressure which favors filtration and is calculated as the difference between the outward and inward forces.
GFR = $K_f [(P_{GC} - P_T) - (\pi_{GC} - \pi_T)]$
GFR = $12.5 (45 - 10) - (25 - 0)$
     = $12.5 \times 10 = 125$ mL/min

h. **Other factors affecting GFR:**
   - Sympathetic stimulation of renal vessels lead to marked vasoconstriction and thereby decreases GFR
   - Hormones like norepinephrine, endothelin and angiotensin II cause intense vasoconstriction and thereby decrease renal blood flow (RBF) and GFR. Angiotensin II at low concentrations cause only constriction of efferent arteriole and thereby increases GFR. ANP, dopamine, nitric oxide, Prostaglandins cause vasodilatation and increase RBF and GFR.

8. Actions of growth hormone.

- Growth hormone (GH) is a polypeptide hormone
- It is a major growth promoting hormone
- It has direct and indirect actions
- It acts directly to catabolize substrates and to supply energy in starvation
- Its anabolic actions are direct on epiphysis and indirect through somatomedins (IGF-1).

Indirect Actions

- Effects of GH on growth, cartilage and protein metabolism is mediated through insulin-like growth factors (IGF)
- Also called as somatomedins
- They are growth factors synthesized in the liver.

Effect on Growth

- Effect on growth is direct or indirect through somatomedins
- Stimulates growth by acting on epiphyseal cartilage of long bones
- It stimulates proliferation of chondrocytes in epiphyseal plates in the ends of long bones
- It stimulates collagen formation in cartilage
- It also stimulates proliferation of osteoblasts and promotes its activity to convert cartilage into bone
- It increases thickness of epiphyseal endplate and thereby promotes linear growth
- Bone mass also increases
- It also has anabolic action and therefore increases muscle growth and hypertrophy
- Induces growth of visceral organs.

Effects on Metabolism

Protein Metabolism

- Protein anabolic
- ↑ Amino acid entry into cells
- ↑ RNA and DNA synthesis
- ↑ protein synthesis
- Decreased level of amino acids in blood.

Carbohydrate Metabolism

- It is an hyperglycemic hormone

- Releases glucose from liver by facilitating gluconeogenesis
- Decreases glucose uptake by skeletal muscles and adipocytes for energy production
- Decreases insulin sensitivity.

Lipid Metabolism
- Causes lipolysis and increases FFA in plasma
- Promotes ketogenesis
- Increased FFA and ketones provide the energy during stress.

Effect on Water and Electrolyte Metabolism
- ↑ plasma Ca^{2+}, by increasing the reabsorption from kidneys
- Causes Na^+ retention and also retention of potassium and chloride
- It maintains ECF volume by stimulating renin-angiotensin-aldosterone pathway
- Also supresses ANP release.

9. Testosterone.

- Testosterone, a C_{19} steroid produced in the testis is the major androgen in the males
- It is synthesized by the Leydig cells in the testis. Also the adrenal cortex produces testosterone from androstenedione
- The secretion of testosterone is under the control of luteinizing hormone (LH). LH in turn is under negative feedback control of testosterone
- Normal secretion rate is 4–9 mg/dL in normal adults. Most of it is transported in bound form. Total plasma level is 300-1000 ng/dL in adult male. Some of the testosterone is converted to estradiol and most of it is converted to 17-ketosteroids and excreted in urine.

Mechanism of action: Testosterone being a steroid hormone has an intranuclear receptor. On binding to the receptor the hormone complex binds to DNA and facilitates transcription of various genes.

Actions of Testosterone
- Developmental effects—Responsible for the development of vas deferens and related structures from the Wolffian duct. The metabolite of testosterone, dihydrotestosterone induces formation of male external genitalia in the fetus
- Development of secondary sexual characteristics—
  a. Enlargement of penis and scrotum, pigmentation of scrotum
  b. Internal genitalia—enlargement of seminal vesicle and secretion of fructose, enlargement of prostate and bulbourethral glands
  c. Larynx enlarges and becomes thicker and the voice becomes deeper
  d. Beard starts appearing, scalp hairline recedes anterolaterally, hair appears on chest, general body hair increases, pubic hair grows in male pattern
  e. Male type of behavior—aggressiveness, active attitude, attraction to opposite sex
  f. Shoulders broaden, muscles enlarge
  g. Sebaceous gland secretion thickens and increases and may predispose to acne.
3. Anabolic action—anabolic effect on protein leads to growth and development of muscles and bones, retention of Na^+, K^+, water, Ca^{++}, sulfate and phosphate and also increases kidney size
4. Role in spermatogenesis—high levels of local testosterone in testis is needed for spermatogenesis. The exact action is not known. But for maturation from spermatids to spermatozoa androgen is needed
5. Other actions—negatively inhibits secretion of gonadotropin-releasing hormone (GnRH), LH and follicle-stimulating hormone (FSH). It also stimulates erythropoiesis.

10. Milk ejection reflex.

- It is a neuroendocrine reflex
- In this type of reflex the afferent limb of the reflex is neural and the efferent limb is humoral or endocrine (refer Fig. 11).

Oxytocin is a hormone secreted from the hypothalamus and released from posterior pituitary gland. It acts on the myoepithelial cells lining the ducts of breast and expels milk through a reflex.

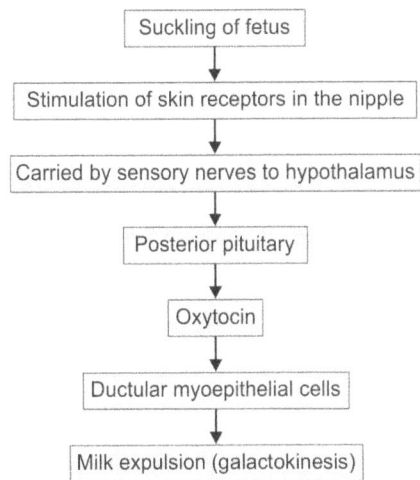

Fig. 11: Milk ejection reflex.

- The receptors for this reflex are touch receptors around the nipple. When the infant suckles at the breast the touch receptors are stimulated
- Impulses are relayed through somatic afferent pathways to the supraoptic (SO) and paraventricular (PV), nuclei of hypothalamus
- These nuclei secrete the hormone. Oxytocin which is transported through blood and acts on the myoepithelial cells lining the ducts of the breast resulting in expulsion of milk.

11. Accommodation for near vision.

When the eye is focusing on a close object the curvature of the lens increases to get a clear image on retina.

Accommodation of Lens

- This occurs due to contraction of ciliary muscles
- Results in increase of curvature of lens – adds 12 diopters to the power of the lens, power of lens increases (> 70 D)
- Near point – 10 cm in young adult
- Presbyopia – Near point increases (83 cm).

Other changes of accommodation are:
- Constriction of pupil
- Convergence of eyeball.

Accommodation Reflex Pathway

Impulses from retina for near vision
↓
Optic nerve
↓
Optic chiasma
↓
Optic tract
↓
Lateral geniculate body
↓
Visual cortex (area 17)
↓
Frontal eyefield
↓
Edinger-Westphal nuclei of both sides (parasympathetic fibers)
↓
Efferents go through the oculomotor nerves → Medial rectus → Convergence of eyeball
↓
Ciliary ganglion
↓
Supplies the sphincter pupillae and the ciliary muscles
↓
Constriction of pupil and anterior curvature of lens increases
↓
Accommodation of eye

12. Visceral pain.

- Visceral pain is poorly localized
- It is very unpleasant
- It is associated with autonomic symptoms like sweating, nausea, vomiting, hypotension, etc.
- Followed by reflex contraction of anterior abdominal wall muscles—Guarding
- Pain is radiated or referred to a somatic structure
- Causes are: Inflammation of viscera, over distension of hollow viscera, spasm of hollow viscera, ischemia, etc.
- Receptors for visceral pain – free nerve endings of unmyelinated C fibers (in sympathetic and parasympathetic)

- Tract carrying visceral pain is—lateral spinothalamic tract
- Pain in the viscera may be radiating or referred.

  Radiating pain—pain in a viscera is associated with pain at the location of the viscera as well it appears to radiate to nearby structure, e.g. in myocardial infarction pain is felt over the heart and it also radiates to the left shoulder, hand till the little finger.

Referred Pain

Irritation of a vicus or viscera usually produces pain which is not usually felt in the location of the viscus but in a somatic structure that is in a distance from the viscus. This is REFERRED PAIN.

For example:
- Cardiac pain is usually referred to the inner aspect of the left arm or to the neck
- When there is an irritation of central region of diaphragm there is pain in the tip of the shoulder
- Pain in the testicle due to distension of ureter as in ureteric calculus.

Theories of Referred Pain

The pain in viscera is usually referred to a somatic structure that has developed from the same embryonic segment or dermatome as the structure in which the pain originates - **Dermatomal rule**.

Theories of referred pain are—convergence theory and facilitation theory

Convergence Theory
- Peripheral nerve fibers from the somatic and visceral structures converge on the same second order neuron present in lamina V of dorsal gray horn (refer Fig. 12)
- The second order neuron is common for impulses from somatic and visceral structures
- So the tract carrying pain sensation from somatic structures also carry pain fibers from visceral structures
- Cortex sometimes cannot differentiate from somatic and visceral inputs and so pain from visceral structure is referred to the somatic structure.

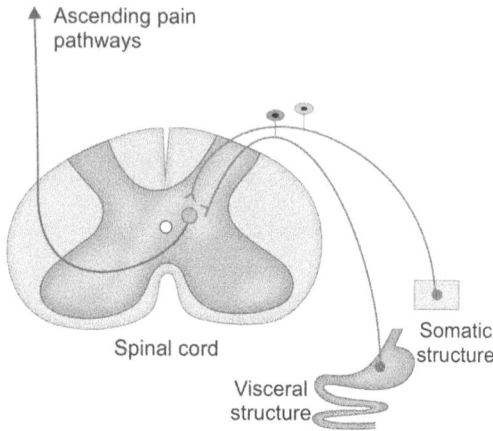

Fig. 12: Convergence theory of Referred pain. Note the afferents from somatic and visceral structures converge on the same second order neuron.
(*Source:* GK Pal)

Facilitation Theory
- The visceral afferent fibers on entering spinal cord give collaterals to afferents coming from the somatic structures
- So impulses coming from the visceral afferents facilitate and strengthen the impulses coming from the somatic structure
- So a minor activity in the somatic afferents is facilitated by the visceral afferents and therefore pain is referred to the somatic structure.

13. Sensory cortex.

Sensory Areas in Cortex

There are various sensory areas in the parietal cortex. They are:
1. **Somatosensory area I** (SS1)—area 3, 2 and 1
2. **Somatosensory area II** (SS2)—inside sylvian fissure
3. **Sensory association areas**—area 5 and 7 (Fig. 13).

Connections of Somatosensory Areas
- SS1 makes reciprocal and specific point to point connection with ventral posterolateral nucleus (VPLN) of thalamus

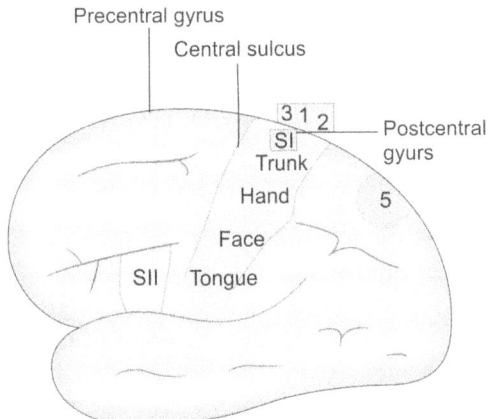

Fig. 13: Sensory areas in cerebral cortex.
(*Source:* GK Pal)

- SS 2 areas receive inputs from venterobasal nucleus of thalamus
- SS 1 and SS2 have reciprocal connections
- SS1 and SS2 of one side is connected with other cortex through corpus callosum
- SS1, SS2 and area 5 have connections with precentral gyrus and are involved in regulation of movement.

Functions of the Sensory Cortex

- SS1 receives information about conscious perception. It is involved in initial information processing
- SS1 → Motor cortex—helps in planning motor activity based on sensory information (e.g. Proprioception)
- SS1 → SS2 and opposite SS II—synthesis of sensory information from two sides of the body
- SS1 → Association areas—combines sensory inputs from various areas to give a meaningful interpretation, e.g. stereognosis.

Effect of Lesion of Various Areas

Lesion of SS1

- Pain and temperature sensations intact
- Loss of fine touch and proprioception
- Cortical sensations are lost
- Lesion on one side cortex affects opposite half of the body

- Lesion of area 3—failure to learn discriminative task
- Lesion of area 1 - Inability to discriminate hard-soft, smooth-rough textures.

Lesion of SS2

- Deficit in learning based on tactile discrimination.

Lesion of Association Cortex

- The main function is to coordinate relationship of the body to extrapersonal relationship like hand-eye coordination
- Lesion of this area results in inability to relate to extrapersonal space. They express constructional apraxia and hemineglect syndrome.

14. Total peripheral resistance in vascular system.

- There is a resistance to blood flow in the peripheral circulatory system and it is said to be the peripheral resistance
- Arterioles are the site of major resistance to blood flow in the vascular system. Therefore, they are called as the 'Resistance vessels'
- The walls of the arterioles are having more of smooth muscles than elastic tissue and these muscles are supplied by noradrenergic fibers and they are in partial contraction at rest—*vasomotor tone*
- The constriction and relaxation of the arterioles in any organ is responsible for the effective tissue perfusion
- The resistance is decided by the vasoconstriction or dilatation. There are other factors also which decide the total peripheral resistance (TPR)
- Important factors responsible for TPR are—radius of the vessel and viscosity of blood.

Radius of the Vessel

- Radius of the vessel is decided by the sympathetic nerves
- Decrease in radius increases TPR and increase in radius decreases TPR
- Even a decrease in resistance by half will increase the TPR 16 times

- When the radius is doubled the resistance is reduced by 6% of its previous value.

Viscosity of Blood

- Viscosity of blood also affects TPR
- But the most commonly occuring change in TPR is due to change in the radius of blood vessel
- Viscosity of blood is decided by the cellular components of blood especially RBCs and composition of plasma and resistance of cells to deformation. Temperature also affects viscosity
   a. **Hematocrit:** Viscosity of blood is mostly dependent on the hematocrit. In large vessels increase in hematocrit largely increases viscosity. In smaller vessels the effect of viscosity on TPR is less due to difference in nature of blood flow. So the net effect of viscosity of blood on TPR is less in vivo than in vitro, unless there is severe polycythemia. In anemia, TPR is decreased as viscosity of blood is decreased
   b. **Composition of plasma:** Viscosity is increased in diseases where there is marked increase in plasma proteins as in multiple myeloma
   c. **Effect of deformed cells:** There is rise viscosity in hereditary spherocytosis
   d. **Effect of temperature:** Increase in body temperature decreases viscosity and decrease in body temperature increases viscosity.

15. Acclimatization to high altitude.

Physiological Changes at High Altitude

- Effects of high altitude is due to low barometric pressure → ↓ Partial pressure of inspired O2 (P_{IO2})
- Hypoxic symptoms appear at an altitude of 10,000 ft and are severe at 15,000 to 18,000 ft
- There are various compensatory mechanisms by which the O_2 supply to tissue is increased. They are:
   - First and foremost—hyperventilation
   - In high altitude, there is no drive for ventilation till PO_2 is <60 mm Hg (at 14,000 ft) and on reaching <60 mm Hg, there is hyperventilation because:
      - **1st stage:** Hypoxia acts on peripheral chemoreceptors (PCR) → stimulation of ventilation → CO_2 blow out →↓ PCO_2 →↑ Arterial pH →↓ ventilation
      - **2nd stage:** Ventilation slowly decreases and then increases and becomes stable after 8–10 hours, due to pH of CSF is more alkaline in the acute phase. But later ventilation increases by ↓ pH, by movement of HCO_3^- out of CSF.
   - There is renal compensation for the alkaline nature because the kidneys excrete more HCO_3^- into the urine →↓ pH.

Acclimatization to High Altitude

- When a person ascends to high altitudes and stays there for sometime he gets adapted
- It starts by 12 hours and takes several days
- The maximum height upto which acclimatization possible is 18,000 ft.

Changes During Acclimatization to High Altitude

- **Respiratory changes:**
   - Initial changes:

   Hyperventilation by hypoxia stimulating peripheral chemoreceptor
   ↓
   CO_2 washout
   ↓
   Renal compensation and HCO_3^- excretion out of CSF
   ↓
   Stimulates central chemoreceptors and ventilation
   ↓
   After 4 days, ventilation slowly increases and is dependent on altitude

- **Hematological changes:**
   - Hypoxia stimulates erythropoietin production by kidneys →↑ RBC production (starts after 3 days) →↑O_2 delivery to tissues

- There is also increase in 2, 3-DPG levels in RBC →↑O_2 delivery to tissues.
- **CVS changes:**
  - There is ↑ in heart rate (HR), cardiac output (CO) and BP due to activation of sympatho-adrenal activity →↑ CO and ↑ HR →↑ blood flow
  - Vasodilatation due to hypoxia →↑ blood flow.
- **Changes in tissues:**
  - ↑ In number of capillaries
  - ↑ In number of mitochondria in cells
  - ↑ In activity of oxidative enzymes like cytochrome oxidase
  - ↑ In myoglobin content
  - Angiogenesis.

16. Compliance of lungs.

- Stretchability or the recoiling tendency due to the elastic property of the lung is said to be the compliance
- Compliance of the respiratory system is defined as the change in the lung volume per unit change in the airway pressure
- It is given as $C = \Delta V/\Delta P$
  C = Compliance
  ΔV = Change in volume
  ΔP = Change in pressure
  It is expressed in L/cm H_2O.

Compliance in Respiratory System is Given under Two Headings

1. Compliance of lungs only
2. Compliance of lungs and thoracic wall.

Compliance of Lungs and Thoracic Wall

Both the lungs and thoracic wall are elastic and viscous in nature and therefore each of them has their own recoiling tendencies.

Normal value of compliance of thoracic wall and lungs together is 0.13 L/cm H_2O.

It means when there is an increase in airway pressure by 1 cm H_2O the volume of the lungs increase by 0.13 Liters.

Compliance of Lung Alone

Normal value is around 0.22 L/cm H_2O.

So compliance of lung is twice that of lung and thoracic cavity together.

Measurement of Compliance of Lungs and Chest Wall

- The interaction of recoiling of lung and chest wall is demonstrated in living subjects by using spirometer
- After clipping the nose, the subject is asked to breathe in from a spirometer from end expiratory position in increments of volumes
- There is a valve beyond the mouth piece, through which he breathes and also a pressure recording device is attached to the mouthpiece
- The person inhales a given volume of air and the valve is shut and the person is asked to relax the respiratory muscles and the change in airway pressure is noted
- This procedure is repeated after inhaling and exhaling various volumes of air and also recording of airway pressures
- The airway pressures are plotted against the lung volumes to get the relaxation pressure curve of the respiratory system (Fig. 14)

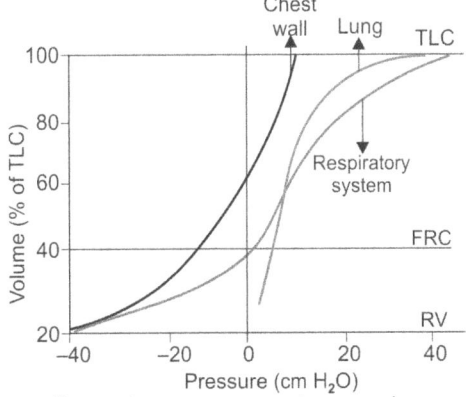

Transpulmonary pressure, transmural pressure across chest wall, pressure across respiratory system

Fig. 14: Relaxation pressure-volume curve of lung and chest wall. It gives the realation between intrapulmonary pressure and volume. Curve in red color is the curve of total respiratory system. At FRC, the transmural pressure is zero and above it the pressure is positive and below it, negative. (TLC: Total lung capacity; FRC: Functional residual capacity; RV: Residual volume)
(*Source:* GK Pal)

- From the curve it is noted that at zero pressure the lung volume is equal to functional residual capacity (FRC) and this volume is said to be the relaxation volume
- It is the volume at which the recoiling of lungs is exactly balanced by the recoiling of the thoracic wall
- The measurement of compliance can be made by using the curve especially where it is the steepest
- Above the relaxation volume as the volume increases the pressure also increases and it reaches about + 30 mm Hg
- Below the relaxation volume as the volume decreases the pressure also decreases and reaches – 30 mm Hg.

Factors Affecting Compliance of Lungs and Chest Wall

- Compliance when decreased shifts the pressure-volume curve to the right and downwards, as in: Pulmonary edema, congestion and pulmonary fibrosis
- Compliance when increased the curve is shifted to the left and above as in: Emphysema and in old age.

Measurement of Compliance of Lungs Alone

- The compliance of lungs alone can be measured by measuring the intrapleural pressures (IPP) at various lung volumes (Fig. 15)
- IPP gives an idea about the distensibility of the lungs
- As the lung expands the IPP becomes more negative as the recoiling forces are more
- IPP can be recorded by measuring intra-esophageal pressures
- The person is asked to breathe in from a spirometer from the end expiratory position upto end inspiratory position and holds the breath
- The IPP is measured in this manner for various lung volumes inhaled and exhaled, and inspiratory and expiratory compliance curves are obtained respectively on the graph.

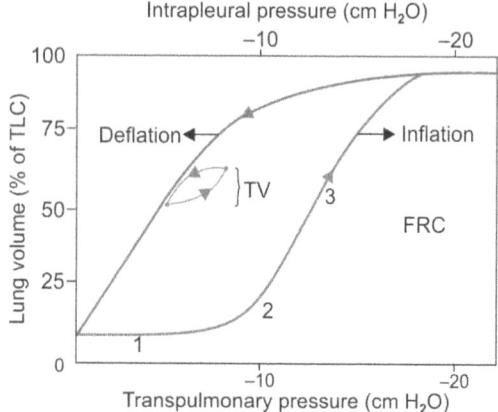

Fig. 15: Pressure-volume relations in the lungs. Pressure changes in inflation and deflation are different.
(TV: Tidal volume; FRC: Functional residual capacity)
(*Source:* GK Pal)

- The inspiratory and expiratory compliance curves are not similar and they form a loop, called the 'Hysteresis loop'
- The observation is that the curves of change in pressure to change in volume is different for inspiration and expiration and is curved
- The curve depicts that at similar IPP, the lung volume is less in inspiratory phase than in expiratory phase.
- The difference in pressure volume-relationship in inspiration and expiration is due to viscous resistance and airway resistance
- Compliance is greater when measured during deflation than when measured during inflation
- Lung compliance is calculated by taking a point on the graph at the end of inspiration when there is no air flow and so there is no viscous and elastic resistance
- Lung compliance is calculated as $\Delta V/\Delta P = 0.22 L/cm\ H_2O$
- This amount of lung compliance is affected by the elastic tissues in the lungs and also the surface tension of the fluid lining the alveoli
- The contribution of each factor is studied by removing the lungs of an experimental animal and distending them with air and

water alternately, while measuring the intrapulmonary pressure
- While distension with air, the pressure-volume curve measures both tissue elasticity and surface tension, whereas while using saline surface tension becomes zero and the curve measures only tissue elasticity
- In the curve with saline there is not much difference in inspiratory and expiratory curves. The elasticity due to surface tension is much smaller at small lung volumes than at large lung volumes. This may be due to the effect of surfactant.

Factors Affecting Lung Compliance Alone
- Lung volume—a person with one lung will have half the change in volume to change in pressure
- Compliance is more during deflation of lung than while inflating the lungs
- Due to effect of gravity in standing position compliance is less in the apex of the lung.

Specific Compliance
- As mentioned above, in a person with one lung (even though compliance of that lung is normal) the compliance is decreased as the lung volume is decreased. To overcome this, compliance can be calculated as a function of FRC
- Specific compliance = Compliance/FRC.

17. Functions of middle ear.

- Middle ear—it is an air filled cavity in temporal bone. It starts at the tympanic membrane and ends at oval window
- Contains - 3 ossicles (malleus, incus and stapes), 2 small muscles (tensor tympani and Stapedius), Ligaments, nerves, blood vessels, etc.

Functions

- **Tympanic reflex:** It is a protective reflex. When a loud sound is transmitted through the ossicles in middle ear a reflex is initiated with a latent period of 40 - 80 msec. Contraction of stapedius and tensor tympani pulls the tympanic membrane medially and membrane covering oval window laterally. This makes the ossicular system rigid and there is reduction in transmission of sounds. This reduces the intensity of sound by 30-40 decibels. It is also called as Attenuation reflex

Functions of this reflex:
a. This reflex protects the cochlea from damaging loud sounds
b. It filters the low frequency sounds
c. It prevents hearing ones own speech.
- Transmission of sound waves from external ear to internal ear
- **Impedence matching:**
  - As the sound waves travel from rarer (air in external and middle ear) to denser medium (fluid in the inner ear) they are dampened (by 30 db)
  - This loss in sound energy is prevented in the middle ear by impedence matching which is by:
    a. **Area difference** - Area of tympanic membrane is greater than foot plate of stapes and therefore there is convergence of sound and pressure is increased by 17 times
    b. **Lever action of the Ossicles** increases pressure by 1.32 times
    c. **Buckling factor** - Tympanic membrane is conical in shape and the handle of malleus is attached to the umbo. As the tympanic membrane moves in and out, the buckling of membrane moves the handle of malleus less and this increases the force and decreases the velocity.

18. Associative learning.

Associative learning means an organism learns about the relation of one stimulus to the other.

They are of two types - Classical conditioning and Operant conditioning

Classical Conditioning or Conditioned Reflex

- A conditioned reflex is a reflex response to a stimulus that previously elicited little or no response, acquired by repeatedly pairing the stimulus with another stimulus that normally produces the response

- An example of this reflex is Pavlov's classic experiment. When meat is placed in the dog's mouth there is salivation. This is an Unconditioned reflex and meat in the mouth is the Unconditioned stimulus (US)
- Usually ringing of bell does not produce any response; salivation, in the dog. But when the bell rings every time before the meat is placed in the mouth and repeated many times, the dog starts to salivate when the bell was rung even without placing meat. This is conditioned reflex. Ringing bell is the conditioned stimulus (CS)
- After pairing US and CS many times the CS was able to evoke a response (salivation) originllay evoked only by US. So learning has happened by associating the two stimuli
- If the CS is repeated many times without pairing with US gradually the response is lost. This is said to be "Internal inhibition"or "Extinction"
- If the animal is disturbed everytime after the CS the response may not appear, "External inhibition"
- Conditioned reflex can happen if the US is associated with a pleasant or unpleasant effect. If it is with pleasant stimulus it is Positive reinforcement. If it is with unpleasant US it is Negative reinforcement.

Operant Conditioning

- In this type of conditioning it is not just learning an association, but the animal learns to perform a task in order to obtain a reward or prevent a punishment
- Conditioned motor response that allows the animal to avoid an unpleasant event is said to be "Conditioned avoidance reflex". For example the animal learns to press a bar to avoid an electric shock.

19. Righting reflexes.

- Phasic or dynamic reflexes help to make rapid adjustments in the posture and are short-term and produce transient changes
- They are also called as righting reflexes
- They help to keep the head upright and in alignment with the body
- These reflexes are integrated in the nuclei of midbrain
- Righting reflexes are demonstrated in experimental animals when the transection is done at the upper border of midbrain.

The reflexes are:

a. *Labyrinthine righting reflexes:*
   - When the animal is held by its body and tipped from side to side, the animal holds the head erect in response to stimulus (gravity) from the otolithic organ (receptors).

b. *Neck righting reflex:*
   - It acts on neck muscles and corrects the position of head to that of the body
   - It happens when the body is in the lateral position and head is erect
   - **The stimulus** is stretch of neck muscles
   - **Receptor** is muscle spindle in neck muscles
   - **Center** is midbrain
   - **Response** is the body gets gradually righted, starting from righting of thorax, shoulders, abdomen and pelvis.

c. *Body on head righting reflex:*
   - It happens when the body is laid on the side and even if the otolithic organs are destroyed, the pressure effect of the body initiates righting of the head
   - **Stimulus** is pressure on the side of the body
   - **Receptor** is exteroceptors
   - **Center** is midbrain
   - **Response** is righting of head.

d. *Body on body righting reflexes:*
   - This happens when the head is prevented from righting, therefore the impulses from the body surface can right the body
   - **Stimulus** is pressure on side of the body
   - **Receptors** are exteroceptors
   - **Center** is midbrain
   - **Response** is righting of body even if body is prevented from righting.

e. *Optical righting reflexes:*
   - Even in the absence of stimuli from labyrinth or body stimulation there can be righting of head due to visual or optical cues. But this needs an intact cerebral cortex. In intact humans, this reflex helps to maintain the head in stable position despite the movements of the body
   - **Stimulus**—visual cues
   - **Receptors**—eyes
   - **Center**—cerebral cortex
   - **Response**—righting of head.
f. *Limb righting reflexes:*
   - *Placing reaction:* It is integrated in cerebral cortex
     - When the snout of a suspended blind-folded animal touches a surface it immediately places both the forepaws on the surface. Exteroceptors are reponsible for the placing reaction
     - If a blind-folded animal is suspended in air with one foot touching the surface it can place the foot firmly on the supporting surface. Labyrinthine and exteroceptors are responsible for the placing reaction
     - If an animal is thrown into air it can land firmly with four limbs. It is due to visual, labyrinthine and exteroceptor cues.
   - *Hopping reaction:*
     - When a standing animal is pushed laterally, hopping movements help to support the body and rights the posture
     - **Stimulus** is lateral displacement of the body
     - **Receptors** are muscle spindles
     - **Center** is cerebral cortex
     - **Response** is hopping, maintains limb in position to support body.

20. Control of food intake.

- Appetite and food intake is controlled by hypothalamus
- In hypothalamus there are feeding and satiety centers
- There are 2 groups of neurons involved in food intake:
  1. Venteromedial nucleus (satiety center)
  2. Lateral nucleus (feeding center).
- Feeding center stimulates appetite and increases food intake and satiety center inhibits feeding center and brings satiety
- Feeding center is chronically active and its activity is transiently inhibited by activity in the satiety center after ingestion of food
- Lesion of feeding center causes severe anorexia
- Lesion of satiety center leads to hyperphagia and overeating results in hypothalamic obesity
- There are various hormones and neurotransmitters regulating the appetite
- The following are:
  - **Hormones increasing food intake:**
    - Neuropeptide Y
    - Orexins
    - Ghrelin
    - Melanin concentrating hormone (MCH)
    - Agouti related peptide (AGRP)
    - Galanin
    - Growth hormone releasing hormone (GHRH).
  - **Hormones decreasing food intake:**
    - Leptin
    - Estrogen
    - Dopamine
    - Melanocyte stimulating hormone (MSH)
    - Cocaine—and amphetamine regulated transcript (CART)
    - Corticotrophin releasing hormone (CRH)
    - Gut hormones
    - Cholecystokinin (CCK)
      * There are 4 hypotheses by which appetite is regulated by action of the above hormones and neurotransmitters on the feeding and satiety centers.

They are:

- Glucostatic hypothesis—blood glucose level affects the appetite. The neurons

in the satiety center are activated by the blood glucose levels. When the blood glucose levels are low the neuronal uptake of glucose decreases and the feeding center is stimulated resulting in hunger and food intake. When glucose utilzation increases, the satiety center is activated and feeding center is inhibited
- Lipostatic hypothesis—the amount of adipose tissue affects the food intake by a proportional amount of humoral signal, the hormone leptin. As the leptin level increases it decreases the appetite and food intake and increases energy output and vice versa
- Gut-peptide theory—food in the gastrointestinal tract causes release of one or more polypeptides like CCK-PZ which acts on the hypothalamus to inhibit food intake
- Thermostatic theory—a fall in body temperature below the set point stimulates appetite and a rise above the set point inhibits appetite.

MBBS Examination 2004

ANSWER ALL QUESTIONS

I. Essay questions (15 Marks each)

1. Describe the mechanism of concentration of urine.
2. Describe the actions and regulation of secretion of glucocorticoids. Write a note on its applied physiology.
3. Describe the mechanism of oxygen transport in the body. Explain Oxygen dissociation curve with a suitable diagram.
4. Draw and explain the visual pathway. Discuss the effects of lesion at various levels along its course.

II. Short notes (5 Marks each)

1. What are plasma proteins? Mention their types and discuss their function.
2. Describe the pharyngeal stage of deglutition.
3. Intercellular connections.
4. Nerve action potential.
5. Physiological effects of thyroid hormone.
6. Contraceptive methods.
7. Neuroendocrine reflex.
8. Small intestinal movements.
9. Discuss the morphology and functions of platelets.
10. Cell-mediated immunity.
11. Respiratory changes during moderate exercises.
12. Describe the origin and spread of cardiac impulse.
13. Fetal circulation.
14. Refractory errors of the eye.
15. Cochlea.
16. Neuroglia.
17. Discuss the functions of limbic system.
18. Mechanism of memory.
19. Describe the humoral regulation of blood pressure.
20. Artificial respiration.

I. ESSAY QUESTIONS

1. Describe the mechanism of concentration of urine.

Humans have the ability to excrete a dilute urine (30 mOsm/L) or concentrated urine (1400 mOsm/L) to regulate the extracellular fluid (ECF) volume and osmolality.

Concentration of urine involves interaction of two entities, countercurrent mechanism and action of antidiuretic hormone (ADH) on collecting duct of nephron.

Countercurrent Mechanism in Kidneys

Countercurrent mechanism refers to a system in which the inflow of fluid runs parallel to, counter to and in close proximity to the outflow for some distance in two tubes placed close to each other. An U-tube system is used for this countercurrent mechanism.

In the kidney it is formed by

1. Countercurrent multiplier (loop of Henle)
2. Countercurrent exchanger (vasa recta).

The role of countercurrent mechanism is to **create** a hyperosmolar medullary interstitium in the kidneys and to **maintain** the osmolar gradient in medullary interstitium.

Hyperosmolality in the interstitium along with action of ADH is essential for concentration of urine.

Medullary Interstitial Osmolarity

- The medullary interstitial fluid osmolality is important in concentrating the urine, because it provides the driving force for reabsorbing water from both the descending thin limb of loop of Henle (LOH) and collecting duct (CD)
- The principal components for creating the hyperosmolarity of the medullary interstitial fluid are NaCl and urea
- At the junction of medulla with cortex, the interstitial osmolality is approximately 300 mOsm/kg H_2O with virtually all osmoles attributable to NaCl
- The concentrations of both NaCl and urea increase progressively as the tubular fluid moves deeper into the medulla to 1,200 mOsm/kg H_2O with each contributing 600 mmol/L
- NaCl in interstitium is got from its reabsorption in thick ascending limb of LOH (TAL of LOH) through the active transporter, Na^+ K^+ $2Cl^-$ symporter and passive reabsorption from thin ascending limb of LOH. This creates a gradient of 200 mOsm/kg H_2O across the tubular lumen and interstitium and this effect is called the **Single effect**
- Urea is filtered and reabsorbed in descending and ascending limb of LOH and medullary CD. The last part is favored by antidiuretic hormone (ADH). Urea also contributes interstitial hyperosmolarity.

Countercurrent Multiplier (Fig. 1)

Countercurrent multiplier operating in the LOH generates hyperosmolarity and creates osmolar gradient in the interstitium by:
- Origin of single effect (already mentioned above)
- Multiplication of the single effect.

Multiplication of Single Effect

- Hyperosmolarity of medullary interstitium is generated by multiplication of the single effect
- **Multiplication happens due to the following characteristic features of the tubule:**
  - High permeability of descending thin segment to water
  - Impermeability to water and active reabsorption of NaCl in TAL of LOH, which creates a osmolar gradient of 200 mOsm/kg H_2O across the tubule
  - In renal medulla, all other tubular structures other than TAL of LOH are in osmotic equilibrium with interstitium
  - The descending limb acquires the osmolality of the surrounding interstitium
  - The effect is multiplied when more and more isosmolar filtered fluid from proximal convoluted tubule (PCT) enters into descending limb and forces the concentrated fluid to the tip of the loop.

Steps in Countercurrent Multiplication

- As iso-osmolar fluid passes into PCT, solutes and equal amounts of water are reabsorbed

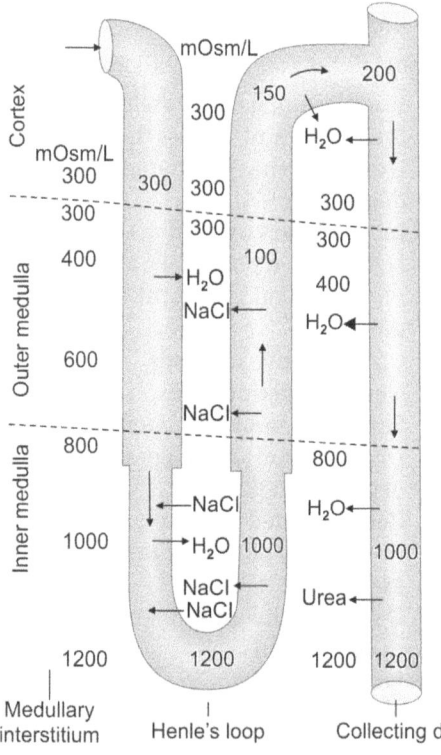

Fig. 1: Countercurrent multiplier formed by Loop of Henle (descending and ascending limbs) and collecting duct.
(*Source:* Sembulingam)

and therefore the osmolality of tubular fluid is unaltered here and is 300 mOsm/L
- In the descending limb as the fluid passes, only water is reabsorbed as the limb is impermeable to solutes, but NaCl enters the tubule
- Now the tubular fluid concentration increases and as it reaches the tip of the loop, it reaches 1200 mOsm/L
- Next the hyperosmolar fluid moves into the thin ascending limb where NaCl is reabsorbed passively and in the TAL of LOH the same is reabsorbed by active transport
- This makes the fluid in TAL hypo-osmolar (200 mOsm/L) and increases the medullary interstitial osmolality to 400 mOsm/L
- Formation of this 200 mOsm/L gradient is the 'single effect'
- This segment and distal convoluted tubule (DCT) are impermeable to water and permeable to NaCl, so the fluid now becomes hypo-osmolar and attains the osmolality of 100 mOsm/L
- All other segments of the tubule, except TAL of LOH, and the interstitium are all in osmolar equilibrium and their osmolality are the same
- This is the mechanism by which the hyperosmolar interstitium is created
- By this time more iso-osmolar filtrate enters the PCT and this process repeats and there is multiplication of creation of the gradient
- Urea also contributes to the osmolality. It is reabsorbed across the CD and LOH and helps in creating the hyperosmolality in the interstitium. This effect is greater in presence of ADH.

Countercurrent Exchanger (Fig. 2)

- Vasa recta is the countercurrent exchanger
- These are capillaries formed from efferent arterioles and are U shaped resembling the LOH. Because of their U shape, they are able to maintain the solute concentration in medullary interstitium and remove water into general circulation
- The flow of blood in vasa recta is very slow which also helps to maintain the gradient

- **Descending limb of vasa recta:** As the descending limb dips into the medulla there is a progressive increase in the osmolality from 300–1200 mOsm/kg of H_2O
- Here the solutes move into the capillary and water moves out into the interstitium and enters the ascending limb. The osmolality of blood is in equilibrium with the surrounding interstitium
- **Ascending limb of vasa recta:** From the point of ascending where the osmolality is 1200 mOsm/kg H_2O, it starts dropping to 300 mOsm/kg H_2O as water from interstitium enters the ascending limb
- From this limb, solutes move out into the interstitium and then into descending limb and water moves into the capillary
- Thus the water moves from here to the general circulation and solutes are circulating within the medullary interstitium and hyperosmolality is maintained.

Role of ADH in Concentration of Urine

- ADH acts through V2 receptors on the principal cells of collecting duct and

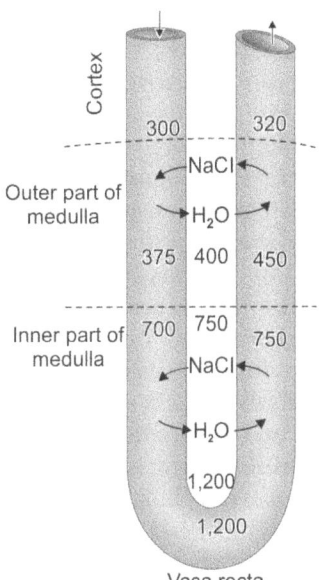

Fig. 2: Countercurrent exchanger (vasa recta)
(*Source:* Sembulingam)

inserts aquaporin 2 on the luminal membrane of the principal cells
- The presence of hyperosmolar medullary interstitium (created by countercurrent mechanism) provides the gradient for water reabsorption through the aquaporins
- When there is dehydration, ADH secretion from the posterior pituitary increases and it helps in reabsorption of water resulting in passing a very low volume of urine (500 mL/day) of 1400 mOsm/L osmolality
- In conditions like alcohol intake or excessive water intake the urine volume may increase upto 23 L/day of 30 mOsm/L osmolality
- Thus the presence of countercurrent mechanism and ADH help in concentrating the urine.

2. **Describe the actions and regulation of secretion of glucocorticoids. Write a note on its applied physiology.**

Metabolic actions of glucocorticoids are:

a. **Effects on Carbohydrate metabolism:**
   - Increases gluconeogenesis in liver → increased glycogen stores
   - Antagonizes the action of insulin on muscle and adipose tissue—prevents glucose uptake
   - This spares glucose for the brain
   - Increases glucose output from liver
   - Results in hyperglycemia.

b. **Effects on Protein metabolism:**
   - It is proteolytic in action
   - Breaks down proteins into aminoacid (AA) and inhibits protein synthesis
   - Amino acids are used for gluconeogenesis
   - Therefore increased cortisol levels drains the protein stores in the body

c. **Effects on Lipid metabolism:**
   - Cortisol is permissive for the lipolytic action of catecholamines
   - But high cortisol levels increase total body fat by 2 mechanisms:
     1. Cortisol stimulates appetite → obesity due to increased caloric consumption
     2. High cortisol → ↑ blood glucose → ↑ insulin secretion → lipogenesis.
   - Pattern of fat distribution - **centripetal** - concentrated in trunk, but wasting is seen in arms and legs.

Permissive Action

Cortisol amplifies effects of certain processes of other hormones where it does not act directly. Examples:

A. It does not induce glycogenolysis itself but augments glycogenolysis by glucagon

B. It also augments vaso responsiveness of blood vessels to catecholamines.

A. Actions on bones

Increases bone resorption by:
Cortisol decreases renal and gastrointestinal tract (GIT) absorption of calcium
↓
Lowers serum calcium levels
↓
Parathyroid hormone secretion stimulated
↓
Mobilizes calcium from bone by resorption and demineralization

- Also inhibits action of osteoblasts and suppresses collagen formation. Hence, high cortisol levels results in **osteoporosis.**

B. Actions on cardiovascular system (CVS)

- Cortisol is permissive for the vasopressor effects of catecholamine and angiotensin II
- Hence it is necessary for the maintenance of normal blood pressure (BP)
- Stimulates erythropoietin synthesis and so increases red blood cell (RBC) production.

C. Actions on connective tissue

Cortisol inhibits fibroblast proliferation and collagen formation:

So excess cortisol levels
↓
Thinning of skin and walls of capillaries
↓
Easy damage to skin and easy bruising of capillaries
↓
Intracutaneous hemorrhage

D. Action on kidneys
- Cortisol inhibits ADH secretion and action, so in the absence of cortisol a water load leads to water intoxication
- Cortisol also has a weak mineralocorticoid action →↑ Na+ and H_2O reabsorption
- **Increases glomerular filtration rate (GFR):**
  i. By increasing cardiac output
  ii. By direct action on kidneys.

E. Action on muscles
- Cortisol has complex action on muscles
- Excess cortisol results in muscle weakness due to:
  i. Proteolysis
  ii. Hypokalemia.

F. Actions on GIT
- Cortisol has a trophic action on GIT
- It also increases appetite → weight gain in hypercortisolism
- Increased acid secretion → acidity, gastritis.

G. Action on CNS
- Glucocorticoids alters mood and behavior
- REM sleep ↓, but slow wave sleep ↑
- In excess – insomnia, elevated or depressed mood, ↓ memory
- Frank psychosis occurs with excess or reduced cortisol levels
- Dampens the acuity to olfactory, gustatory, auditory and visual stimuli.

H. Action in fetus
- Facilitates maturity of CNS, retina, skin, GIT, and lungs
- During the last week of pregnancy the synthesis of surfactant is stimulated by cortisol
- So if premature delivery suspected weekly doses of cortisol given to mother till delivery.

I. Action on inflammation and immune system
- Cortisol is frequently used clinically for its anti-inflammatory property
- It inhibits synthesis of mediators of inflammation
- Inhibits migration of leukocytes to the site of injury
- Decreases the number of circulating eosinophils
- Inhibits fibroblast proliferation at inflammatory site which is a defense mechanism in the body to prevent spreading of infection
- Excess cortisol inhibits normal defense mechanisms of body against infection.

J. Effect on immune response
- Cortisol inhibits immune response in the body
- At high doses it decreases the number of T lymphocytes (helper t-cells) and their migration to antigenic site
- B lymphocytes and antibody production are not affected directly
- Because of these effects, glucocorticoids are used for immunosuppression after organ transplantation.

K. Effect on stress
- Protects the body against stress
- During stress there is increased secretion of corticotropin-releasing hormone (CRH) from hypothalamus
- This increses the secretion of adrenocorticotropic hormone (ACTH) from anterior pituitary
- Therefore glucocorticoid secretion increases
- Cortisol facilitates lipolysis by catecholamine and increases release of free fatty acids which supplies the energy needed to cope up with stress
- It is also permissive for the vasoconstriction induced by catecholamines which is needed for maintaining BP during stress.

Regulation of Glucocorticoid Secretion
- Secretion of cortisol is regulated by ACTH from anterior pituitary (Fig. 3)
- ACTH secretion is in turn is stimulated by CRH from hypothalamus
- Free cortisol levels negatively inhibit ACTH
- All types of stress stimulates hypothalamus →↑ CRH →↑ ACTH →↑ cortisol

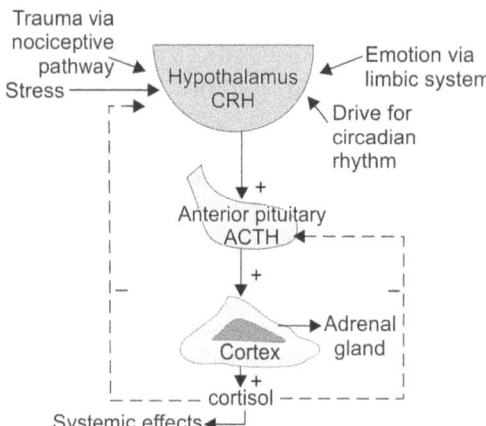

Fig. 3: Regulation of secretion of glucocorticoids. (CRH: Corticotrophin-releasing hormon; ACTH: adrenocorticotropin hormone)

- Circadian rhythm alters ACTH secretion and also affects cortisol secretion.

Applied Aspects of Glucocorticoids

a. Hypersecretion of glucocorticoids— Cushing's syndrome:

Causes:
i. Pharmacological use of exogenous glucocorticoids—ACTH levels are low
ii. ACTH secreting pituitary tumor (Cushing's disease)—ACTH levels high, skin pigmentation present
iii. Primary hypercortisolism due to adrenal tumor—ACTH levels low

Symptoms:
- Obesity with characteristic centripetal distribution of fat, sparing the limbs
- Face is rounded and cheeks are red due to polycythemia
- Loss of bone mass (osteoporosis)—vertebral fractures and necrosis of hip
- Loss of connective tissue integrity—fragile capillaries, easy bruisability and purple striae in abdomen.
- ↑ Protein catabolism—atrophy and weakness of skeletal muscles
- Poor wound healing and response to infection
- Disturbances in glucose metabolism—glucose intolerance, insulin resistance, hyperglycemia or even diabetes mellitus
- Mineralocorticoid activity of glucocorticoids leads to Na^+ and H_2O retention → hypertension
- Excess androgen secretion in women → hirsuitism, male pattern baldness, clitorial enlargement.

Diagnosis:
- Elevated plasma cortisol or urinary free cortisol levels
- Loss of diurnal pattern of secretion
- Loss of suppressive effect of exogenous dexamethasone.

b. Primary adrenal insufficiency (Addison's disease): In this condition there is deficiency of both glucocorticoid and mineralocorticoid.

Causes:
- Autoimmune destruction of adrenal gland
- Tuberculosis
- Malignancy

Symptoms:
- **Symptoms due to Cortisol deficiency:**
  - GIT
    - Anorexia, nausea, vomiting, diarrhea, abdominal pain, weight loss.
  - CNS
    - Confusion, psychosis.
  - Metabolic
    - Hypoglycemia on fasting and stress
    - Impaired gluconeogenesis
    - Increased insulin sensitivity.
  - CVS and Renal
    - Impaired free water clearence
    - Impaired pressor response to catecholamines
    - Hypotension.
  - Pituitary
    - Increased ACTH
    - Hyperpigmentation.
- **Symptoms due to Aldosterone deficiency:**
  - Inability to conserve sodium
  - Decreased extracellular fluid volume
  - Decreased blood volume
  - Weight loss
  - Increased renin production
  - Hypotension
  - Shock

- Impaired renal secretion of potassium and hydrogen
- Hyperkalemia
- Metabolic acidosis.

Addisonian Crisis

- Severe hypotension and shock
- Treated with excess glucocorticoids.

---

3. **Describe the mechanism of oxygen transport in the body. Explain Oxygen dissociation curve with a suitable diagram.**

Transport of O_2

- O_2 is transported in blood in 2 forms
- They are—dissolved form (2%) and as oxyhemoglobin (98%)
- As O_2 enters the blood it gets saturated in plasma as dissolved O_2 and then there is a gradient between plasma and RBC → leads to entry of O_2 into RBC → as PO_2 increases inside the RBC, O_2 saturates Hb.

Dissolved O_2

- Dissolved O_2 is measured by the following equation:
  Dissolved O_2 = Solubility of O_2 (0.003 mL/mm Hg) × arterial PO_2 (100 mm Hg)
  = 0.3 mL/dl
- Partial pressure of O_2 (PO_2) in blood is decided by the dissolved O_2 content of blood.

Oxy-hemoglobin

- Hemoglobin is an O_2 carrying protein in RBC
- It increases the O_2 carrying capacity of blood by 70 times
- Iron in the Hb is in ferrous form (Fe^{2+}) and combines with O_2 in appropriate affinity
- O_2 + Hb ↔ Hb O_2—oxygenation reaction (it is not oxidation reaction)
- If Fe^{2+} gets oxidized to Fe^{3+} methemoglobin is formed which does not release O_2
- When the binding of O_2 with hemoglobin happens, affinity of Hb for O_2 increases gradually
- Initially, Hb is in a tense configuration (T), as one molecule of O_2 combines, the Hb changes to Relaxed configuration (R) and the affinity to O_2 increases to maximum when the 3rd O_2 molecule has combined.

O_2 Carrying Capacity of Blood

- Each gram of Hb carries 1.34 ml of O_2
- Maximum amount of O_2 carried by Hb is the **O_2 carrying capacity of blood**
- In a healthy individual, it is 20 mL/100 mL of blood. (15 × 1.34 mL = 20.1 mL/dl)
- O_2 **content** is the amount actually bound to Hb
- % **saturation of O_2 (SO_2)** = Hb O_2 content/ HbO_2 capacity × 100
- Normally in arterial blood % SO_2 is 98%.

O_2-Hb Dissociation Curve

- This curve compares the Partial pressure of O_2 and % saturation of Hb with O_2
- It is sigmoid in shape (Fig. 4)
- The shape is sigmoid because of the change in configuration of hemoglobin from T to R state and therefore there is gradual increase in affinity for O_2 and then it gets saturated
- It has a steep and plateau phase
- About 90% saturation of Hb takes place at a PO_2 of 60 mm Hg
- P_{50} is the partial pressure at which 50% of the hemoglobin is saturated with oxygen
- P_{50} is inversely related to the affinity of hemoglobin for oxygen

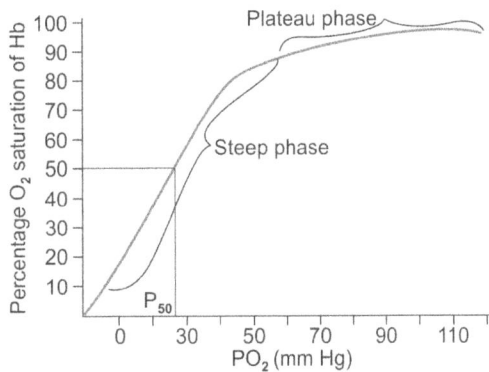

Fig. 4: Oxygen-hemoglobin dissociation curve. P_{50} is the partial pressure of O_2 at which 50% of hemoglobin is saturated with O_2. It is around 27 mm Hg. There are two phases: Steep phase and plateau phase.
(Source: GK Pal)

- The **steep phase** denotes the unloading zone where even a minimum drop in PO_2 results in unloading of large amounts of oxygen to the tissues
- The **plateau phase** denotes the loading zone, where O_2 is taken up by hemoglobin in the lungs and once all the four sites in Hb are loaded with O_2 there is no further uptake and thereby a plateau phase is reached
- The curve gets shifted to right are left in conditions of decreased or increase in affinity of hemoglobin for O_2, respectively.

Conditions where O_2-Hb Dissociation Curve is Shifted to Right (Fig. 5)

- Hypoxia
- ↑ PCO_2
- ↑ Temperature
- ↑ 2, 3-DPG levels in RBC
- ↑ H^+ concentration (acidosis).

Conditions where O_2-Hb Dissociation Curve is Shifted to Left (Fig. 5)

- High PO_2
- Low PCO_2
- Low body temperature
- Presence of fetal hemoglobin
- Alkalosis
- Low 2, 3-DPG levels in RBC
- Carbon monoxide poisoning.

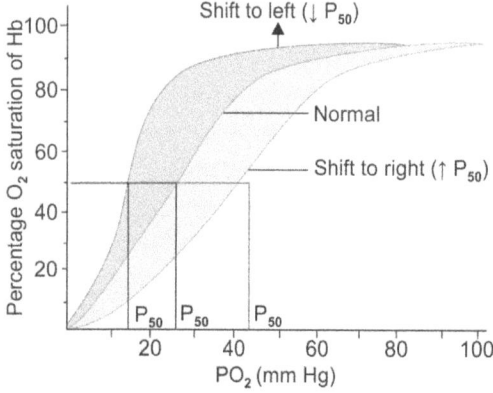

Fig. 5: Right and Left shift of O_2-Hb dissociation curve. P_{50}, PO_2 at which Hemoglobin is 50% saturated is 27 mm Hg. Right shift denotes decrease in hemoglobin affinity for O_2 and left shift increased affinity for O^2.
(*Source:* GK Pal)

4. Draw and explain the visual pathway. Discuss the effects of lesion at various levels along its course.

Visual Pathway

- The visual pathway starts in the retina
- Retina has ten layers. Rods and cones are in the innermost close to choroid
- The light passes through all the layers and fall on rods and cones
- The layer close to vitreous chamber is made of ganglion cells. The axons of these cells form the optic nerve
- The optic nerve leaves the eye through the optic disc, blind spot
- The fibers from temporal part of retina receive impulses from nasal field of vision and travels in the lateral half of the nerve and the fibers from nasal part of retina receive impulses from temporal field of vision and travels in medial half of the nerve (Fig. 6)
- The optic nerves cross in the optic chiasma. The medial fibers alone cross-over and join the uncrossed fibers of the opposite optic nerve
- On each side medial crossed fibers and lateral uncrossed fibers join to form the optic tract
- The optic tract reaches the lateral geniculate body (LGB) of the thalamus and relays there
- The next order of fibers which originate in the LGB is termed the geniculocalcarine fibers and they reach the primary visual area in the occipital cortex (area 17)
- From here impulses reach the visual association areas (areas 18 and 19).

Lesions

Injury in the visual pathway leads to visual field defects. The type of lesion depends on the site of lesion.

Loss of vision in one visual field—**Anopia**
Loss of vision in one half of the visual field—**Hemianopia**

a. **Lesion in optic nerve** – There is complete loss of vision (anopia) on the same side visual field.

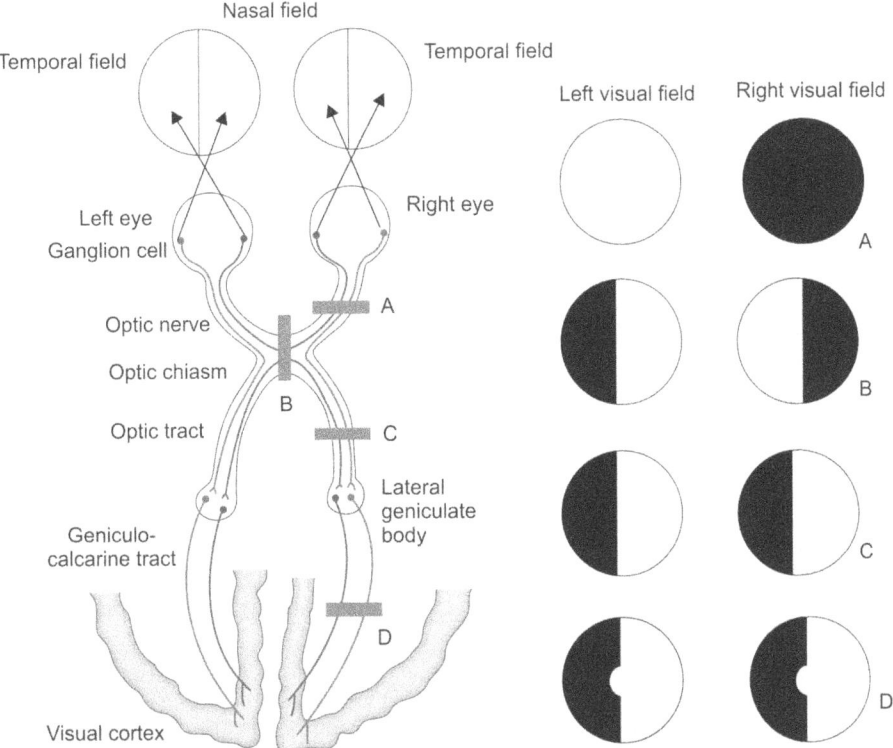

Fig. 6: Visual pathway and lesions. A—Lesion in right optic nerve causes right anopia. B—Lesion of nasal fibers of optic chiasma causes bitemporal heteronemous hemianopia. C—Lesion of right optic tract, causes left homonymous hemianopia. D—Lesion in geniculocalcarine tract causes left homonymous hemianopia with macular sparing. (*Source:* GK Pal)

b. **Lesion in optic chiasma:**
   - **Crossed fibers:** Bitemporal hemianopia
   - **Uncrossed fibers:** Damage happens due to carotid artery aneurysm. Leads to binasal hemianopia.
c. **Lesion in optic tract** - Lesion in one side will cause homonymous hemianopia of the opposite side, like lesion in left optic tract will cause right homonymous hemianopia.
d. **Lesion in geniculocalcarine tract**—homonymous hemianopia
e. **Optic radiation (medial fibers)**—homonymous lower quadrantinopia
f. **Optic radiation (lateral fibers)**—homonymous upper quadrantinopia.
g. **Lesion in visual cortex**—homonymous hemianopia with macular sparing. Macula is spared because it has a larger area of representation in the visual cortex.

II. SHORT NOTES

1. What are plasma proteins? Mention their types and discuss their function.

Plasma proteins are the major solutes in plasma.

Plasma proteins are categorized as albumin (55%), globulin (38%) and fibrinogen (7%).

They are classified based on their electrophoretic pattern.

Albumin

- Their levels are 4.8 g/dL
- Molecular weight is the least and is 69,000
- They are synthesized in the liver
- They regulate plasma colloidal oncotic pressure
- It helps in transport of bilirubin, hormones, ions, fatty acids, metals, etc.
- It also helps in regulating acid-base balance.

Globulin

- Normal level is 2-3g/dL
- Their molecular weight is 90,000-156,000
- There are α, β and γ globulins with subtypes for each one
- There are different forms of globulins—glycoprotein, lipoprotein, transferrin, haptoglobins, ceruloplasmin and Immunoglobulins
- They act as transport proteins as in transferrin transports iron, Ceruloplasmin copper, lipoproteins lipids, etc.
- The immunoglobulins provide immunity
- The normal albumin: globulin ratio is 1.5-2.5:1 ratio.

Fibrinogen

- Normal value is 0.3g/dL
- Their molecular weight is 500,000
- It has the highest molecular weight
- It helps in coagulation of blood and provides viscosity of blood
- There are other plasma proteins like prealbumin, prothrombin, etc.
- There are nearly 100s of plasma proteins
- All the above proteins are amphoteric in nature since they have both the NH_2 and COOH groups, they act as buffers for both acids and bases.

2. Describe the pharyngeal stage of deglutition.

Deglutition is the Process of Swallowing

- It is a reflex response integrated in the medulla in nucleus tractus solitarius (NTS) and nucleus ambiguus (NA)
- Afferents pass through the cranial nerves V, IX and X
- Efferents come through cranial nerves V, VII and XII nerves to the tongue and pharynx.

There are 3 phases of deglutition:

1. Oral or voluntary phase
2. Pharyngeal or involuntary phase
3. Esophageal phase.

Pharyngeal Phase

- It starts when food enters pharynx
- Soft palate is elevated and closes the nasopharynx and prevents food from entering the nose
- Larynx rises, vocal cords approximate and epiglottis closes the laryngeal opening and prevents food from entering the trachea
- Deglutition apnea follows
- Palatopharyngeal folds approximate for selective material to move into the esophagus
- Cricopharyngeus (upper esophageal sphincter) relaxes and bolus enters upper esophagus
- On entering of food into esophagus, the cricophargeus closes, vocal cords open and air entry is allowed.

3. Intercellular connections.

The intercellular connections play basically two roles:

1. They attach the cells together in a tissue
2. They allow passage of substances across the cells (see Table 1 and Fig. 7).

4. Nerve action potential.

- Resting membrane potential (RMP) of a neuron is -70 mV. On excitation of a neuron the change in RMP can be of two types—graded potential and action potential
- Action potentials are brief, rapid and large changes in the membrane potential (100 mv) following a threshold stimulus, conducted for a long distance along the axon in all or none fashion with the same shape and amplitude (Fig. 8)
- It takes the membrane potential from -70 mV to +35 mV
- They occur in a small patch of membrane
- In a motor neuron it originates in the "initial segment"
- They are due to opening up of voltage-gated Na^+ and voltage-gated K^+ channels.

Phases of Action Potential

When a stimulus is given there is deflection in the baseline which is due to leakage of current from stimulating electrodes—**Stimulus artifact.**

Table 1: Intercellular connections, their location and functions.

Intercellular connections	Organization	Location	Functions
Tight junctions or zonula occludens	They are thickening of cell membranes of adjacent cells and there is no space in between	Present in the apical membranes of epithelial cells of intestines and renal tubules	• They prevent the movement of the membrane proteins in the plane of membrane • Allows passage of extracellular solutes and water
Zonula adherens	These are continuous band like structures below the tight junctions. Microfilaments are attached	Present in epithelial cells	Holds cells together
Desmosomes	They are seen as patches—thickening of membrane of adjacent cells	Present in epithelial cells	Holds cells together
Hemidesmosomes and focal adhesion molecules	Looks like half desmosomes	Present between the cells and basal lamina	Attaches the cell to basal lamina
Gap junctions	They are pores between adjacent cells surrounded by a protein—Connexon	Present between cells as in cardiac myocytes, smooth muscle cells	• Allows passage of chemical messengers, ions between cells • Also transmits electrical impulses between cells

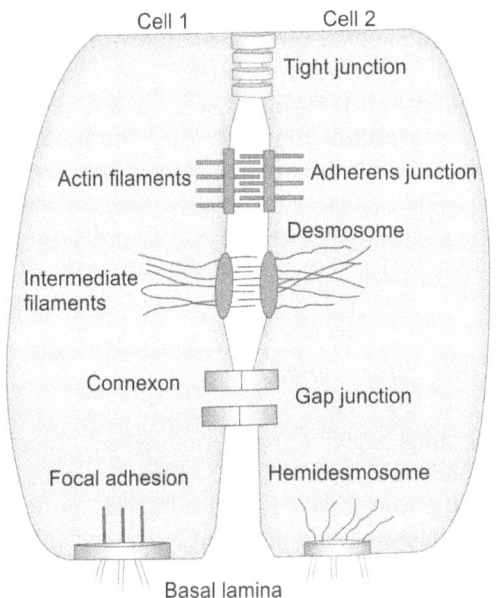

Fig. 7: Intercellular connections
(*Source:* Sembulingam)

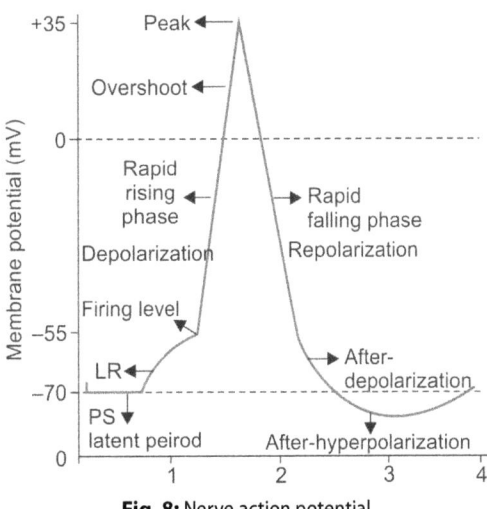

Fig. 8: Nerve action potential.
(PS: Point of stimulus; LR: Local response)
(*Source:* GK Pal)

Latent period: Following the stimulus artifact, there is an isopotential line, the latent period just before the AP.

It is due to the time taken for the impulse to travel from the stimulating to the recording electrode. Its duration is proportionate to the distance between stimulating and recording electrode. It also depends on the type of nerve.

Phase of depolarization: Following latent period there is phase of slow depolarization (*Local response*) due to slow opening of Na^+

channels. On reaching − 55 mV, the firing level, there is a phase of rapid depolarization.

This is due to the rapid opening of voltage-gated Na^+ channels. There is rapid inrush of Na^+ ions (5000 fold increase) taking the membrane potential to +35 mV. On reaching this potential there is inactivation of sodium channels within a fraction of millisecond.

Phase of repolarization: On reaching a potential of +35 mV, the potential reverses and starts falling rapidly to resting level. On completion of 70% repolarization there is decrease in rate of repolarization, it is said to be *after-depolarization*.

The repolarization is due to inactivation of voltage-gated Na^+ channels and opening of voltage-gated K^+ channels and the third reason for repolarization is on reaching +35 mV, there is reversal of electrical gradient for Na^+ movement and so no more sodium influx happens.

After-hyperpolarization: On reaching the RMP, the membrane potential hyperpolarises beyond RMP for a short period. It is called as after-hyperpolarization. It is due to closure of K^+ channels after a millisecond delay.

RMP: The membrane potential comes back to −90 mV due to the action of sodium-potassium pump.

Properties of Action Potential

A. All or None Law

When given a threshold stimulus the action potential is produced at the maximum amplitude. If a subthreshold stimulus is given action potential is not produced and also if a suprathreshold stimulus is given the amplitude and duration of action potential (AP) remains the same as the one generated by giving a threshold stimulus.

B. Threshold Stimulus

The minimum intensity of stimulus given for a particular time and can excite a nerve is said to be the threshold stimulus. If a weaker stimulus is given it has to be given for a longer period. The relationship between the strength and duration

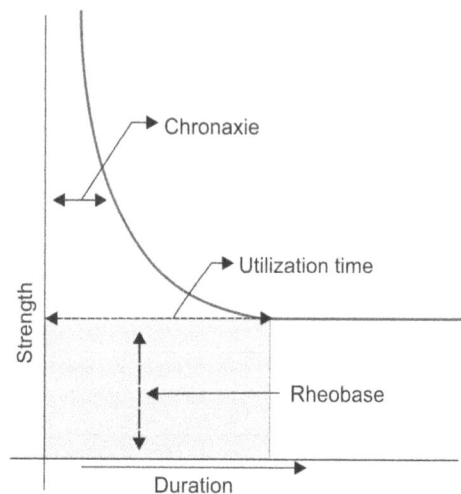

Fig. 9: Strength-duration curve.
(Source: GK Pal)

of the stimulus needed to excite a nerve is given as the *strength-duration curve (Fig. 9)*.

Rheobase is the minimum strength of a stimuls given for a particular time and is able to excite a tissue. The time for which the rheobase current should be given is said to be the *utilization time.* The time duration for which double the strength of rheobase current should be given to excite a tissue is said to be the *Chronaxie.* Chronaxie is an indicator of tissue excitability. Shorter the chronaxie for a tissue, excitability is better. Smooth muscles have the longer chronaxie.

C. Refractory period

There is a time period during AP, if a second stimulus is given, the stimulated part of the membrane is not excited again. It is said to be the membrane is in a refractory period. The refractory period is divided into absolute refractory period and relative refractory period.

Absolute refractory period (ARP) is the time period during an action potential, if a second stimulus is applied, however strong the stimulus is and for any duration it is applied, the nerve does not get excited. It happens from the firing level to 1/3rd completion of repolarization. It is because of the state of the gates of voltage-gated Na^+ channels.

Voltage-gated sodium channels: These channels have two gates, inactivation gate (along the exterior of the membrane) and the activation gate (along the interior of the membrane). At **resting state**, the inactivation gates are open and activation gates are closed. During an AP, on reaching the firing level, the activation gates also open and the rapid inrush of Na⁺ produces the spike potential (**activated state**). On reaching +35 mV, the inactivation gates close rapidly and the Na⁺ influx comes to a halt (**inactivated state of the channel**). This starts the repolarization phase.

These voltage-gated channels reach their resting state when the RMP is reached (−90 mV). Only on reaching the resting state, the channels can be reactivated. So during ARP the channels are in the inactivated state, so they are refractory to the second stimulus.

Relative refractory period (RRP) is the period after ARP when the membrane can be excited by a suprathreshold stimulus. This phase is from the end of ARP to after-depolarization.

During this phase, some of the channels would have reached the resting state, some may be still in inactivated state. When a suprathreshold stimulus is given it spreads to larger area of membrane and it can activate the channels which have reached the resting state.

D. Conductivity

The AP in a motor neuron is generated at the initial segment. Once the AP is generated it is conducted towards the axon terminal. The conductivity depends on two factors: myelination and diameter of the axon.

Impulse conduction is faster in a myelinated axon and in a larger diameter axon.

Impulse conduction in unmyelinated axons: The neuronal membrane is polarized at rest with negative charges lined on the interior and positive charges on the exterior. When an AP is generated at a location, the inside of the membrane reverses its polarity and positive charges flow into the depolarized site from either sides of the membrane. These are called the "current sinks". These current sinks excite the membrane ahead of the site of AP and also the site behind the AP. But since the area behind is in refractory period the current sinks travel in one direction only. Now the area excited ahead reaches a threshold and it can fire an AP (Fig. 10A).

Impulse conduction in myelinated axon: In a myelinated axon, the voltage-gated Na⁺ channels are concentrated in the nodes of Ranvier and the myelin sheath acts as an insulator. So the current sinks move from one node to another node rather than exciting the neighboring area as in unmyelinated axon. This type of impulse conduction is called as saltatory conduction. Since the impulses jump across nodes it can travel faster (Fig. 10B).

Larger diameter axons: In larger axons as the resistance for movement of ions is less the impulse transmission is faster.

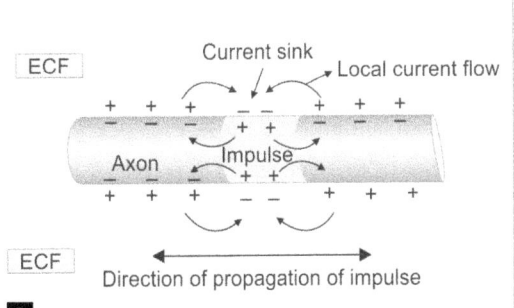 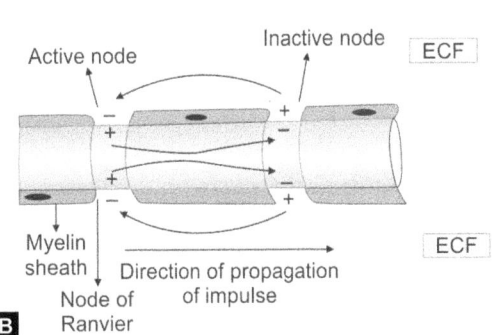

Figs. 10A and B: Conduction of impulses in (A) Unmyelinated neuron and (B) Myelinated neuron.
(*Source:* GK Pal)

E. Accommodation

When a stimulus of slow rising nature is given it does not excite the nerve as the nerve adapts to the applied stimulus and it is called as accommodation.

The cause for this is when there is no rapid depolarization the gradual influx of sodium is balanced by the efflux of K^+ through the slow opening of voltage-gated K^+ channels.

5. Physiological effects of thyroid hormone.

The actions of thyroid hormone are grouped as:
1. Metabolic actions
2. Developmental effects
3. Effects on various systems.

1. Metabolic Actions

- Calorigenesis
- Regulation of intermediary metabolism (carbohydrate, lipid and protein metabolism)
- Vitamin metabolism.

Calorigenesis

- It increases heat production
- The major role of thyroid hormone is to increase O_2 cosumption and basal metabolic rate (BMR). In hyperthyroidism, BMR and O_2 consumption increases by 50–100% and in hypothyroidism it decreases by 30–40%.

Effect on Protein Metabolism

- Thyroid hormone (TH) stimulates protein synthesis and degradation
- TH increases cellular uptake of amino acids and formation of proteins
- In hypothyroidism small doses of TH helps in protein anabolism
- High levels of TH increase protein catabolism.

Effect on Carbohydrate Metabolism

- Thyroid hormone acts on all aspects of carbohydrate metabolism
- Increases glucose uptake from GIT
- Increases insulin resistance and degradation
- Glycogen synthesis and degradation is also affected
- Increases gluconeogenesis.

Effects on Lipid Metabolism

- Thyroid hormones affect all aspects of lipid metabolism—lipogenesis, fat mobilization and lipolysis
- TH increases cholesterol synthesis and also its clearance by increasing low density-lipoprotein (LDL) synthesis
- So in hypothyroidism serum cholesterol levels increase and in hyperthyroidism it is decreased.

Effect on Vitamin Metabolism

- Thyroid hormones are needed for the conversion of β-carotene to vitamin A
- In hypothyroidism carotene accumulate in blood and give yellow discoloration – CAROTENEMIA.

2. Effects on Growth, Development and Maturation

Thyroid hormone has an important action on growth and maturation. This effect has been evidenced in metamorphosis of tadpoles. Thyroid hormone levels increase sharply just before the major step of metamorphosis.

In hypothyroid humans puberty is delayed or absent. The bone maturation is also delayed.

3. Effects on Other Systems

Effects on Skeletal System

Thyroid hormone stimulates linear growth of bone and maturation of epiphyseal center.

Growth hormone (GH) secretion and actions are potentiated by TH. Adequate thyroid hormones are needed for normal growth.

Effects on Respiratory System

The respiratory rate, minute ventilation and response to hypercapnia and hypoxia are increased. O_2 carrying capacity is increased by increase in red cell mass.

Effects on Cardiovascular System

The main action on CVS is to increase blood supply to tissues to deliver more O_2.

1. **In hyperthyroidism**
   - Heart rate and stroke volume increases. Thereby there is increase in cardiac output

- Systolic BP ↑ and diastolic BP ↓→ widened pulse pressure
- Diastolic BP is decreased due to decreased peripheral resistance (due to increase in body temperature and vasodilatation).

2. **In hypothyroidism**
   - Heart rate and stroke volume decrease
   - Peripheral resistance is usually increased
   - The cutaneous vasoconstriction is responsible for the cold skin in hypothyroids.

Effect on Nervous system
- Thyroid hormones are important for the growth and development of the brain in fetal and neonatal period. So TH deficiency in this period leads to irreversible brain damage and mental retardation
- The parts in CNS mostly affected are cerebral cortex, basal ganglia and cochlea. Many actions of excessive TH resemble increased sympathetic activity like: Tachycardia, tremor, increase in metabolism.

6. **Contraceptive methods.**

Contraception is prevention of pregnancy.

The needs for prevention of pregnancy are:
- To control population explosion
Certain methods prevent transmission of sexually transmitted diseases like AIDS.

The methods can be:
- Temporary methods
- Permanant methods.
The methods are described as contraceptive methods in males and females.

Contraceptive Methods in Males

I. Temporary Methods
a. Natural method
b. Barrier method
c. Pills.

a. *Natural method or Coitus interruptus:* Withdrawal of penis before ejaculation prevents deposition of semen in the vagina. This method needs practice and timing is very important. The disadvantages are that the precoital secretions may contain sperms and it can lead to pregnancy

b. *Barrier method:* Condoms are the widely used barrier method in males. It is made of fine latex sheet. It prevents deposition of semen in the vagina and prevents fertilization of ovum. It can be used to prevent transmission of sexually transmitted diseases

c. *Pills:* Drugs are used to inhibit spermatogenesis.
Gossypol and testosterone are used.
Gossypol—it is derived from cottonseed oil. It decreases sperm count.
Testosterone—high testosterone levels inhibit sperm production.

II. Permanent Methods

Vasectomy—a small portion of vas deferens is removed after clamping. Both the open ends are ligated and sutured.

Contraceptive Methods in Females

I. Temporary Methods
a. Rhythm method
b. Barrier method
c. Oral contraceptive pills
d. Intrauterine contraceptive device.

a. Rhythm method
- This method can be followed in females with regular menstrual cycles of 28–30 days
- During a normal menstrual cycle, ovulation happens on 14th day of the cycle
- The ovum stays viable for 48–72 hours after ovulation
- After ejaculation, sperm stays viable in female reproductive tract for 24–48 hours
- So pregnancy can happen if intercourse happens within this period
- So the days are calculated from first day of menstrual cycle and intercourse should be avoided in this period
- 5–6 days after the bleeding phase and 5–6 days before the next menstruation is considered to be the "safe period"

- It can be utilized by females with regular cycles and who can keep a record of their time of ovulation by checking basal body temperature.

b. Barrier method
- Barriers can be mechanical or chemical barriers. They basically prevent the meeting of sperm and ovum
- Mechanical barrier—diaphragm and cervical caps
- Chemical barrier—spermicidal agents in the form of creams, foam or jelly are placed in the female reproductive tract before coitus. It can be used along with a mechanical barrier.

c. Oral contraceptive pills
- By pills we mean the oral contraceptive pills used for female contraception
- They are usually synthetic preparation of estrogen, progesterone or combination of both.
- *The pills can be of different types:*
  1. Combined pill or Classical pill
  2. Sequential pill
  3. Minipill
  4. Post-coital pill.

Combined pill
- It is a combination of estrogen and progesterone pill
- It contains a strip of 21 tablets and is consumed for 21 days from 5th day of menstrual cycle
- After 21 days, on stopping the tablets, withdrawal bleeding happens
- Again from 5th day, next cycle is started.

It:
- Prevents ovulation, as the high estrogen levels disorganize the LH and FSH secretions
- Prevents implantation of fertilized ovum
- Progesterone makes the cervical mucus thick and prevents sperm penetration.

Sequential pill
- It has high dose of estrogen and minimal amounts of progesterone
- It is not used nowadays as the high estrogen may induce endometrial cancer or breast cancer.

Minipill
- It is progesterone only pill
- It does not affect ovulation but makes the cervical mucus thick and prevents sperm penetration.

Postcoital pill
- It is used within 72 hours of unprotected intercourse
- It has high doses of estrogen and is given for 4-6 days
- High estrogen prevents implantation of the fertilized ovum.

Depot preparation
- These are implants of progesterone and they are subdermally implanted and prevent pregnancy for 5 years
- The only problem is it can cause amenorrhea and irregular cycles.

d. Intrauterine contraceptive devices
- These are small devices made of plastic or copper and placed in the uterus to prevent implantation of fertilized ovum

Lippes loop
- It is a simple S-shaped plastic device with nylon threads
- Under aseptic precautions, the loop is inserted into the uterus and the thread is present in the vagina
- The loop is also impregnated with a small amount of barium sulphate for checking its presence by radiographs.

Copper-T
- It is a T-shaped device made of copper with nylon threads
- They are inserted during the first 10 days of menstrual cycle
- Copper prevents implantation of fertilized ovum by stimulating an aseptic inflammation of the endometrium.

- Disadvantages of IUCD: Chances of ectopic pregnancy, pelvic inflammation, menorrhagia and dysmenorrhea. Spontaneous expulsion of the device can also happen.

II. Permanent Method
Tubectomy
- It can be done by an open surgery or by laparoscopic surgery

- Here the fallopian tubes are cut and ligated and buried.

7. **Neuroendocrine reflex.**
- In this type of reflex the afferent limb of the reflex is neural and the efferent limb is humoral or endocrine
- Examples of this reflex are milk ejection or milk let down reflex and the parturition reflex.

Milk ejection reflex: Oxytocin is a hormone secreted from the hypothalamus and released from posterior pituitary gland. It acts on the myoepithelial cells lining the ducts of breast and expels milk through a reflex as shown in Figure 11.
- The receptors for this reflex are touch receptors around the nipple. When the infant suckles at the breast the touch receptors are stimulated
- Impulses are relayed through somatic afferent pathways to the supraoptic (SO) and paraventricular (PV) Nuclei of Hypothalamus
- These nuclei secrete the hormone. Oxytocin which is transported through blood and acts on the myoepithelial cells lining the ducts of the breast resulting in expulsion of milk (Fig. 11).

Parturition reflex (Fig. 12):
- Towards the term of pregnancy, estrogen levels in the blood rise and increases the sensitivity of oxytocin receptors in the uterine myometrium to oxytocin
- As a result of action of oxytocin, the uterus contracts and fetal head is pushed down stretching the cervix. There are stretch receptors in the cervix
- As the cervix is stretched the stretch receptors are stimulated and impulses are transmitted through sensory afferent fibers to SO and PV nuclei of hypothalamus
- These nuclei secrete oxytocin
- Oxytocin binds to the receptors in the uterine myometrium and induces further contractions. This further pushes the fetal head down, further streching the cervix and more oxytocin is released

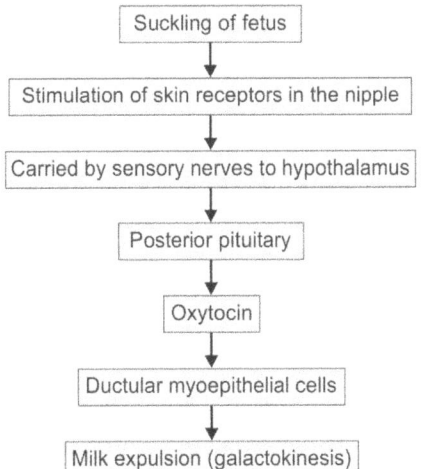

Fig. 11: Milk ejection reflex.

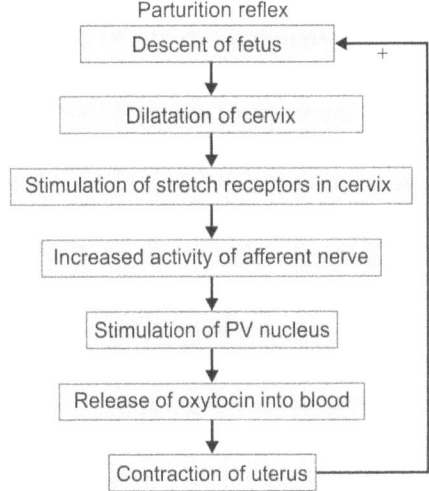

Fig. 12: Parturition reflex.
(PV: paraventricular)

- This continues as a positive feedback mechanism till the fetus is born.

8. **Small intestinal movements.**

Movements of the Small Intestines

Five Types of Movements in the Normal State
1. Peristalsis—propulsive movement
2. Mixing movements—segmentation contraction and tonic contraction
3. Migrating motor complexes (MMC)
4. Movements of villi
5. Contractions of muscularis mucosa.

Abnormal movements: Peristaltic rushes.

Migrating Motor Complexes

- Migrating motility complexes are motility present in the interdigestive period
- These are bursts of electrical and mechanical activities in GIT
- It starts in the esophagus and spreads through the stomach and ileum to the ileocecal valve
- Occurs once in 90 minutes and lasts for 10-20 minutes
- It clears the GIT for the next meal
- Occurs in 3 phases—Pases I, II and III
- Phase I—no spike potential, no contractions
- Phase II—irregular spike potentials and contractions
- Phase III—regular spike potentials and contractions.

Mixing Movements

Segmentation Contractions (Fig. 13)

- These are ring like contractions present in short segments of the intestine of 1-2 cm
- They are present in regular intervals
- Their frequency matches the slow wave frequency
- Slow waves are waves generated in the pacemaker cells located in the wall of duodenum and it spreads through the muscular wall of the intestines
- Strength of the contraction depends on the spike waves superimposed on the slow waves
- These ring like contractions appear in one segment and the nearby segment relaxes, this is followed by another set of contractions in the segments between the previous contractions
- These contractions appear sausage shaped and they cut into the bolus and move it to and fro and increase their exposure to the absorptive surface of the mucosa
- Therefore, these contractions help in mixing the bolus with digestive juices and in digestion, and absorption of food.

Tonic Contractions

- These are prolonged contractions of one segment of intestine and the segment appears to be isolated from rest of the ileum
- Segmentation and tonic contractions delay the passage of chyme and thereby allow contact of chyme with enterocytes and favor absorption.

Peristalsis

- This is a type of propulsive movement which helps to move the chyme forward. It is a reflex initiated by the stretch of the intestinal wall following the entry of food
- Stretch of the intestinal wall initiates a ring of constriction behind the bolus and a relaxation in front of the bolus (refer Fig. 13)
- The ring of contraction behind pushes the bolus to the relaxed segment in front of the bolus
- Next ring of contraction now appears in the previous relaxed segment and the bolus is pushed further
- These waves always propel the contents from the oral to caudal direction and never in the opposite direction - *Law of the gut*
- These waves appear even in the absence of nerve supply but they can be modified by the autonomic nerves, parasympathetic nerves increase the activity and sympathetic nerves decrease the activity

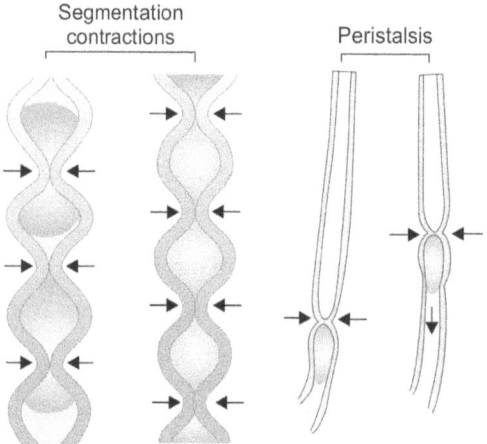

Fig. 13: Segmentation contractions and peristalsis. (*Source:* Sembulingam)

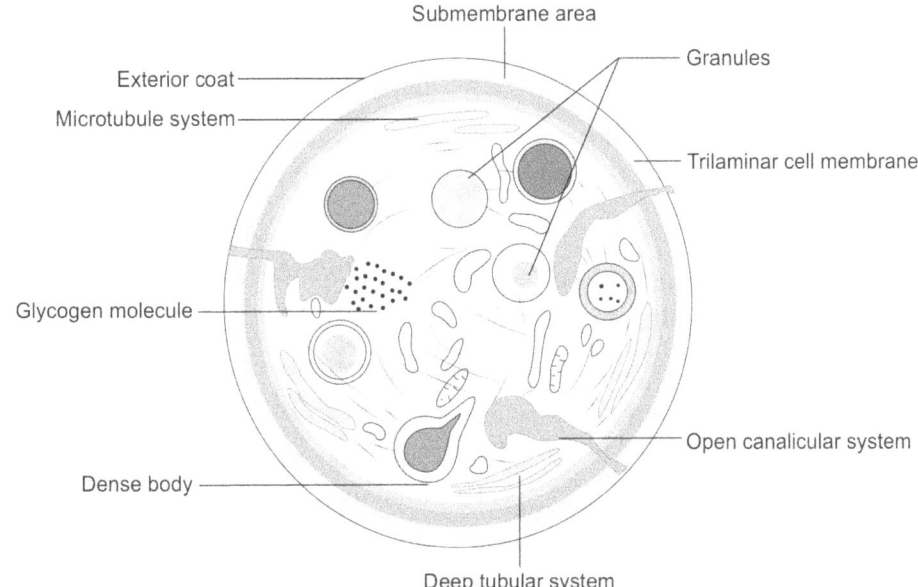

Fig. 14: Structure of platelets.
(*Source:* GK Pal)

- The propelling speed varies from 2–25 cm/s
- Sometimes the peristaltic waves can be very fast and they empty the contents faster—**peristaltic rushes** seen in acute diarrhea
- Antiperistalsis happens in vomiting.

Contractions of Muscularis Mucosa

- Irregular in nature
- Occurs at a frequency of 3/min
- It helps in mixing the contents and in absorption.

Contraction of Villi

- The type of contraction seen as elongation and shortening of the villi
- It helps in emptying of central lacteals of the villi and increases the absorptive surface area
- It is stimulated by the hormone Villikinin.

Functions of Movements of Small Intestine

- Mixing the chyme with the digestive juices and helps in digestion
- Propelling the chyme forward
- Presenting the chyme to absorptive surface and helps for absorption.

9. **Discuss the morphology and functions of platelets.**

- Platelets are flat and disc shaped structures which are involved in the process of hemostasis (Fig. 14)
  - Platelets are in a diameter of 2–4 µm. They are colorless, disc shaped and do not have nucleus.

  The membrane of platelets is made of lipids, cholesterol, carbohydrates, proteins and glycoproteins. There are many receptors present in the cell membrane for collagen and fibrinogen.
- Below the cell membrane microtubules made of tubulin is present and helps in regulating the shape of the platelets.

Cytoplasm

- Organelles like endoplasmic reticulum, golgi apparatus and mitochondria are present in the cytoplasm
- It also contains contractile proteins like actin, myosin and thrombasthenin and are responsible for contraction of platelets which causes clot retraction
- Cytoplasm contains two types of granules—dense granules and alpha granules
- Alpha granules contain—Von Wille brand factor (VWF), platelet derived

growth factor (PDGF), platelet activating factor (PAF), fibronectin, plasminogen, thrombospendin, etc.
- Dense granules—nonprotein substances like serotonin, adenosine diphosphate (ADP), calcium, adenosine triphosphate (ATP) and pyrophosphate.

Functions of platelets are
- **Role in primary hemostasis or temporary platelet plug formation:** Damage to the endothelial lining of the blood vessels exposes collagen which activates the platelets and results in adhesion and aggregation of platelets to the injured vessel and thereby seals the injured vessel. Platelets have receptors for collagen, ADP and VWF which favor adhesion of platelets
- **Role in secondary hemostasis:** Formation of clot is said to be the secondary hemostasis. The platelets release platelet phopholipid and platelet factor II which activates prothrombin to thrombin
- **Role in clot retraction:** Platelets have contractile proteins like actin, myosin and thrombasthenin. Once the platelets and other blood cells are trapped in the fibrin mesh, these contractile proteins contract and the clot shrinks. This squeezes out the serum from the clot. Clot retraction happens only in the presence of functional platelets and it helps in sealing the wound in the blood vessel
- Platelets **store and release** serotonin (5HT) which is a potent vasoconstrictor
- Platelets also store and release platelet derived growth factor which mutiplies endothelial cells and fibroblasts and thereby **help in wound healing**
- Platelets are also involved in **mild phagocytosis**. They ingest carbon particles, immune complexes and viral particles.

10. Cell-mediated immunity.
- It is mediated by T Lymphocytes
- T Lymphocytes are formed in the bone marrow and they are processed in the thymus (Fig. 15).

Stages of Cell-mediated Immunity

a. **Antigen presentation:** Cells like macrophages, mast cells and dendritic cells act as antigen presenting cells (APCs).

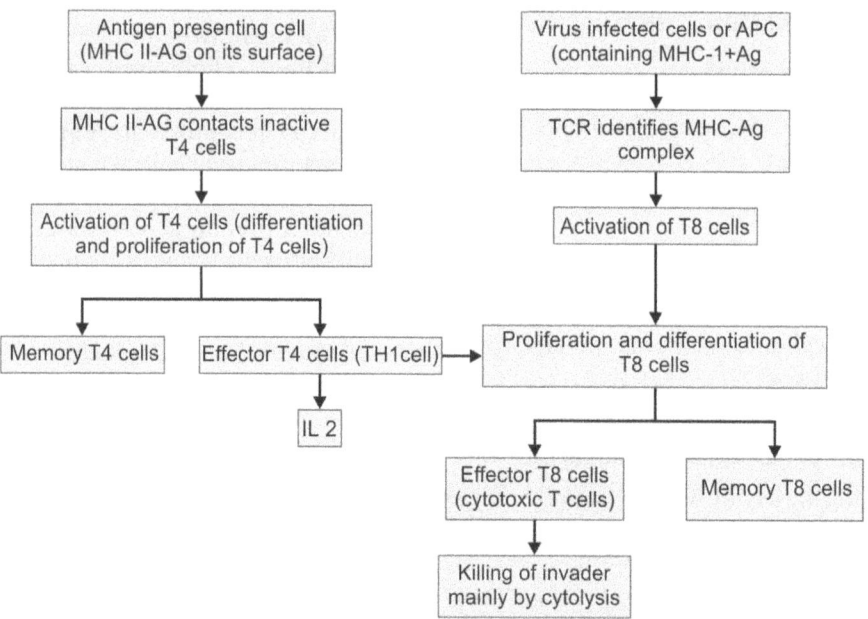

Fig. 15: Mechanism of Cell-mediated immunity.
(MHC-Ag: Major histocompatibility complex-antigen; APC: Antigen-presenting cells; TCR: T cell receptors.)
(*Source:* GK Pal)

Once the antigens enter the body they are phagocytosed by the macrophages and are broken down to peptide fragments. The antigenic fragment forms a complex with the major histocompatibility complex (MHC) II protein formed by the macrophages. The antigen and MHC II complex are expressed on the membrane of macrophage.

b. **Antigen recognition by lymphocytes**: The APC with the antigen-MHC II complex is recognized by the T lymphocytes with the receptors for that antigen. T cells become activated if it binds to the antigen and is co-stimulated by cytokines like IL-2. Once 2 stimulations have happened, the lymphocyte is activated. The activated T cells enlarge and begin to proliferate and differentiate to form a clone of similar T cells. This happens in the secondary lymphoid organs like lymph nodes.

c. **Types of T cells:** There are 3 main types of T cells—helper T cells (CD4 cells), cytotoxic T cells (CD8 cells) and memory T cells.

   1. *Helper T cells*: Helper T cells or CD4 cells recognize the antigen presented along with MHC II and cytotoxic or CD8 cells recognize the antigens presented with MHC I.

      After co-stimulation of helper T cells, they secrete many cytokines. The most important cytokine is IL-2 which is needed for all the immune responses and is the major stimulator for T cell proliferation. IL-2 is also the co-stimulator for resting helper T cells and cytotoxic T cells. It also enhances activation and proliferation of B cells and natural killer cells.

   2. *Cytotoxic T cells:* The T cells that express CD8 develop into cytotoxic T cells. They recognize foreign antigens expressed along with MHC I on the membranes of body cells infected by viruses, tumor cells and cells of tissue transplant. But to get activated into a killer cell it needs co-stimulation by IL-2 produced by helper cells. Therefore for maximal activation of cytotoxic T cells it needs antigen presentation with MHC I and II.

   3. *Memory T cells:* The T cells for a specific antigen which remain in the lymph organ after the immune response is over are termed as memory T cells. If the same pathogen is encountered for the second time, these cells get activated and they initiate a swift and fast immune response. The second response is faster and vigorous and the pathogen is eliminated even before any symptom develops.

Elimination of the pathogens:

The killing of the pathogen is done by the cytotoxic T cells.

a. The activated CD8 cells synthesize and secrete proteins called "perforins" which are inserted into the membrane of the pathogen. The perforins are water channels which allow influx of water and thereby swelling of the microbe and cause its lysis.

b. Release of lymphotoxins by activated T cells. These cytokines destroy the microbes.

c. Cytotoxic T cells secrete interferons which will favor the phagocytic activity of the neutrophils and macrophages by promoting opsonization.

Role of Cell-mediated Immunity

- It is activated against intracellular pathogens like viral infections and bacterial infections like *Mycobacterium tuberculosis*
- It removes the tumor cells
- It is responsible for rejection of transplanted tissues
- It is responsible for hypersensitivity reactions.

11. Respiratory changes during moderate exercises.

Changes in the Respiratory System (RS)

- Changes happening in RS during exercise is to supply the extra amount of O_2 needed

by the muscles and to remove the extra CO_2 put out by the working muscles
- Hyperventilation during exercise helps to achieve this demand and also to maintain pO_2 and pCO_2 at normal levels in arterial blood.

Increased Ventilation during Exercise

- Increase in ventilation matches the energy requirement of working muscles
- Increase in ventilation is by increasing the depth and rate of respiration
- Normal rate of respiration is 12–18 cycles/min and the depth of respiration is assessed by the tidal volume and it is 500 mL at rest. So the minute ventilation is around 6 L/min
- During exercise, tidal volume (TV) and rate increases, initially both are increased and once TV reaches its saturation, further increase is by increasing the rate of respiration. It can be increased to 80–100 L/min
- The **pattern of increase in ventilation** is by an abrupt increase in the beginning followed by a small pause then a gradual increase and after stopping the exercise there is an abrupt decrease in ventilation followed by a gradual decline to baseline level
- The initial abrupt increase is due to psychic stimuli from the cortex followed by neural stimuli arising from the proprioceptors in muscles, joints and tendons
- The gradual increase in ventilation is due to the chemical changes happening in the PO_2, PCO_2 levels and pH in arterial blood
- Arterial PO_2 and PCO_2 levels remain the same, even in severe exercise, but the stimulation of chemoreceptors happen because of increase in sensitivity of the chemorecptors for the normal fluctuations in the levels of PO_2 and PCO_2
- The other important mechanism by which ventilation increases is due to increase in body temperature
- Increase in plasma K^+ levels in blood following its release from the exercising muscles also stimulates respiration.

Increase in O_2 Uptake

- O_2 uptake increases following exercise from 250 mL/min to 4,000 mL/min
  This is happening because of:
  a. **Increased blood flow to lungs** as the cardiac output increases, due to increase in heart rate and stroke volume.
  b. **Increase in PO_2 gradient** between the alveolus and pulmonary arterial blood. Exercising muscles extract more O_2 from arterial blood and therefore the venous blood reaching the pulmonary artery has low PO_2. This increases the gradient for O_2 movement.
  c. **Increase in diffusion capacity** of the respiratory membrane. Most of the pulmonary capillaries remain closed in resting states. During exercise these capillaries also open up and therefore the surface area across which exchange happens increases.

---

12. Describe the origin and spread of cardiac impulse.

Conducting System of the Heart (Fig. 16)

- Ability to conduct an impulse (action potential)
- Conduction of impulse is by sequential depolarization of adjacent membrane
- In the heart there is a specialized conducting system

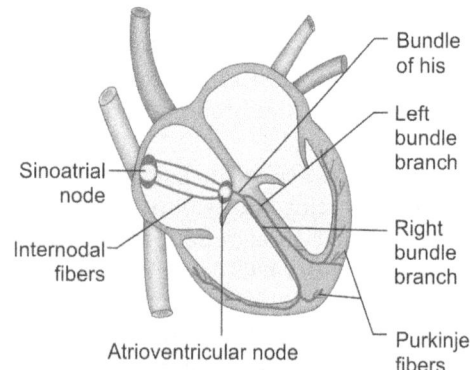

Fig. 16: Conducting system of the heart.
(Source: Sembulingam)

- It starts in the SA Node and reaches the ventricles
- It consists of the sinoatrial (SA) node, internodal tracts, atrioventrical (AV) node, bundle of His, right and left branches of bundle of His, Purkinje fibers and ventricular muscles.

Sinoartrial Node

- It is located in the wall of the right atrium close to the opening of superior vena cava (SVC)
- It is made up of modified muscle fibers with more rounded cells with indistinct borders and less striations. They are called as P cells
- Such cells are present in the AV node also
- In the heart, SA node, AV node, His bundle and ventricles can generate their own impulses
- But SA node is called the pacemaker as it generates impulses at a faster rate than the other tissues
- The pacemaker cells do not have a stable resting membrane potential
- They tend to depolarize and repolarize in a continuous fashion in spite of nerve supply
- The potential developed here is called as the pacemaker potential.

Pacemaker potential:

- The resting membrane potential (RMP) in SA node is around –55 to –60 mV
- But it is not a stable potential. There is a slow depolarization till – 40mV. Once – 40 mV is reached there is a rapid depolarization (Phase 0) to +5 mV and there is a rapid repolarization to – 55 mV (Phase 3)
- Then it reaches the RMP (Phase 4)
- Once again there is a slow depolarization, the process continues
- This slow rising phase before the rapid depolarization is called as the prepotential or pacemaker potential (Fig. 17).

Ionic events responsible for pacemaker potential:

- The prepotential is divided into 3 sections based on the ionic events—the first part of slow depolarization is due to decay of K+ current (closure of K+ channels), followed by Na+ influx through 'h' or 'f' channels and the last part is due to Ca^{2+} influx through transient type Ca^{2+} (T-type) channels
- The rapid depolarization which starts at –40 mV is due to Ca^{2+} influx through Long lasting Ca^{2+} channels (L-type)
- Rapid repolarization is due to K+ efflux through K+ channels resulting in repolarization to –55 to –60 mV.

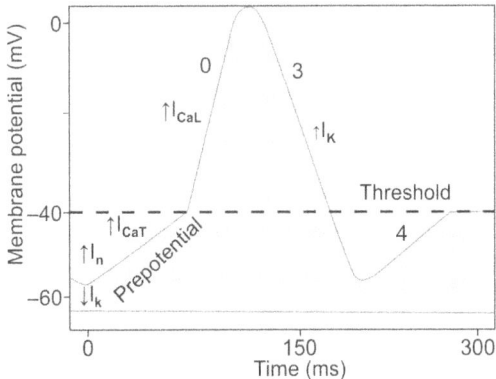

Fig. 17: Pacemaker potential. Slope of pacemaker potential (Phase 4), the prepotential is due to 3 events; first part of depolarisation is due to closure of K+ channels, 2nd part is due to Na+ influx through sodium channel and last part of depolarisation is due to Ca^{2+} influx through T-type Ca^{2+} channels. Rapid depolarisation (Phase 0) is due to opening of L-type Ca^{2+} channels and repolarisation (Phase 3) due to opening of K+ channels.
(*Source:* GK Pal)

Conducting Pathway

- These impulses originated in the SA node are conducted down through the specialised conducting system as mentioned above
- The impulses from SA node are transmitted to the AV node through 3 internodal bundles which are specialized tissues for conduction of impulses from SA node to AV node in a faster way
- The atrial tissues also conduct impulses but they are slower.

The internodal bundles are:

1. Anterior internodal tract of Bachman

2. Middle internodal tract of Wenckebach
3. Posterior internodal tract of Thorel.

Through these bundles the impulses reach the AV Node.

Interatrial Tract of Bachman

- This bundle starts in the SA node and ends in the left atrium
- The left atrium is also depolarized simultaneously.

Atrioventricular Node

- It is located beneath the endocardium on the right side of lower part of atrial septum near the tricuspid valve
- The conduction velocity through the atrioventrical node (AVN) is very slow because the fibers are smaller with less number of gap junctions
- There is a delay of 0.1 s
- The delay provides time for atrial contraction and final ventricular filling
- It also prevents transmission of all impulses from atria to ventricles in supraventricular tachycardia
- It is supplied by sympathetic and parasympathetic nerves which alter the conduction rate.

Atrioventricular Bundle of His

- This bundle starts in the AV node and descends down the fibrous skeleton and divides into right and left branches and they supply the right and left ventricles
- The bundles divide into many small branches, the Purkinje fibers.

Purkinje Fibers

They are present in the endocardium and reaches all parts of ventricles.

Ventricles:

- The spread of depolarization in the ventricular muscles are from the AVN to the His bundle → Purkinje fibers → ventricles
- The conduction velocity of the AP through ventricular muscles are 0.3-0.4 msec
- This results in depolarization of both ventricles at the same time and leads to contraction of both ventricles at the same time
- In ventricle, the spread of depolarization is from endocardium to epicardium.

In humans depolarization of ventricle starts in the left side of interventricular septum
↓
Then moves to right side across the mid-portion of the septum
↓
Then the wave spreads downwards to the apex of the heart
↓
Then it turns back along the ventricular muscle towards the AV groove from endocardium to epicardium
↓
The last part to be depolarized are the posterobasal part of left ventricle, pulmonary conus and uppermost portion of the septum
↓
Repolarization proceeds from the epicardium to endocardium in the ventricle

- Repolarization starts in the epicardium and spreads towards endocardium
- Ability to contract follows the excitation of atrial and ventricular myocardium
- The function of conducting system is to excite the myocardium following which intracellular calcium is increased and thereby contraction of the muscle follows.

13. Fetal circulation.

- Fetal circulation is different from circulation in postnatal life. In postnatal life the circulation between right and left heart is in series and in fetal life it is parallel in many sites (Fig. 18)
- The fetal lung is not functioning and the placenta behaves like the fetal lung and the fetus derives O_2 and nutrients from placenta through umbilical vessels
- Fetus receives blood from the placenta through umbilical veins and is 80% saturated with oxygen
- Blood from umbilical vein enters the liver and mixes with portal blood and some amount is diverted to the inferior vena cava through 'ductus venosus'

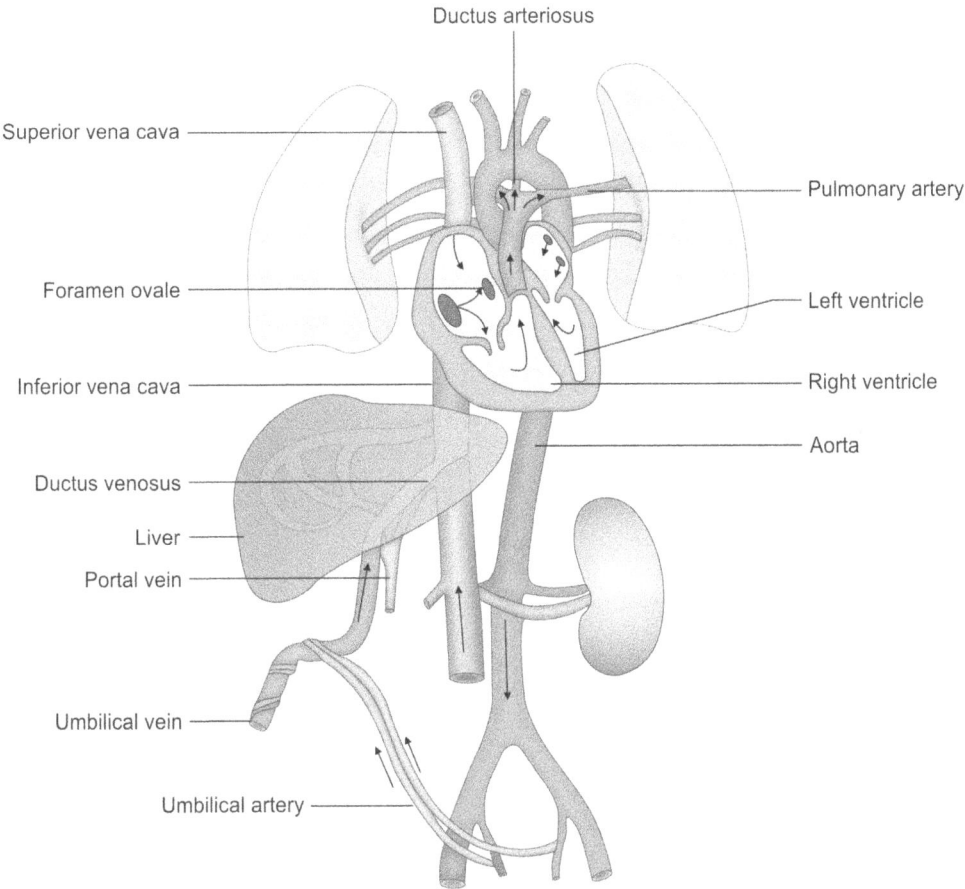

Fig. 18: Fetal circulation.
(*Source:* Sembulingam)

- The portal and systemic venous blood in fetus is 26% saturated with O_2 and the saturation of mixed blood in inferior vena cava (IVC) is around 67%
- Most of this blood entering the right atrium through IVC is directed into left atrium through Foramen ovale
- Blood from superior vena cava (SVC) enters the right ventricle and is sent into the pulmonary artery
- But the fetal lung is collapsed and therefore resistance in pulmonary artery is higher than in the aorta
- Most of the blood in pulmonary artery is pushed into the aorta through 'ductus arteriosus'
- In this fashion relatively unsaturated blood is diverted to the trunk and lower parts of the body and head of the fetus receives better saturated blood from left ventricle
- From aorta some of the blood is pumped into the umbilical artery and back to the placenta.

Changes Happening at Birth

- At birth, placental circulation is cut off and the pressure in aorta rises more than that in the pulmonary artery
- Since no supply comes from placenta the fetus suffers from asphyxia and it gasps for breath and cries which causes expansion of lungs
- As the lung expands the pulmonary resistance falls and blood starts flowing into the pulmonary vessels

- Blood returning to left atrium rises the left atrial pressure and it closes the foramen ovale
- Ductus arteriosus constricts within few hours after birth and permanent closure happens due to intimal thickening by 24–48 hours.

14. Refractory errors of the eye.

Myopia – short-sightedness

Eyeball may be elongated and therefore parallel rays of light from a distant object are brought to focus in front of the retina (Fig. 19). It may be genetic or acquired. It can be corrected by using biconcave lenses. The lens diverges the light rays before they strike the cornea and then they are converged by the lens in the eye, so that the object is focussed on the retina. It is the most common error of refraction.

Hypermetropia – Farsightedness

Here the parallel rays of light from a distant object are brought to focus behind the retina (Fig. 19). It occurs due to decrease in anteroposterior diameter of the eye. It can be corrected by using biconvex lenses so that they converge the light rays before they fall on the cornea and therefore the light rays fall on the retina.

Astigmatism

The problem here is the corneal surface is not sperical. One meridian of the cornea is different from the other. So the parallel rays of light are not able to converge to a point of focus as there is unequal refraction from the different meridians. So a blurred image is seen. It can be corrected by using cylindrical lenses.

Presbyopia

It is commonly seen in aged people above the age of 40 years.

The near point has receded beyond the normal reading distance due to increased hardness of the lens which results in loss of accommodation property of lens. It is corrected by using convex lens for near work

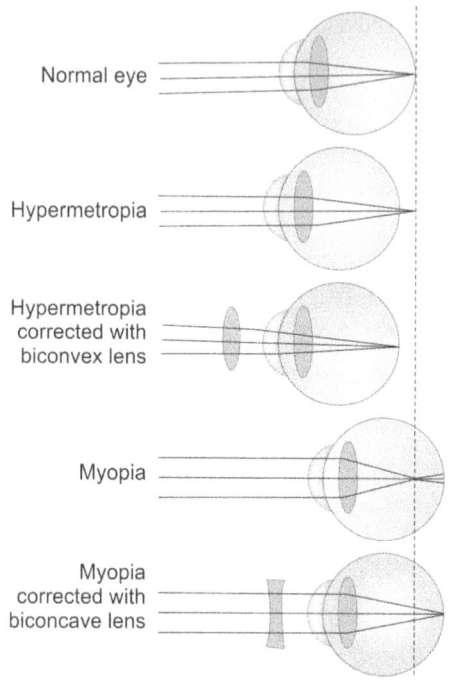

Fig. 19: Refractory errors of with corrections. Hypermetropia is corrected with convex lens and myopia is corrected with concave lens.
(*Source:* GK Pal)

and plain glasses for far work and it is given as the bifocal lenses.

15. Cochlea.

Components of Inner Ear

Cochlea and vestibular apparatus.

Cochlea has the following Components

- It has a bony component and a membranous component. Bony part is a curved structure in temporal bone. Membranous part is a tube like structure within the bony labyrinth
- It is 35 mm in length and is snail like with 2 ¼ turns
- It has a base and apex
- Base is close to oval window and apex is said to be helcotrema
- It is divided into 3 fluid filled compartments by two membranes – Reissner's membrane and basilar membrane
- The compartments are – scala vestibuli, scala media and scala tympani

- Scala vestibuli is above Reissner's membrane and is filled with perilymph a fluid resembling plasma. At the apex it continues with scala tympani
- Scala media is between Reissner's membrane and basilar membrane and is filled with endolymph secreted by stria vascularis present in the lateral wall of scala media. Endolymph is rich in K^+. This duct is triangular in shape and houses the organ for hearing, the organ of Corti (Fig. 20)
- Scala tympani—this is the space below basilar membrane and is filled with perilymph. This part is seperated from middle ear by round window and is covered by secondary tympanic membrane
- Receptor organ of hearing in cochlea—organ of Corti
- Receptor cells for hearing—hair cells in organ of Corti.

Organ of Corti

- The organ of Corti is the organ of hearing and is present in the inner ear in Cochlea
- It is placed on the basilar membrane and contains the receptors for hearing - hair cells
- The organ of Corti consists of the hair cells, supporting cells, tunnel of corti, basilar membrane, tectorial membrane and reticular lamina
- There are two groups of hair cells—the inner hair cells and outer hair cells seated on the basilar membrane seperated by the rods of Corti
- There is a tringular space between the rods—tunnel of Corti (Fig. 20).

Hair Cells

- The inner hair cells are 3,500 in number and are arranged in a single row along the entire length of cochlea
- There are 20,000 outer hair cells and are arranged in 3 rows
- At the bases of the hair cells are the nerve endings which later become the cochlear division of vestibulocochlear nerve
- The apical ends of the hair cells contain the cilia that pass through the reticular lamina
- The cilia of outer hair cells are embedded in the thin gelatinous tectorial membrane
- The hairs of the inner hair cells do not touch the membrane
- When the sound waves reach the organ of Corti it acts as the transducer to convert sound waves into action potentials which travel through the cochlear nerve to reach the auditory area in the cortex.

16. Neuroglia.

Neuroglial cells are the supporting cells in the CNS. They are 50 times more than the neurons. They are of 4 types (Fig. 21):
1. Astrocytes—helps in forming the blood brain barrier

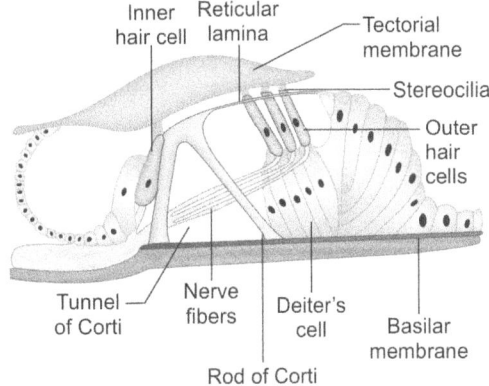

Fig. 20: Organ of Corti with hair cells.
(*Source:* GK Pal)

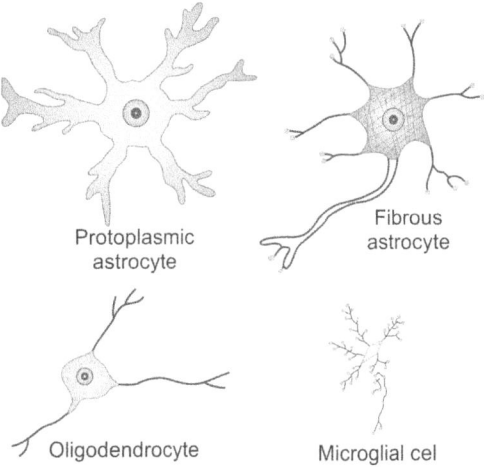

Fig. 21: Neuroglial cells.
(*Source:* Sembulingam)

2. Oligodendrocytes—myelination of neurons in the CNS
3. Microglia—scavenger cells belong to macrophage type cells
4. Schwaan cells—myelination of neurons in peripheral nervous system (PNS).

General Functions of Neuroglial Cells

- They help to maintain the appropriate levels of ions and neurotransmitters in the synapse
- They produce substances that are trophic to neurons
- They are supportive to the neurons.

17. Discuss the functions of limbic system.

Functions of Limbic System

Limbic system (Fig. 22) is involved in functions of emotions and memory.

It has functions in motivation, addiction, emotional features like rage and placidity, sexual behavior and autonomic responses.

Role in Motivation

- There are areas in the brain when stimualted induces pleasurable sensation and is said to be the 'reward center'
- The reward center is situated in between the ventral tegmental area to nucleus accumbens
- The neurotransmitter involved in reward system or approach system is dopamine
- Similarly there are areas in brain when stimulated produces sensation of fear and displeasure. It is said to be the 'avoidance system'
- It is in the lateral portion of posterior hypothalamus, dorsal midbrain and entorhinal cortex.

Role in Addiction

- Addiction is a compulsive behavior to use a particular substance in spite of knowing the negative impact of the substance on health
- Addiction happens for opiates, cocaine, amphetamine, ethyl alcohol, nicotine, etc.
- The reason for addiction is increase in dopamine levels in reward area, the nucleus accumbens
- Dopamine acting on D_3 receptor is responsible for addiction behavior.

Role in Emotions

- Fear—fear is produced on stimulation of hypothalamus and amygdala. Amygdaloid nucleus also encodes memories that induce fear. Damage to amygdala abolishes fear
- Anxiety—it is a normal emotional reaction to a stimulus which creates uncertainity about future. But excessive anxiety for any event is abnormal. Seat of anxiety is frontal part of temporal lobe
- Rage and placidity—rage is anger to even a minor stimuli and placidity is opposite to rage and the person does not react to even major irritating stimuli. Lesion of

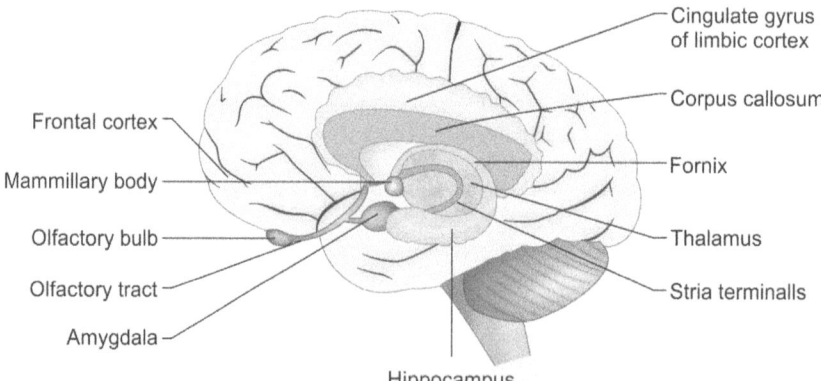

Fig. 22: Structures in limbic system.
(*Source:* Sembulingam)

amygdaloid leads to placidity and lesion of neocortex, venteromedian hypothalamus and septal nuclei causes rage
- Aggression—it is the violent form of rage. Male hormone testosterone can induce aggression and castration reduces aggression. Stimulation of hypothalamus and amygdala can induce aggression and bilateral removal of amygdala causes placidity.

Role in Sexual Activity

- Sexual behavior is controlled by limbic system. But in humans it is controlled by cortex
- In males, lesion of neocortex inhibits sexual behavior. This shows that there is a need for integration between limbic system and cortex in sexual behavior
- Bilateral lesion of piriform cortex overlying amygdala and destruction of amygdala results in hypersexuality
- In females, anterior hypothalamus is responsible for sexual behavior and lesion in this area abolishes sexual activity.

Role in Autonomic Activity

- Hypothalamus is said to be the "Head ganglion of ANS"
- Autonomic responses to emotional activities are controlled by amygdala
- Parts of limbic system that project to brainstem and spinal cord areas control autonomic responses.

18. Mechanism of memory.

- **Memory** is the process by which acquired information is stored and retrieved
- An experience to become a memory should produce a structural and functional change in the brain
- Types of memory—short-term or long term memory
- Short-term memory—ability to recall ongoing experiences for a few seconds
- Brain areas involved are hippocampus, mamillary bodies and two nuclei of thalamus
- If the information is repeatedly used it results in reinforcement of the synaptic pathway and results in long-term memory
- Reinforcement that results from frequent retrieval of a piece of information is called memory consolidation
- Long-term memories are stored in wide regions of cerebral cortex
- Memories for motor skill are stored in basal ganglia and cerebellum
- Several conditions that inhibit electrical activity of brain affect the memory.

Mechanism of Memory is by:

- Alteration in strength of synapses
- Development of new neuronal circuits by the development of new synapses
- Deoxyribonucleic acid (DNA) and ribonucleic acid (RNA) molecules have a part to play in the development of memory
- New proteins are synthesized
- These molecules store memory and RNA molecules increase when memory develops.

Mechanism of Short-term Explicit Memory

- Brain areas involved are hippocampus and other parts of medial temporal lobes
- Physiological processes involved are:
  - Continuous neural activity in reverberating circuits
  - Activation of presynaptic facilitation
  - Accumulation of Ca^{2+} in axon terminals leading to enhanced synaptic output.

Mechanism of Long-term memory

- Areas involved are many areas of neocortex.
  Process of consolidation involves expression of genes and synthesis of new proteins leading to structural changes like:
  - Increase in number of synaptic vesicle releasing sites
  - Increase in number of vesicles
  - Increase in number of synaptic terminals
  - Change in shape or number of post-synaptic spines.

19. Describe the humoral regulation of blood pressure.

There are many vasodilator and vasoconstrictor hormones which regulate blood pressure.

Vasoconstrictors

- Epinephrine
- Norepinephrine
- Antidiuretic hormone (ADH)
- Renin-angiotensin-aldosterone system
- Endothelins.

Vasodilators

- Nitric oxide
- Kinins
- Prostacyclin
- Substance P
- Histamine
- Atrial natriuretic peptide (ANP)
- Vasoactive intestinal peptide (VIP).

1. Catecholamines—they are released from adrenal medulla during hypotension and they cause vasoconstriction, increase heart rate and cardiac output and thereby increase in BP.
2. ADH/vasopressin—decrease in blood volume and blood pressure releases ADH from posterior pituitary. ADH acts on the collecting duct and increases water reabsorption and thereby increases blood volume and blood pressure. ADH is also a potent vasoconstrictor.
3. Renin-angiotensin-aldosterone system—decrease in BP and blood volume stimulates secretion of renin from juxtaglomerular (JG) cells. It converts angiotensinogen in plasma to angiotensin I and angiotensin I is converted to angiotensin II by angiotensin converting enzyme. Angiotensin II acts on adrenal cortex to synthesize aldosterone which increases salt and water reabsorption and thereby increase in blood volume and pressure. Angiotensin II also stimultes thirst center and increases water intake. Angiotensin II also directly acts on proximal convoluted tubule (PCT) to increase salt and water reabsorption.
4. Endothelins—these are potent vasoconstrictors released from endothelium. It also increases heart rate and cardiac output.
5. Nitric oxide—it is synthesized by endothelial cells from arginine. It causes potent vasodilatation and thereby decreases blood pressure. It is also called as endothelium derived relaxing factor (EDRF). It mediates vasodilatory effects of acetylcholine, bradykinin, VIP and substance P.
6. Atrial natriuretic peptide—when blood volume increases there is stretch of right atrium and there is release of ANP. ANP induces diuresis and natriuresis. It causes vasodilation and thereby decreases BP.
7. Kinins - Bradykinin and lysyl-bradykinin cause vasodilataion and thereby decreases BP. It acts via nitric oxide (NO).
8. Histamine—it is also a potent vasodilator. It is secreted from mast cells during allergy. This causes vasodilatation and decrease in BP.

20. Artificial respiration.

- When there is respiratory deficiency or respiratory arrest artificial respiration is given.

Conditions

- Drowning, gas poisoning, electric shock, anesthesia, accidents, etc.

Methods

- Instrumental and manual methods.

Instrumental Methods

- Used when there is a need for prolonged support
- **Three types:**
  1. Positive pressure method
  2. Negative pressure method
  3. Boyle's apparatus.

Positive pressure method:

- Used in operation theaters
- Here air or O_2 mixture is used to inflate the lungs at positive pressures either continuously or intermittently
- It impairs venous return.

Negative pressure method:
- Achieved by alternate compression and relaxing the chest wall
- They are:
  1. Drinker's method (iron lung chamber)
  2. Braggpaul method—use of hollow elastic rubber bag
  3. Others

Drinker's method (iron lung method):
- The instrument contains an airtight iron chamber with a bellow on one side of the instrument
- When the bellow moves in and out it creates a rise and fall of pressure inside the chamber
- The person is placed inside the chamber with the head and neck outside the chamber
- When the pressure rises inside the chamber expiration happens for the patient and when the pressure falls in the chamber there is inspiration.

Braggpaul method:
- Here an elastic rubber bag is tied around the chest of the patient
- The bag is connected to a pump which can inflate and deflate the bag
- When the bag is inflated it compresses the chest and air is expired
- When the pressure is released the chest enlarges passively and air is drawn in.

Boyel's apparatus: This apparatus is used in the hospitals for artificial ventilation. It is an automatic instrument in which rate and depth of ventilation and composition of inspired can be altered.

Manual Methods
- **Holger-Neilson method (Fig. 23):**
  - The subject is made to lie prone and the head is turned to one side (Fig. 23A)
  - The shoulder is abducted and flexed at the elbow and the hands are placed under the cheek
  - The operator is in kneeling position at the head of the patient and he places his hands spread on the back of the subject and bends forward to press on his back (Fig. 23B)
  - The pressure on the back of the subject and compresses on the chest and expels the air out (Fig. 23C)
  - Then he holds the arm above the elbow of the subject and pulls the arm forward (Fig. 23D)
  - This enlarges the chest and results in inspiration. It is repeated 12/min. This is an exhaustive method from the examiner.
- **Eve's rocking method:**
  - Here the subject is made to lie prone on board which is rocketed on a pivot so that it can move up and down like a see-saw
  - When the board is tilted head down the abdominal organs push on the diaphragm resulting in decrease

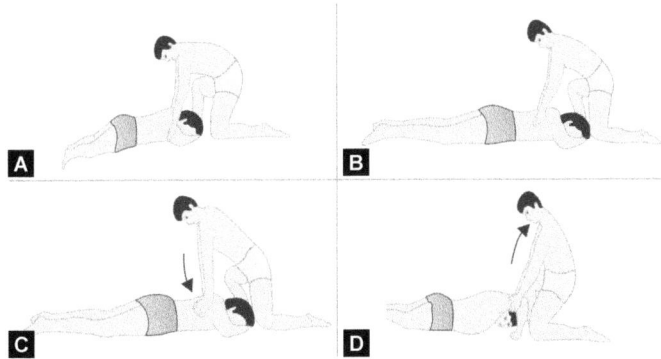

Fig. 23: Hoger-Neilson method of artificial respiration
(*Source:* GK Pal)

in thoracic volume and expiration happens
- When the board is tilted in the opposite direction inspiration happens.

- **Mouth to mouth respiration:**
  - It can be direct or indirect method. In direct method, the operator places his mouth directly on the subject's mouth and in indirect method it is done with a small tube
  - The subject is made to lie supine; the airway is kept clean from vomitus, foreign body, etc.
  - The subject's head is extended, the operator sits on the side of the subject holds the lower jaw with his left hand and opens the mouth and with his right hand and clips the nostrils
  - The operator then inhales deeply and places his mouth on the subject's mouth or the tube placed in the subject's mouth and blows into the subject's mouth smoothly, volume twice that of the tidal volume
  - This inflates the lungs of the subject and then the examiner removes his mouth from the subject's mouth and the lungs recoil resulting in expiration
  - It is repeated 12 times a minute.

  Advantages: Can be applied immediately, can achieve large tidal volumes, CO_2 stimulates respiration, simple technique.

  Disadvantage: Infection may spread, volunteer may get exhausted.

MBBS Examination 2005

ANSWER ALL QUESTIONS

I. Essay Questions   (15 Marks each)

1. Mention the composition of gastric juice. Describe the mechanism of secretion of hydrochloric acid. Give a note on the regulation of gastric secretion.
2. Define glomerular filtration rate (GFR). Describe in detail the factors affecting GFR. Give a note on inulin clearance.
3. Define cardiac cycle. Describe the pressure changes in left ventricle, left atrium and aorta during cardiac cycle. What is second heart sound?
4. What is stretch reflex? Describe in detail the structure and functions of muscle spindle. Add a note on reciprocal inhibition.
5. Enumerate the hormones of the pituitary gland. Describe the mechanism of action of the growth hormone at the cell level. Add a note on acromegaly.
6. Discuss the role of platelets in coagulation.
7. What are chemoreceptors? Describe the chemical control of respiration. Add a note on Cheyne-stokes breathing.
8. What are otolith organs? Explain their mechanisms of action and the physiological functions.

II. Short Notes   (5 Marks each)

1. Carrier-mediated transport.
2. Action potential and its ionic basis.
3. Determination of plasma volume.
4. Actions and regulation of secretion of aldosterone.
5. Mechanism of parturition.
6. Extrinsic mechanism of coagulation.
7. Actions and regulation of secretion of parathormone.
8. Myasthenia gravis.
9. Mechanism of action of insulin.
10. Succus entericus.
11. Regulation of coronary blood flow.
12. Hypoxic hypoxia.
13. Decompression sickness.
14. Definition and measurement of functional residual capacity.
15. Role of hypothalamus on hunger perception.
16. Mechanism of accommodation for near vision.
17. Structure and functions of middle ear.
18. Taste pathway.
19. Chloride shift.
20. Stages of asphyxia.
21. Saltatory conduction in nerve fibers.
22. Phagocytosis.
23. Humoral immunity.
24. Functions of saliva.
25. Actions of pancreatic juice.
26. Hypothalamic thermostat.
27. Cystometrogram.
28. Myxedema.
29. Negative feedback mechanism in hormonal regulation.
30. Female contraceptive methods.
31. Pacemaker potential.
32. Maximum breathing capacity (MBC).
33. Parkinson's disease.
34. Draw an ECG. Mention the cause of each wave.
35. Excitation-contraction coupling.
36. Dark adaptation.
37. Color vision.
38. Basal ganglia.
39. Endorphins.

I. ESSAY QUESTIONS

1. **Mention the composition of gastric juice. Describe the mechanism of secretion of hydrochloric acid. Give a note on the regulation of gastric secretion.**

Composition of Gastric Juice

- 2–2.5 L/day
- pH 1–2
- Water—99.45%
- Solids—0.55%
- Electrolytes—Na^+, K^+, Mg^{2+}, Cl^-, HCO_3^-, HPO_4^-, SO_4^-
- Enzymes—pepsin, lipase, gelatinase
- Mucus—insoluble and soluble
- Intrinsic factor.

Mechanism of HCl Secretion

- In stomach, hydrochloric acid is secreted by the parietal cells which are present in the main gastric glands in body of the stomach
- Pure secretion from the parietal cell has a pH of 0.82 and is isotonic (150 mEq of H^+ and 150 mEq of Cl^+)
- Parietal cell is polarized with an apical side facing the lumen and basolateral side facing the interstitium
- There are many tubulovesicular structures in the parietal cell which are studded with H^+-K^+ ATPase which pump H^+ into the lumen in exchange for K^+
- These cells are highly metabolizing and they put out lot of CO_2. The cell is also rich in the enzyme carbonic anhydrase.

HCl secretion from the Parietal cells happens in 2 steps:
1. Secretion of H^+ into the lumen
2. Secretion of Cl^- into the lumen.

The steps involved in HCl secretion:
1. CO_2 in the cell is hydrated in the presence of carbonic anhydrase, $CO_2 + H_2O \rightarrow H_2CO_3$
2. $H_2CO_3 \rightarrow H^+ + HCO_3^-$
3. The H^+ is pumped into the lumen by the H^+-K^+ ATPase pump on the apical side. For one H^+ pumped out of cell, one K^+ is taken into the cell which later diffuses back into the lumen
4. HCO_3^- is extruded in the basolateral side through an anion exchanger in exchange for one Cl^-
5. The Cl^- which enters the cell will diffuse across the apical membrane into the lumen
6. So for every H^+ secreted, one Cl^- is also secreted into the lumen and one HCO_3^- is absorbed into the blood (Fig. 1).

So when gastric secretion is increased after a meal, the HCO_3^- getting added to the blood is increased, thereby raising the pH of blood—*postprandial alkaline tide*.

Regulation of Gastric Secretion
Refer 2003 paper.

2. **Define glomerular filtration rate (GFR). Describe in detail the factors affecting GFR. Give a note on Inulin clearance.**

Glomerular Filtration Rate
Refer 2003 paper.

Inulin Clearance

- Clearance is defined as the quantity of plasma cleared of a particular substance per unit time
- Clearances of various substances are used to assess the functions of the kidneys
- Clearance of a substance, which is excreted from the body by only filtration

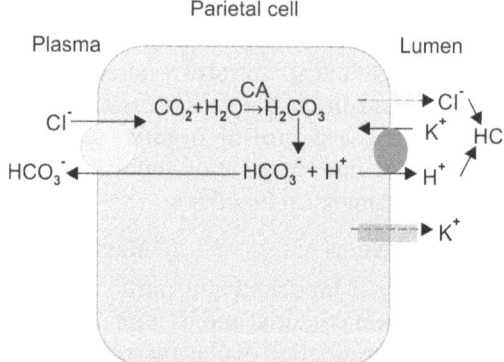

Fig. 1: Mechanism of HCl secretion. (CA: Carbonic anhydrase)

and is neither reabsorbed or secreted or metabolized, is used to measure GFR
- It should be also non-toxic
- Inulin is a polymer of fructose and meets the above criteria.

Methodology
- A loading dose of Inulin is administered intravenously followed by a continuous infusion to maintain its plasma arterial levels
- After equilibration of inulin in plasma, a timed sample of urine and a sample of plasma are collected half way through
- Plasma and urine concentrations of inulin are calculated
- Clearance of inulin is calculated by the formula:

$C_{IN} = U_{IN} \cdot V/P_{IN}$
U_{IN} = Urinary concentration of inulin
V = Volume of urine excreted
P_{IN} = Plasma concentration of inulin.

---

3. **Define cardiac cycle. Describe the pressure changes in left ventricle, left atrium and aorta during cardiac cycle. What is second heart sound?**

Definition
- Cardiac cycle is defined as the cycle of mechanical and electrical events taking place from beginning of one heart beat to the beginning of next heart beat
- It is given as the changes in volume, pressure and flow in different cardiac chambers, the electrical activities occurring (through ECG) and coinciding heart sounds (using PCG) in various phases of cardiac cycle
- Duration of a cardiac cycle is 0.8 s when heart rate is 75/min.

Phases of Cardiac Cycle and their Duration
1. Atrial systole—0.1 s
2. Atrial diastole—0.7 s
3. Ventricular systole—0.3 s
4. Ventricular diastole—0.5 s
- Atrial diastole merges with ventricular systole
- So the phases described here are atrial systole, ventricular systole and diastole

- **Ventricular systole: 2 phases – 0.3 sec**
  1. Isovolumetric contraction phase— 0.05 s
  2. Phase of ejection—0.25 s
     a. Phase of rapid ejection—0.1 s
     b. Phase of reduced ejection—0.15 s
- **Ventricular diastole: 0.5 s**
  1. Protodiastole—0.04 s
  2. Isovolumetric relaxation phase—0.06s
  3. Rapid ventricular filling—0.11 s
  4. Diastasis—0.19 s
- **Atrial systole: 0.1 s.**

Atrial Systole
- Duration is 0.1 sec
- This follows the phase of diastasis
- Begins from peak of "P" wave in ECG to peak of "QRS" complex
- Atria contracts and increases intra-atrial pressure. Blood is pumped into ventricles
- Final filling of Ventricle takes place here (Last 25–30% of filling)
- Already the ventricles are in diastole and 75% of filling is complete
- 4th heart sound is recorded in Phono-cardiogram.

Ventricular Systole
- **Isovolumic contraction phase:**
  - Starts at peak of 'QRS' complex. Duration is 0.05 sec
  - Rise in ventricular pressure closes the AV valves and semilunar valves have not yet opened
  - 1st heart sound (S1) is heard, due to closure of AV valves
  - Ventricular pressure rises (> 80 mm Hg) steeply and ventricular volume remains same (refer Fig. 2)
  - There is bulging of AV valves into the atria due to ventricular contraction. This creates 'C' wave in JVP curve
  - Phase ends with opening of semilunar valves and ejection of blood.
- **Ventricular ejection**
  - Rapid ejection phase: (0.1s)
    - Semilunar valves open and blood is rapidly ejected (2/3rd of stroke volume) into aorta/pulmonary artery

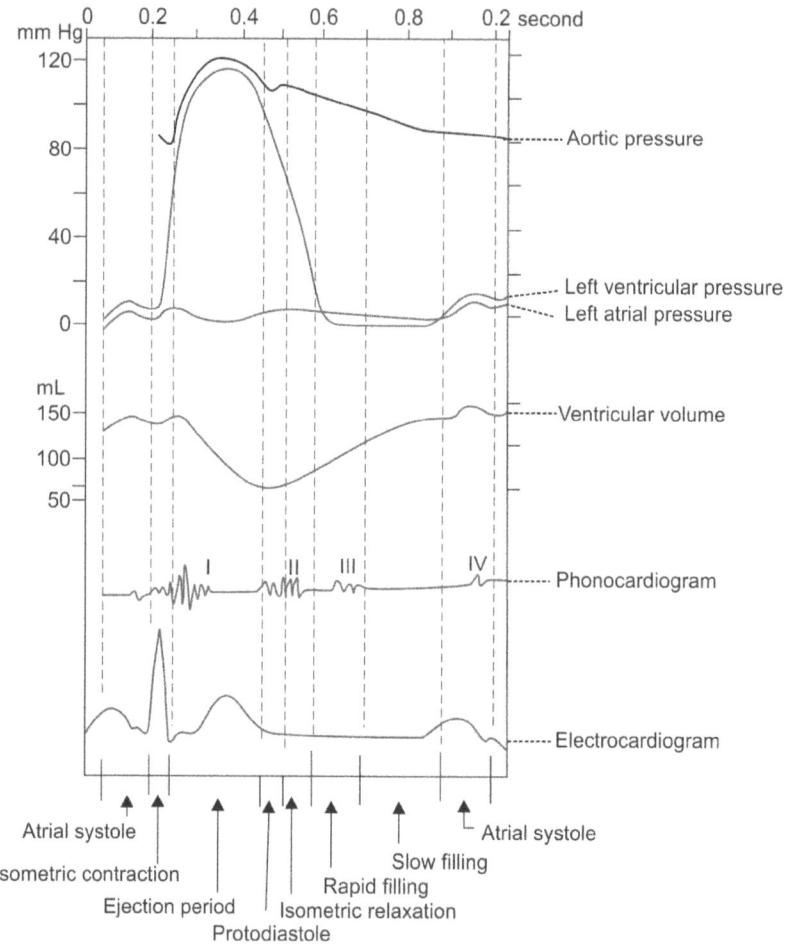

Fig. 2: Cardiac cycle with pressure volume changes in aorta, left ventricle, left atrium, ECG and phonocardiogram. (*Source: Sembulingam*)

- Steep fall in ventricular volume and steep increase in aortic flow
- Ventricular pressure increases to a peak (120 mm Hg in the left and 25 mm Hg in the right)
- Aortic pressure also increases
- Corresponds to ST segment in ECG.
- Reduced ejection phase: (0.15s)
  - Duration is 0.15 sec
  - Ventricular and aortic pressure decreases but aortic pressure is greater
  - Aortic blood flow decreases. Only 1/3rd of stroke volume is ejected here
  - Ventricular volume further decreases
  - Momentum keeps blood flowing into aorta
  - 'T' wave appears in ECG.

Ventricular Diastole—0.5 s

a. Protodiastole—0.04 s
b. Isovolumetric relaxation—0.06 s
c. Phase of rapid ventricular filling—0.11 s
d. Phase of reduced filling or diastasis—0.19 s
e. Phase of second rapid filling—0.1 s.

a. Protodiastole

- Duration is 0.04 sec
- As the reduced ejection phase ends, the ventricles start relaxing

Heart sounds	Events responsible	Duration	Frequency	Others
First sound (S_1)	Due to vibrations set by sudden closure of AV valves at the onset of verticular systole	0.15 sec	25–45 Hz In PCG recorded as 9–13 waves	Soft and long, heard as "LUBB"
Second sound (S_2)	Associated with closure of aortic and pulmonary valves after the end of ventricular systole	0.12 sec	50 Hz In PCG recorded as 4–6 waves	Normally S2 can be split due to early closure of aortic valve, heard as "Dubb"
Third sound (S_3)	Is heard in diastole due to rapid filling of ventricle due to vibrations set by inrush of blood		0.1 sec In PCG recorded as 1–4 waves	Normally audible only in children and young adults
Fourth sound (S_4)	Heard just before (S_1). Occurs during atrial contraction. Due to ventricular filling		20 cyc/sec In PCG recorded as 1–2 waves	Rarely heard in normal adults. Heard in ventricular hypertrophy and congestive cardiac failure (CCF)

Fig. 3: Heart sounds.

- Intraventricular pressure drops
- This phase ends when aortic valve closes.

b. Isovolumetric relaxation phase

- Duration is 0.06 sec
- This phase is between closure of semilunar valves and opening of AV valves
- Second heart sound (S2) appears due to closure of semilunar valves (refer Fig. 3)
- Closure of semilunar valves creates 'Dicrotic Notch' in aortic pressure curve
- Ventricular volume remains the same and pressure drops steeply as the ventricles relax (2–3 mm Hg)
- When intraventricular pressure drops below atrial pressure, AV valves open.

c. Rapid ventricular filling

- Duration is 0.11 sec
- As the AV valves open there is rapid inrush of blood into ventricles
- This is because the atria are filled with venous return and pressure is high here
- This vibration of ventricular wall creates the 3rd (S3) heart sound
- Major filling takes place here.

d. Diastasis

- Duration 0.19 sec
- This is a slow filling phase
- Ventricular volume rises slowly
- Ventricular and atrial pressures reduce and remain same (Little > 0 mm Hg)
- Nearly 75% of filling has occurred.

e. Last rapid filling

- Duration 0.1 sec
- Atria contracts and pumps the last 25% of blood into ventricles
- At rest, this volume is not essential
- But in tachycardia (as in exercise) when the duration of diastole decreases this volume assumes importance.

4. **What is stretch reflex? Describe in detail the structure and functions of muscle spindle. Add a note on reciprocal inhibition.**

Stretch Reflex

It is a monosynaptic reflex integrated at the level of spinal cord and helps in regulating the length of the muscle. The components of the reflex arc are:

- Stimulus: Stretch of the muscle
- Receptor: Muscle spindle
- Afferent nerve: Ia and II sensory fibers
- Center: Spinal cord
- Efferent nerve: Alpha motor nerve fiber
- Effector: Extrafusal muscle fiber
- Response: Contraction of extrafusal fibers.

Muscle Spindle

- Muscle spindle is also called as the intrafusal fibers
- They are placed parallel to the extrafusal fibers

- They are the receptors for stretch reflex
- They are of two types: Nuclear bag (NB) and Nuclear chain (NC) fibers.

  They are supplied by:
  - *Afferents:*
    - Type **Ia fibers: Aα (also known as annulospiral fibers)**
    - Type **II fibers: Aβ nerves**
    - Type Ia fibers are stimulated on stretch of extrafusal and intrafusal fibers
    - Ia fibers supply both NB and NC fibers. Type II supplies only NC fibers (refer Fig. 4).
  - *Efferents:*
    - γ **Motor neurons**
    - β **Efferents**
    - Stimulation of γ efferents, increases sensitivity of Ia fibers to stretch. (They get stimulated when the muscle contracts)
    - β efferents supply both intra and extrafusal fibers. Their role is not known.

Stretch Reflex

- When a muscle is stretched, the intrafusal fibers in parallel, also stretch → stimulates Ia fibers – Afferent impulse reaches α motor neuron supplying the same muscle → contraction of muscle—**Monosynaptic Stretch Reflex (Fig. 5)**
- When the α motor neurons discharge (to contract a muscle) the spindles shorten and stop firing. Information to CNS comes to a halt. But for posture maintenance, this should not happen
- Therefore when α motor neurons fire they also send impulse to γ motor neurons → Impulses are sent to the ends of NB fibers → they contract (as there are contractile proteins only in the ends of NB fibers) – there is maintained stretch in the center of NB fibers (sensitivity increased). Therefore spindles respond not only in stretch of a muscle but also during contraction of a muscle—α-γ linkage
- Muscle spindles respond in both conditions (Stretching and Contraction of the extrafusal fibers). It is essential to maintain posture in a steady state.

Two Types of Response: Dynamic and Static

- **Dynamic response**: The nerves from nuclear bag region discharge most rapidly

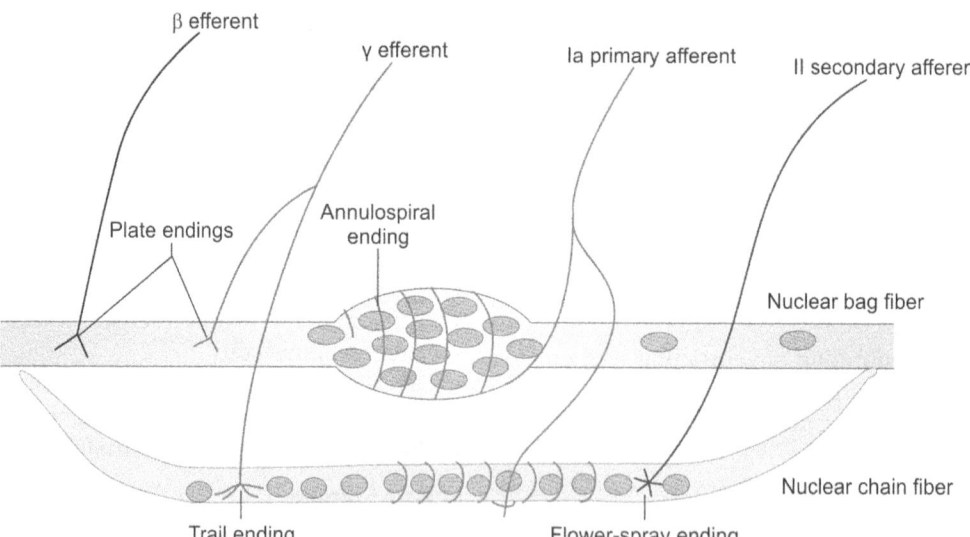

Fig. 4: Muscle spindle with its nerve supply. Nuclear bag and Nuclear chain fibers are present in the muscle spindle. Afferents to muscle spindles are Ia primary afferents and II secondary afferents. γ-efferents supply the contractile ends of the fibers. (*Source:* GK Pal)

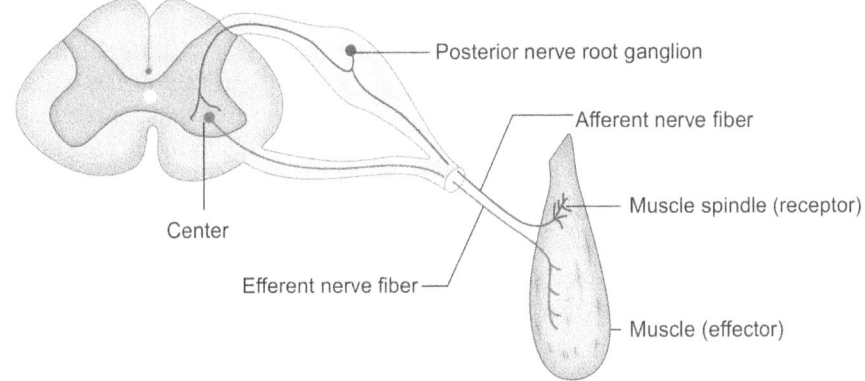

Fig. 5: Stretch reflex pathway.
(*Source:* Sembulingam)

while being stretched and less rapidly during sustained stretch
- **Static response**: The nerves from the nuclear chain fibers discharge at an increased rate during sustained stretch
- Thus, the primary endings respond to both changes in length and changes in the rate of stretch.

Functions of Muscle Spindle

- It is the receptor for stretch reflex and therefore it is responsible for stretch reflex
- It helps in regulation of muscle length
- Stretch reflex in antigravity muscles regulates muscle tone and therefore posture and therefore muscle spindles are responsible for regulation of tone and posture
- Monitors velocity of muscle contraction
- Concerned with conscious perception of joint position and movement.

This is in turn essential for:

- Maintenance of posture
- Facilitates locomotion
- Smoothens voluntary activity.

Reciprocal Inhibition

- When an agonist muscle is stretched the impulses from the muscle spindles within the muscle reaches the spinal motor neuron of the motor units supplying the same muscles
- This induces excitatory postsynaptic potential (EPSP) in the postsynaptic

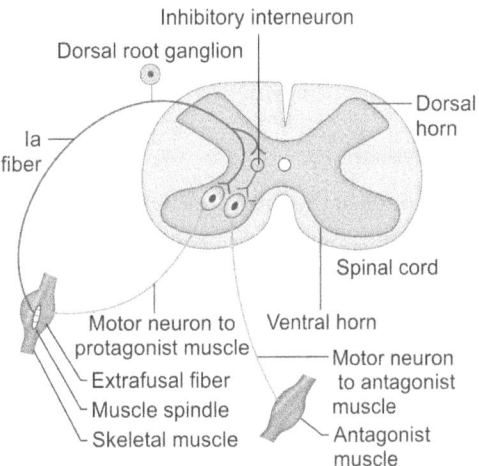

Fig. 6: Inverse stretch reflex or reciporocal inhibition.
(*Source:* GK Pal)

neurons and causes contraction of the extrafusal fibers
- At the same time inhibitory postsynaptic potential (IPSP) are produced in the motor neurons supplying the antagonist muscle
- This response is mediated by branches of the afferents ending on the inhibitory interneurons in the anterior horns, which secrete glycine at the synapse with the motor neurons supplying the anatagonist muscles (Fig. 6)
- Therefore the impulses from the muscle spindle excite the motor neurons supplying the agonists and at the same time inhibit motor neurons supplying the antagonists
- This type of inhibition is Reciprocal Inhibition.

5. Enumerate the hormones of the pituitary gland. Describe the mechanism of action of the growth hormone of the cell level. Add a note on acromegaly.

Hormones of the Pituitary Gland

Hormones of the anterior pituitary gland are:

- Thyroid stimulating hormone (TSH)
- Adrenocorticotrophic hormone (ACTH)
- Growth hormone (GH)
- Luteinizing hormone (LH)
- Follicle stimulating hormone (FSH)
- Prolactin.

Hormones of the posterior pituitary gland are:

- Antidiuretic hormone (ADH) or vasopressin
- Oxytocin.

Hormones of the intermediate lobe are:

- Melanocyte stimulating hormone
- Lipotrophin.

Mechanism of Action of Growth Hormone at the Cell Level

- On reaching target organ GH binds with GH receptor on the cell membrane
- The receptor has an extracellular, transmembrane and intracellular domains
- It is a tyrosine kinase associated receptor
- Growth hormone has 2 binding sites for receptors and when it binds to one of the receptor subunit the other binding site attracts another subunit
- There is homodimerisation of the receptor subunits
- On dimerisation it activates the intracellular JAK2-STAT pathway
- JAK 2 is a member of the Janus family of cytoplasmic tyrosine kinases
- STATs (for signal transducers and activators of transcription) are a family of inactive cytoplasmic transcription factors
- On phosphorylation by the JAK kinases the STATs migrate to the nucleus and activate various genes (Fig. 7).

Acromegaly

- Acromegaly is a clinical condition due to excess secretion of Growth hormone (GH) in the adults (After the fusion of the epiphyseal plates in the long bones)
- It is usually due to a tumor of the Growth hormone producing cells (Somatotrophs) in the Anterior pituitary gland
- Rarely, it can also be due to hypothalamic tumors secreting growth hormone releasing hormone (GRH)
- There is no increase in height of the individual
- But because of the excess levels of GH there is thickening of bones and proliferation of soft tissues like connective tissue and skin
- This leads to coarse disfigured appearance. "Acro" means extremity and "megaly" is large.

Clinical features are:

Excess GH levels lead to:

- Acromegalic face: Jaw and cheek bones become more prominent, lips are thickened, Nose is broad and thick, enlarged brows and coarse skin
- Prognathism: Protrusion of the lower jaw due to elongation and thickening of mandible
- Enlarged spade like hands, broad fingers and large feet
- Body hair is increased
- Kyphosis: Since the vertebral bones continue to grow the person has kyphosis
- They develop osteoarthritis
- Organomegaly: Internal organs like heart, liver, spleen and kidneys are enlarged
- High levels of GH decreases insulin sensitivity in the tissues and the patient has hyperglycemia and are prone to develop Diabetes Mellitus.

Effect of tumor on neighboring structures:

- The tumor in the anterior pituitary compresses the optic chiasma resulting in visual disturbances
- There will be enlargement of sella turcica and headache.

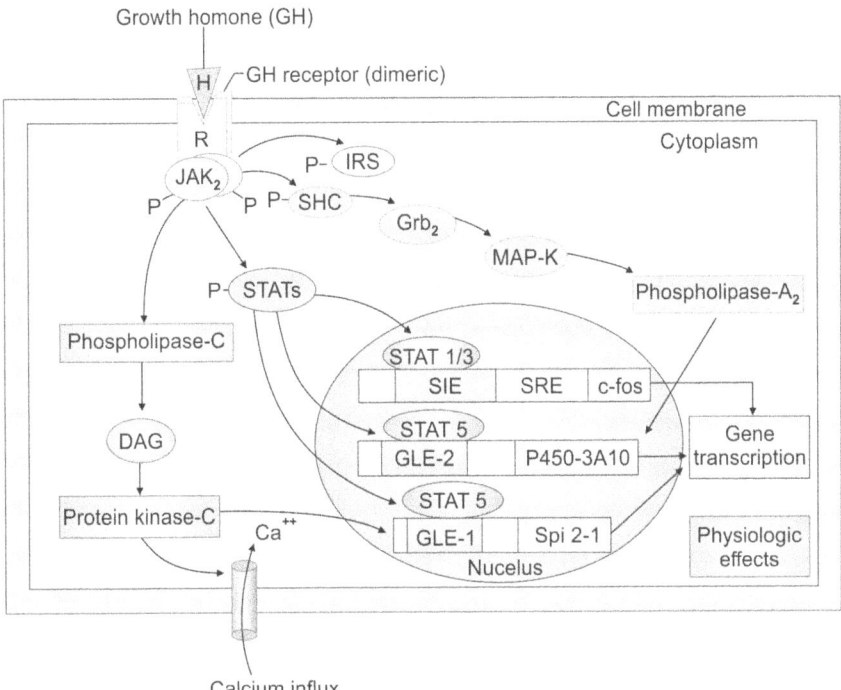

Fig. 7: Mechanism of action of growth hormone. Binding of GH with receptor activates JAK-STAT pathway and subsequent gene transcription.
(JAK: Jannus kinase; STATs: Signal transduction and activator of transcription factors; IRS: Insulin receptor substrate; SIS: Sis induced element; SRE: Serum response element; GLE: Interferon-activated response element; SHC and Grb2: Intracellular protein; MAP-K: Mitosis activated proteinkinase; DAG: Diacylglycerol)
(Source: GK Pal)

6. Discuss the role of platelets in coagulation.

- Hemostasis is the spontaneous arrest of bleeding from the damaged blood vessels by physiological processes
- There are 3 steps involved in hemostasis:
  - Vasoconstriction
  - Formation of temporary platelet plug
  - Formation of a definitive clot – Clotting or coagulation.

The first two steps are involved in temporary hemostasis and the platelets play a major role in the temporary hemostasis. Following temporary hemostasis the definitive clot is formed. Platelets take active part in the coagulation process also.

Coagulation of Blood

- Blood while flowing in the vessels is fluid in nature, but when the vessel wall is injured or the blood is removed from the body and collected in a test tube it becomes a jelly like mass—the clot
- Clotting or coagulation of blood involves a series of cascade of events in which many clotting factors (proteins in the plasma) are activated in a serial manner (refer Fig. 8). There are many such clotting factors.

They are:
- Factor I—fibrinogen
- Factor II—prothrombin
- Factor III—thromboplastin
- Factor IV—calcium
- Factor V—labile factor or proaccelerin
- Factor VI—non-existant
- Factor VII—stable factor or proconvertin
- Factor VIII—antihemophilic factor
- Factor IX—Christmas factor or Plasma thromboplastic component (PTC) or Antihemophilic factor B

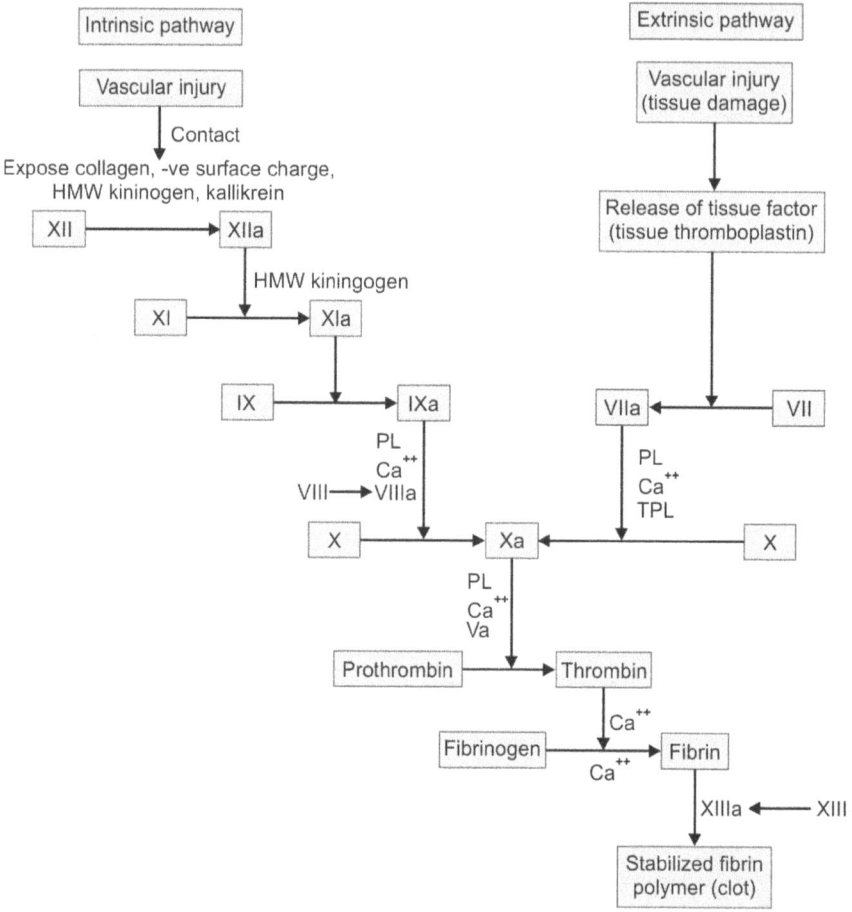

Fig. 8: Mechanism of clotting.
(TPL: Tissue phospholipid; PL: Platelet phospholipid)
(*Source:* GK Pal)

- Factor X—Stuart-Prower factor
- Factor XI—plasma thromboplastin antecedent (PTA) or antihemophilic factor C
- Factor XII—Hageman factor or Glass factor or Contact factor
- Factor XIII—Laki Lorand factor or Fibrin stabilizing factor
- HMW-K—high molecular weight kininogen or Fitzgerald factor
- Pre-Ka (Prekallikrein or Fletcher factor)
- Kallikrein—Ka
- PL—Platelet phospholipid.

The coagulation process involves three major steps:

- Formation of prothrombin activator
- Conversion of prothrombin to thrombin
- Conversion of fibrinogen to fibrin.

Formation of prothrombin activator is by two pathways - Intrinsic and Extrinsic pathways.

Formation of Prothrombin Activator is by 2 Mechanisms

- Extrinsic pathway
- Intrinsic pathway.

Extrinsic Pathway

The extrinsic pathway is triggered when the injury involves damage to the blood vessels and the surrounding tissues. The damaged tissue releases tissue thromboplastin, a protein-phospholipid mixture which

activates Factor VII. This triggers the extrinsic pathway.
- Inactive factor VII is activated to active factor VIIa
- VIIa in the presence of Ca^{++}, Platelet phospholipid (PL) and Tissue thromboplastin, activates factors IX and X
- Active factor Xa, Va, Ca^{++} and PL, forms the prothrombin activator
- Prothrombin activator converts prothrombin to thrombin
- Thrombin catalyzes the conversion of fibrinogen to fibrin.

Intrinsic Pathway

This pathway is activated when there is injury to vessel wall and exposure of collagen or blood itself.

Steps involved are:

- Injury to vessel wall exposes collagen activates Factor XII to XIIa
- Factor XIIa activates Factor XI to XIa
- Factor XIa activates Factor IX to IXa
- Factor IXa in the presence of VIII, Ca^{2+} and platelet phospholipids (PPL) activates factor X to Xa
- The activated factor Xa, platelet phospholipids, factor Va and Ca^{2+} forms the Prothrombin Activator.

Conversion of Prothrombin to Thrombin

Prothrombin activator in the presence of Ca^{2+} converts prothrombin to thrombin. This happens at the surface of platelets. Thrombin is a proteolytic enzyme.

Conversion of Fibrinogen to Fibrin

- Thrombin, a proteolytic enzyme removes two pairs of polypeptide chains from each fibrinogen molecule and converts it to fibrin monomer
- The fibrin monomers now polymerize to form long fibrin threads. The fibrin is initially a loose mesh of interlacing strands. This meshwork traps the blood cells
- It is later converted to a dense tight aggregate by formation of covalent cross-linkages. This is catalyzed by Factor XIII

and Ca^{2+}. The stabilized fibrin mesh with the trapped blood cells forms the Clot.

Role of Platelets in Coagulation

- Platelet activation during temporary hemostasis activates its role in clotting
- Platelets release platelet factor 4 which helps in coagulation
- Platelets take part in intrinsic and extrinsic pathways
- Platelet phospholipids present in the membrane of platelets enhance the activation of factors V, VIII and IX to Va, VIIIa and IXa in the intrinsic pathway. It also is a component of prothrombin activator needed for activation of prothrombin to thrombin
- Along the extrinsic pathway they also enhance the activation of X to Xa in the presence of VIIa
- Thus in through both the pathways platelets enhance formation of thrombin from prothrombin.

Role in Clot Retraction

- Within 15-30 minutes the clot formed shrinks and exudes serum. This process is called clot retraction. It is an important function of platelets
- Platelets have contractile proteins like actin and myosin which can change the shape of platelets and make them contractile
- This shrinking of all the platelets trapped in the fibrin mesh makes the clot a firm structure and also brings the injured walls closer so that healing happens faster
- Since clot retraction is a function of platelets the clot retraction time is used for assessing platelet function.

---

7. **What are chemoreceptors? Describe the chemical control of respiration. Add a note on Cheyne-Stokes breathing.**

- Chemical regulation of respiration is also through the modulation of activities of neural centers through chemoreceptors
- There are 2 sets of chemoreceptors responding to changes in arterial PO_2, PCO_2 and pH

- They are Peripheral and Central Chemoreceptors.

Peripheral Chemoreceptors

- Carotid and aortic bodies (Fig. 9)
- They have high blood flow (2000 mL/100 g /min) and high metabolic rate
- Their metabolic needs are met by dissolved O_2
- So they are highly sensitive to $\downarrow PO_2$, $\uparrow PCO_2$ and $\downarrow pH$
- These receptors are not stimulated in anemia or carbon monoxide poisoning (Since PO_2 is normal)
- They are stimulated in $\downarrow PO_2$, vascular stasis and cyanide poisoning
- They have 2 types of cells—Glomus and Sustentacular cells.

Sensitivity of Peripheral Chemoreceptors (PCR)

- Glomus cells are the sensors (refer Fig. 10)
- Hypoxia is the major stimulus. Neurotransmitter is Dopamine
- PCRs also responds to $\uparrow PCO_2$ and $\downarrow pH$
- When $PO_2 < 100$ mm Hg there is $\uparrow$ firing rate of the nerves supplying them (9th and 10th cranial nerves)
- Response is maximum when PO_2 falls < 60 mm Hg
- Effect of hypoxia is less when $PO_2 > 60$ mm Hg because:
  a. Hypoxia → Hyperventilation → CO_2 blow out →$\downarrow$ arterial PCO_2 ($PaCO_2$) →$\downarrow$ ventilation
  b. Deoxy-Hb has more affinity for H^+ →$\downarrow$ arterial $[H^+]$ →$\downarrow$ ventilation.

Mechanism of Hypoxia Stimulating PCR

Hypoxia inhibits K^+ channels by:

O_2 sensor in the glomus cell is a heme containing protein and is associated with O_2. In hypoxia the lack of O_2 inhibits the K^+ channels and there is decreased K^+ efflux. This depolarises the cell and causes Ca^{++} influx and triggers neurotransmitter release followed by excitation of afferent nerves (Fig. 11).

Effect of CO_2 on PCR

Integrated effects of arterial - PCO_2, PO_2 and pH on ventilation, by stimulating PCR (refer Fig. 12)

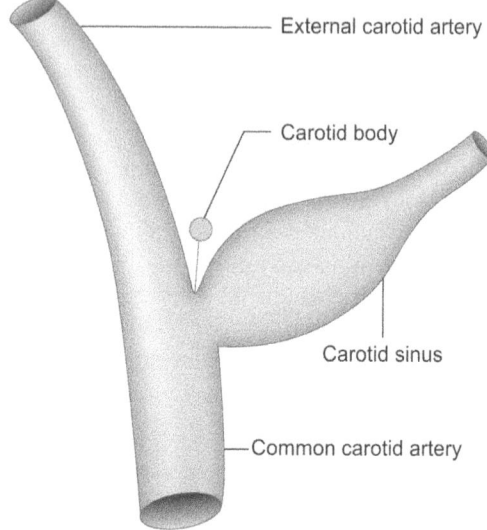

Fig. 9: Location of peripheral chemoreceptors at bifurcation of common carotid artery; the carotid body. Carotid sinus is the dilatation in internal carotid artery; the baroreceptor. (Source: GK Pal)

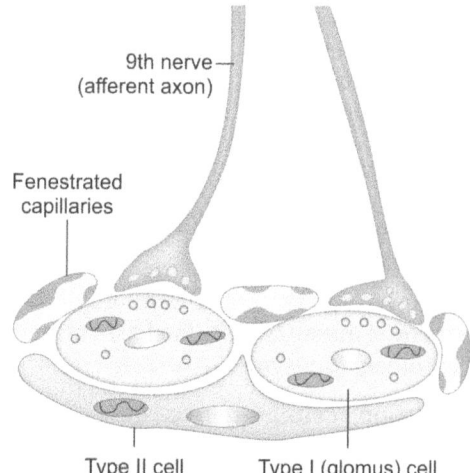

Fig. 10: Cells in carotid body – Type I (Glomus cells) and Type II (Supporting cells). Glomus cells are supplied by 9th cranial nerve and are close to fenestrated capillaries. (Source: GK Pal)

- At low $PaCO_2$ level with hypoxia, ventilation is not stimulated till $PO_2 < 60$ mm Hg
- High $PaCO_2$ levels (as in $\uparrow$metabolic rate/ breathing CO_2 mixtures) →$\uparrow$ ventilation. But if CO_2 content in breathed air is >7% → CNS depression → CO_2 Narcosis

- Hypercapnia with hypoxia, shifts the CO_2 curve to left and slope is increased
- Acidosis by itself (as in Diabetic ketoacidosis) can stimulate ventilation by stimulating PCR. (Even in absence of hypoxia or hypercapnia).

Central Chemoreceptors (CCR)

- Located in the medulla and is different from the other respiratory neurons (Fig. 13)
- There are also other such CCR in and around the brainstem nuclei—Nucleus tractus solitarius, nucleus ambiguus
- They respond maximally to changes in [H^+] in brain CSF and ISF which is in turn decided by $PaCO_2$ and HCO_3^- of CSF.

↑Arterial PCO_2
↓
↑Brain ECF CO_2 level
↓
$CO_2 + H_2O \rightarrow H_2CO_3 \rightarrow H^+ + HCO_3^-$
↓
Increase in brain ECF H^+ level
↓
Stimulation of CCR
↓
Stimulation of medullary inspiratory center
↓
Firing of neurons supplying diaphragm and external intercostal muscles
↓
Increase in ventilation

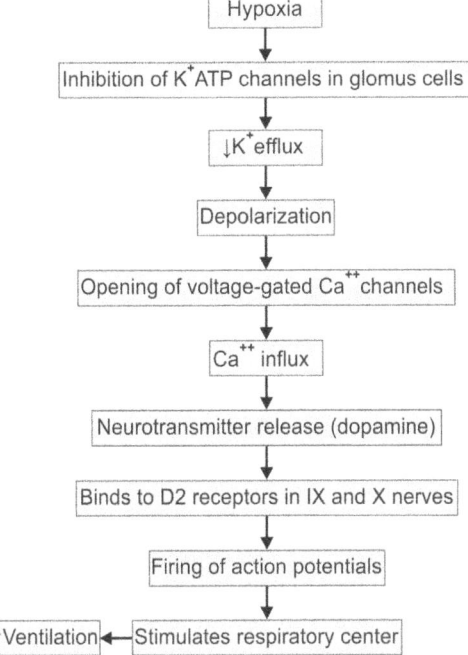

Fig. 11: Effect of hypoxia on peripheral chemoreceptors.

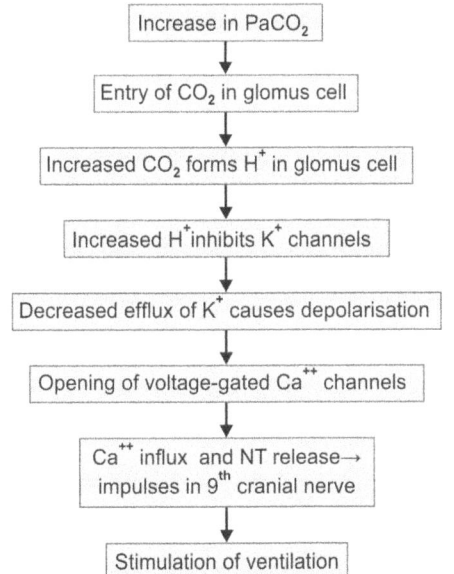

Fig. 12: Effect of hypercapnia on peripheral chemoreceptors.

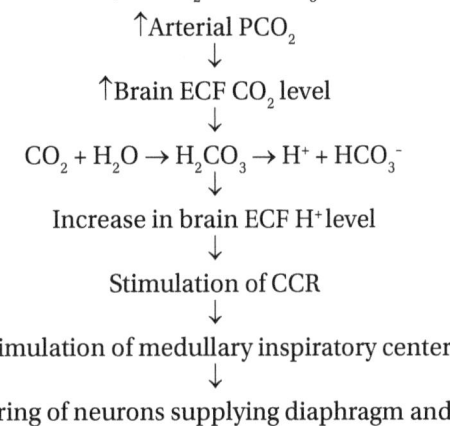

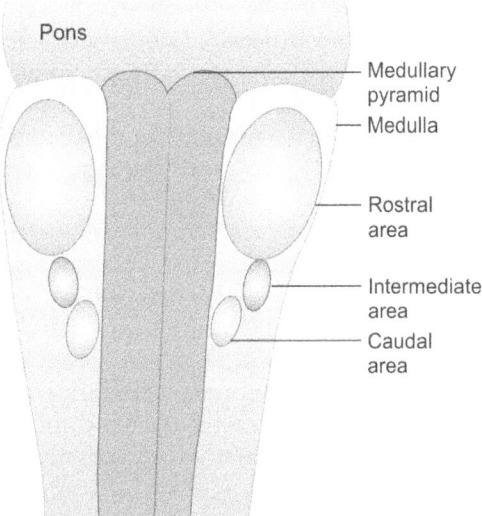

Fig. 13: Location of central chemoreceptors in ventral medulla. There are rostral, intermediate and caudal centers. (*Source:* GK Pal)

Periodic breathing means respiratory activity alternating with apnea. There are alternating periods of apnea and hyperpnea.

Cheyne-Stokes Respiration

- It is an abnormal respiratory pattern with waxing and waning of respiration seperated by periods of apnea
- Duration of each cycle is 1 minute
- Arterial PO_2 and PCO_2 levels fluctuate in different phases of respiration
- Seen in conditions like drug overdosage, brain diseases, congestive cardiac failure, uremia and hypoxia due to other causes
- It is also seen in physiological conditions like—sleep and during voluntary hyperventilation, also in persons with increased sensitivity to CO_2
- There is usually disruption of neural pathways that inhibit respiration.

Cheyne-Stokes Respiration in Voluntary Hyperventilation

Following hyperventilation there is apnea → accumulation of CO_2 → Stimulation of respiratory center → Gradual increase in respiration → as PCO_2 decreases → CO_2 is blown out → Apnea.

Cheyne-Stokes Respiration in CCF

- In patients with heart failure the circulation time of blood is longer (as the pumping of heart is inefficient)
- So it takes a longer time for the changes in blood PCO_2 to reach the respirtaory centers
- As these patients hyperventilate the PCO_2 levels are lowered and since the circulation time is prolonged it takes time for this lowered PCO_2 levels to be detected
- By the time the PCO_2 levels are further lowered in pulmonary capillaries and when this blood reaches the brain, the low PCO_2 inhibits respiratory center producing apnea.

Therefore the respiratory control system oscillates because the negative feedback loop between brain and lungs is lengthened.

8. What are otolith organs? Explain their mechanisms of action and the physiological functions.

- Otolith organs are two sac like structures in the vestibular apparatus, the utricle and saccule (refer Fig. 14)
- Utricle communicates with saccule and saccule communicates with cochlea through ductus reuniens
- Their receptor cells, hair cells are located in the receptor organs maculae of both the utricle and saccule.

Macula

- The macula consists of the hair cells and the supporting cells
- The hairs of these cells are embedded in a gelatinous mass containing crystals of calcium carbonate – the Otoliths or Otoconia
- So these organs are called as otolithic organs
- The hairs of the cells are arranged in ascending order. The tallest hair is the Kinocilia and the others are called as stereocilia
- The hairs are embedded in the otolith membrane
- Macula of utricle is in the horizontal plane, its hairs are directed vertical and macula of saccule is in vertical plane and its hairs are in horizontal plane
- From the base of the hair cells, the nerve fibers arise and they become the Vestibular branch of VIIIth cranial nerve

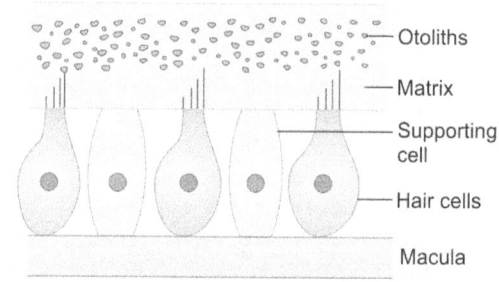

Fig. 14: Otolithic organ.
(*Source:* GK Pal)

- Movement of head bends the hairs and when the smaller hairs bend towards kinocilia there is depolarisation in the nerves and when the hairs bend in opposite direction there is hyperpolarisation in the nerves.

Functions and Mechanism of Action of Otolith Organs

- Utricle and saccule are concerned with detection of linear acceleration—horizontal and vertical
- Utricle responds for horizontal acceleration and saccule for vertical acceleration
- In utricle, the hairs are arranged vertically and movement in horizontal direction will allow the endolymph to move along but the otoconia being heavier lags behind and cause bending of the hairs resulting in stimulation of hair cells
- Impulses from the hair cells reach vestibular nuclei, cerebellum and reticular nuclei
- From these areas impulses reach the appropriate muscles to maintain equilibrium and posture during the movement
- Similar informations are transmitted from the saccule during vertical acceleration and equilibrium and posture is maintained
- Otolith organs discharge at rest, even without acceleration or head movement due to the gravitational pull on the otoconia and they give information about position of head
- The impulses generated from these receptors are partly responsible for righting reflexes and other postural reflexes.

II. SHORT NOTES

1. Carrier-mediated transport.

- This type of transport across cell membrane is done with the usage of membrane-bound carrier proteins
- The carrier proteins bind to the molecule to be transported and changes its configuration to move the molecule from one side of the cell membrane to the other side (From ECF to ICF or ICF to ECF)

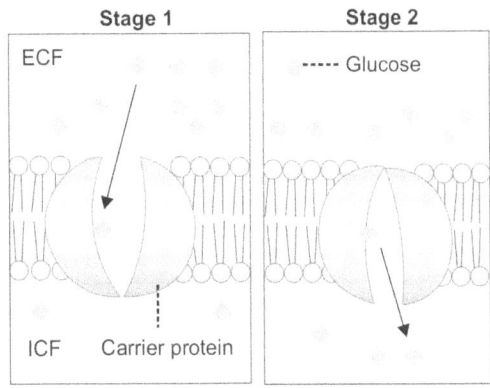

Fig. 15: Facilitated diffusion. A uniport transporting glucose molecules.
(*Source:* Sembulingam)

- Facilitated diffusion is a type of diffusion where carrier proteins transport substances along the concentration or electrical gradient (downhill transport), without energy expenditure (refer Fig. 15), e.g. GLUT, a transporter of glucose across skeletal muscles and adipose tissues etc.
- There are also other types of carrier-mediated transports where substances are moved uphill, i. e. against the concentration and electrical gradients. They are active transporters – Primary (Na^+-K^+ ATPase) and secondary active transporters (Na^+-Glucose symport).

Characteristics of the carrier-mediated transporters are – They are, highly selective, specific and faster in transport of substances. They also have saturation kinetics.

- ***Faster rate***: Even though it reaches saturation, movement of substances through carriers are faster than simple diffusion
- ***Specificity***: Each carrier is specific for the substances it carries. GLUT for transport of glucose
- ***Saturation***: The number of carrier proteins in a membrane are limited therefore as the carrier binding sites are occupied, the transport of substances get saturated and reaches a plateau.

Types of Carrier Proteins

- Uniport: Transports only one substance across the membrane (GLUT)

- Symport: Transports two substances along same direction of the membrane (Na⁺-Glucose symport)
- Antiport: Transports two substances in opposite directions across the membrane (Na⁺-H⁺ exchanger).

2. **Action potential and its ionic basis.**

Refer 2004 Paper.

3. **Determination of plasma volume.**
- Plasma is a component of ECF. It is the fluid part of blood and it contributes around 5% of the body weight
- Plasma volume can be measured by using substances which always stay in the plasma like Evan's blue, a dye which binds to plasma proteins or serum albumin bound to radioactive iodine
- It can be measured by indicator dilution method
- Suitable volume of the injected solution (dye or radiolabelled albumin) and the plasma sample after injecting the solution are taken and are counted in a scintillation counter. Based on the dilution factor the plasma volume is measured. It is around 3500 mL in an adult weighing 70 kg
- The other method of measuring plasma volume is by subtracting hematocrit from total blood volume. To find the red cell volume (Hct), the red blood cells are tagged with a radioactive isotope of chromium, ^{51}Cr, radioisotopes of iron (^{59}Fe) and phosphorus (^{32}P). Antigenic tagging is also employed. This is done by injecting tagged RBCs into the blood and after mixing of the tagged cells have occurred the fraction of red cells that are tagged is measured
- Plasma volume = 100 − Hct/100 × Blood volume.

4. **Actions and regulation of secretion of aldosterone.**

Actions of Aldosterone

Physiological Actions of Aldosterone
- Promotes Na⁺ and water reabsorption and K⁺ and H⁺ excretion from collecting duct (CD) and DCT
- It acts mainly on the Principal cells (P Cells) of CD and DCT, sweat and salivary glands and colon
- Controls only 3% of total Na⁺ reabsorption
- **This is done by:**
  - Insertion of epithelial sodium channels (ENaC) on apical membrane of P cells of collecting duct
  - Stimulates Na⁺-K⁺ pumps on basolateral side of P cells
  - Stimulates ATP generation to activate the pump
  - As Na⁺ is reabsorbed, Cl⁻ follows and water is reabsorbed by osmosis.

It is classified as rapid and slow effect.
- **Rapid effect:**
  - Increased insertion of ENaC on the luminal membrane of cells from a cytoplasmic pool
  - It also binds to cell membrane and increases Na⁺-K⁺ exchanger
  - On the basilar membrane Na⁺-K⁺ pump activity is also increased.
- **Slower effect:**
  - Increases synthesis of ENaCs
  - As a result of this, Na⁺ reabsorption increases with K⁺ and H⁺ secretion into urine
  - Along with Na⁺, Cl⁻ and H_2O is also reabsorbed.

Regulation of Secretion

Regulatory Mechanisms
- Angiotensin ll
- High potassium
- ACTH
- Posture
- Circadian rhythm
- ANP.

Stimuli that Increase Aldosterone Secretion

1. High potassium intake
2. Low sodium intake
3. Constriction of inferior vena cava in thorax
4. Standing
5. Secondary hyperaldosteronism
6. Hemorrhage
7. Surgery
8. Physical trauma
9. Anxiety.

Stimuli that Decrease Secretion

1. Expansion of ECF volume
2. Hypernatremia
3. Hypokalemia.

5. Mechanism of parturition.

- Parturition is the delivery of a full term fetus
- Throughout pregnancy the uterine musculature remains relaxed and helps in maintaining the pregnancy. It is due to the action of the hormone progesterone
- During pregnancy there is production of estrogen and progesterone by the fetoplacental unit. Towards the term period the estrogen levels rise
- Estrogen increases the excitability of the myometrium
- Relaxin produced by the placenta softens the cervix and aids in its dilatation
- The oxytocin receptor sensitivity and number also increases towards term and later oxytocin levels increase and the labor starts by a reflex – The parturition reflex.

Parturition Reflex

Refer answers to 2004 paper.

6. Extrinsic mechanism of coagulation.

Conversion of fluid blood into a jelly like mass is called coagulation or clotting of blood.

Following are the steps in clotting:

1. Formation of prothrombin activator
2. Conversion of prothrombin to thrombin
3. Conversion of fibrinogen to fibrin.

Formation of prothrombin activator is by two pathways—intrinsic and extrinsic pathways

The **extrinsic pathway** is triggered when the injury involves damage to the blood vessels and the surrounding tissues (Fig. 16).

The damaged tissue releases tissue thromboplastin, a protein-phospholipid mixture which activates Factor VII. This triggers the extrinsic pathway.

1. Inactive factor VII is activated to active factor VIIa
2. VIIa in the presence of Ca^{2+}, Platelet phospholipid (PL) and Tissue thromboplastin, activates factors IX and X

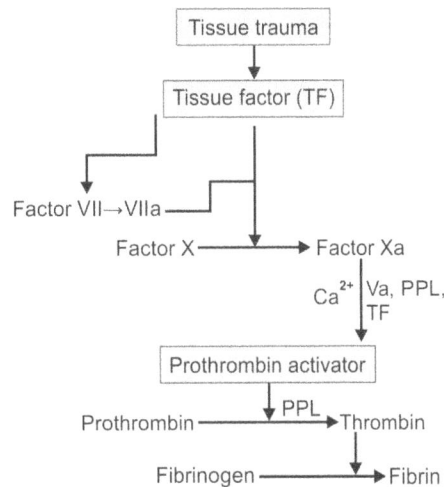

Fig. 16: Extrinsic pathway of clotting.
(PPL: platelet phospholipid; TF: tissue factor;
Va: active factor V)

3. Active factor Xa, Va, Ca^{2+} and PL, forms the prothrombin activator
4. Prothrombin activator converts prothrombin to thrombin
5. Thrombin catalyzes the conversion of fibrinogen to fibrin
   - Fibrinogen a soluble glycoprotein in plasma is converted to insoluble fibrin
   - Fibrin forms a mesh and traps the blood cells
   - This is facilitated by the Fibrin stabilizing factor (Factor XIII)
   - The stabilized fibrin mesh with entrapped blood cells forms the clot. This pathway involves fewer steps in the clot formation and therefore is a faster pathway than the intrinsic pathway.

7. Actions and regulation of secretion of parathormone.

- Parathormone (PTH) is a Polypeptide hormone with 84 amino acids (AA) secreted by the Chief cells of the Parathyroid gland
- The main actions of PTH are to increase blood calcium levels and decrease Phosphate levels.

a. Effect on Bones

- It increases activity of both osteoclasts and osteoblasts

- But the osteoclastic activity is the major effect resulting in resorption of bone and release of calcium and phosphates into the ECF
- PTH stimulates the differentiation of precursors into osteoclasts, increases their numbers and size. The products of resorption are present in blood and are excreted in urine
- PTH increases calcium resorption from the bones in 2 phases—rapid phase and slow phase
- **Osteolytic activity:** PTH causes demineralization of bone and there is transport of calcium from the bone fluid into the osteocytes and from there to the Osteoblasts through gap junctions. Osteoblasts pump calcium into surrounding matrix and then into ECF. This process is termed Osteocytic osteolysis
- **Action on osteoclasts:** This effect comes into action after a few days of exposure to PTH. The number and activity of osteoclasts are increased. Osteoclasts increase bone resorption and thereby increases calcium and phophate levels in the blood. Also levels of hydroxyproline and hydroxylysine are increased
- **Action on osteoblasts:** At low doses PTH increases osteoblastic activity but in high doses it inhibits action of osteoblasts.

b. Action on Kidneys

- There are 3 major actions on the kidneys:
  1. Increased reabsorption of calcium in the thick ascending limb of loop of Henle and DCT. 25 - 30% of the filtered Ca^{2+} is reabsorbed in the DCT and Loop of Henle by the action of PTH. 65% of filtered Ca^{2+} is reabsorbed in the PCT
  2. Decreases reabsorption of phosphate in the kidneys by its action on the PCT and induces phosphaturia. Serum phosphate levels are lowered by the action of PTH
  3. Stimulates the formation of 1, 25 Dihydroxycholecalciferol (Calcitriol) by the kidneys. PTH stimulates the 1α hydroxylation of 25 hydroxycholecalciferol to form the active form of Vitamin D3. Calcitriol in turn increases reabsorption of calcium from GIT and kidneys.

Regulation of Parathormone Secretion

- There are two factors regulating PTH secretion–plasma calcium levels and 1, 25, dihydroxycholecalciferol (Calcitriol)
- Plasma Ca^{2+} levels are the major regulators of secretion of PTH. As the levels of ionized plasma calcium fall there is increased secretion of PTH and if calcium levels increase PTH levels decrease
- Calcitriol inhibits formation of PTH by decreasing prepro PTH mRNA
- Increased plasma phosphate levels increase PTH secretion by lowering plasma Ca^{2+} levels and inhibiting formation of calcitriol
- Magnesium is needed for normal PTH response.

8. Myasthenia gravis.

- It is an autoimmune disease
- Antibodies are formed against the Nicotinic ACh receptors in neuromuscular junction
- There is weakness, fatigue and the muscles become weak with repeated use and therefore symptoms worsen towards the evening
- The antibodies not only combine with ACh for the receptors but they also flatten the post-synaptic membrane and cause endocytosis of ACh into presynaptic membrane
- Because of these effects, the muscle response to repeated stimulation gradually decreases
- Symptoms improve after rest and are better on getting up in the morning
- The extraocular and facial muscles are the first to be affected and ptosis and diplopia are present.

Treatment

a. Acetylcholine esterase (ACh E) inhibitors: ACh E inhibitors increase the amount of ACh in the NMJ and they can displace the antibodies and improve functions

b. Thymectomy: Decreases the immune response by inhibiting T cell activation
c. Immunosuppressants
d. Plasmapheresis.

9. Mechanism of action of insulin.

- Insulin being a peptide hormone has a membrane bound receptor
- The insulin receptors are present in different cells in the body including the ones in which it does not increase glucose uptake
- The receptor is a tetramer with 2α and 2β subunits which are glycoproteins
- The intracellular part of β subunit has tyrosine kinase activity
- On binding of insulin to the receptor triggers the tyrosinekinase activity of β subunit and it leads to autophosphorylation of the β subunit
- Following this there is phosphorylation of other cytoplasmic proteins which is needed for exerting the actions of insulin
- The activated tyrosine kinase phosphorylates Insulin receptor substrates (IRS 1 and 2)
- Phosphorylation of IRS leads to translocation of GLUT to cell membrane and also induction of certain genes to form intracellular proteins
- On insertion of GLUTs on the cell membrane glucose entry is facilitated into the cells
- It also inserts many channels for influx of proteins and amino acids, potassium, phosphates etc.

10. Succus entericus.

- Secretions of small intestine is called as Succus entericus
- It is isotonic in nature
- Daily secretion rate is 1000–2000 mL/day.

Composition

1. **Mucus:**
   - Secreted by Brunner's glands in duodenum and goblet cells in mucosa of small and large intestines
   - Stimulated by cholinergic stimulus, chemicals and physical irritation
   - Protective against HCl and chyme from damaging the mucosa.
2. **Enzymes:**
   - They are brush border enzymes and not secreted into the lumen
   - The brush border enzymes are – peptidases (proteolytic enzymes), disaccharidases (carbohydrate digesting enzymes), intestinal lipases and enterokinase.
3. Water and electrolytes.

Regulation of Secretion

1. Vagal stimulation increases secretion
2. Local distension and irritation of mucosa increases secretion
3. Hormones like vasoactive intestinal peptide (VIP) also increase the secretion.

Functions of Succus Entericus

- Proper mixing of chyme to favor its digestion and absorption
- Brush border enzymes digest nutrients
- Mucus in the secretion protects mucosa and also traps bacteria
- Mucus also contains Ig A for providing mucosal immunity
- Brunner's gland secretions protect duodenum from damage due to stomach acid.

11. Regulation of coronary blood flow.

Regulation of coronary blood flow is by autoregulation, neural regulation and by metabolic regulation.

Autoregulation

- Well developed in heart but autoregulation falls when the BP falls below 70 mm Hg and coronary blood flow is decreased
- Autoregulation is between 70–110 mm Hg.

Neural Regulation

By sympathetic and parasympathetic nerves.

Sympathetic stimulation: Norepinephrine secreted from sympathetic nerve terminal acts on α and β adrenergic receptors. There is a direct effect and an indirect effect following stimulation of sympathetic nerves to heart.

a. **Direct effect:** It is the effect of norepinephrine (NE) on α receptors - resulting in vasoconstriction and thereby decreases coronary blood flow
b. **Indirect effect:** Effect of NE on β receptors leads to—↑HR and contractility → production of vasodilator metbolites → Vasodilatation → Increased blood flow in coronary vessels.

Effect of parasympathetic stimultion: Decreased heart rate → No metabolites formed → Decreased blood flow in coronary vessel.

Metabolic Regulation

- This is the most important mechanism by which coronary blood flow is regulated
- Metabolic regulators are—↓PO_2, ↑PCO_2, ↑H^+, Prostaglandins, ↑Lactate, Adenosine and Adenine nucleotides
- Adenosine is a major factor regulating blood flow. Adenosine is released from myocardium during hypoxia and it causes vasodilation
- ↓PO_2 - Directly produces vasodilatation.

Regulation by Endothelium

- Endothelium derived relaxing factors like Nitric Oxide, Prostaglandins, prostacyclin and endothelium derived hyperpolarizing factors (EDHF) also cause vasodilatation and increase coronary blood flow.

12. Hypoxic hypoxia.

Hypoxic Hypoxia

Arterial pO_2 is low, therefore tissue pO_2 is less.

Mechanism of Hypoxia

pO_2 of arterial blood is low due to either ↓O_2 in inspired air or disease of respiratory apparatus.

Conditions

- Low pO_2 in inspired air (as in high altitude)
- Hypoventilation as in airway obstruction, paralysis of respiratory muscles
- Diffusion defects as in pulmonary edema
- Ventilation/perfusion mismatch
- A-V shunt as in congenital cyanotic heart disease.

13. Decompression sickness.

- Also called as "Dysbarism, The bends, Caissons disease, Divers palsy"
- This happens when a person breathing compressed air ascends up rapidly (from high barometric pressure to low barometric pressure)
- At high pressures, N_2 dissolves in body fluids and stays dissolved
- When the person ascends up to sea level gradually N_2 is converted to air gradually and is blown out
- But when he ascends up rapidly the dissolved N_2 does not have enough time to be converted to air and to be blown out and therefore it stays in the tissues as N_2 bubbles
- N_2 dissolved in tissues form bubbles while escaping from tissues due to rapid ascent
- Gas bubbles block the blood vessels and stay in tissues to create symptoms.

Symptoms

- Pain in joints and muscles of legs or arms
- Sensation of numbness
- The chokes—shortness of breath, pulmonary edema etc.
- Paralysis of muscles
- Coronary ischemia
- Neurological symptoms.

Treatment

Recompression in pressurized chamber followed by slow decompression.

14. Definition and measurement of functional residual capacity.

- It is the volume of air remaining in the lung at the end of tidal expiration
- It is equal to Residual volume + Expiratory reserve volume
- Normal value is 2.5 L.

Measurement of FRC

It can be measured by two methods.
a. Nitrogen washout method
b. Helium dilution method.

a. Nitrogen Washout Method

- It is based on the fact that alveoli contain 80% N_2 (Got from breathing atmospheric air which has 80% N_2)
- The subject is asked to breathe 100% O_2 for 5 minutes
- Then he is asked to expire into the Douglas bag (Which is washed with 100% O_2)
- The volume of air expired and the concentration of N_2 in the expired air is measured and with these values FRC is calculated

For example:
The volume of air expired into the bag = 40L
N_2 concentration is 5%
So 100 mL of air contains 5 mL of N_2 and therefore 40,000 mL of air will contain
= 5 × 40,000/100
= 2000 mL of N_2
The 2000 mL of N_2 has been washed out from the alveoli and there is 80% N_2 in the air, i.e. 80 mL of N_2 in 100 mL of air.
So 2000 mL would have been present in =
2000 × 100/80 = 2500 mL
2500 mL is the FRC.

b. Helium Dilution Technique

- Here the subject is made to breathe from the spirometer containing a mixture of air and helium
- He is asked to exhale, till the tidal expiration and then he breathes in and out of the spirometer continuously till the amount of helium in spirometer and lungs are equilibriated.

Then FRC is calculated by using the formula:

- Initial volume (V_1) × Initial concentration of helium (He_i) = Final volume (V_1 + FRC) × Final concentration of helium (He_f)
- Therefore FRC = V_1 (He_i - He_f) / He_f
- If V_1 = 2000 mL
- He_i = 12%
- He_f = 5%
- Then FRC = 2000 (12 - 5) /5 = 2000 × 7/5 = 2800 mL
- FRC = 2800 mL.

Significance of FRC

1. FRC acts as a buffer and allows continuous exchange of gases in inspiration as well as expiration
2. Without FRC, the pO_2 in alveoli will increase to 150 mm Hg in inspiration and in expiration it may reach even zero
3. Presence of FRC maintains pO_2 at 100 mm Hg
4. FRC dilutes the toxic gases, as the FRC (2300 mL) is always present in lungs
5. Helps in breath holding
6. Work of breathing is minimised by the FRC as the presence of this volume of air in lungs prevent the collapse of the alveoli
7. FRC prevents collapse and thereby decreases pulmonary vascular resistance.

15. Role of hypothalamus on hunger perception.

Refer 2003 paper.

16. Mechanism of accommodation for near vision.

Refer answers to 2003 paper.

17. Structure and functions of middle ear.

Refer answers to 2003 paper.

18. Taste pathway.

The taste receptors are present in the taste buds which are located on the tongue in the papillae (Fig. 17).

- There are 10,000 taste buds
- Taste buds are located in: Fungiform, foliate and vallate papillae
- Cells in taste buds: Type 1 and 2—supporting cells
- Type 3 cells: Receptor epithelial cells have microvilli projecting into taste pore
- The receptors are replaced constantly in 10 days
- Each bud is innervated by 50 nerves at bases of receptor cells
- Each nerve innervates 5 taste buds
- The sensory fibers from the taste buds travel through 3 nerves – Chorda tympani branch of facial nerve (from anterior 2/3rd

- From here the second order neurons travel along with medial lemniscus to reach ventral posteromedial nucleus of ipsilateral thalamus
- Some fibers from medulla go to the vomiting center, hypothalamus, limbic system and salivary nucleus
- The 3rd order neurons arise from the thalamus and they reach the foot of Postcentral gyrus on the same side (area 43)
- From there impulses are also transmitted to the insula and lateral orbitofrontal cortex.

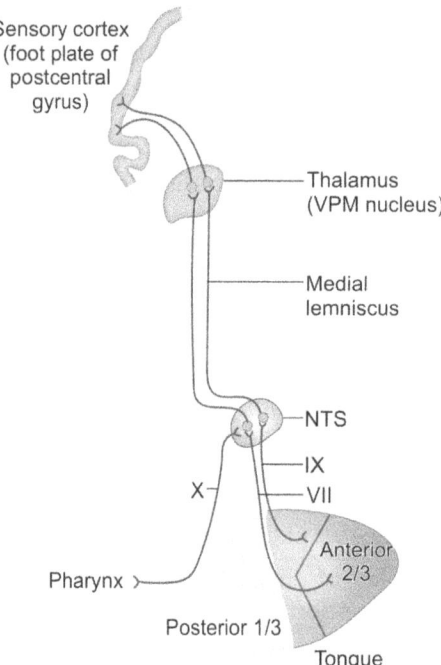

Fig. 17: Taste pathway. Sensation of taste is carried through VIIth cranial nerve from anterior 2/3rd of tongue, by Glossopharyngeal nerve (IX) from anterior 1/3rd of tongue, from pharynx, epiglottis by Vagus Nerve (X) to Nucleus tractus solitarius (NTS).
(*Source:* GK Pal)

of the tongue), Glossopharyngeal nerve (from posterior 1/3rd of the tongue) and Vagus nerve from epiglottis, pharynx and palate
- They all reach the medulla and terminate on Nucleus Tractus solitarius of the same side

19. Chloride shift.

1. The major part of CO_2 (70%) is transported as HCO_3^- in plasma. CO_2 diffuses from the tissues and enters the interstitial tissue and from there it enters the RBC due to the pressure gradient in these areas (Fig. 18)
2. Inside the RBC the enzyme carbonic anhydrase (CA) is present
3. CO_2 enters RBC and combines with H_2O in presence of CA to form H_2CO_3
4. H_2CO_3 dissociates immediately and splits into H^+ and HCO_3^-
5. HCO_3^- levels increase within the RBC and the excess of HCO_3^- leaves the cell in exchange for an anion, Cl^- through the anion exchanger, band 3 protein
6. This exchange is called **Chloride shift or Hamburger shift**
7. For each molecule of CO_2 added to a red cell there is an increase of one osmotically active particle in the cell—either Cl^- or HCO_3^-

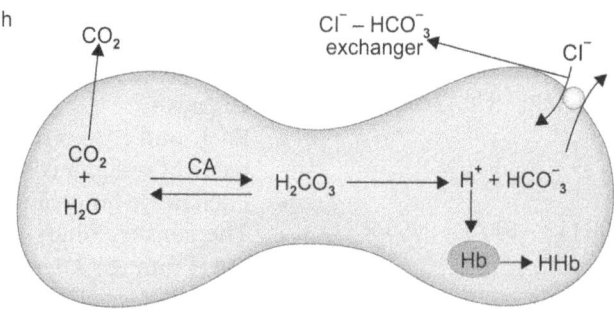

Fig. 18: Chloride shift in RBC.
(*Source:* GK Pal)

8. Therefore the RBC takes up water and swells up and increases in size
9. This increases the hematocrit of venous blood by 3% than the arterial blood.

20. Stages of asphyxia.

- It is a condition produced by occlusion of airways
- There is acute hypoxia and hypercapnia
- It is seen in conditions like strangulation, foreign body in trachea or larynx, drowning and traumatic compression of chest
- Artificial respiration should be started immediately; if not cardiac arrest happens in 4-5 minutes.

It happens in 3 stages:

- Stage of hyperpnea or exaggerated breathing: It exists for 1 minute. There is hyperpnea due to hypoxia and hypercapnea. It is followed by dyspnea and cyanosis. Eyes become prominent
- Stage of convulsions: There is violent respiratory efforts followed by muscular convulsions. BP and Heart rate rises. This stage lasts for 1 minute. Loss of consciousness occurs
- Satge of collapse: It happens due to severe hypoxia. It lasts for 3-5 minutes. Disappearence of convulsions, CNS depression and gasping happens. Pupils dilate and the pulse is feeble and death occurs.

21. Saltatory conduction in nerve fibers.

- In myelinated axons, the action potentials are generated only at the nodes of Ranvier. This part of the axon is exposed to ECF (Fig. 19)
- Voltage-gated Na^+ channels are concentrated in the Nodes of Ranvier and the myelin sheath in the subsequent area acts as an insulator
- So the current sinks move from one node to another node rather than exciting the neighboring area as in unmyelinated axon
- This type of impulse conduction is called as Saltatory conduction
- Since the impulses jump across nodes it can travel faster and impulses are conducted 50-100 times faster than the unmyelinated fibers.

22. Phagocytosis.

It is a process of engulfing and destruction of solid particles/microbes by cells.

Neutrophils and macrophages are the phagocytic cells.

It involves the following stages:

Margination, emigration, diapedesis, chemotaxis, opsonisation, engulfing, degranulation and degradation stage.

Steps in Phagocytosis

a. *Margination:* At the site of infection, neutrophils get marginated towards the

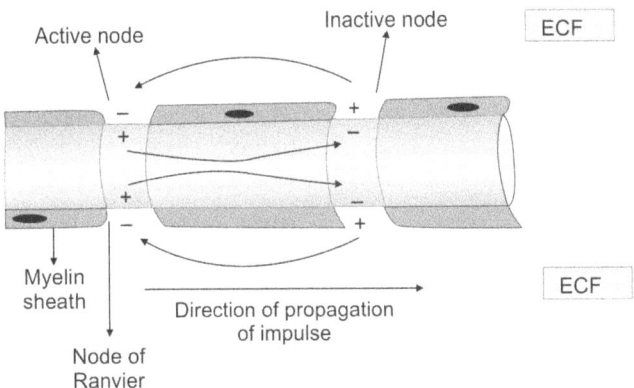

Fig. 19: Saltatory conduction.
(*Source:* Sembulingam)

wall of the vessel and they get attached to the endothelium through proteins called selectins which are present on the endothelial cell membranes

b. *Emigration and diapedesis:* The marginated neutrophils move out of the capillary wall through the junctions between endothelial cells. Walking out of the WBCs is called as Diapedesis (Fig. 20)

c. *Chemotaxis:* It is the process of attraction of neutrophils to site of infection. The chemotactic substances are released by endothelial cells and damaged tissue. They are called chemokines. Leukotrienes and proteins in complementary pathway are some of the chemokines

d. *Opsonisation:* It is the process of coating the infective agent with opsonins to make it tastier for neutrophils to engulf it. Some of the opsonins are IgG and complementary proteins

e. *Engulfment stage:* Once the neutrophils come in contact with the microbe it puts out pseudopodia and engulfs it. The microbe now surrounded by a vesicle (Phagosome) enters the neutrophil and is attached to lysosomes to form phagolysosome. The lysosome releases its proteolytic enzymes and destroys the microbe. The phagocytes also have oxidative enzymes in them which form lethal oxidative metabolites like—O_2^-, H_2O_2 and hypochlorites. Antimicrobials - *Defensins* in phagocytes kill the micoorganisms

f. *Degradation stage:* The destroyed microbe is now extruded as a residual body from the neutrophil.

23. Humoral immunity.

- B lymphocytes mediate humoral immunity
- Humoral immunity provides protection against extracellular pathogens, takes part in immediate hypersensitivity reactions type I, II and III.

Stages of Humoral Immunity

- Antigen processing and presentation
- Activation of B cells
- Differentiation of B cells to plasma cells
- Proliferation of plasma cells
- Formation of antibodies by plasma cells
- Destruction of pathogens by antibodies
- Formation of memory B cells.

Antigen processing and presentation: Antigen on entering the body is engulfed by macrophages and is broken to fragments and the antigenic fragments are attached to the MHC II protein and inserted on the cell membrane of macrophage. Macrophage with the antigen and MHC II are presented to the lymphocytes—**antigen presentation**.

Activation of B cells: B cells in the lymph nodes which have the receptor for the antigen recognizes it and binds with the receptor. This is said to be antigen recognition and activation. Activation is further stimulated when it is co-stimulated by Helper T cells. T helper cells secrete interleukin—2, 4 and 5 which stimulates B cells.

Differentiation of B cells to plasma cells: Activated B cells become enlarged and looks like a blast cell. It then gets transformed into plasma cells. Plasma cells are larger and have lot of endoplasmic reticulum and they secrete antibodies. Co-stimulation by T helper cells help in transformation.

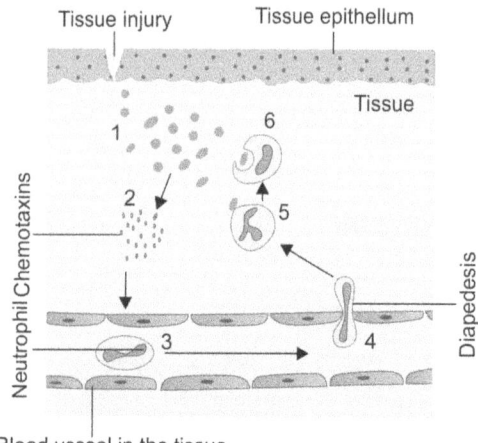

Fig. 20: Steps in phagocytosis; Margination of WBCs, diapedesis, chemotaxis and engulfing of microbe.
(*Source: GK Pal*)

Proliferation of plasma cells: Activated plasma cells undergo proliferation to form millions of similar cells. This is called clonal selection of plasma cells.

Formation of antibodies: The plasma cells secrete antibodies which are called as Immunoglobulins. Each cell can form 2000 immunoglobins (Ig) in a second. The Igs formed are very specific to the antigen which stimulated the B cells (Fig. 21).

Destruction of pathogens: Antibodies do the killing of antigens by the following mechanisms:
a. Neutralization of antigens
b. Precipitation of antigens
c. Activation of complemetary pathway
d. Opsonization of antigens and facilitates phagocytosis
e. Prevent mobilization of microbes.

Formation of memory B cells: Some of the plasma cells get differentiated into memory B cells and they stay inactive in the lymph nodes till the second encounter with the same pathogen. On exposure for the second time, they produce a rapid, swift and strong response to the antigen – Seconday immunological response.

24. Functions of saliva.

Refer 2003 paper.

25. Actions of pancreatic juice.

Pancreatic juice contains enzymes for digestion of lipids, proteins and carbohydrates.

A. Digestive Function of Pancreatic Juice

Digestion of Lipids

a. Pancreatic lipase is the major fat digesting enzyme. It digests triglycerides into monoglycerides and fatty acids
b. Colipase: It exposes the active sites of pancreatic lipase and facilitates its lipolytic action
c. Phospholipase A2: It acts on phospholipids and converts it to fatty acids and lysophospholipids

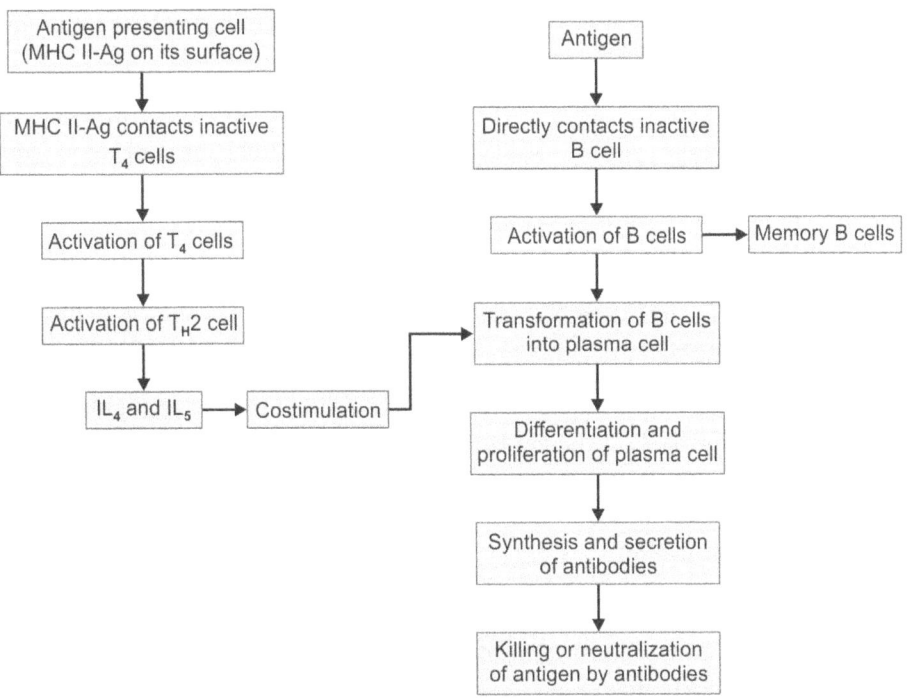

Fig. 21: Mechanism of humoral immunity.
(*Source:* GK Pal)

d. Cholesterol ester hydrolase acts on cholesterol esters and splits it into cholesterol and fatty acids.

Digestion of Proteins

Proteolytic enzymes are secreted in the inactive forms: Trypsinogen, chymotrypsinogen, proelastase and procarboxypeptidase A and B.
a. Trypsinogen on secretion into duodenum is activated to trypsin by the enzyme enterokinase in the intestine
   Trypsinogen → Trypsin, happens in presence of intestinal enzyme, enterokinase.
b. Chymotrypsinogen → Chymotrypsin, happens in presence of trypsin
c. Proelastase and procarboxylase → elastase and carboxylase, in presence of trypsin
d. Trypsin and chymorypsin act on proteins and polypeptides and cleaves the peptide bonds in basic and aromatic amino acids
e. Elastase acts on elastin and some other proteins
f. Carboxypeptidases also act on proteins and polypeptides
g. Nucleases split ribose and deoxyribose nucleotides
h. Collagenase digests collagen.

Digestion of Carbohydrates

Pancreatic α amylase: It is secreted in active form and just like salivary amylase it hydrolyzes glycogen, starch and other complex carbohydrates to form disaccharides.

B. Regulation of Intestinal pH

- Pancreatic juice is rich in HCO_3^- and therefore alkaline in nature
- HCO_3^- is secreted by the ductal cells of pancreas
- The alkalinity created by HCO_3^- neutralizes the HCl derived from gastric juice as it enters the intestine.

26. Hypothalamic thermostat.

- Humans need to maintain body temperature at 37°C
- Hypothalamus is the most important area to control body temperature
- Preoptic region of anterior hypothalamus is said to be the hypothalamic thermostat. This area is sensitive to local changes in temperature
- Warmth in this area stimulates vasodilatation and sweating and when this area is cooled it causes vasoconstriction and heat conservation. So this area is considered to maintain the hypothalamus temperature to a set point
- Posterior hypothalamus is concerned with integrating mechanisms which correct the deviation of the set point
- Preoptic region of anterior hypothalamus has a role in regulation of body temperature in warmth. When body temperature goes above set point it stimulates heat dissipating mechanisms like vasodilation and sweating
- Posterior hypothalamus acts in cool temperature and involved in heat conserving mechanisms like vasoconstriction, piloerection and sympathetic stimulation.

Afferent Impulses to Regulate Temperature by these Areas are by Two Mechanisms

- Direct mechanism: When the environmental temperature is high the warm blood stimulates the hypothalamus and causes vasodilatation and sweating. In cold conditions the cool blood stimulates the hypothalamus to conserve heat and also to generate heat. Therefore in any external conditions the body temperature is maintained normal
- Impulses from skin: Skin has thermoreceptors. Afferent nerves from the skin carry impulses to hypothalamus and the temperature regulation is done through autonomic nerves (sweating, vasoconstriction, vasodilatation etc.) and somatic nerves (shivering, other muscle activities etc.).

27. Cystometrogram.

- Smooth muscles which make up the urinary bladder show the property of plasticity, a property when a muscle is stretched, the tension initially developed is not maintained. So there is no length-

tension relationship in the bladder wall muscle
- A study is done to assess the relation between the intravesicular pressure and intravesicular volume. The bladder is catheterised and fully emptied. Then volumes of fluid in increments of 50 mL are filled into the bladder through the catheter. This test is said to be the **Cystometry**
- A graph is plotted relating the intravesicular volume and intravesicular pressure, this is the cystometrogram
- There are 3 components in this graph – Ia, Ib and II (Fig. 22)
  - **Ia:** There is an initial rise in the pressure of 10 cm of H_2O when the bladder is filled with the first 100 mL of fluid
  - **Ib:** Further increments of fluid upto 300–400 mL produces not much rise in the pressure and a flat segment is seen in the cystometrogram. This segment is said to follow the Law of Laplace which states that the distending pressure (P) in a spherical viscus is equal to twice wall tension (T) divided by the radius (r). $P = 2T/r$. As the bladder gets filled, the wall tension increases, so does the radius of the bladder and therefore the pressure increase is less till the organ is full
  - **II:** As the volume in the bladder reaches 400 mL there is a sharp rise in the pressure resulting in initiation of the micturition reflex.
- Beyond 600 mL, the urge to empty the bladder is unbearable.

28. Myxedema.

Hypothyroidism in Adults is Myxedema

- ↓ BMR, hypothermia and cold intolerance, skin is dry and cold.

CNS Symptoms

- They are dull and lethargic, speech and mentation slow, reflex time is prolonged
- Depression, excess sleep, Frank psychosis (myxedema madnesss).

CVS Symptoms

- Bradycardia, ↓ myocardial contractility, cardiac output ↓, hypertension is present
- Serum cholesterol and TGL levels ↑ - leads to atherosclerosis.

Skin

- Non-pitting edema (myxedema) is seen
- Hoarseness of voice, thick skin, thick facial features, enlarged tongue, hair is brittle, thin, coarse and lacks lustre.

GIT Symptoms

- ↓ Appetite and food intake, constipation, BMR and caloric use ↓ → wt gain
- Amenorrhea is present, conception is difficult, stillbirths and abortion are common.

29. Negative feedback mechanism in hormonal regulation.

- Most of the control systems in the body are negative feedback regulations
- In negative feedback regulation, if a particular activity is increased or decreased, the control system initiates a chain of actions by which the activity returns back to normal

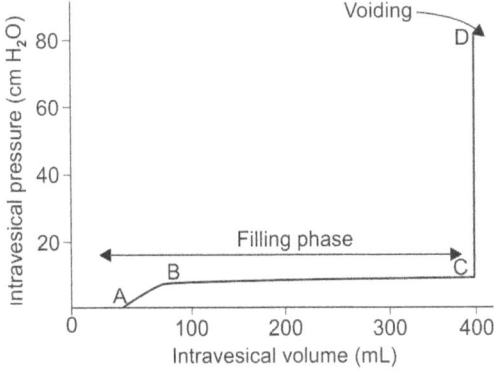

Fig. 22: Cystometrogram, Phases 1a (Mild increase in pressure when 100 mL of water is infused into bladder), Phase 1b (Not much rise in pressure from 100–400 mL intravesicle volume) and Phase II (Steep rise in pressure when intravesicular volume reaches 400 mL and stimulates micturition reflex).
(*Source:* GK Pal)

- So the control system has a sensor to sense the change, a control center that receives signals from the sensor and sends command to the effector which will bring about the change.

Examples:

Body temperature regulation, regulation of pH, regulation of blood glucose levels, regulation of thyroid hormone secretion.

Blood pressure regulation:

Increase in mean arterial pressure
↓
Sensed by baroreceptors
↓
Impulses are carried by IXth and Xth cranial nerves
↓
Inhibits vasomotor center and stimulates cardiac vagal center
↓
Decreases heart rate and stroke volume
↓
Decreases cardiac output
↓
Decreases mean arterial pressure

30. Female contraceptive methods.

Refer 2004 paper.

31. Pacemaker potential.

Refer answers to 2004 paper, short note 12.

32. Maximum breathing capacity (MBC).

- It is the maximum volume of air which can be breathed in and out of the lungs in one minute by maximum voluntary effort
- Normal value—90-170 L/min
- It needs the co-operation of the patient
- It can be recorded with a spirometer with writing pen or by using a Douglas bag.

MBC is dependent on:
- Respiratory muscle strength
- Compliance of the lung
- Airway resistance.

MBC is decreased in:
- Emphysema
- Airway obstruction
- Respiratory muscle weakness.

33. Parkinson's disease.

- Also called as Paralysis Agitans
- Due to destruction of Nigrostriatal Dopaminergic neurons (Fibers to Putamen is mostly affected) of basal ganglia.

Characterized by:
- Hyperkinetic features:
  - Rigidity: Lead-pipe or cogwheel
  - Tremors: Resting tremors, 6-8 Hz frequency.
- Hypokinesia
  - Weakness of movements and lack of initiation of movements—akinesia
  - Bradykinesia.
- Lack of automated movements
- Mask like face without expression
- Festinant or short shuffling gait.

34. Draw an ECG. Mention the cause of each wave.

Normal ECG in Lead II

- Lead II is a bipolar limb lead between right arm (negative electrode) and left arm (positive electrode)
- The ECG tracing in Lead II shows both negative and positive deflections equally and therefore used as a standard recording
- There are intervals and segments in the ECG.

ECG waves:

- There are positive and negative waves or deflections in the ECG tracing
- There are 4 waveforms—P wave, QRS complex, T wave and U wave
  1. *P wave:* This is the first positive wave in ECG and is due to atrial depolarisation. Duration is 0.1 second
  2. *QRS complex:* Consists of a negative Q wave, positive R wave and negative S wave. This complex is due to ventricular depolarisation. Normal duration is 0.08 seconds
  3. *T wave* is a positive deflection following QRS complex and is due to ventricular repolarisation. Normal duration is 0.27 seconds

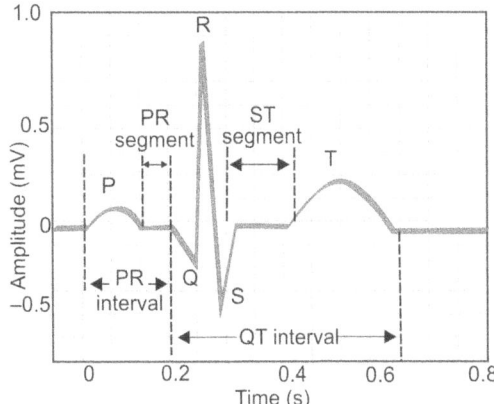

Fig. 23: Normal ECG in Lead II with waves, segements and intervals.
(*Source:* GK Pal)

4. ***U wave*** is also positive deflection and is normally not seen. It is seen in slow depolarisation of the papillary muscle. Duration is 0.08 seconds (Fig. 23).

ECG segments:
- These are isoelectric lines seen in between the ECG waves
- There are two segments – PR segment and ST segment
  1. ***PR segment:*** It starts at the end of P wave to beginning of QRS complex
  2. ***ST segment:*** It begins in the end of QRS complex and is upto the beginning of T wave.

ECG intervals:
- Intervals in ECG include waves and segments
- The intervals are: PR interval, QT interval, ST interval, PP interval and RR interval
- ***J point:*** This is an indicator of end of ventricular depolarisation and start of ventricular repolarisation. It is at the end of QRS and is at the isoelectric line
  1. ***PR interval:*** It is between beginning of P wave to beginning of Q wave
     - The normal duration is 0.12–0.2 Sec (Average 0.18 sec)
     - This denotes atrial depolarisation and conduction to AV node
     - Prolonged PR interval signifies AV conduction block
  2. ***QT interval:*** It starts at Q wave and ends with T wave
     - Normal duration is 0.4 seconds
     - It denotes the systolic phase of the ventricle
     - It is prolonged in ventricular conduction defects, hypocalcemia and myocardial ischemia.
  3. ***ST interval:*** It is from the end of S wave to the end of T wave
     - Normal duration is 0.32 seconds
     - It denotes ventricular repolarisation.
  4. ***PP interval:*** It is the interval between two successive P waves
     - It denotes the diastolic phase of the atria.
  5. ***RR interval:*** It is the interval between two successive R waves
     - It is used to calculate the heart rate.

35. Excitation-contraction coupling.
Refer 2003 paper.

36. Dark adaptation.
- When a person moves from a brightly illuminated place to a dark environment he is not able to see anything. But gradually the eyes get accommodated to the darkness and his vision improves. This is said to be Dark Adaptation (Fig. 24). Complete adaptation happens in 20 minutes
- The changes happening in the eye in darkness are: Dilatation of pupil, shifting of cone vision to rod vision and regenertaion of rhodopsin in darkness
- The changes happening are discussed under neural adaptation and chemical adaptation.

Neural Adaptation
- The dark adaptation happens in two phases
- The first phase is due to cone adaptation and it happens in the first 5-10 minutes
- This increases the retinal sensitivity to light 100 times

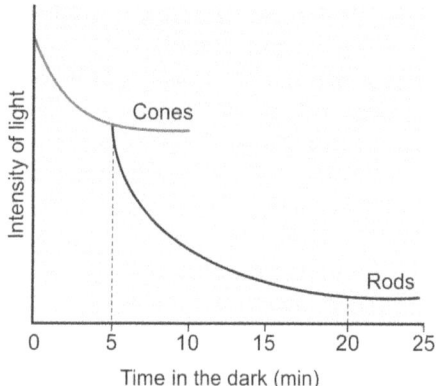

Fig. 24: Dark adaptation curve. There are two curves, red curve shows cone adaptation and violet curve shows rod adaptation.
(Source: GK Pal)

- In the second phase of adaptation the rod sensitivity to light increases and the retinal sensitivity increases by 1000-10,000 times
- Once rod adaptation has happened even a single photon of light is visible to the eye.

Chemical Adaptation

- When a person stays in bright light, the rod pigment rhodopsin is bleached and is converted to all-trans-retinal and opsin
- Therefore rods are insensitive to light and do not respond to light
- The rod sensitivity can increase only when the rhodopsin is re-synthesized and this takes several minutes to happen
- That is why the dark adaptation by rods takes 20 minutes
- The rods are present in the retina 15–20 degrees away from the fovea. That is the reason there is dilatation of the pupil to expose the retina rich in rods to light
- The time taken for dark adaptation depends on the degree of brightness of light to which the eye is exposed and for how long it is being exposed
- Brighter the light and longer the duration later it takes for dark adaptation.

37. Color vision.

- Color has 3 attributes—hue, intensity and saturation
- Each color has a complementary color and when it is mixed with it, produces white color
- Cones are the receptors for color vision
- There are 3 primary colors—red wavelength (723 - 647 nm), green (575 - 493 nm), blue (492 - 450 nm)
- Young-Helmholtz have postulated that there are 3 types of cones each responding to a particular wavelength of light
- They are maximally sensitive to each of the primary colors due to presence of 3 types of Photopigments and therefore 3 types of cones - S (Blue), L (Red) and M (Green) cones (Fig. 25)
- The L, M and S cones show maximal response to wavelengths of 560 nm, 530 nm and 420 nm respectively
- Different color sensations are perceived by determining the relative frequencies of impulses from each cone system
- The color perceived is also dependent on the level of illumination and also the background color
- Different shades of colors perceived also depend on the intensity of the color

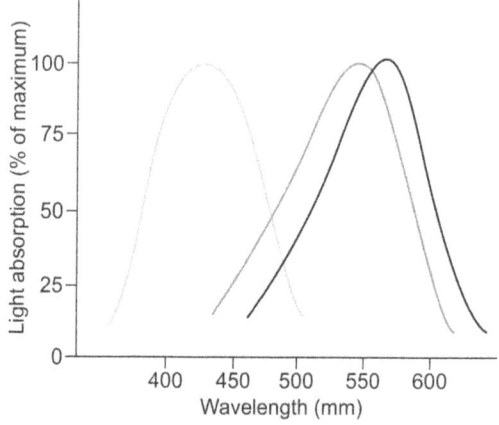

Fig. 25: Three cones and their sensitive wavelength.
(Source: GK Pal)

- Based on young-Helmholtz theory, for perceiving a colour atleast two cone types are needed
- The visual cortex compares the relative frequency of action potentials in the activated cone pathways and finds the wavelength and thereby identifies the color
- Change in intensity is appreciated by change in wavelength
- Color vision is a function of fovea as it has densely packed cones and this can get details of the object rather than discrimination of colors
- Gene for Rhodopsin is on chromosome 3 and gene for S cone pigment is on chromosome 7 and for green and red pigment it is on X chromosome.

Neural Mechanisms

- Color impulses are mediated by P type of Ganglion cells by subtracting input from one cone type to other
- From Lateral geniculate body (LGB) impulses travel to cortex in 3 pathways:
    1. A red-green pathway: Signals differences between L and M cones
    2. A blue-yellow pathway: Signals differences between S and sum of L and M cones
    3. Luminance pathway: Signals sum of L and M cones.
- They project to 4C layer and Blobs in layer 2 and 3 of Area 17 (V1) → then projects to V8
- **Color blindness** may be only for some colors – due to absence of one or more types of cones
- The suffix 'anopia' is used for color blindness
- The suffix 'anomaly' is used to denote color weakness
- The prefixes 'Prot, deuter, trit' are used to for 'red, green and blue' colors
- If only 2 cones are present and one cone is absent (**Dichromats**) – **Protanopia** (red blindness), **Deutranopia** (green color blindness) or **Tritanopia** (blue color blindness)
- **Trichromats**: Have all 3 cones, but one is weak
- **Monochromats** are individuals with only one cone system. They do not appreciate any colours. They see only black, white and shades of grey.

38. Basal ganglia.

Basal ganglia is a groups of nuclei in the forebrain and upper part of brainstem underlying the cortical mantle.

They are:
1. Caudate nucleus
2. Putamen
3. Globus pallidus
4. Subthalamic nucleus
5. Substantia nigra.

Caudate nucleus + Putamen: **Striatum**
Putamen + Globus pallidus: **Lenticular nucleus**
Globus pallidus: **Internal and external segments**
Substantia nigra: **Pars reticulata and pars compacta.**

Connections of Basal Ganglia

- **Afferents**: All afferents enter basal ganglia via striatum. They are from most of the cortex and thalamus. Also receives from Raphe magnus nucleus (RMN) and pedunculopontine region of brainstem:
    1. Corticostriate projections: Originate from many areas of cortex, premotor, Somatosensory area I (SSI) and supplementary motor cortex
    2. Thalamostriate fibers: Arise from centeromedian nucleus and end on striatum
    3. Rapestriatal projection: Serotonergic fibers from raphe nucleus in reticular formation (RF)
    4. Pedunculostriate projection: Arises from pedunculopontine nucleus of brainstem.
- **Efferent connections:**
    – Output from basal ganglia is through Internal segment (IS) of Globus pallidus

and Pars reticulata (PR) of Substantia nigra (SN)
- **From IS of GP:**
  1. Via thalamic fasciculus to ventrolateral (VL) and ventroanterior (VA) and centeromedian nuclei of thalamus → Prefrontal and premotor cortex
  2. Via ansa lenticularis fibers go to subthalamic nucleus, substantia nigra and red nucleus of midbrain and reticular formation of brainstem.
- **From PR of SN to:**
  1. VL and VA nuclei of thalamus
  2. To Pedunculopontine nucleus, Habenula and Superior colliculus
- Output from IS of GP to thalamus is inhibitory whereas from thalamus to cortex is excitatory
- Efferents to red nucleus → Rubrospinal tract.

Motor Loop

The connection between basal ganglia and cortex is forming a motor loop.

Various areas of cerebral cortex projects to striatum → Striatum projects to IS of globus pallidus → Thalamic nuclei → back to cortex.

Internuclear Connections

1. Dopaminergic Nigrostriatal system – From SN to striatum
2. GABA-ergic inhibitory projections
   a. Striatum to PR of Substantia nigra
   b. Striatum to IS and External segment (ES) of GP
   c. ES of GP to STN.
3. Excitatory Glutaminergic projections from STN:
   a. To IS and ES of GP
   b. To PR of SN.

Neural Pathways through Basal Ganglia: Direct and Indirect Pathways

Direct pathway in basal ganglia: Cerebral Cortex → Striatum (Caudate and Putamen) → internal segment (IS) of Globus Pallidus (GP) → Thalamus → Motor cortex.

Cortex excites striatum (Glutamate)
↓
Striatum inhibits IS of GP (GABA)
↓
IS of GP inhibits the inhibition of thalamus via thalamic fasciculus (goes to VA and VL nuclei of thalamus) (GABA)
↓
Impulses from thalamus to Prefrontal and premotor cortex and the final effect is disinhibition.

Indirect Pathway

Cortex → Striatum → ES of GP → STN → IS of GP → Thalamus → cortex

- Striatum inhibits ES of GP
- Inhibition by ES of GP on STN is removed
- STN activates IS of GP
- So stimulation of striatum activates IS of GP
- The final effect of this pathway is inhibition of thalamocortical fibers by the IS of GP
- Nigrostriatal projections have important effects on both pathways
- Dopaminergic connections of PC to striatum has an excitatory effect on direct pathway and inhibitory effect on indirect pathway
- In health there is a balance between the two pathways
- Alteration of either of them results in imbalance in motor output
- So BG disorders may have both hypo and hyperkinetic movement disorders.

Functions of Basal Ganglia

1. Basal ganglia is involved in planning and programming of voluntary movement. The neurons of basal ganglia fire impulses even before the movement starts. Caudate loop is involved in planning of movements (direct pathway through caudate nucleus)
2. Controls muscle tone through inhibition of motor cortex and inhibitory medullary RF. The pathway involved is cortex –

striatum – GP – SN – Medullary RF – Spinal cord via reticulospinal tract. In lesion of BG there is hypertonia
3. Controls the limb movements. In diseases of BG unpurposeful limb movements appear
4. Controls automated associative limb movements like swinging of arms while walking. Putamen circuit (direct pathway through putamen nucleus) is involved in control of subconscious movements
5. Timing the movements is also a role of BG
6. BG exerts an inhibitory effect on spinal reflexes which help to regulate posture
7. Somatic movements associated with emotions are controlled by BG
8. Provides muscle tone for skilled movements
9. Functions in motivated behavior
10. Caudate nucleus plays a role in cognition because of its connections with associative cortex. Lesion leads to deficits of performance based learning
11. Because of its connections with RF, GP has a role in arousal mechanism
12. Lesion of head of left caudate nucleus leads to dysarthric aphasia.

Disorders of Basal Ganglia

BG disorders are associated with movement disorders like:
- Hyperkinetic movements
  - Rigidity
  - Chorea
  - Athetosis
  - Ballismus
  - Rest tremors.
- Hypokinetic movements
  - Akinesia
  - Bradykinesia.

Parkinson's Disease

- Also called as Paralysis Agitans
- Due to destruction of Nigrostriatal Dopaminergic neurons, to Putamen is mostly affected
- Causes:
  - Primary or idiopathic
  - Complication of drugs: Phenothiazines.
- Characterized by:
  - Hyperkinetic features:
    - Rigidity: Lead pipe or cogwheel
    - Tremors: Resting tremors, at 6–8 Hz frequency.
  - Hypokinesia
    - Weakness of movements and lack of initiation of movements: Akinesia
    - Bradykinesia.
  - Lack of automated movements
  - Mask like face without expression
  - Festinant or short shuffling gait: Patient walks in an attitude like he is going to catch the center of gravity.
- Treatment:
  - Treatment with L-Dopa rather than Dopamine as it cannot cross the Blood brain barrier.
  - Bromocryptine, a dopamine agonist can also be used
  - Anticholinergics like atropine, tries to reduce the acetylcholine levels in basal ganglia and regulates the ratio between dopamine and acetylcholine
  - L-deprenyl
  - Dopamine agonists like bromocryptine
  - Transplantation of adrenal medulla in BG
  - Implantation of fetal BG.

Chorea

- Due to disease of the caudate nucleus
- Characterized by rapid, irregular, involuntary movements of short duration
- Seen in Huntington's disease, rheumatic fever in children.

Athetosis

- Due to lesion in Lenticular nucleus
- Characterized by continuous, slow, twisting movements. Movements are worm like writhing movements of extremities like the fingers and wrist.

Hemiballism

- It is due to damage to Subthalamic nucleus, due to hemorrhage in it
- Characterized by spontaneous attacks of uncoordinated movements affecting whole of opposite side of body.

Huntington's Disease

- Genetic disorder inherited as an autosomal dominant disease
- There is damage to GABAergic and cholinergic neurons of striatum
- Loss of GABAergic neurons leads to hyperkinetic movements
- Early sign is a jerky trajectory of the hand when reaching to touch a spot especially towards the end of the target
- Later hyperkinetic choreiform movements appear and may later incapacitate the patient
- Speech becomes slurred and incomprehensible and later dementia sets in and death happens in 10-15 years
- There is no effective treatment.

Wilson's Disease

- Also called as hepatolenticular degeneration
- It is due to accumulation of copper in brain and liver
- Cirrhosis of liver is seen
- In brain the damage is more in lenticular nucleus especially putamen and symptoms of Parkinsonism is seen.

Kernicterus

Damage to GP following deposition of unconjugated bilirubin.

It is usually seen in hemolytic disease of newborn.

Symptoms are—rigidity, chorea, athetosis, mental defeciency and may lead to death.

39. Endorphins.

- Presence of opioid receptors in the body has led to the search for endogenous opioids. These are endogenous opioids and and their precursors have been identified in the body
- There are precursors for opioids identified, which form opioid peptides.

The first one to be recognised is Enkephalins:

- Met-enkaphalin and Leu-enkephalin
- They are found in the nerve endings of GIT and in brain. They are also present in substantia gelatinosa of spinal cord where gating of pain happens
- It is also present in the brain stem
- They bind to the δ and μ opioid receptors.

β-endorphin

- It is an opioid peptide and is a part of Proopiomelanocortin produced from the anterior and intermediate lobe of pituitary gland
- It has 31 amino acid residues
- It is present in the brain and the blood coming from the pituitary gland.

The next precursor is Prodynorphin,

- It contains **Dynorphins** and α and β **Neoendorphins**
- Dynorphins are present in the duodenum, posterior pituitary and hypothalamus
- **Neoendorphins** are also present in the hypothalamus
- Endorphins bind only to μ receptors whereas other opioids bind to various receptors.

Effect of Stimulation of the Following Opioid Receptors

μ **receptor:** They get activated on binding to opioids and results in activation of second messengers. This leads to K^+ conductance and thereby hyperpolarises the neurons.

Effects on stimulation are: Analgesia, Respiratory depression, constipation, euphoria, sedation, increased secretion of growth hormone and prolactin and miosis.

κ **receptor:** Is bound by dynorphins. Activation of these receptors results in closure of Ca^{2+} channels.

Effect of stimulation: Analgesia, diuresis, sedation, miosis and dysphoria.

δ **receptor:** Bound by all the above types of opioids. Activation of these receptors results in closure of Ca^{2+} channels.

Effect of stimulation: Analgesia.

MBBS Examination 2006

ANSWER ALL QUESTIONS

I. Essay Questions (15/20 Marks each)

1. Describe stages of erythropoiesis and factors controlling it. (15 marks)
2. Describe steps of synthesis, regulation and functions of cortisol. (15 marks)
3. Define blood pressure. Give normal value. Describe regulation of blood pressure. (15 marks)
4. Describe connections and functions of cerebellum. (15 marks)
5. Enumerate the hormones of adrenal cortex. Describe the functions and regulations of glucocorticoids. Add a note on Cushing's syndrome. (20 marks)
6. Describe the composition, function and regulation of secretion of pancreatic juice. (15 marks)
7. Write an essay on immunity. (15 marks)
8. Define cardiac cycle. Describe the pressure and volume changes in the left ventricle during the cardiac cycle with a suitable graph. (20 marks)
9. Name all the descending tracts. Describe the corticospinal tract and mention the diffrences between UMN and LMN lesions. (15 marks)
10. Discuss the mechanics of pulmonary ventilation. (15 marks)

II. Short Notes   (5 Marks each)

1. Ultrastructure of skeletal muscle.
2. Deglutition.
3. Give composition and functions of gastric juice.
4. Erythroblastosis fetalis.
5. Describe nerve supply to urinary bladder and micturition.
6. Thrombocyte.
7. Ovarian cycle.
8. Describe the hormones acting on the breast.
9. Describe functions of skin.
10. Thyrotoxicosis.
11. Spirogram.
12. Dysbarism.
13. Hypoxia.
14. Heart sounds.
15. Triple response.
16. Berger's rhythm.
17. Decerebrate rigidity.
18. Errors of refraction.
19. Aqueous humor.
20. Cochlear microphonic potential.
21. Fate of hemoglobin after hemolysis.
22. Movements of small intestine.
23. Steps involved in formation of urine.
24. Spermatogenesis.
25. Neuroendocrinal reflex.
26. Adrenogenital syndrome.
27. Conducting system of the heart.
28. Referred pain and its theories.
29. EEG changes during sleep.
30. Excitation-contraction coupling in skeletal muscles.
31. Classification of sensory receptors and their properties.
32. Clinical classification of reflexes with examples and their significance.

I. ESSAY QUESTIONS

1. Describe stages of erythropoiesis and factors controlling it.

- Erythropoesis is production of RBCs. Life span of RBCs are 120 days

- Hence continuous destruction and production of RBCs take place at a constant rate.

Site of Erythropoiesis

a. **Mesoblastic stage:** In the embryonal stage RBC production is from yolk sac
b. **Hepatic stage:** Later in the fetal stage upto 5 months RBCs are produced in liver, spleen, thymus and lymph nodes
c. **Myeloid stage:** 3 months before birth—produced in red bone marrow of all bones
d. **Adult life:** Red bone marrow of flat bones and epiphysis of long bones are the site of erythropoiesis.

Changes during Maturation

- Gradual reduction in cell size
- Cytoplasm increases in amount
- Cytoplasm changes from basophilic to polychromatophilic to acidophilic due to gradual appearance of hemoglobin
- Nucleus and nucleoli decreases in size and are extruded.

Stages of Erythropoiesis

The stages of development and maturation of RBCs are - Pluripotent stem cell, Myeloid stem cell, Colony forming unit - E (CFU-E), Blast forming unit (BFU-E), Proerythroblast or Pronormoblast, Early normoblast, intermediate normoblast, late normoblast, reticulocyte and mature RBC.

CFU-E & BFU-E are progenitor cells of erythroid series and they give rise to the precursor cell for RBC, the Pronormoblast.

a. **Pronormoblast:**
- Large cell, diameter—20–25 μm
- Cytoplasm is less and is basophilic
- Large nucleus with multiple nucleoli
- Hemoglobin is not formed
- Mitosis is present.

b. **Early normoblast:**
- Diameter of cell is 15–18 μm
- Cytoplasm is increased in amount and is basophilic
- Nucleus with nucleoli occupies 3/4th of cell
- Open chromatin is present
- Mitosis is present.

c. **Intermediate normoblast:**
- Cytoplasm volume increases and is polychromatophilic due to appearance of hemoglobin
- Nucleus decreases in size
- Nucleoli is absent
- Mitosis is still present.

d. **Late normoblast:**
- Cell is smaller in size and is 8–10 μm
- Cytoplasm is markedly increased and presence of hemoglobin has made it orthochromatophilic.
- Hemoglobin content increases
- Nucleus is very small and cartwheel appearance of chromatin is seen
- Mitosis stops here.

e. **Reticulocyte:**
- Cell size is 7.8 μm
- Nucleus is extruded
- Hemoglobin is present
- Chromatin reticulum is seen.

f. **Mature RBC:**
- Cell size is 7.5 μm
- RBC is biconcave in shape
- Chromatin reticulum disappears.

The whole process of maturation from pronormoblast to reticulocyte takes 7 days. It takes 2 days for reticulocyte to mature as an RBC (refer Fig. 1).

Regulation of Erythropoiesis

There are general and special factors regulating erythropoiesis.

General Factor – Hypoxia

- Major function of RBC is to carry oxygen to the tissues
- So when there is decrease in tissue oxygen levels, it induces production of RBCs
- Hypoxia stimulates the interstitial cells of the kidneys to synthesize the hormone Erythropoietin
- It acts on bone marrow to stimulate the erythropoietin sensitive stem cells to

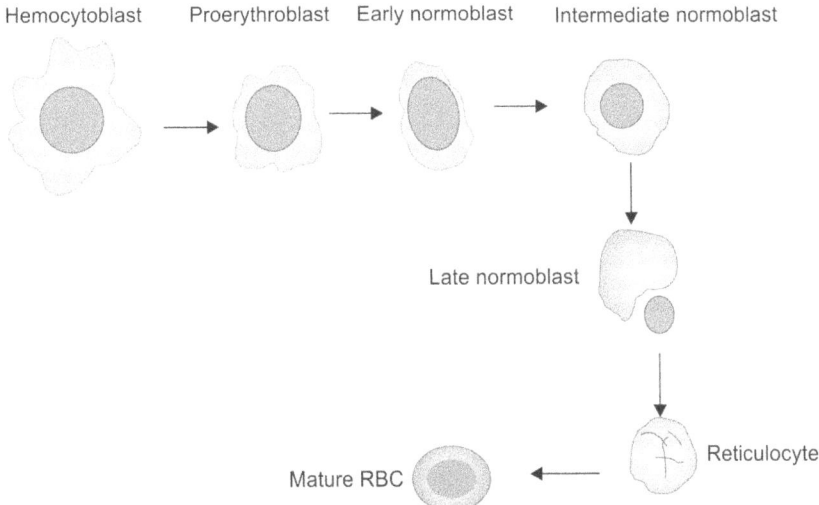

Fig. 1: Stages of erythropoiesis.

become proerythroblasts and thereby stimulates formation of RBCs
- It also increases the release of reticulocytes from the bone marrow
- It increases all aspects of hemoglobin synthesis.

Factors Increasing Erythropoietin Production

- Hypoxia
- Catecholamines
- Thyroxine
- Testosterone
- Catecholamines
- ACTH
- Prolactin
- cAMP, NAD.

Special Maturation Factors

Dietary factors:

- Proteins help in globin formation
- Iron helps in heme formation
- Copper, cobalt and nickel also helps in heme formation
- Calcium helps in absorption of iron from GIT
- Vitamin C also helps in iron absorption
- Vitamin B12 and folic acid helps in synthesis of nucleic acids and final maturation of RBC
- Intrinsic factor synthesized in the stomach by the parietal cells help in absorption of Vitamin B12.

2. **Describe steps of synthesis, regulation and functions of cortisol.**

Synthesis of Glucocorticoids

- Cortisol is produced in zona fasiculata and zona reticularis layers of adrenal cortex, due to the presence of the enzyme 17-α hydroxylase
- Steroidogenesis in zona fasiculata and zona reticularis is regulated by adrenocorticotropic hormone (ACTH)
- **Cholesterol** is the precursor for synthesis of all adrenocortical steroid hormones
- Cholesterol for synthesis is got from either the circulation (80%) or formed in the cells from acetate (20%)
- LDL receptors are present on the cell membrane
- On binding of low-density lipoprotein (LDL) with receptor the complex is internalized and cholesterol is esterified and stored
- On stimulation, esterified cholesterol is hydrolyzed and free cholesterol transferred to mitochondria
- Cholesterol is transported across outer mitochondrial membrane to inner membrane
- Cholesterol is converted to pregnenolone. The reaction is catalyzed by cholesterol

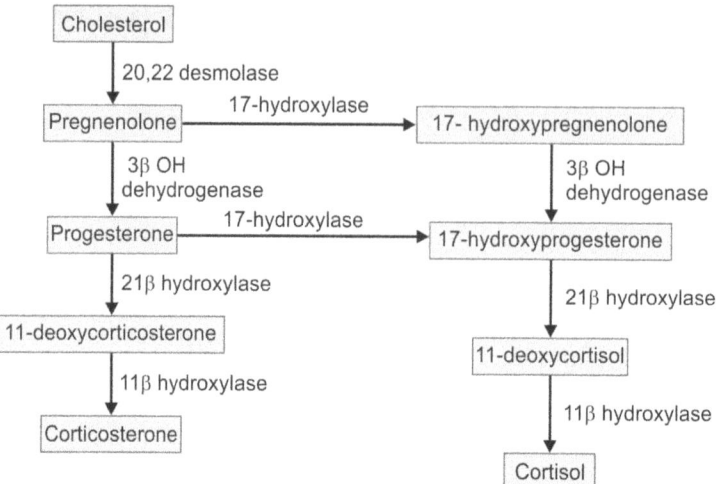

Fig. 2: Synthesis of glucocorticoids.

side-chain cleavage (SCC) enzyme, also called 20, 22-desmolase (refer Fig. 2)
- Pregnenolone is converted to 11-deoxycortisol by successive steps in endoplasmic reticulum
- 11-deoxycortisol is transferred back to mitochondria (MC) and hydroxylated at 11th position to form cortisol
- Cortisol once formed, rapidly diffuses out of the cell.

Regulation of Secretion of Glucocorticoids
- Secretion of cortisol is regulated by ACTH from anterior pituitary (refer Fig. 3)
- ACTH secretion in turn is stimulated by corticotropin-releasing hormone (CRH) from hypothalamus
- Free cortisol levels negatively inhibit secretion of ACTH and CRH
- All types of stress stimulates hypothalamus → ↑ CRH → ↑ ACTH → ↑ cortisol
- Circadian rhythm alters ACTH secretion and also affects cortisol secretion.

Functions of Glucocorticoids
Refer answers in August 2004 paper.

3. Define blood pressure. Give normal value. Describe regulation of blood pressure.

Refer answers to 2003 paper (Definition, normal value, regulation by baroreceptors).

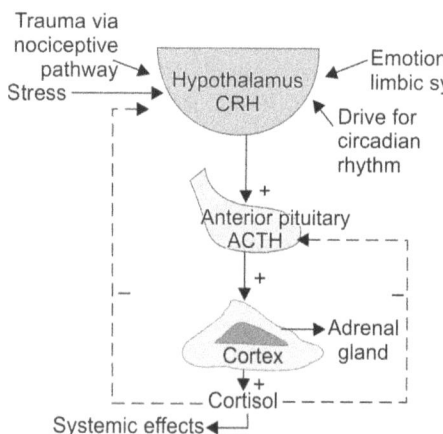

Fig. 3: Regulation of glucocorticoids.

b. Chemoreceptor reflex
- Chemoreceptors are located in the carotid and aortic bodies
- They sense the change in PO_2, pH and PCO_2 in arterial blood and stimulate respiration
- They are supplied by IX and X cranial nerves
- They usually project to respiratory centers and also to cardiovascular centers in medulla
- They also send inputs to VMC and CVC and regulate BP
- They are active within a range of 40–100 mm Hg mean arterial pressure (MAP).

Decrease in MAP (40–100 mmHg)
↓
Decreased blood flow to chemoreceptors
↓
Stimulation of chemoreceptors
↓
Impulses carried through IXth and Xth cranial nerves to medulla

Respiratory center	VMC	Cardiac vagal center (CVC)
↓	↓	↓
Hyperventilation, Tachycardia (TC)	Vasoconstriction, TC, Release of catecholamines	Bradycardia (BC)

- **The net effect is mild tachycardia and vasoconstriction → increase in BP.**

c. CNS ischemic response

- It is activated when MAP falls below 40 mm Hg. It is said to be the "last ditch stand", the last effort put up by the body to try to correct the fall in BP.

Severe hypotension
↓
Decreased cerebral blood flow
↓
Hypoxia and hypercapnia at VMC
↓
Strong stimulation of VMC
↓
Intense vasoconstriction
↓
↑BP

Intermediate Regulation of BP

- They come into play after several minutes and reach full effect in few hours
- They act for few days
- They alter the blood volume and try to correct BP
- **They are:**
  1. **Capillary fluid shift mechanism:** Capillary hydrostatic pressure is dependent on arterial blood pressure and therefore when BP increases the capillary hydrostatic pressure increases and there is filtration of fluid into the interstitium resulting in decrease in ECF volume and thereby the decrease in BP. It is more effective than short term regulatory mechanisms but it takes longer time to bring BP back to normal
  2. **Stress-relaxation mechanism:** When there is increase in ECF volume as in IV infusion of fluids, the blood flow to visceral organs like spleen, liver and lungs increase, resulting in relaxation of blood vessels of the viscera by local mechanisms and blood is pooled here. The blood volume decreases and BP decreases
  3. **Reverse stress relaxation mechanism:** It is the opposite of stress-relaxation process. In conditions of fall in BP, the vessels in the visceral organs tighten and push the stored blood back into circulation. By this ECF volume and BP increase.

Long-term Regulation of BP

- These mechanisms are slow to begin and last for a longer duration. It continues for years to months
- They bring the BP back to normal. It is done by the kidneys.

It is by 2 mechanisms:

a. Direct mechanism:

- Kidneys directly control the blood volume and thereby regulate the BP
- Also called as the renal fluid mechanism or ECF volume mechanism

Decrease in BP
↓
↓ Blood flow to kidneys
↓
↓ GFR
↓
Reabsorption of water and electrolyte is increased

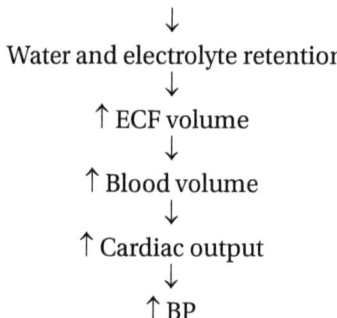

↓
Water and electrolyte retention
↓
↑ ECF volume
↓
↑ Blood volume
↓
↑ Cardiac output
↓
↑ BP

b. **Indirect mechanism:**
- Here hormones are secreted which in turn acts through the kidneys to regulate BP
- It is by the Renin-Angiotensin-Aldosterone mechanism.

Decreased Blood pressure
↓
Renal ischemia
↓
Renin is secreted from JG cells
↓
Angiotensinogen → Angiotensin I
↓ ACE
Angiotensin II
↓

- Increases reabsorption of water and electrolytes from PCT
- Induces potent vasoconstriction
- Stimulates adrenal cortex to secrete aldosterone.

Aldosterone

- It acts on the DCT and collecting duct to increase water and salt reabsorption
- Thereby increases ECF volume and increases BP.

4. Describe connections and functions of cerebellum.

Anatomically each hemisphere of cerebellum is divided into 3 lobes by two transverse furrows—anterior lobe, posterior lobe and flocculonodular lobes.

Functional Divisions

- The main functions of cerebellum are to maintain posture and balance and coordinate voluntary movements

- Based on the functions it is divided into three parts (refer Fig. 4):
  1. **Vestibulocerebellum:** Made up of the Flocculonodular lobe
  2. **Spinocerebellum:** Consists of vermis and the intermediate part of the cerebellar hemispheres (paravermal portion)
  3. **Neocerebellum:** Consists of the lateral parts of the hemispheres.

Connections and Functions of Cerebellum

- Connections include the afferents and efferents to cerebellum which enter cerebellum and leave, through the cerebellar peduncles
- There are 3 cerebellar peduncles: Superior, inferior and middle cerebellar peduncles.

Afferent Connections

The afferents to cerebellum come through the Climbing fibers and Mossy fibers.

Climbing fibers:
- They contain the olivocerebellar tract which arises from the inferior olivary nucleus in medulla
- The olivary nucleus in turn receives proprioceptive inputs from all over the body
- The climbing fibers end on the dendrites of Purkinje cells and they make one-to-one connection with the Purkinje cells and excite them (refer Fig. 5)
- Collaterals from climbing fibers also excite the golgi cells and the deep nuclei of cerebellum
- Climbing fibers enter the cerebellum through the inferior cerebellar peduncle. This peduncle brings in most of the other afferent fibers to cerebellum.

Mossy fibers:
- Mossy fibers include all the other afferents entering the cerebellum other than Olivocerebellar tract
- It includes – Dorsal and ventral spinocerebellar tracts, vestibulocerebellar tract, reticulocerebellar tract, cuneocerebellar tract, tectocerebellar tract, rubrocerebellar tract and pontocerebellar tract

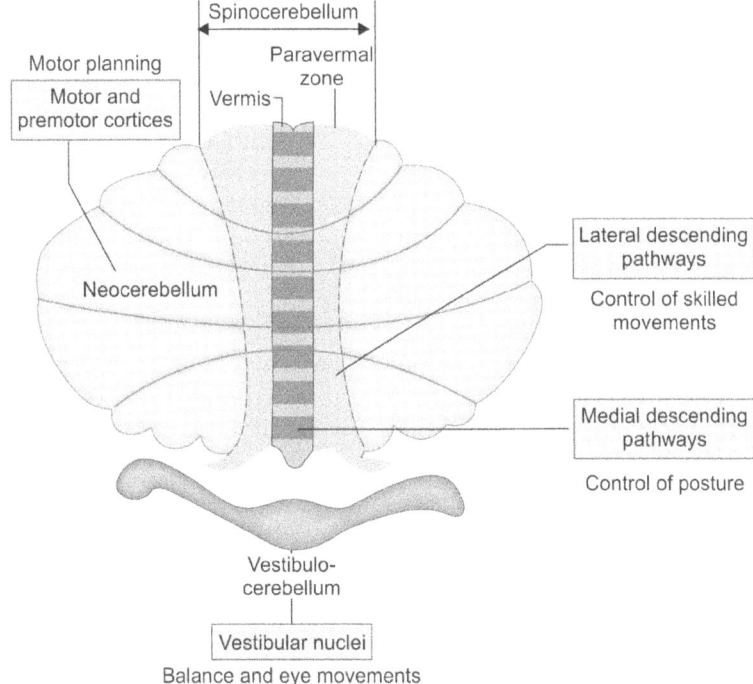

Fig. 4: Functional divisions of cerebellum with their connections and functions.
(*Source:* GK Pal)

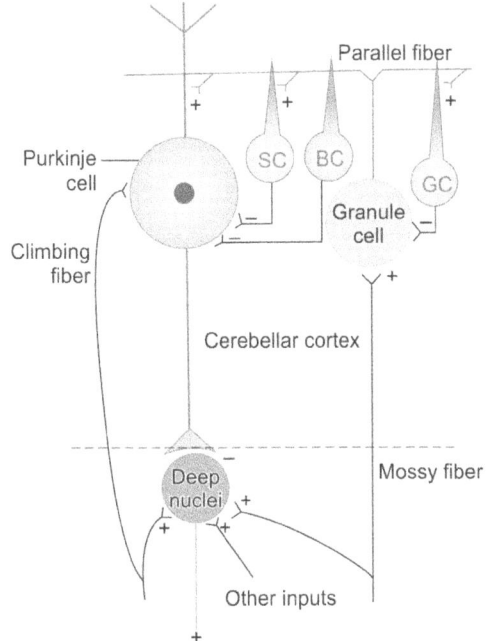

Fig. 5: Afferents to cerebellum through Climbing and Mossy fibers.
(SC: Stellate cells; BC: Basket cells; GC: Golgi cells; (–): Inhibition; (+): Stimulation)
(*Source:* GK Pal)

a. *Dorsal spinocerebellar tract:* It carries unconscious proprioceptive inputs and exteroceptive inputs from limbs and trunk of same side and they enter cerebellum through ipsilateral inferior cerebellar peduncle. It ends on the spinocerebellum

b. *Ventral spinocerebellar tract:* It carries cutaneous and proprioceptive inputs from opposite side of the lower limbs and enters cerebellum through ipsilateral superior cerebellar peduncle and they are distributed to the hind limb area of spinocerebellum

c. *Vestibulocerebellar tract:* It carries impulses from the same side vestibular nucleus about information regarding the position of head in relation to body posture. It enters the cerebellum through ipsilateral inferior cerebellar peduncle. It ends in the flocculo-nodular lobe (Vestibulocerebellum)

d. *Reticulocerebellar tract:* It arises from the lateral reticular nucleus and enters through inferior cerebellar peduncle and is distributed to all areas of cerebellar cortex

e. *Cuneocerebellar tract:* It arises from external arcuate nucleus and carries proprioceptive information from head, neck, upper limb and upper part of the body. It enters through ipsilateral inferior cerebellar peduncle and distributed to spinocerebellum

f. *Tectocerebellar tract:* It carries visual and auditory information from superior and inferior colliculi. It enters through superior cerebellar peduncle

g. *Rubrocerebellar tract:* It arises from the red nucleus. It contains information from cerebral cortex. It has both crossed and uncrossed fibers. It enters through superior cerebellar peduncle and ends on dentate nucleus (one of the deep nuclei of cerebellum)

h. *Pontocerebellar tract:* These are fibers arising from motor area of cerebral cortex and end on pontine nuclei. From here they arise to form the pontocerebellar fibers. They cross to opposite side and enter through the opposite middle cerebellar peduncle and are distributed to all areas of cerebellar cortex.

Efferent Connections

- All the efferents from cerebellar cortex are through the Purkinje fiber output which ends on the deep cerebellar nuclei. Purkinje cell output is inhibitory in nature
- The deep nuclei are: Dentate, Emboliform, Fastigial and Globose. Emboliform and globose are together called as Nucleus interpositus (refer Fig. 6)

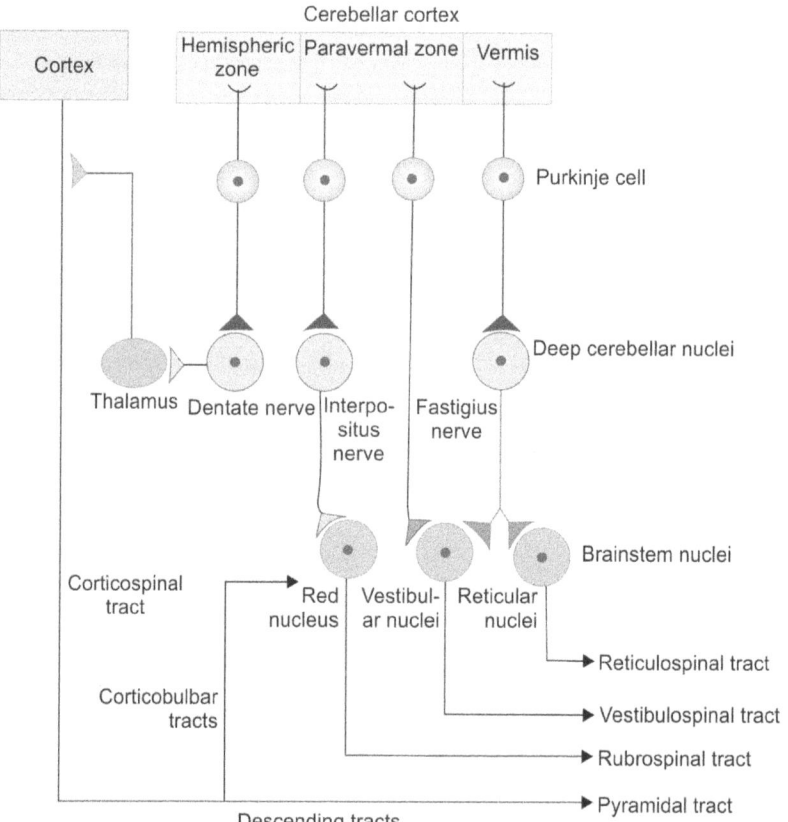

Fig. 6: Efferent connections from cerebellum through deep nuclei to brainstem. They are vestibulospinal tract, reticulospinal tract, rubrospinal tract. Through thalamic connections controls corticospinal tract.
(*Source:* GK Pal)

- The deep nuclei also receive collaterals from climbing and mossy fibers and both are excitatory in nature
- The net effect of output from deep nuclei is excitatory to brain stem and thalamus
- All parts of cerebellum, except the vestibulocerebellum exit the cerebellum through deep nuclei
  a. **Cerebellovestibular pathway-Vestibulospinal tract:** It leaves the vestibulocerebellum and projects to the vestibular nuclei directly. It controls the activity of vestibulospinal tract
  b. **Cerebelloreticular pathway-Reticulospinal tract:** The vermal portion of spinocerebellum projects to pontine reticular formation through fastigial nucleus. From here the reticulospinal tract arises and through this tract cerebellum controls the anterior horn cells
  c. **Paravermal portion** of spinocerebellum project to nucleus interpositus and this in turn projects to the red nucleus. Thereby cerebellum controls the rubrospinal tract
  d. **Dentatothalamo-cortical pathway:** Impulses from cerebrocerebellum end on dentate nucleus and from here it goes through thalamus and reaches motor cortex. From motor cortex corticospinal tract arises and ends on alpha motor neurons. Through this pathway cerebellum fine tunes the activity of corticospinal tract.

Functions of Cerebellum

a. **Control of posture and equilibrium:**
   - Vestibulocerebellum or the flocculonodular lobe controls posture and equilibrium
   - It receives inputs from vestibular apparatus directly and also through vestibular nuclei about position of head and body
   - It sends efferents to vestibular nuclei from which the vestibulospinal tract arises to regulate posture
   - Vestibulocerebellum is also concerned with regulating vestibulo-ocular reflex.

b. **Control of muscle tone and stretch reflex:**
   - Spinocerebellum influences the muscle tone through its output via fastigial nucleus which in turn controls the vestibulospinal and reticulospinal tract (arisisng from pontine reticular formation)
   - The major influence of cerebellum on tone is facilitatory
   - Vestibulospinal tract is facilitatory to α motor neurons and reticulospinal tract is facilitatory to γ motor neurons
   - Since control of cerebellum is on both α and γ motor neurons it has an important role in α-γ linkage.

c. **Control of voluntary movements:**
   - Paravermal portion of spinocerebellum controls skilled voluntary movements
   - It does not initiate movements but it coordinates voluntary movements
   - Coordination of movements is by regulating the time, rate, range, force and direction of movements

All three functional divisions of the cerebellum work together as "comparator of servo mechanism".

Comparator servo mechanism:
- Impulses for voluntary movements are planned and programmed in the premotor cortex and it is sequenced in primary motor area and the command to skeletal muscles is sent through the corticospinal tract
- A copy of the plan or intended movement is also sent to the spinocerebellum
- Cerebellum also gets feedback from the proprioceptors about the actual movement performed by the muscles and joints
- It also receives other sensory inputs from eye, ear and vestibular apparatus
- Now the cerebellum compares the intended movement and the executed movement along with other sensory inputs mentioned above
- It thereby modifies appropriately the ongoing movement

- If any corrections have to be done in programming of movements the error signals are sent to the motor cortex.
d. **Control of body movements of one side:**
   - Motor cortex of one side is connected to opposite cerebellum through a closed feedback loop; Cerebral-cerebellar-cerebral circuit, the cortico-ponto-dentato-thalamo-cortical pathway
   - So each cerebellar hemisphere controls the opposite cerebral cortex
   - But the corticospinal tract descending down from the motor cortex decussates in medulla and controls the opposite side of the body
   - Since there is double decussation it is that cerebellum controls same side of the body.
e. **Planning and programming of movements:** Cerebrocerebellum has extensive connections with motor cortex and therefore is involved in planning and programming of movements.
f. **Learning of skills:**
   - Cerebellum always tends to make changes in ongoing movements and therefore it improves by learning
   - Another eveidence is that there are increased activities in the climbing fibers when a new skill is learnt
   - So cerebellum has a great role in learning skills.
g. **Eyeball movement:** Pyramis of cerebellum is concerned with eyeball movement.

---

5. **Enumerate the hormones of adrenal cortex. Describe the functions and regulations of glucocorticoids. Add a note on Cushing's syndrome.**

Hormones secreted from adrenal cortex are:
- Mineralocorticoids: C_{21} Steroids (secreted by zona glomerulosa)
  - Aldosterone
  - Deoxycorticosterone.
- Glucocorticoids: C_{21} Steroids (secreted by zona fasiculata and zona reticularis)
  - Cortisol
  - Cortisone
  - Corticosterone.
- Adrenal androgens: C_{19} steroids (secreted by zona reticularis and zona fasiculata)
  - Dehydroepiandrosterone
  - Androstenedione.

Functions and Regulation of Glucocorticoids
Refer above in same paper.

Cushing's Syndrome
It is due to hypersecretion of glucocorticoids.

Causes
- Pharmacological use of exogenous glucocorticoids: ACTH levels are low here
- ACTH secreting pituitary tumor - Cushing's disease: ACTH levels are high, skin pigmentation present (because of MSH like activity of ACTH)
- Primary hypercortisolism due to adrenal tumor: ACTH levels are low.

Symptoms
- Obesity with characteristic centripetal distribution of fat, sparing the limbs
- Face is rounded and cheeks red due to polycythemia
- Loss of bone mass → osteoporosis → vertebral fractures and necrosis of hip
- Loss of connective tissue integrity → fragile capillaries, easy bruisability and purple striae in abdomen
- Increased protein catabolism → atrophy and weakness of skeletal muscles
- Poor wound healing and response to infection due to loss of protein
- Disturbances in glucose metabolism - Blood glucose levels are high resulting in glucose intolerance, insulin resistance, hyperglycemia or even diabetes mellitus
- Mineralocorticoid activity of glucocorticoids leads to Na^+ and H_2O retention → Hypertension
- Excess androgen secretion in women → hirsuitism, male pattern baldness, clitorial enlargement.

Diagnosis
- Elevated plasma cortisol or urinary free cortisol levels
- Loss of diurnal pattern of secretion of cortisol

- Loss of suppressive effect of exogenous dexamethasone.

6. **Describe the composition, function and regulation of secretion of pancreatic juice.**

Composition of Pancreatic Juice

- Rate of secretion—1200-1500 mL/day
- Specific gravity—1.010-1.018
- pH—7.8-8.4, due to high concentration of HCO_3^-
- 99.5% is water and 0.5% solids
- *Organic constituents:* Contains enzymes like amylase, lipase, protease, trypsin inhibitor and traces of albumin and globulin
- *Inorganic constituents:*
  - Cations like—Na^+, K^+, Ca^{++}, Mg^{++} and Zn^{2+}
  - Anions like—HCO_3^-, Cl^-, SO_4^{2-} and HPO_4^{2-}.

Functions of Pancreatic Juice

Digestive Function of Pancreatic Juice

a. **Digestion of lipids:**
   - Pancreatic lipase is the major fat digesting enzyme: It digests triglycerides into monoglycerides and fatty acids
   - Colipase: It exposes active sites of pancreatic lipase and facilitates its action
   - Phospholipase A_2: It acts on Phospholipids and converts it to fatty acids and lysophospholipids
   - Cholesterol ester hydrolase acts on cholesterol esters and splits it into cholesterol and fatty acids.

b. **Digestion of proteins:**
   - Proteolytic enzymes are secreted in the inactive forms: Trypsinogen, chymotrypsinogen, proelastase and procarboxypeptidase A and B
   - Trypsinogen on secretion into duodenum is activated to trypsin by the enzyme enterokinase in the intestine
   - Trypsinogen → Trypsin, happens in presence of enterokinase
   - Chymotrypsinogen → Chymotrypsin, in presence of trypsin
   - Proelastase and procarboxylase → Elastase and carboxylase, in presence of Trypsin
   - *Trypsin and chymorypsin* act on proteins and polypeptides and cleaves the peptide bonds in basic and aromatic amino acids
   - *Elastase* acts on elastin and some other proteins
   - *Carboxypeptidases* also act on proteins and polypeptides
   - *Nucleases* split ribose and deoxyribose nucleotides
   - *Collagenase* digests collagen.

c. **Digestion of carbohydrates:** *Pancreatic α amylase:* It is secreted in active form and just like salivary amylase it hydrolyzes glycogen, starch and other complex carbohydrates to form disaccharides

d. **Trypsin inhibitor** secreted from pancreas inhibits activation of trypsinogen and thereby prevents autodigestion of pancrease by trypsin.
   Trypsin if activated initiates a chain of reaction and activates other proteolytic enzymes and can digest the pancreas.

Regulation of Intestinal pH

- Pancreatic juice is rich in HCO_3^- and therefore alkaline in nature
- HCO_3^- is secreted by the ductal cells
- The alkalinity created by HCO_3^- neutralizes the HCl derived from gastric juice as it enters the intestine.

Regulation of Pancreatic Secretion

- Pancreatic secretion is regulated by neural and humoral mechanisms
- Neural regulation is by vagal efferents supplying exocrine pancreas
- Hormonal regulation is by the hormones—secretin, cholecystokinin (CCK), gastrin and somatostatin
- Regulation is discussed under the headings—cephalic phase, gastric phase and intestinal phase.

Regulation in Cephalic Phase

- This phase is under the reflex vagal stimulation
- Regulation of this phase starts even before the food enters stomach

- It happens by unconditioned reflex (presence of food in mouth and actions of mastication and swallowing) and conditioned reflexes (by sight, smell and thought of food).

Regulation in Gastric Phase
- This phase starts when food enters the stomach
- It is stimulated by distension of stomach
- It is under the influence of vagus stimulation and by the hormone gastrin.

Regulation in Intestinal Phase
- This phase starts when the food enters duodenum and jejunum
- It stimulates secretion of pancreatic juice rich in bicarbonate
- It is under the control of intestinal hormones – Secretin and CCK.

Role of secretin:
- Secretin is secreted by the 'S' cells of duodenum and jejunum
- Its secretion is stimulated by presence of acid in the intestine
- It acts on the pancreatic ductal cells and stimulates secretion of large volume of watery bicarbonate rich pancreatic juice
- It also stimulates bicarbonate rich bile secretion from hepatocytes in liver.

Role of cholecystokinin:
- It is secreted from 'I' cells of the duodenum and jejunum
- Its secretion is stimulated by presence of products of amino acids and fatty acids in the intestine
- CCK is secreted into blood and it acts on the pancreatic acini and stimulates secretion of enzyme rich pancreatic juice.

7. **Write an essay on immunity.**
- **Innate or non-specific immunity** is present since birth and offer protection against wide variety of pathogens and foreign substances. Non-specific means there is no specific response for specific invaders; protective mechanisms function the same way regardless of the type of invaders
- **Acquired immunity or specific immunity**, the ability of the body to defend against specific invading agents such as bacteria, toxins, viruses and foreign tissues, is called as specific resistance or immunity and it develops after exposure to the antigen
- It has two properties—specificity and memory
- Specificity for particular antigen which involves distinguishing self from non-self molecules
- Memory for previously encountered antigen is present and when a second encounter happens there is a swift and rapid response
- It includes two types—**cell-mediated and humoral immunity.**

Cell-mediated Immunity

Refer cell-mediated immunity in 2004 paper.

Humoral Immunity

Refer humoral immunity in 2005 paper.

8. **Define cardiac cycle. Describe the pressure and volume changes in the left ventricle during the cardiac cycle with a suitable graph.**

Refer from 2005 Paper.

9. **Name all the descending tracts. Describe the corticospinal tract and mention the diffrences between UMN and LMN lesions.**

a. There are descending tracts arising from cerebral cortex and ending on spinal cord motor neurons—corticospinal tract. They pass through the pyramid in medulla oblogata. Also called as Pyramidal tract

b. They are of two types—lateral corticospinal tract and anterior corticospinal tract. Fibers originating from cerebral cortex ends on cranial nerves—corticobulbar tract.

c. Extrapyramidal tracts: Fibers which do not descend down through pyramidal tract from cerebral cortex but ends on nuclei in brainstem. From there they descend down

to end on spinal cord motor neurons. They are:
1. Rubrospinal tracts
2. Vestibulospinal tract
3. Reticulospinal tract
4. Tectospinal tract
5. Olivospinal tract
6. Medial longitudinal fasciculus.

Pyramidal Tract

Origin of CST

Corticospinal tract (CST) arises from the following areas in the cerebral cortex:
- 30% fibers arise from the Primary motor area (Area 4)
- 30% fibers arise from Premotor area (Area 6)
- 40% fibers arise from Somatosensory area 1 (Area 3, 1, 2) (refer Fig. 7).

Course of CST

- The fibers, after originating from the above areas pass through the Corona radiata and then pass through the posterior limb of internal capsule
- In corona radiata the fibers are spread out and appear fan-like
- On entering the internal capsule (IC) they are arranged in a very compact manner.

Internal Capsule (IC)

In IC, CST is present in the anterior 2/3rd of the posterior limb of the capsule. The whole body is represented here from anterior to posterior aspect.

Midbrain

CST passes through pes pedunculi and occupies the middle 3/5th of it. Here the representation of body is, head in the medial aspect and legs laterally and trunk in the middle.

Pons

In pons, the fibers are dispersed as they pass through the pontine nuclei and pontocerebellar fibers.

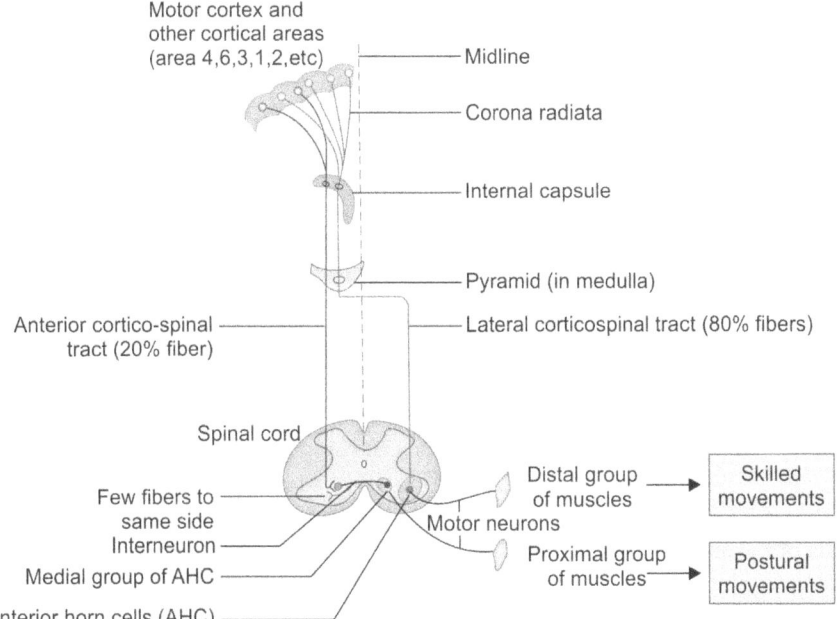

Fig. 7: Origin, course and termination of pyramidal tract. Lateral corticospinal tract supplies distal limb muscles and anterior corticospinal tract supplies proximal limb and trunk muscles.
(*Source:* GK Pal)

Medulla oblongata

- The split fibers reunite here to form a single bundle which appears as a bulge in the anterior aspect and which is said to be the Pyramid. Therefore it gets the name—pyramidal tract
- In medulla, 75% of the fibers cross over to the opposite side and forms the lateral corticospinal tract (LCST). 25% of the fibers descend down on the ipsilateral side as the anterior corticospinal tract (ACST).

Spinal Cord

The crossed and uncrossed fibers descend down in spinal cord (SC) as the ACST and LCST. The *LCST fibers* end on the internuncial neurons in SC, which in turn synapse with anterior horn cells (α motor neurons) and they supply the distal limb muscles and are responsible for the *fine voluntary movements*.

Uncrossed *ACST fibers* reach the respective spinal segment and they cross over at the segment to opposite side and end on internuncial neurons which in turn synapse on the anterior horn cells. ACST fibers supply the proximal limb muscles and trunk muscles and are responsible for *regulation of posture and tone*.

- There are many inputs which converge on the spinal motor neurons. These supra segmental inputs come from other spinal segments, brainstem and cerebral cortex. These neurons which converge on the anterior horn cells of spinal cord are the **upper motor neurons**. It includes the Pyramidal and extrapyramidal tracts
- Anterior horn cells and their fibers which supply the muscles form the **lower motor neurons**. So they are called as the **"final common pathway"**.

Functions of Pyramidal Tract

a. LCST supplies the distal limb muscles and therefore they control voluntary fine movements like writing, stitching etc.
b. VCST supplies axial and proximal limb muscles and they control posture and gross movements like balancing, climbing etc.
c. LCST facilitates superficial reflexes and in its lesion, superficial reflexes are lost.
d. CST facilitates muscle tone.
e. CST also communicates with other areas controlling motor activites like basal ganglia, cerebellum and brainstem.
f. Some fibers from the cortex also terminate on cranial nerve nuclei (corticobulbar fibers) and therefore suppies facial muscles.

Effects of Lesions of Pyramidal Tract at Various Levels

Lesion in Motor Area

Whole body is represented in this area and the area of representation for each organ is based on their skilled activity. So the neurons controlling each part are widely distributed and therefore a lesion in this area usually produces monoplegia in the contralateral side.

Lesion in Corona Radiata

Monoplegia.

Lesion in Internal Capsule

Here fibers are densely packed and therefore lesion in small region induces a greater damage. The patient usually presents with contralateral hemiplegia (paralysis of one half of the body).

In lesions of larger areas, hemiplegia is associated with sensory loss and also visual symptoms as these fibers are also present close to CST here. Patient presents with hemiplegia, hemianaesthesia and homonymous hemianopia.

Midbrain

Here again the fibers are closely kept and therefore lesion in midbrain results in hemiplegia and since the 3rd cranial nerve nuclei are present here, contralateral hemiplegia is seen with ipsilateral 3rd nerve palsy.

Pons

Contralateral hemiplegia and ipsilateral 7th nerve palsy as the facial nerve nuclei are present in the pons.

Medulla Oblongata
Contralateral hemiplegia and ipsilateral 12th nerve palsy on same side.

Spinal Cord (Upper Level)
Quadriplegia and respiratory paralysis.

Thoracic and Lumbar Level Spinal Cord
Paraplegia.

Differences between UMN and LMN Lesions

S. No	Upper motor neuron lesion	Lower motor neuron lesion
1.	Damage to motor tracts above anterior horn cell	Damage to the anterior horn cells and below
2.	Muscles affected in groups	Individual muscles affected
3.	Spastic type of paralysis	Flaccid type of paralysis
4.	Deep reflexes are exaggerated	Deep reflexes are lost
5.	There is no muscle atrophy	Paralysed muscles are atrophied
6.	Babinski's sign is positive	Plantar reflex is normal
7.	Muscle tone is increased (hypertonia)	Muscle tone is decreased (hypotonia)
8.	Common site of lesion is at the internal capsule	Injury to peripheral nerves, poliomyelitis
9.	No involuntary movements	Fasiculations are present
10.	Nerve conduction study is normal	Nerve conduction velocity is decreased

10. Discuss the mechanics of pulmonary ventilation.

Pulmonary ventilation comprises of two processes—inspiration and expiration.

All physical properties involved in the process of respiration are discussed here.

Respiration is dependent on active participation of respiratory muscles, changes in intrapleural and transpulmonary pressures and elastic tendencies of lung.

So mechanics of respiration is given as:
- Muscles of respiration
- Pressure changes during respiration
- Compliance of lungs.

Muscles of Respiration

Muscles of Inspiration
Normal inspiration is an active process and it includes active contraction of inspiratory muscles.

When the muscles of inspiration contract they expand the thoracic cavity and make the intrapulmonary pressure lower than atmospheric pressure and thereby allows enrty of air.

Major muscles of inspiration are diaphragm and external intercostal muscles. **Diaphragm** is a dome shaped muscle, with fibers arising from xiphisternum, lower six ribs and lumbar vertebrae. It is present between the thorax and abdomen. As the diaphragm contracts the dome flattens downwards and the vertical diameter increases. The diaphragmatic muscle fibers inserted to lower ribs, when they contract the lateral diameter is also increased (pump handle movement). The convexity of the dome is towards thorax and as the muscle contracts during quiet respiration it pulls the dome downwards. This increases the vertical diameter by 1.5 cm at rest and in forced expiration it can be increased up to 7 cm (refer Fig. 8).

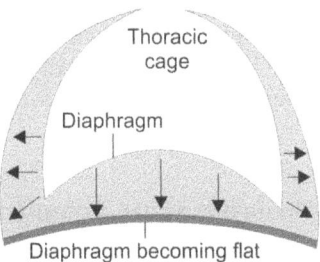
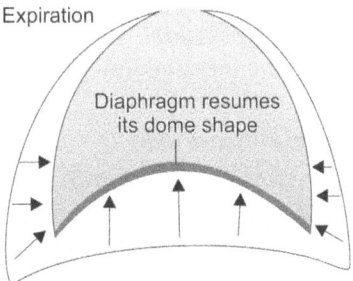

Fig. 8: Movement of diaphragm during inspiration and expiration.
(*Source: Sembulingam*)

External intercostal muscles: Fibers of this muscle are attached to the outer side of the rib and they slope downward and forward as that when they contract they pull the rib cage forward and upward increasing the lateral and anteroposterior diameter.

There are other accessory muscles of inspiration, the scalene muscle, sternocleidomastoid, neck and back muscles.

Abductors of vocal cords pull them apart and help during inspiration.

Muscles of Expiration

Expiration in quiet breathing is a passive process.

The contracted inspiratory muscles relax and the thoracic cage drops to normal position and lungs recoil. This increases intrapulmonary pressure and causes expiration. This happens in quiet breathing.

But during forced expiration muscles of expiration come into action. The major muscles of expiration are anterior abdominal wall muscles and internal intercostal muscles.

Contraction of anterior abdominal wall muscles presses on the abdomen and increase the intra-abdominal pressure and pushes the diaphragm above. The intrapleural pressure rises and causes expiration.

The internal intercostal muscles when they contract pull down the rib cage and decrease the thoracic volume transversely and anteroposteriorly. Thereby it favors expiration.

Pressure Changes during Respiration

The changes in the following pressures affect respiration:
- Intrapleural pressure
- Transpulmonary pressure
- Alveolar pressure.

Intrapleural Pressure (IPP)

- IP space is the space between visceral and parietal pleura
- Pleural fluid between the two layers helps in lubricating the movement of lungs and thoracic cavity during respiration
- The IP pressure is negative due to the recoiling tendencies of the lung and thoracic cavity. Lungs have the tendency to recoil inward and the thoracic cage has the tendency to recoil outward
- This creates a relative vacuum in the pleural cavity and the IPP is negative
- Normal IPP at rest is −2.5 mm Hg. It is the pressure at which both the opposing (recoiling) forces of lungs and thoracic cavity oppose each other. This is the pressure at which the lung is held at equilibrium volume or at functional residual capacity (FRC) (refer Fig. 9)
- During inspiration as the thoracic cage expands the IPP becomes −6 mm Hg. This pulls the lungs to expansion and the alveolar pressure drops, sucking in air

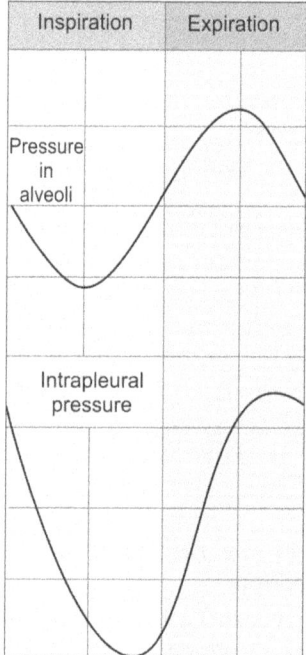

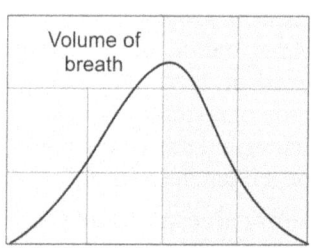

Fig. 9: Alveolar and intrapleural pressure and volume changes in quiet inspiration and expiration.
(Source: GK Pal)

- During expiration as the lung recoils the IPP becomes –2.5 mm Hg
- During forced inspiration IPP becomes even –30 mm Hg and during forced expiration it becomes more negative.

Transpulmonary Pressure

- It is the pressure difference between Intrapulmonary pressure (IPP) and alveolar pressure
- It is the pressure that keeps the lungs inflated and prevents it from collapsing. It is always positive in normal respiration.

Intrapulmonary Pressure

- It is the pressure inside the alveoli and therefore said to be the alveolar pressure. The flow of air into and out of the alveoli is dependent on the pressure gradient between alveoli and atmosphere (transairway pressure)
- At the end of inspiration and end of expiration and when the glottis is open there is no movement of air and the pressure in all respiratory passages are equal and alveolar pressure is zero
- During inspiration as the inspiratory muscles contract and intrathoracic volume decreases and intrapulmonary pressure decreases to 1 mm Hg below atmospheric pressure, the gradient derived results in inflow of air
- During expiration as the lungs recoil the intrapulmonary pressure rises above atmospheric pressure (+1 mm Hg) there is an outward gradient for the air from the alveoli.

Compliance of Lung

The ability of lungs to stretch or recoil is said to be compliance.

Compliance is represented by volume change per unit change in pressure. It is given as:

Compliance = $\Delta V/\Delta P$
ΔV = Change in volume
ΔP = Change in pressure

Compliance of the lungs is dependent on two factors (refer Fig. 10):

- Elastic tissue in lungs and arrangement of collagen fibers in lung parenchyma
- Elastic forces caused by surface tension of fluid lining alveoli.

The force of pull exerted by water molecules at an air-liquid interface is said to be the surface tension. This interface in the alveoli is a major factor responsible for lung compliance. The water molecules at the air-water interface are attracted to each other by surface tension and they are pulled together. This pulls the alveoli inward and results in collapse of alveoli. But this action of surface tension if not balanced will cause complete collapse of alveoli and during the next inspiration much effort has to be applied by respiratory muscles to expand the lungs and so work of breathing will be increased. To prevent this, a surface tension lowering agent is synthesized by Type II pneumocytes, the Surfactant. The role of surfactant in lowering surface tension is more during expiration than inspiration. That is why the pressure volume curves recorded to see the effect of surface tension in expiration and inspiration on compliance is in the shape of a hysteresis loop and not a linear one.

The other factor affecting compliance is the lung size. Smaller lung size as in lower animals or removal of one lung may decrease the compliance.

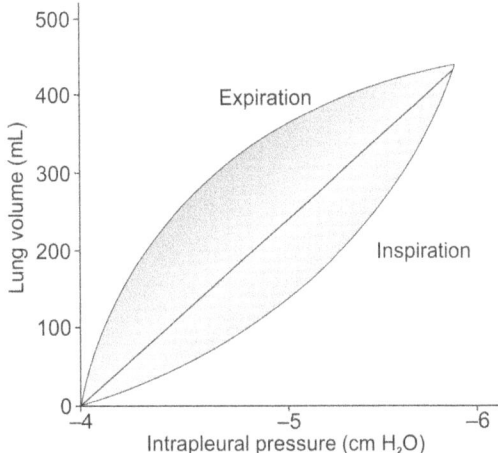

Fig. 10: Pressure-volume curve.
(*Source:* Sembulingam)

Diseases which affect lung compliance as in fibrosis of lung the lung distensibility is decerased as the elastic tissue is replaced by fibrous tissue and a normal tidal volume may not be achieved.

II. SHORT NOTES

1. Ultrastructure of skeletal muscle.

Structure of Skeletal Muscle

- Skeletal muscle is made up of muscle fibers, which are the basic unit of muscles and the surrounding connective tissues
- Each muscle fiber is surrounded by connective tissue—endomysium
- Many muscle fibers are bundled up to form fasciculi and each fasciculus is surrounded by—perimysium
- The fasiculi are bundled to form the muscle and it is surrounded by - Epimysium
- All these connective tissues join to form the tendon (refer Fig. 11)
- Each muscle fiber has many myofibrils and the muscle fiber is surrounded by sarcolemma—the cell membrane (refer Figs. 12A and B)
- The myofibrils have thick and thin filaments

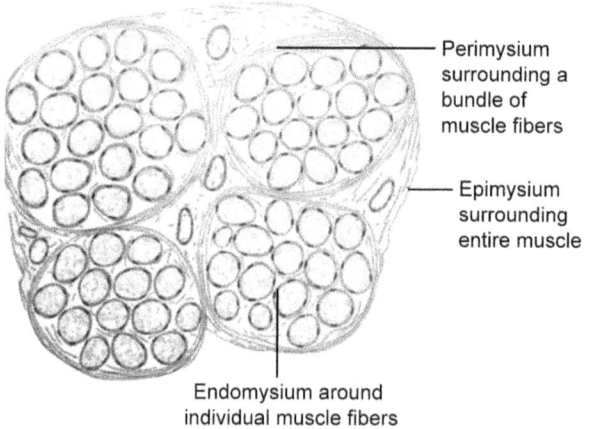

Fig. 11: Skeletal muscle with the surrounding connective tissues.
(*Source:* GK Pal)

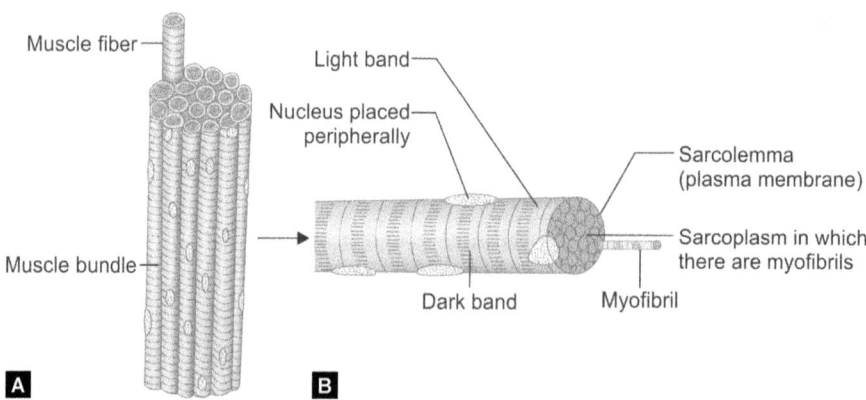

Figs. 12A and B: Structure of muscles; Muscle bundle (A) and muscle fiber (B). Arrangement of thick and thin filaments in the muscle fiber (B).
(*Source:* GK Pal)

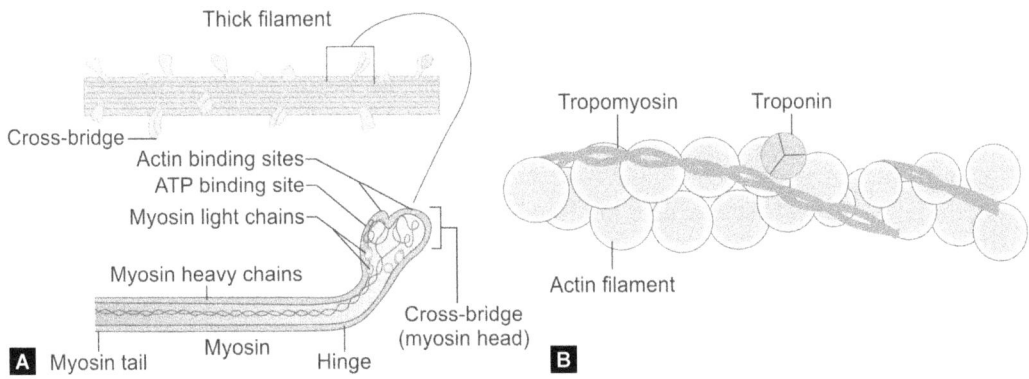

Figs. 13A and B: Structure of myosin in thick filament (A) and Structure of actin, tropomyosin and troponin molecules in thin filament (B).
(*Source:* GK Pal)

- The filamants are made of proteins—actin, myosin, troponin and tropomyosin (refer Figs. 13A and B)
- Actin and myosin are the contractile proteins and troponin and tropomyosin are regulatory proteins
- The arrangement of thick and thin filaments appears as light and dark striations (bands) under light microscope due to the refractive indices of the various parts
- The **dark band** is A band and is 1.5 μm in length and is made of **thick filaments and overlapping thin filaments**. The center of A band has a lighter H zone with a M line in the middle of it. H zone is the area where thin filaments do not overlap thick filaments and therefore appears as lighter area. The thick filament is made of myosin molecules
- The **light band** is made of **thin filaments** with a dark line—Z line in the middle of it. The thin filament is made of the proteins —actin, tropomyosin and troponin with 3 subunits—I, C and T.

Sarcomere

- The segment of myofibril between two Z lines is the **Sarcomere**
- It includes ½ of I band and A band and ½ I band
- It is 2.5 μm in length
- This forms the structural and functional unit of the muscle fiber

- On contraction of the muscle, the length of sarcomere decreases and on relaxation it is increased.

Thick Filament

- Under electron microscope, a transverse section of the A band, it is seen that each thick filament is surrounded by 6 thin filaments in a hexagonal pattern
- The type of myosin in skeletal muscle is Myosin II. Myosin has two globular heads and a tail
- It is made of 2 heavy chains and 4 light chains. The light chains and the amino terminals of heavy chains form the head. The rest of the heavy chains are wound on each other to form the tail
- Each head of the myosin molecule has two binding sites, one for actin and the other is the ATPase site which hydrolyses ATP
- The myosins are arranged symmetrically in the thick filament and in the center part, on either sides of M line there is a small zone where there is absence of myosin heads and it appears lighter. It is the Pseudo H zone
- M line is the site of revesal of polarity of myosin molecules in each of the thick filaments.

Thin Filament

- It is made of actin, troponin and tropomyosin
- There are 300–400 actin molecules present in each thin filament. The actin molecule

is made of two chains of globular units of G actin. The chain is said to be F-actin. The actin forms a double helix
- There are 40–60 tropomyosin molecules in each thin filament. It is in the form of strands and lies in the groove between the actin helix. It covers the myosin binding site on actin
- Troponin molecules are globular units which are present on tropomyosin at intervals. There are 3 subunits—troponin T, I and C
- Troponin T—attaches other components of troponin to tropomyosin
- Troponin I—inhibits myosin head binding with actin
- Troponin C—binds to calcium ion following which muscle contraction is initiated.

Other Proteins in Skeletal Muscle
- There anchoring proteins: Actinin, Titin and Desmin.

Sarcotubular System
- Under electron microscope, the myofilaments in sarcoplasm are surrounded by vesicles and tubules which make up the sarcotubular system (refer Fig. 14)

- This system is made up of T-tubules and the sarcoplasmic reticulum (SR)
- T-tubules are invaginations of sarcolemma
- Sarcoplasmic reticulum covers the myofibrils and they enlarge as cisterns and are in contact with the T-tubules at the junction of A-I bands
- The T-tubule with the cistern of SR on either side forms the **Triad**
- T-tubule helps in spread of impulse into the muscle membrane and causes release of Ca^{2+} from SR.

2. Deglutition.
Refer answers to 2003 paper.

3. Give composition and functions of gastric juice.
Refer answers to 2005 paper.

4. Erythroblastosis fetalis.
Refer answers to August 2003.

5. Describe nerve supply to urinary bladder and micturition.

Nerve Supply of Urinary Bladder
- Urinary bladder is a triangular-shaped sac like structure. The bladder extends down as the urethra

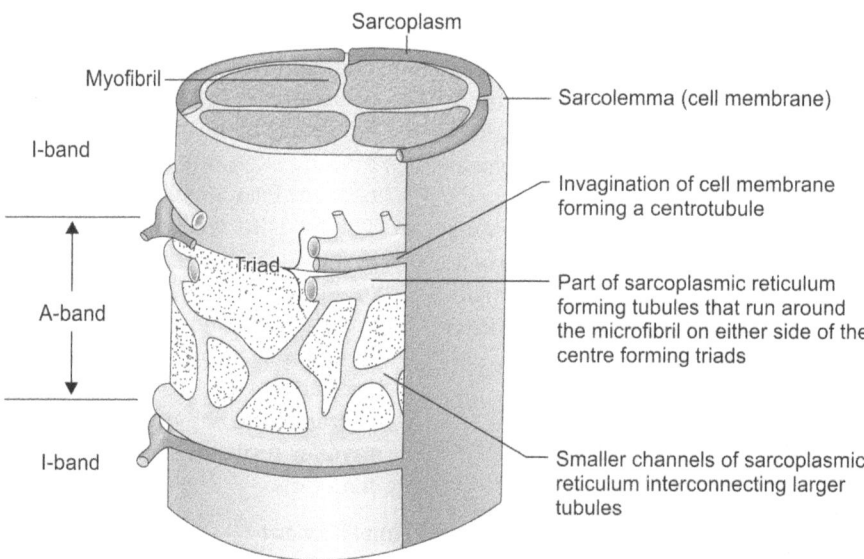

Fig. 14: Arrangement of Sarcotubular system in the myofibril.
(*Source:* GK Pal)

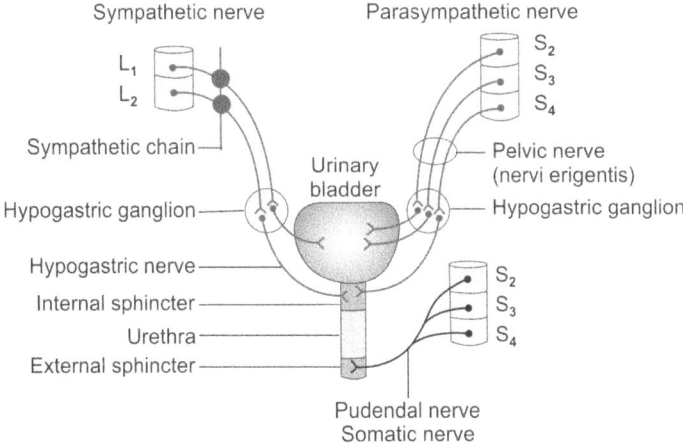

Fig. 15: Nerve supply of urinary bladder.
(*Source:* Sembulingam)

- The bladder wall is made of detrusor, a smooth muscle and there are two sphincters—internal and external urethral sphincters
- Internal sphincter is at the neck of the bladder and is made of smooth muscle. It is supplied by sympathetic and parasympathetic nerves
- External sphincter is made of skeletal muscle and is supplied by somatic motor nerve (pudendal nerve)
- The bladder wall is also supplied by sympathetic and parasympathetic nerves
- Parasympathetic nerves (Pelvic nerve) has both afferent and efferent components and they supply the bladder wall and the internal sphincter (refer Fig. 15)
- The sympathetic nerves (hypogastric nerve) also have afferents and efferents and they arise from L1–L3 segments of spinal cord. They also supply the bladder wall and internal sphincter. When stimulated, they cause relaxation of bladder wall and contraction of internal sphincter and therefore helps in filling of bladder
- Somatic nerve (pudendal nerve) to external shincter arises from S2–S4 segments of spinal cord and have control from higher centers. It is under voluntary control
- Once urine enters the renal pelvis, it flows through the ureters and enters the bladder, where urine is stored.

Micturition Reflex

- Micturition is the process of emptying the urinary bladder
- Two processes are involved:
  1. The bladder fills progressively until the tension in its wall rises above a threshold level, and then
  2. A nervous reflex called the micturition reflex occurs that empties the bladder.

The micturition reflex is an automatic spinal cord reflex; however, it can be inhibited or facilitated by centers in the brainstem and cerebral cortex.

The Reflex Pathway (refer Fig. 16)

- **Initiation:** Reflex initiated by stimulation of stretch receptors in bladder wall
- **Stimulus:** Filling of bladder upto 300–400 mL
- **Afferents:** Through pelvic nerves (parasympathetic) to reach S2–S4 segments in spinal cord
- **Efferents:** PS motor fibers from S2–S4 end in the detrusor muscle (excitatory) and internal sphincter (inhibitory)
- **Response:** Causes contraction of bladder wall and relaxation of internal sphincter.

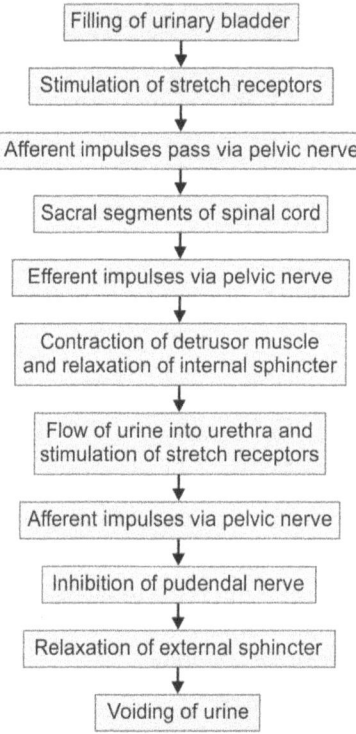

Fig. 16: Micturition reflex.
(*Source:* Sembulingam)

Once it becomes powerful another reflex through pudendal nerve relaxes the ES → voiding.

6. Thrombocyte.
Refer answers to 2004 Paper.

7. Ovarian cycle.

Ovarian Changes during the Monthly Cycle

There are 3 phases of ovarian changes during the cycle.

They are:
1. Follicular phase
2. Ovulatory phase
3. Luteal phase.

Follicular Phase
- In the female fetus, at the time of birth there are millions of primordial follicles. Inside each follicle there is an immature ovum
- At the start of each menstrual cycle 6–12 primordial follicles start to grow in size and mature

- This is due to the increase of FSH and LH release from the anterior pituitary gland. FSH levels are more than LH levels (refer Fig. 17A)
- After 5–7 days, one follicle continues to grow and mature (Dominant follicle), while the other follicles start to degenerate and undergo atretic changes
- The follicle, which will mature and become dominant, will be based on the ability of it to secrete estrogen.

Changes happening in the maturing follicle are:
- Ovum inside the follicle grows in size and the surrounding granulosa cells multiply in number—**primary follicle**
- Outer to the granulosa cell layer, spindle shaped cells in the interstitium of the ovary develop into theca cells. They get differentiated to theca interna and theca externa cells—**preantral follicle**
- The granulosa and the theca cells start secreting estrogen. Granulosa cells secrete a follicular fluid which gets accumulated as the antrum—**early antral follicle**
- Till this phase, growth of the follicle is due to high levels of FSH. The FSH and estrogen together increase the LH receptors on the granulosa cells (Fig. 17B)
- As estrogen levels in the follicle increase, follicular growth is increased at a greater rate. The antrum increases in size and ovum also enlarges. The ovum is pushed to one pole surrounded by granulosa cells—**mature Graafian follicle**
- Mature follicle reaches the size of 1 to 1.5 cm
- The cycle reaches the 14th day.

Ovulatory Phase
- In a female with a 28 days cycle, Ovulation occurs on the 14th day
- Just before ovulation, outer wall of the follicle swells and a small protrusion, the Stigma is seen
- After a few minutes a fluid starts oozing out followed by the release of ovum along with the corona radiata around it.

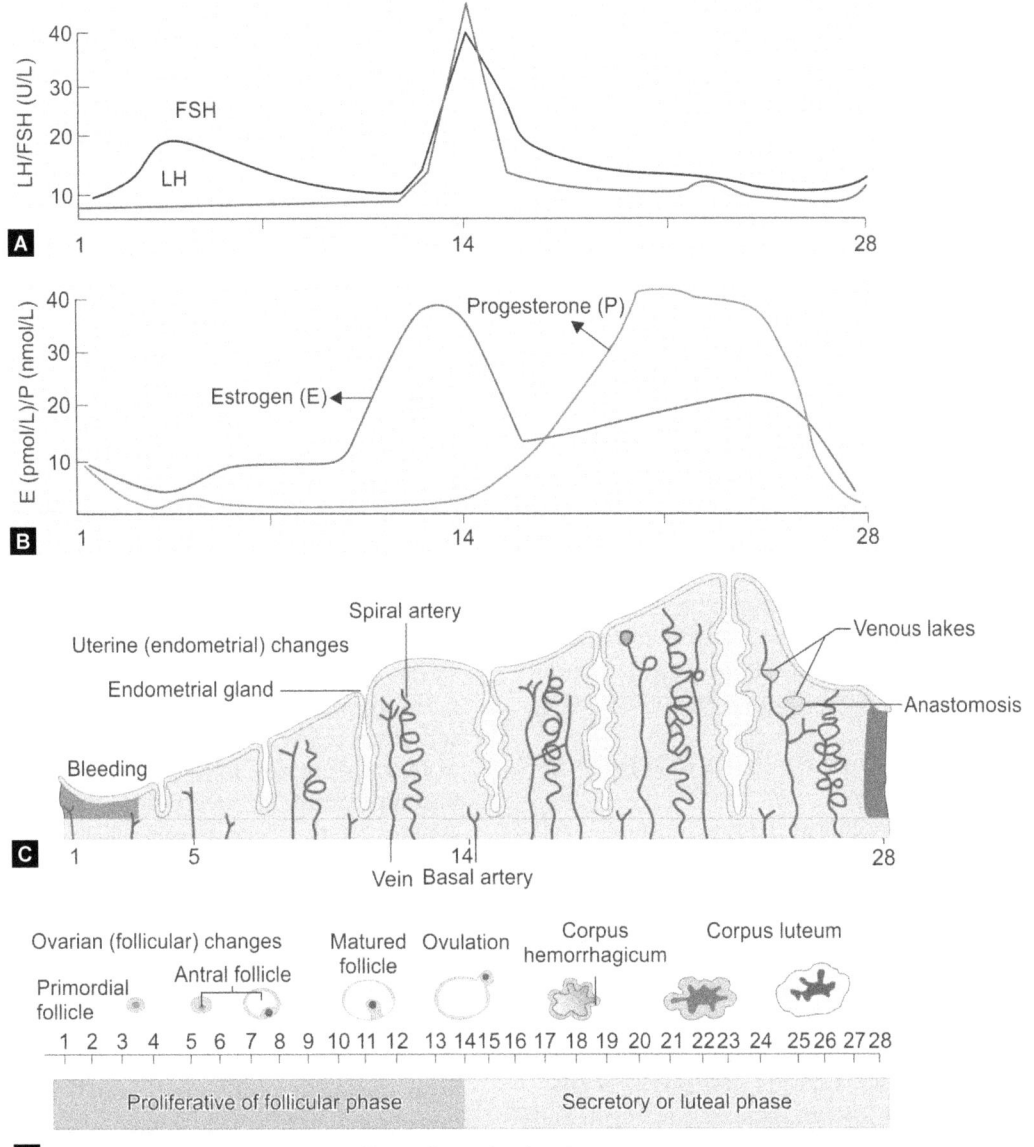

Figs. 17A to D: Sequential changes in the hormone levels in menstrual cycle along with the ovarian and endometrial changes.
(*Source:* GK Pal)

Hormonal changes:
- 2 days before ovulation, estrogen levels increase and there is a positive feedback regulation of estrogen on LH secretion
- LH levels reach 6–10 times the normal value and peaks 10–12 hours before ovulation (Fig. 17A)
- High LH levels are essential for the final growth, maturation and ovulation
- LH acts on the granulosa cells to increase progesterone secretion.

This causes:
- Theca externa cells to release proteolytic enzymes from lysosomes, which will

- dissolve the follicular capsule and degeneration of stigma
- Blood vessels grow rapidly into the follicle and prostaglandins are secreted into the follicle
- Both these events cause the follicle to swell and break the stigma and release the ovum.

Luteal Phase

- As soon as the follicle is ruptured and ovum released, the Follicle is filled with blood—**corpus hemorrhagicum (Fig. 17D)**
- The granulosa and theca cells are laiden with fat droplets and are leutinized, the cells are now in yellow color—**corpus luteum**
- LH induces leutinization of the follicle and favors its hormonal function
- The corpus luteum starts producing estrogen and progesterone, progesterone levels are more than estrogen levels (Fig. 17B)
- Corpus luteum continues to grow for the next 7-8 days
- High estrogen and progesterone levels negatively inhibit the LH and FSH secretion from anterior pituitary
- Also inhibin released from corpus luteum inhibits FSH secretion
- If ovum is not fertilized, as the FSH and LH levels decrease, by 26th day of the cycle, the corpus luteum completely involutes and becomes a scar tissue—**corpus albicans**
- As corpus luteum regresses, estrogen and progesterone levels decrease suddenly and the inhibition on FSH and LH is removed. FSH and LH levels start rising and a new set of follicles start developing and the next cycle starts
- If the ovum is fertilized, corpus luteum continues to secrete progesterone under the influence of hCG till the placenta takes over the secretion of progesterone.

8. Describe the hormones acting on the breast.

- Breast gland is a modified apocrine gland
- It is divided into lobes, lobules and alveoli
- They are drained by alveolar ducts and lobular ducts to drain the milk in the nipple
- Ducts are lined by myoepithelial cells
- Many hormones act on the breasts during the development and also during pregnancy and lactation.

Hormones Acting on the Breast

- *Estrogen:* Induces growth and development of the ducts of the breast
- *Progesterone:* Growth and development of the lobules are promoted by progesterone
- *Prolactin:* Acts on estrogen and progesterone primed breast during pregnancy. It initiates milk secretion from 5th month of pregnancy. But the actions of prolactin are kept inhibited till the time of delivery and when estrogen levels drop at the time of delivery of fetus, milk secretion starts—*lactogenesis*
- *Galactopoiesis:* Maintenance of milk secretion is by prolactin. After delivery of fetus prolactin levels come down to baseline value. But every time the baby suckles at the breast there is a surge of prolactin secretion, increasing milk secretion
- *Oxytocin:* When the infant suckles at the breast the touch receptors around the nipple are stimulated and impulses are carried through sensory nerves to hypothalamus. Oxytocin is released from posterior pituitary. It acts on the myoepithelial cells of the ducts and causes expulsion of milk—*galactokinesis*
- Other hormones acting on the breast are: Insulin, cortisol, hCG, hPL, thyroxine, growth hormone.

9. Describe functions of skin.

- It forms a **protective covering** for the body and prevents entry of micro-organisms and other toxic substances from the environment
- Helps in **body temperature regulation**
  – Evaporation of sweat from skin and the

- loss of water by insensible perspiration help in temperature regulation
- It is the **largest sensory organ** in the body as it has many receptors in the skin and hair follicle
- **Synthesis of 1, 25 Dihydrocholecalciferol** – By the action of sunlight on the skin 7-dehydrocholesterol is formed from Vitamin D. It is the precursor for 1, 25 Dihydrocholecalciferol
- **Protects the body from U-V radiations** due to the presence of Melanin pigment
- It is a form of **innate immunity** and thereby provides resistance against infections
- Helps in regulation of water balance
- Acts as a reservoir of blood as the skin vasculature can store blood
- Has excretory functions also.

10. Thyrotoxicosis.

- Grave's disease or toxic goitre is said to be thyrotoxicosis
- There is hypertrophy and hyperplasia of the gland and increased secretion of thyroid hormones
- Grave's disease is an autoimmune disorder
- It accounts for 60–80% cases of hyperthyroidism
- It is more common in women
- Thyroid stimulating antibodies are formed against TSH receptors and the antibodies act like TSH
- Therefore it results in enlargement of the gland and excess secretion of thyroid hormones
- But the high levels of T3 negatively inhibit secretion of TSH and TSH levels are low.

Symptoms

- Goitre is present
- Due to action of excess TH on tissues:
  - BMR and body temperature are increased
  - Heat intolerance
  - Heart rate is increased. Palpitations and fine tremors are present
  - Muscle weakness is present
  - Nervousness, irritability and anxiety
  - Exaggeration of deep tendon reflexes
  - Increased frequency of defecation
  - Increased appetite
  - Weight loss
  - Moist and warm skin
  - Bruit is heard over thyroid
  - Pretibial myxedema is present
  - Fatigue is present
  - Impotence in males
  - Oligomenorrhea or amenorrhea in females
  - Eye problem—exophthalmos is seen.
- Exophthalmos is protrusion of eyeballs
- This is due to increase in retro-orbital contents
- In the retro-orbital region, fibroblasts proliferate and develop into adipocytes, which have receptors for circulating TSH Ab → gets activated → release cytokines → inflammation and edema → Accumulation of fluid causes, protrusion of eyeball.

Treatment

- The condition is treated with either antithyroid drugs or with radioactive iodine
- Subtotal thyroidectomy can also be done

11. Spirogram.

- Spirogram is a graphic recording of the various lung volumes and capacities other than residual volume, functional residual capacity and total lung capacity
- The instrument is the spirometer
- Spirometry is the recording of volume changes during the breathing events
- There are two types of spirometers—simple spirometer or a computerised spirometer
- The spirogram shows the various lung volumes and capacities (refer Fig. 18)
- Capacities are two or more lung volumes.

Tidal Volume (TV)

- It is the volume of air inspired or expired with each breath during normal breathing
- Normal value—500 mL.

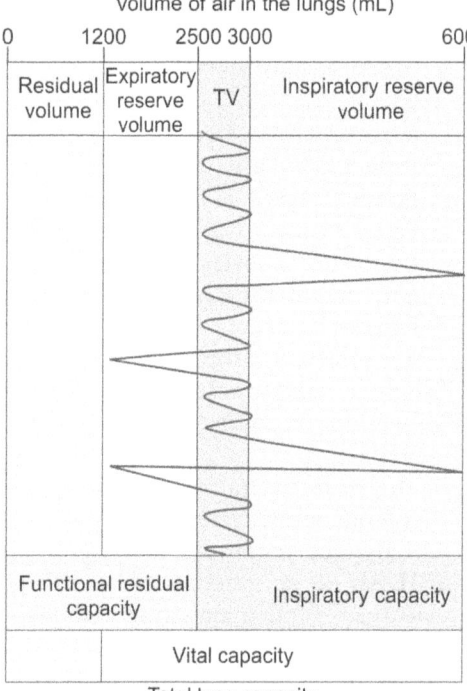

Fig. 18: Spirogram: Lung volumes and capacities. (*Source:* GK Pal)

Inspiratory Reserve Volume (IRV)

- It is the maximal volume of air inspired with effort in excess of tidal volume
- Normal value—2000 to 3200 mL.

Expiratory Reserve Volume (ERV)

- It is the maximal volume of air exhaled from the resting end-expiratory level. (volume expired by active expiration after passive expiration)
- Normal value—750 to 1000 mL.

Residual Volume (RV)

- It is the volume of air remaining in the lungs at the end of maximal expiration. Normally it accounts for about 25% of TLC
- Normal value—1200 mL
- This volume cannot be measured with spirometer
- It is calculated from subtracting ERV from FRC

- FRC is measured by Helium Dilution technique.

Inspiratory Capacity (IC)

- It is the maximal volume of air inspired from resting expiratory level
- Normal value—3000 to 3500 mL.

Functional Residual Capacity (FRC)

- It is the volume of air remaining in the lungs at the end of resting (normal) expiration. NV—2500 mL
- FRC = RV + ERV
- It is measured by nitrogen washout technique or helium dilution technique
- **Significance of FRC:**
  - This volume of gas in the lung helps in continuous exchange of gases between breaths
  - Helps to Buffer the levels of concentration of O_2 and CO_2 in blood

Total Lung Capacity (TLC)

- It is the total volume of air within the lung after maximum inspiration (Maximum volume of air that the lung can contain)
- NV—**6000 mL**
  TLC = FVC + RV
  Or
  TLC = RV + ERV + TV + IRV
- TLC Increased in airway narrowing with air trapping (bronchial asthma).

Vital Capacity

- Maximum volume of air completely expired from the lungs following a maximal inspiration
- NV – 4800 mL (in males) and 3200 mL (in females)
  VC = TLC - RV or
  VC = IRV+TV+ERV

Factors that Influence VC

- Respiratory muscle power
- Airway patency
- Compliance of the lung
- Elasticity of lung.

Conditions Increasing and Decreasing VC

- Increased in:
  - Swimmers and divers
  - Trained athletes
  - People living in high altitude.
- Decreased in:
  - Old age
  - Lying posture
  - Pregnancy
  - Obesity
  - Diseases like poliomyelitis, pleural effusion, asthma, emphysema etc.

12. Dysbarism.

Refer answers to 2005 paper.

13. Hypoxia.

Hypoxia is defined as deficiency of O_2 at tissue level.

Types

- Hypoxic hypoxia
- Anemic hypoxia
- Stagnant hypoxia
- Histotoxic hypoxia.

Hypoxic Hypoxia

- Arterial pO_2 is low, therefore tissue pO_2 is less
- **Mechanism of hypoxia:** pO_2 of arterial blood is low due to either ↓O_2 in inspired air or disease of respiratory apparatus
- **Conditions:**
  - Low pO_2 in inspired air (as in high altitude)
  - Hypoventilation as in airway obstruction, paralysis of respiratory muscles
  - Diffusion defects as in pulmonary edema
  - Ventilation/perfusion mismatch
  - A-V shunt as in congenital cyanotic heart disease.

Anemic Hypoxia

- It is due to decreased O_2 carrying capacity of blood and so ↓O_2 content in blood. pO_2 is normal
- **Conditions:** Anemia, CO poisoning, presence of altered Hb (methemoglobin) etc.
- In mild anemia the 2, 3-DPG levels increase in the RBC → Easy dissociation of O_2.

Stagnant Hypoxia

- Hypoxia due to decreased blood flow to tissues. Also called as ischemic hypoxia
- **Mechanism:**
  - O_2 content and pO_2 are normal in arterial blood. Hypoxia is due to stagnation of blood → circulatory hypoxia
- **Seen in:**
  - Heart failure
  - Shock
  - Vascular obstruction
  - Hemorrhage.

Histotoxic Hypoxia

- Tissues cannot utilize O_2 inspite of normal O_2 supply as in cyanide poisoning
- Venous pO_2 is high (> 46 mm Hg)
- Cyanide poisoning is treated with Methylene blue or nitrites → Forms Methemoglobin → Reacts with cyanide → Cyanmethemoglobin. It is less poisonous
- Hyperbaric O_2 is also used for treatment.

Types of hypoxia:

Features	Hypoxic hypoxia	Anemic hypoxia	Stagnant hypoxia	Histotoxic hypoxia
Arterial PO_2	Decreased	Normal	Normal	Normal
% O_2 saturation of hemoglobin	Decreased	Decreased	Normal	Normal
Arterial O_2 content (mL/dL)	Decreased	Markedly decreased	Normal	Normal
A-V PO_2 difference	Decreased	Normal	More than normal	Less than normal
Peripheral chemoreceptor stimulation	Present	Absent	Present	Present
Cyanosis	Present	Absent	Present	Absent

Heart sounds	Events responsible	Duration	Frequency	Others
First sound (S_1)	Due to vibrations set by sudden closure of AV valves at the onset of verticular systole	0.15 sec	25–45 Hz In PCG recorded as 9–13 waves	Soft and long, heard as "LUBB"
Second sound (S_2)	Associated with closure of aortic and pulmonary valves after the end of ventricular systole	0.12 sec	50 Hz In PCG recorded as 4–6 waves	Normally S2 can be split due to early closure of aortic valve, heard as "Dubb"
Third sound (S_3)	In heard at 1/3 rd of diastole due to rapid filling of ventricle due to vibrations set by inrush of blood		0.1 sec In PCG recorded as 1–4 waves	Normally audible only in children and young adults
Fourth sound (S_4)	Heard just before (S_1). Occurs during atrial contraction. Due to ventricular filling		20 cyc/sec In PCG recorded as 1–2 waves	Rarely heard in normal adults. Heard in vent hypertrophy and CCF

Fig. 19: Heart sounds: Their causes and characteristics.

14. Heart sounds.

Heart sounds—Causes, features, phonocardiogram recordings refer Fig. 19

Significance of heart sounds:

- 1st sound: Increased in exercise, hyperkinetic states like anemia and decreased in shock, myocardial infarction, pericardial effusion
- 2nd sound: Loud in hypertension, low in aortic and pulmonary stenosis. Splitting is common
- 3rd sound: Increased in mitral regurgitation. Important sign of heart failure
- 4th sound: Always seen in abnormal conditions. Seen in left ventricular hypertrophy.

15. Triple response.

Vascular response of skin to injury with a sharp pointed object—triple response.

Red Reaction

- Occurs within 10 secs when stroked firmly by a sharp object. Seen as a red line
- Due to capillary dilatation.

Wheal

- Swelling within (local edema) few minutes after red reaction
- There is ↑ in permeability of capillaries due to histamine released by the injured tissue.

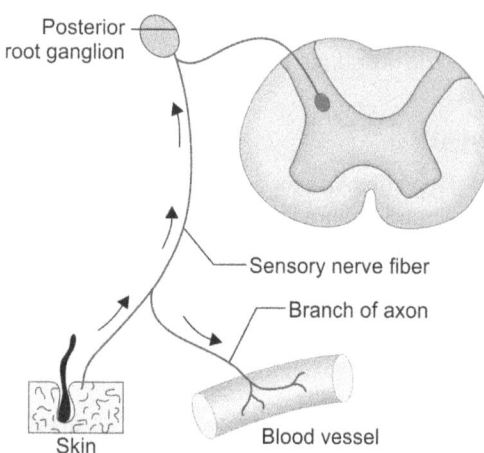

Fig. 20: Axon reflex. Sensory fibers give a branch which travels antidromically to supply arterioles below the skin.
(*Source: Sembulingam*)

Flare

- Spreading out of redness from site of injury
- Due to arteriolar dilatation
- Due to axon reflex.

Axon Reflex

- When there is an injury to skin with a sharp object, impulses from the skin carried by sensory fibers not only go to the spinal cord but also goes antidromically through other branches to the arterioles below the skin (refer Fig. 20)
- The neurotranmitter released here is Substance P

- This causes vasodilatation and extravasation of fluid.

16. Berger's rhythm.

Electroencephalogram

- This is a recording of spontaneous electrical activities generated in the cerebral cortex
- These waves are recorded by placing electrodes on the scalp at various areas and also on the forehead
- Neurons are known to generate impulses like action potentials (AP) and graded potentials—collectively called as Brain waves
- Also called as "Berger's rhythm" (refer Fig. 21)
- **Waves of EEG:**
  - Alpha waves:
    - Occurs at a frequency of 8-13 per second. Amplitude 50-100 µV
    - Present in all normal individuals when they are awake and resting with closed eyes
    - Disappears entirely during sleep
    - It is found in the parieto-occipital region
    - Alpha block: Alpha rhythm disappears on opening the eyes
    - Also called as desynchronization
    - Alpha rhythm is affected by blood glucose levels, body temperature and glucocorticoids.
  - Beta waves:
    - Frequency of the waves is between 14 and 30 Hz
    - Amplitude 5-10 µV
    - These waves appear when the nervous system is active
    - These waves appear in frontal regions.
  - Theta waves:
    - Appear at a frequency of 4-7 Hz. Amplitude is larger
    - Occurs normally in children and in adults at time of emotional stress
    - Found over parietal and temporal areas
    - Also occurs in many disorders of brain.
  - Delta waves:
    - Frequency of these waves is 1-5 Hz
    - Amplitude is 20-200 µV
    - Delta waves occur in sleep in adults but present in infants during wakefulness
    - When present in an awake adult it indicates brain damage.

Uses of EEG

- Used to study normal functions of brain
- To study the changes in brain activity during sleep
- To diagnose various brain disorders like epilepsy, tumors, sites of trauma, degenerative diseases.

17. Decerebrate rigidity.

- Decerebration is a procedure where the medulla is seperated from the brainstem by making a mid collicular transection (between superior and inferior colliculi). It is done experimentally in animals to study the role of medulla in posture regulation
- Muscle tone is exaggerated in the decerebrate animal
- Righting reflexes are lost
- There are no features of shock immediately after the transection
- Immediately after transection there is marked rigidity in the muscles especially

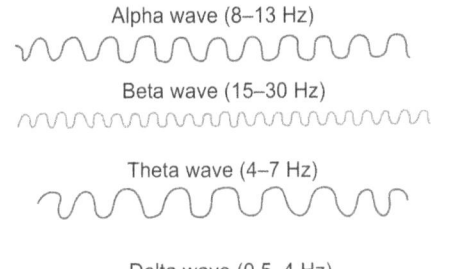

Fig. 21: EEG waves.
(*Source:* Sembulingam)

in the extensor group of muscles and the back muscles
- So limbs and spine are hyperextended
- The rigidity is due to hyperactive stretch reflex in the extensor groups of muscles.

It happens by two mechanisms:
a. Increased excitability of alpha motor neurons supplying the muscles
b. Increased activity in gamma motor neurons supplying the muscle spindles of extensors

- For understanding the cause of increase in activity of the above two groups of neurons we need to understand the higher centers controlling the stretch reflex
- There are two major areas in the brainstem controlling the excitability of anterior horn cells in the spinal cord:
  a. A large facilitatory area in the pontine reticular formation which gives rise to the pontine reticulospinal tract
  b. A small inhibitory area in the medullary reticular formation, giving rise to the medullary reticulospinal tract (refer Fig. 22).
- The facilitatory area discharges spontaneously whereas the inhibitory medullary area is under the control of higher centers—cerebral cortex, basal ganglia and cerebellum
- The basal ganglia acts through cerebral cortex and from the cortex the cortical fibers control the medullary inhibitory area
- So the net effect of stimulation of 3 inhibitory areas and one facilitatory area is overall inhibition of stretch reflex in normal condition
- In midcollicular section two of the inhibitions are removed and the facilitation continues resulting in rigidity and hypertonia.

18. Errors of refraction.
Refer answers to August 2004 paper.

19. Aqueous humor.
- It is present in the anterior and posterior chambers
- It is a protein-free fluid
- It has a refractive index of 1.33, pH is 7.1–7.3.

Formation and Circulation
- It is formed from the ciliary processes in the posterior chamber
- It is formed by processes like active transport, diffusion and ultrafiltration
- It is formed at the rate of 2–3 mm^3/minute
- Its composition resembles that of plasma
- Circulation is from the posterior chamber, through the pupil it flows into the anterior chamber (refer Fig. 23)

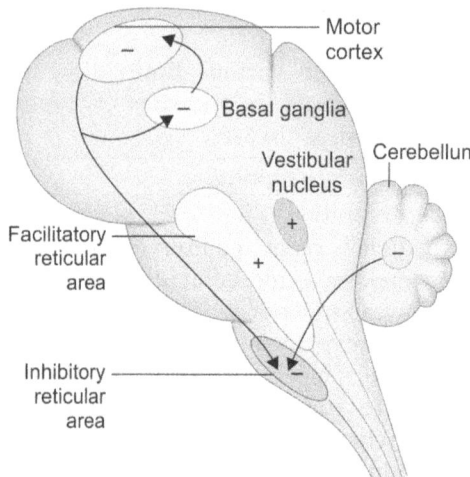

Fig. 22: Higher control of muscle tone: Inhibitory areas—cerebral cortex, basal ganglia, cerebellum and inhibitory medullary reticular area. Facilitatory area—pontine facilitatory reticular formation.
(*Source:* GK Pal)

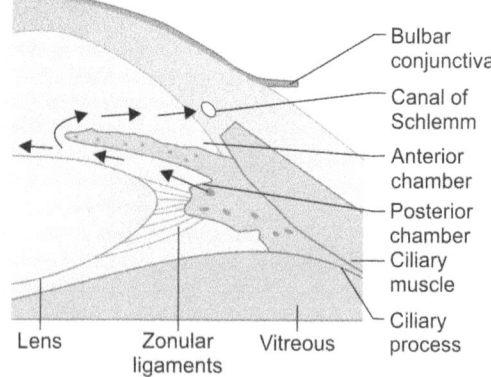

Fig. 23: Formation and circulation of aqueous humor.
(*Source:* GK Pal)

- Then it flows to the angle of the anterior chamber and crosses the meshwork of tissue here, the corneoscleral trabeculae and drains into the canal of Schlemn
- The canal is a venous sinus present in the layers of sclera
- Fluid is then drained into the aqueous vein and then into the ciliary vein
- The pressure of this fluid contributes to the intraocular pressure (along with vitreous humor) (IOP) and it is normally 10-20 mm Hg.

Functions

- It supplies nourishment to the cornea and lens
- Maintains shape of the eyeball
- Maintains and is responsible for intraocular pressure
- Act as a refractive medium for the light rays entering the eye.

Applied Aspects

Glaucoma

- Increase in IOP is mostly due to increase in pressure by the aqueous humor
- It could be due to deficient drainage or increased production of fluid.

There are two types: Primary and secondary glaucoma.

a. **Primary glaucoma** is of two types: Open angle and closed angle glaucoma.
   1. **Open angle glaucoma:**
      - It is bilateral and commonly seen in old age
      - The canal of Schelmm is kept open but the formation of aqueous humor is more.
   2. **Closed angle glaucoma:** Here the angle is closed and therefore the drainage is defective resulting in increased IOP.
b. **Secondary glaucoma:** In this type IOP is raised due to other causes like adhesions, uveitis, cataract etc.

20. Cochlear microphonic potential.

- They are the sum of receptor potentials in the hair cells in cochlea
- It is an oscillatory event and it has the same frequency as that of sound stimulus
- Bending of hairs of the hair cells towards the tallest stereocilia causes depolarisation and bending in opposite direction causes hyperpolarisation
- Depolarisation is due to entry of K^+ in the apical region creating a receptor potential
- The sum of these receptor potentials are recorded by placing one electrode in scala media and one in the scala tympani
- The sum of these potentials is cochlear microphonics
- They do not have latency
- They do not obey all or none law
- They are resistant to ischemia and anesthetics
- Their response increases with the intensity of stimulus
- So they are a type of generator potentials.

21. Fate of hemoglobin after hemolysis.

- The life span of RBC is 120 days. The cell membranes of older RBCs become fragile and are easily lysed when they squeeze through the narrow capillaries in the spleen
- On lysis of RBC, hemoglobin is released and are taken up by the tissue macrophages in the spleen
- Hemoglobin is now split into heme and globin (refer Fig. 24)

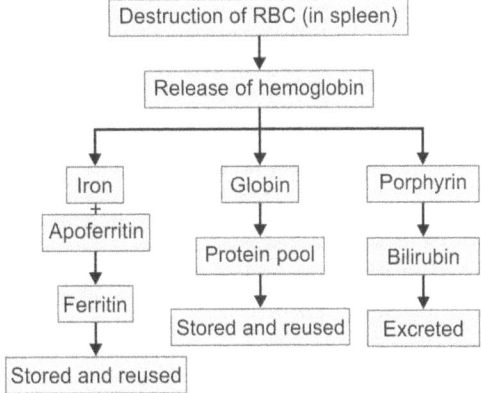

Fig. 24: Fate of hemoglobin.
(*Source: Sembulingam*)

- The macrophages open the porphyrin ring at one of the methine bridges by oxidising it
- This results in a straight chain of pyrrole nuclei
- The first pigment is formed here, biliverdin
- Once biliverdin is formed, iron is split off and is added to the iron pool in the bone marrow or stored in tissues as ferritin
- Biliverdin is converted to bilirubin by the enzyme biliverdin reductase and is released into blood
- Bilirubin is now called as Unconjugated bilirubin or Free bilirubin. This form of bilirubin is lipid soluble and therefore is transported in blood bound with albumin. Even though it is bound to albumin it is said to be Free bilirubin
- Unconjugated bilirubin is taken up by the liver and the albumin is split off and 80% is conjugated with glucoronic acid. The reaction is catalysed by UDP-Glucoronyl transferase. Now the bilirubin is said to be Conjugated bilirubin and is water soluble. It is secreted into bile
- Bilirubin enters the intestine through bile. In the ileum and colon, bilirubin is acted upon by the intestinal bacteria and is converted to urobilinogen. 80% of it is excreted in the stools as Stercobilinogen. The rest of it is absorbed into portal circulation and is taken back into the liver and re-excreted in bile
- Some urobilinogen enters general circulation and is excreted in urine
- Urobilinogen and stercobilinogen are oxidised to urobilin and stercobilin when exposed to air.

22. Movements of small intestine.

Refer February 2004 answers.

23. Steps involved in formation of urine.

- Glomerular filtration
- Tubular secretion
- Tubular re-absorption.

Glomerular Filtration

- **Plasma** is filtered across the glomerular membrane and all constituents except the proteins are present in the filtrate
- The osmolality of the ultrafiltrate is 300 mOsm/L.

Glomerular Membrane

- It is a 3 layered structure
  1. The capillary endothelial cell lining
  2. Epithelium lining the Bowman's capsule, made of Podocytes
  3. Between them, the basement membrane.
- The total area is $0.8 m^2$.

Glomerular Filtration Rate

- GFR is the rate at which the plasma is filtered into the Bowman's capsule by all the nephrons per unit of time
- It is about 125 mL/min or 180 L/day.

Factors Regulating GFR

- Hydrostatic pressure gradient across the capillary wall
- Osmotic pressure gradient across the capillary wall
- Size of the capillary bed
- Permeability of the membrane.

Control of GFR

- $GFR = K_f \times NFP$
  - K_f = Ultrafiltration co-efficient (Membrane factor)
  - NFP (Net filtration pressure)
    $= [(P_{GC} - P_T) - (\pi_{GC} - \pi_T)]$
    (Balance between Starling's forces)

Starling's forces are:

P_{GC} = Glomerular hydrostatic pressure
π_{GC} = Capillary oncotic pressure
P_{BS} = Hydrostatic pressure in Bowman's space
π_{BS} = Osmotic pressure in Bowman's space.

Ultrafiltration is the Balance Between the Starling's Forces

Forces favoring filtration are:

Glomerular capillary hydrostatic pressure = 45 mm Hg.

Forces opposing filtration are:

- Hydrostatic pressure in Bowman's space = 10 mm Hg
- Capillary oncotic pressure = 20 mm Hg
- Net glomerular filtration pressure are = $P_{GC} - P_{BS} - \pi_{GC}$ = 15 mm Hg.

Factors Affecting GFR

- Changes in renal blood flow
- Changes in glomerular capillary hydrostatic pressure: Dependant on systemic blood pressure and afferent and efferent arteriolar constriction. It is directly proportional to GFR
- Changes in hydrostatic pressure in Bowman's space: Dependant on ureteric obstruction and edema of kidney inside tight renal capsule. It is inversely proportional to GFR
- Concentration of plasma proteins decides plasma oncotic pressure. So dehydration and hypoproteinemia affect GFR. Oncotic pressure is inversely related to GFR.
- Factors affecting filtration co-efficient: Changes in glomerular capillary permeability and changes in effective filtration surface area. As the permeability and surface area increase GFR also increases.

Tubular Secretion and Reabsorption

- Transport of substances between filtrate and interstitium by two routes—transcellular and paracellular routes (refer Fig. 25)
- As the filtrate enters the tubule changes happen in each segment—proximal convoluted tubule (PCT), loop of Henle (LOH), distal convoluted tubule (DCT) and collecting duct.

We have discussed the reabsorption as well as secretion happening in each segment.

Events in PCT

- 65% of Na^+, Cl^- are reabsorbed from filtrate
- 80–90% HCO_3^- is reabsorbed
- 100% of Glucose and amino acids filtered are reabsorbed
- H^+ is secreted into the lumen
- 65% water filtered is reabsorbed here due to the osmotic gradient, $2/3^{rd}$—by paracellular, $1/3^{rd}$—by transcellular routes
- Water reabsorption helps to reabsorb Mg^{++}, Ca^{++} by solvent drag.

Events in Loop of Henle (Refer Fig. 26)

- 20% of filtered Na^+, Cl^- are reabsorbed
- 15% of H_2O (in Thin descending limb) and K^+, Ca^{++}, Mg^{++} are reabsorbed
- Some amount of H^+ secretion happens through Na^+-H^+ exchanger
- Descending limb of LOH is permeable to water whereas ascending limb is totally impermeable to water
- Counter-current flow of fluid in the ascending and descending limbs of LOH and Collecting duct helps in concentrating urine by building up an hyper-osmolar medullary interstitium.

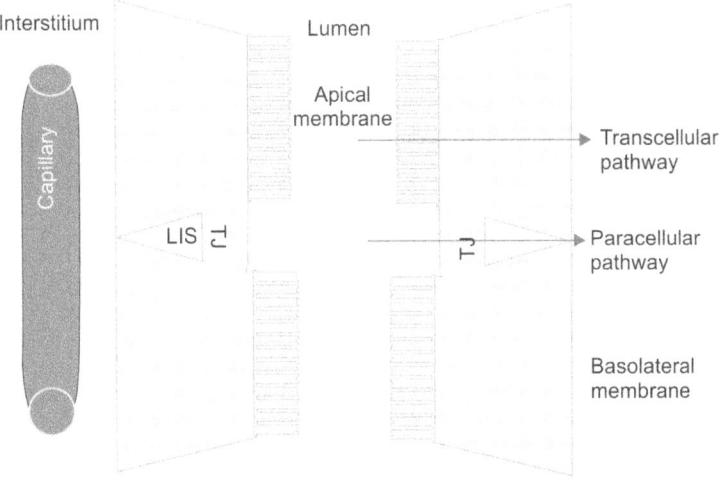

Fig. 25: Transport of substances across the epithelial cells in the nephron.
(LIS: lateral intercellular space; TJ: tight junction)

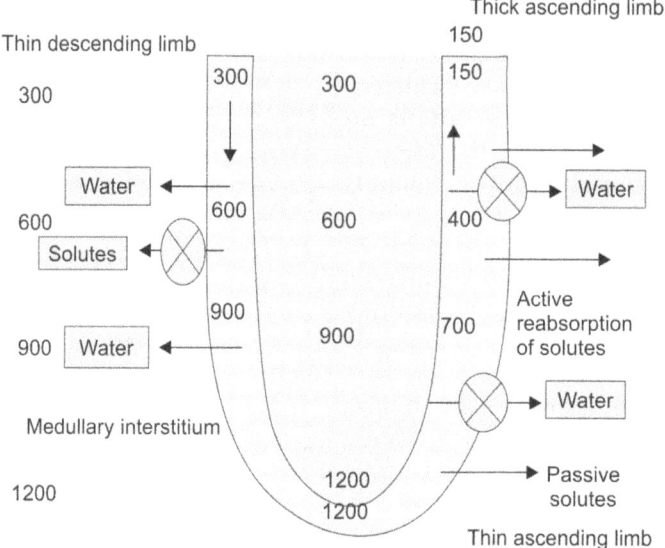

Fig. 26: Movement of solutes and water in the Loop of Henle (The numbers denote the osmolality of the fluids).

Events in Early Part of DCT

- Initial part of DCT is similar to TAL of LOH.
- It is also impermeable to water
- There is a NaCl symporter in the luminal membrane and reabsorbs Na⁺ and Cl⁻
- Nearly 7% of filtered NaCl is reabsorbed here.

Events in Late DCT and Collecting Duct

- In the late part of DCT and CD there are Principal (P) and Intercalated (I) cells
- Aldosterone and ADH act on P cells to increase Na⁺ and H_2O reabsorption respectively
- Aldosterone also stimulates K⁺ secretion
- There are 2 types of I cells (A and B), where H⁺ secretion and HCO_3 reabsorption or vice versa happens respectively.

After the above reabsorptions and secretions have happened in the tubule the final urine of 1-2 L/day of 1200 mOsm/L is excreted in normal conditions.

24. Spermatogenesis.

- The process of formation of mature sperm is called spermatogenesis
- It takes place in the seminiferous tubule. It happens in the wall of the tubule from basal lamina towards the lumen
- The immature cells are present in the basal aspect of the tubule and the maturing cells move toward the adluminal compartment
- Spermatogenesis invoves both mitotic and meiotic divisions and spermiogenesis (refer Fig. 27).

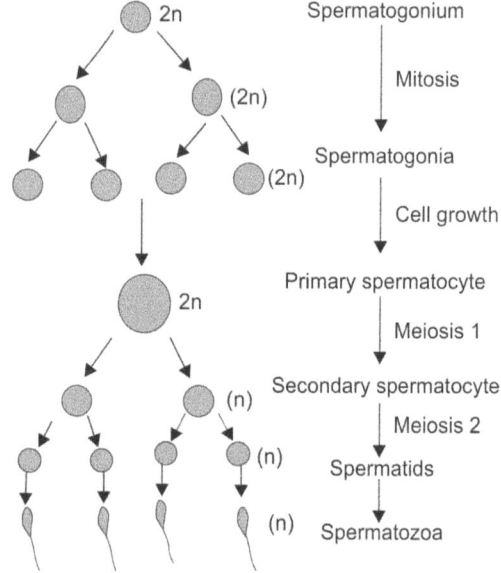

Fig. 27: Steps in spermatogenesis: 2n – Diploid number of chromosomes, n – Haploid number of chromosomes.

Mitotic Division

- The primitive germ cell, spermatogonia, in the basal lamina of the seminiferous tubule undergoes mitotic divisions to form primary spermatocytes
- Each spermatogonium divides 5 times to produce 32 spermatogonia
- 32 spermatogonia (44+X+Y) reach the adluminal side of the tubule and undergo mitosis to become 64 primary spermatocytes (44+X+Y)
- Primary spermatocytes are large cells with diploid number of chromosomes (2n).

Meiotic Divisions

- The primary spermatocytes with diploid number of chromosomes undergo the first meiotic division to form the secondary spermatocyte which is haploid in nature
- The second meiotic division results in formation of spermatids (22+X or Y)
- A total of 512 spermatids are drived from single spermatogonia.

Spermiogenesis

- The spermatids do not undergo further divisions but structural changes takes place as the spermatids mature into sperm—spermiogenesis
- This process happens in the deep folds of Sertoli cells.

The changes taking place are:

- The amount of cytoplasm is reduced in spermatids
- The nucleus elongates to become the head of sperm
- The acrosomal cap is formed
- The tail and middle piece are formed.

Spermiation

- After maturation the sperms stay attached to the sertoli cells
- The release of sperms into the tubule is called spermiation.

Factors Regulating Spermatogenesis

Hormones regulating spermatogenesis are—androgens, gonadotrophins and estrogen

- *Androgens:* A high concentration of testosterone in the tubular fluid is essential for spermatogenesis. LH stimulates Leydig cells to secrete testosterone. Sertoli cells secrete androgen binding protein (ABP) to which testosterone binds and its levels are kept elevated.
  Spermiogenesis is androgen dependent
- *LH:* It stimulates Leydig cells to secerete testosterone and thereby is needed for spermatogenesis
- *FSH:* Stimulates Sertoli cells and sertoli cells help in conversion of spermatids to sperms, secretion of ABP and secretion of inhibin. It also increases LH receptors in Leydig cells. It maintains gametogenic function of testis
- *Estrogen* content is high in the fluid in rete testis and estrogen acts to increase fluid reabsorption and spermatozoa is concentrated. This is essential for fertility of an individual
- *Body temperature:* Spermatogenesis takes place in a temperature less than the inner body temperature. The testis is kept at a temperature of 32°C. If the testis is exposed to higher temperatures the tubular walls degenerate and sterility results.

25. Neuroendocrinal reflex.

Refer answers to 2004 paper.

26. Adrenogenital syndrome.

- Synthesis of sex steroid takes place in zona reticularis (refer Fig. 28)
- Dehydroepiandrosterone (DHEA) and androstenedione are weak androgens
- They are converted into testosterone and estrogen in the periphery
- Small amounts of testosterone and estrogen are also synthesized in zona reticularis
- These adrenal androgens are the major source of androgen in females
- They are responsible for pubic and axillary hair growth in women and also for maintenance of RBC production

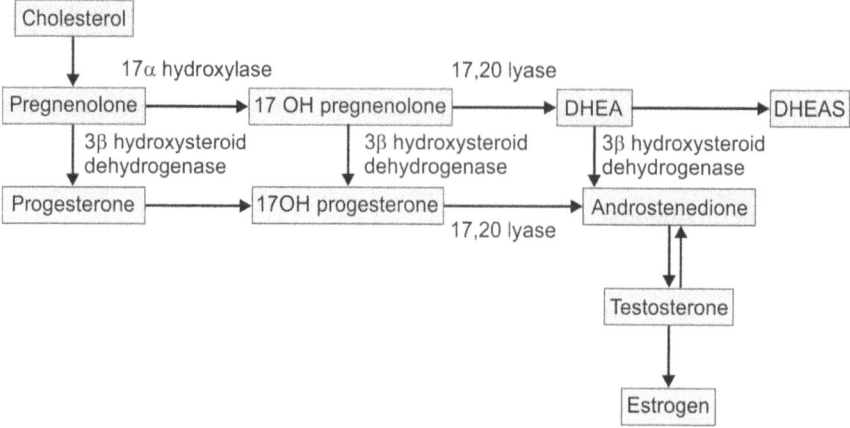

Fig. 28: Synthesis of adrenal androgens.

- In men it is of less importance because of the testicular source of testosterone
- In some pathological conditions where excess adrenal androgen is produced results in masculinization in females and premature puberty in men
- Some amount of testosterone is also converted to estrogen in periphery
- It forms a major source of estrogen in post menopausal women.

Congenital Adrenal Hyperplasia and Adrenogenital Syndrome

- Congenital absence of any enzymes in synthesis of cortisol results in high ACTH levels
- This leads to congenital adrenal hyperplasia (CAH)
- The most common cause of CAH is due to deficiency of the enzymes 21 and 11β hydroxylases
- This deficiency decreases cortisol synthesis
- But it increases the synthesis of the products before the blockage and the products are diverted to form excess of androgens.

Adrenogenital Syndrome due to 21β Hydroxylase Defeciency

- There is deficiency of glucocorticoids and mineralocorticoids
- So ACTH levels are high
- The substrates are diverted for synthesis of androgens resulting in their high levels
- Characterized by virilization and results in adrenogenital syndrome
- In severe case this results in masculinization of genitalia of a female fetus (female pseudohermophroditism)
- They lose Na^+ excessively—salt losing form of congenital virilizing adrenal hyperplasia.

Adrenogenital Syndrome due to 11β Hydroxylase Defeciency

- Decreased synthesis of cortisol
- ACTH levels are high
- Increased synthesis of adrenal androgens
- 11 deoxycorticosterone and 11 deoxycortisol are also in excess
- Salt and water retention is present
- This leads to hypertensive form of congenital virilizing adrenal hyperplasia.

27. Conducting system of the heart.

Refer answers to august 2004 paper.

28. Referred pain and its theories.

Referred Pain

Irritation of a vicus or viscera usually produces pain which is not usually felt in the location of the viscus but in a somatic structure that is in a distance from the viscus. This is **referred pain.**

For example:

1. Cardiac pain is usually referred to the inner aspect of the left arm or to the neck

2. When there is an irritation of central region of diaphragm there is pain in the tip of the shoulder
3. Pain in the testicle due to distension of ureter as in ureteric calculus.

Theories of Referred Pain

The pain in viscera is usually referred to a somatic structure that has developed from the same embryonic segment or dermatome as the structure in which the pain originates— **dermatomal rule**.

Theories of referred pain are— convergence theory and facilitation theory.

Convergence Theory

- Peripheral nerve fibers from the somatic and visceral structures converge on the same second order neuron present in lamina V of dorsal grey horn (refer Fig. 29)
- The second order neuron is common for impulses from somatic and visceral structures
- So the tract carrying pain sensation from somatic structures also carry pain fibers from visceral structures
- Cortex sometimes cannot differentiate from somatic and visceral inputs and so pain from visceral structure is referred to the somatic structure.

Facilitation Theory

- The visceral afferent fibers on entering spinal cord give collaterals to afferents coming from the somatic structures (refer Fig. 30)
- So impulses coming from the visceral afferents facilitate and strengthen the impulses coming from the somatic structure
- So a minor activity in the somatic afferents is facilitated by the visceral afferents and therefore pain is referred to the somatic structure.

29. EEG changes during sleep.

- Sleep is said to be a state of altered consciousness or partial unconsciousness from which a person can be aroused
- Sleep has two components – Non rapid eye movement (NREM) and Rapid eye movement (REM) sleep
- NREM sleep has four stages, each with different EEG activities (refer Fig. 31).

Stage 1

- Stage of transition between wakefulness and sleep
- Lasts for 1–7 minutes
- Person is relaxed with eyes closed and fleeting thoughts

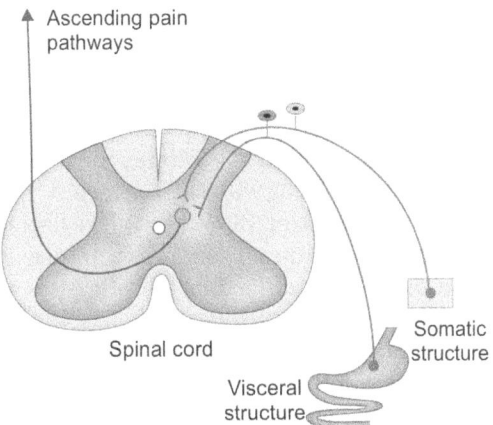

Fig. 29: Convergence theory of referred pain. Note the afferents from somatic and visceral structures converge on the same second order neuron.
(*Source:* GK Pal)

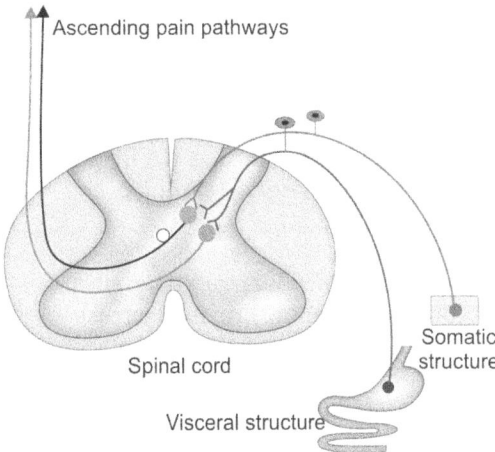

Fig. 30: Facilitation theory of referred pain. Note the visceral afferents give a collateral to second order neurons of somatic structure.
(*Source:* GK Pal)

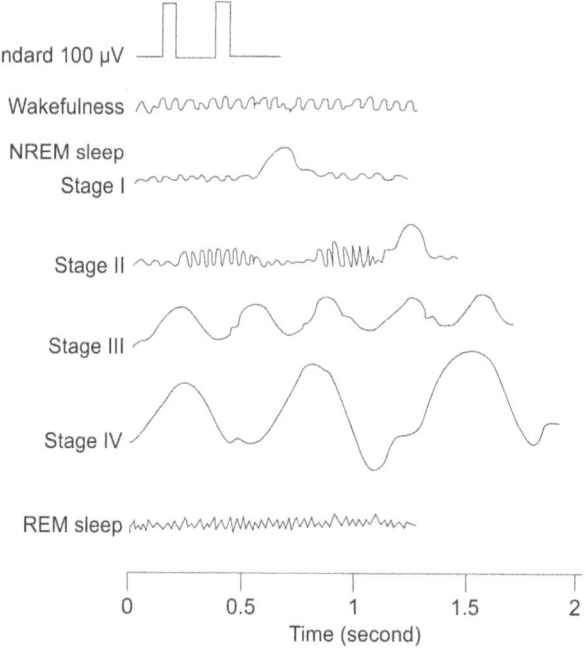

Fig. 31: EEG changes in various stages of sleep.
(*Source: Sembulingam*)

- Alpha waves which were present will diminish
- People when awakened at this stage will say that they were not sleeping.

Stage 2
- Stage of light sleep
- It is little more difficult to wake the person
- Fragments of dreams maybe experienced
- Eyes may role from side to side
- EEG shows sleep spindles – bursts of sharply pointed waves occurring at a frequency of 12–14 Hz and lasts 1–2 seconds.

Stage 3
- Is a period of moderately deep sleep
- Body temperature and BP decrease
- It is difficult to wake the person
- EEG shows mixture of sleep spindles and large, low frequency waves
- This stage occurs 20 minutes after falling asleep.

Stage 4 or Slow Wave Sleep
- Deepest level of sleep
- Brain metabolism drops significantly
- Body temperature slightly falls
- Muscle tone is decreased only slightly
- Reflexes are intact
- EEG shows slow, large amplitude Delta waves.

A person during sleep will go from stage 1–4 in about 1 hour. Then has the REM sleep.

REM Sleep
- In a period of sleep of 7–8 hrs, REM and NREM sleep alternate
- REM sleep occurs 3–5 times during the sleep alternating with NREM sleep
- Initial episode of REM sleep will be lasting for 10–20 minutes. Then with each episode it prolongs and the final episode is for 50 minutes
- In adults REM sleep totals for about 90–120 minutes. With increasing age period of REM sleep decreases
- After the stage 4 slow wave sleep, in REM sleep the large amplitude slow waves are replaced by rapid low voltage waves, as seen in stage 1 sleep

- That is why this phase is also called as paradoxical sleep.

30. Excitation-contraction coupling in skeletal muscles.

Refer answers to 2003 paper.

31. Classification of sensory receptors and their properties.

Receptors are transducers which convert any form of energy into electrical potentials.

There are many types of classifications:

Classifications of Receptors

Based on Source of Stimulus

1. **Exteroceptors:** Receptors which receive stimulus from external environment close to the body. For example, cutaneous receptors—receptors for touch, pain, temperature etc.
2. **Interoceptors:** Receptors which collect informations from within the body. For example, chemoreceptors, baroreceptors, osmoreceptors, proprioceptors etc.
3. **Telereceptors:** Receptors which receive information from a distant stimuli. For example, visual, auditory and olfactory receptors.

Based on Type of Stimulus

1. **Mechanoreceptors:** Responds to mechanical stimuli like touch, pressure etc. They can be cutaneous receptors which sense it from the skin and subcutaneous tissues
2. **Thermoreceptors:** Detects the change in temperature
3. **Chemoreceptors:** Sense the chemical changes in the environment. For example, taste receptors, olfactory receptors, aortic and carotid bodies etc.
4. **Photoreceptors:** Sense light. For example, rods and cones
5. **Nociceptors:** Receptors for pain.

Based on Adaptation to Stimulus

1. **Tonic receptors or slow adapting receptors:** They adapt slowly or do not get adapted at all. For example, receptors for pain
2. **Phasic receptor or fast adapting receptor:** They get adapted quickly to a stimulus. For example, touch receptor.

Properties of Receptors

1. **Specificity:** Receptors are specific to a particular sensory modality and respond to them at a lowest intensity. They can also respond to other stimuli but at a higher threshold. For example, retina responds to light but on deep pressure to eye a sensation of light is generated
2. **Adequate stimulus:** Only on giving an adequate stimulus the receptor is stimulated
3. **Mullers' Doctrine of specific nerve energies:** This gives information about how the sensations are coded. When a nerve fiber from a specific sense organ is stimulated at any point of pathway, the sensation evoked depends on the part of the brain it reaches and the sensation produced is that for which the receptor is specialized
4. **Law of projection:** This codes the location of stimulus. Along the pathway anywhere from the receptor to brain, wherever stimulated, the conscious sensation is referred to the location of receptor. This is one of the cause for phantom limb phenomenon
5. **Adaptation:** Receptors are capable of adaptation. Some are slow adapting, e.g. pain receptors and some are fast adapting, e.g. touch receptor
6. **Localisation of sensation:** This is due to presence of specific receptors in the location
7. **Intensity discrimination:** Based on Weber-Fechner law. This law codes for the intensity of stimulus. There are two ways by which intensity is coded:
   a. By variation in the frequency of action potentials
   b. By variation in the number of receptors stimulated.

   This law states that magnitude of sensation felt is proportional to log of intensity of stimulus.

32. Clinical classification of reflexes with examples and their significance.

Clinical Classification of Reflexes

1. **Superficial reflexes:** These refelexes are obtained by stimulating the receptors in skin or mucous membrane from the surface of the body. Examples are – Plantar reflex, conjunctival reflex, cremastric reflex, abdominal reflex etc. These reflexes are having afferents and efferents travelling in spinal cord and are lost in UMN lesions
2. **Deep reflexes:** These reflexes are obtained by stimulating receptors in the deeper tissues like muscles and joints. Examples are knee jerk, biceps jerk, etc. These reflexes are lost in LMN lesion and are exaggerated in UMN lesions
3. **Visceral reflexes:** Baroreceptor reflex, chemoreceptor reflex, micturition reflex etc. They are obtained by stimulating receptors located in the viscera
4. **Pathological reflexes:** These refelxes are present only in pathological conditions like Babinski's sign or extensor plantar reflex. It is seen in corticospinal tract lesion.

MBBS Examination 2007

ANSWER ALL QUESTIONS

I. Essay questions (15/20 Marks each)

1. Describe glucose homeostasis in detail. Briefly explain GTT. Add a note on diabetes mellitus and physiological basis of treatment. (20 marks)
2. Describe menstrual cycle in detail and explain the hormonal control involved in various phases. Add a note on pregnancy tests. (15 marks)
3. Describe in detail how urine is concentrated in kidneys. Add a note on kidney function tests. (15 marks)
4. Describe a normal ECG recorded from standard limb lead and explain how each wave is produced. Describe ECG changes in abnormal conditions. (20 marks)
5. Describe the connections and functions of basal ganglia in detail. Explain the clinical disorders and physiological basis of management. (15 marks)
6. Describe the refractory errors of eye and explain the physiological basis of their corrections. (15 marks)
7. Define hemostasis. Explain the steps involved in intrinsic mechanism of clotting. Add a note on hemophilia. (15 marks)
8. Describe in detail the phases of deglutition. (15 marks)
9. Classify hypoxia, what are the causes and features of each type? What types respond best to oxygen therapy? (15 marks)
10. Draw and label the visual pathway. What are the effects of lesions at various levels of pathways. (15 marks)

II. Short notes (5 Marks each)

1. Blood groups.
2. Anticoagulants.
3. Micturition reflex.
4. Fat absorption.
5. Plasma proteins.
6. Gastrointestinal hormones.
7. Neural regulation of respiration.
8. Hypoxia.
9. Excitation-contraction coupling.
10. Functions of middle ear.
11. Functions of parietal lobe.
12. Functions of thalamus.
13. Artificial kidney.
14. Feedback mechanisms.
15. Female contraceptives.
16. Nerve action potential.
17. Hypothyroidism.
18. B-lymphocytes.
19. Cytoskeleton.
20. Erythropoietin.
21. Calcitonin.
22. Functions of blood.
23. Korotkov's sound.
24. Heart sounds.
25. Timed vital capacity.
26. Oxygen dissociation curve.
27. Non-respiratory functions of lung.
28. ECG leads.
29. Baroreceptors.
30. Color blindness.
31. Parkinsonism.
32. Middle ear.

I. ESSAY QUESTIONS

1. Describe glucose homeostasis in detail. Briefly explain GTT. Add a note on diabetes mellitus and physiological basis of treatment.

Glucose Homeostasis

- Normal fasting peripheral venous blood glucose level is 70–90 mg/dL
- After food intake, it reaches 110–130 mg/dL and after 2 hours it comes back to normal values. Blood glucose levels are 20 mg/dL higher in arterial blood
- There are hormones which increase blood glucose levels and hormones which decrease blood glucose levels.

Hormones which increase blood glucose levels are:

- Glucagon
- Glucocorticoids
- Catecholamines
- Growth hormone
- Thyroid hormones.

Hormones which decrease blood glucose levels: Insulin.

Mechanisms of Actions of Hormones

Glucagon

- It increases blood glucose levels by various mechanisms like glycogenolysis and gluconeogenesis
- In the liver it activates the enzyme phosphorylase and breaks down glycogen
- Glycogenolysis is favored by activating Phospholipase C and increase in cytoplasmic Ca^{2+} in the hepatocytes. It has no glycogenolytic action on muscles
- It increases gluconeogenesis with the help of pyruvate, lactate, glycerol and amino acids.

Glucocorticoids

- Increases gluconeogenesis in liver → increases glycogen stores
- Antagonizes the action of insulin on muscle and adipose tissue – prevents glucose uptake by these cells
- This spares glucose for the brain
- Increases glucose output from the liver
- Induces hyperglycemia.

Catecholamines

- Adrenaline acts via β and α-adrenergic receptors
- Thereby increases hepatic glucose output by activating the enzyme phosphorylase and induces hyperglycemia
- Phosphorylase is activated in the skeletal muscle also, but glucose-6-phosphate is converted to pyruvate because of the absence of glucose-6-phosphatase
- Pyruvate is converted to lactate which diffuses into circulation and is oxidised in the liver to pyruvate and then to glycogen
- Therefore on stimulation by epinephrine there is initial glycogenolysis followed by glycogen synthesis
- Stimulates gluconeogenesis
- Epinephrine also decreases peripheral utilization of glucose
- Stimulates secretion of glucagon.

Growth Hormone

- Effects of growth hormone are both direct and indirect (through IGF-1)
- It increases hepatic glucose output by stimulating gluconeogenesis
- It has anti-insulin effect and thereby prevents peripheral utilization of glucose by the tissues
- It decreases insulin sensitivity.

Thyroid Hormone

- It increases blood glucose levels by increasing absorption of glucose from intestines
- It also for some extent increases hepatic glucose output and thereby depletion of hepatic glycogen
- Glycogen depletion in hepatocytes induces damage to hepatocytes and decreases glucose uptake
- It also causes degradation of insulin.

Insulin

- Insulin favors glucose storage in the liver. It **enhances glucose entry** into liver cells

by stimulating the enzyme glucokinase which phosphorylates glucose to glucose-6-phosphate thereby maintaining a gradient for glucose entry into hepatocytes
- Insulin stimulates glycolysis in skeletal muscles, adipose tissue and liver by activating the enzyme phosphofructokinase and pyruvate
- **Glycogen synthesis and its storage** are enhanced by stimulation of the enzyme glycogen synthase
- It inhibits glycogenolysis and prevents glucose output from liver
- It also **inhibits gluconeogenesis**
- In skeletal muscles and adipose tissues, insulin facilitates glucose entry into muscle cells by inserting the glucose transporter GLUT 4 and it also stimulates the enzyme hexokinase.

Effect of Exercise

Exercise increases glucose uptake into skeletal muscles by inducing an insulin-independent increase in GLUT transporters in the muscle membrane. The effect of exercise in lowering blood glucose levels lasts for many hours and it can induce hypoglycemia in diabetics with insulin treatment. Therefore the dosage of insulin should be adjusted in diabetics if they are exercising.

Glucose Tolerance Test

- It is a test in which an oral dose of glucose is given and series of blood samples are collected to check how quickly the glucose is cleared from blood. It is usually done to test for diabetes, glucose intolerance etc.
- This test is based on the principle that in diabetics, blood glucose levels rise steeply after food intake. In a diabetic patient, when a glucose load is given, the blood glucose level rises and comes back to baseline level very slowly than in normal individuals.

Methodology
- 75g of glucose in 300 ml of water is given to the adults
- In normal individuals the fasting venous blood glucose level is less than 115 mg/dL. After 2 hours the value is less than 140 mg/dL and none of the values is more than 200 mg/dL
- Impaired glucose tolerance is when the values are above upper normal limit but below the value for diagnosis of diabetes (110-126 mg/dL in fasting and 140-200 mg/dL in peak levels)
- In diabetics, the glucose tolerance curve is abnormal. Fasting blood glucose is >126 mg/dL and after glucose intake peak value reached is >200 mg/dL and takes nearly 4-6 hours to reach baseline value.

Diabetes Mellitus

Defeciency of insulin is Diabetes mellitus.

Causes

Diabetes mellitus occurs due to destruction of β cells of islets in the pancreas or due to decreased sensitivity of receptors for insulin. Based on the causes and features diabetes is classified into two types—Type 1 and Type 2 Diabetes mellitus (**Primary diabetes mellitus**).

Secondary diabetes mellitus: Diabetes is secondary to some other diseases like Cushing's syndrome, acromegaly, pancreatitis etc.

Type 1 diabetes mellitus:
- This is due to autoimmune destruction of β cells and insulin is not secreted
- Plasma insulin levels are low and undetectable
- This condition is treated with only insulin and therefore also called as Insulin dependent diabetes mellitus (IDDM)
- Antibodies are present against β cell surface antigens
- It is usually seen in children and adults of <45 years of age
- They are prone for ketoacidosis and are thin
- Chance of developing the disease in identical twins is 50%

Type 2 diabetes mellitus:
- This is due to decreased sensitivity of insulin receptors for insulin
- Insulin levels are normal or even elevated

- Therefore it is also called as Non-insulin dependent diabetes mellitus (NIDDM)
- The individual with NIDDM are obese and the disease occurs usually after 45 years of age
- This is the most common type of DM
- The chance of developing the disease in identical disease is 100%.

Symptoms of DM

DM is characterized by polyphagia, polydipsia, polyuria, weight loss, hyperglycemia and glycosuria. In severe conditon it leads to ketoacidosis and coma.

a. *Polyphagia:* Increased food intake. This is due to inability of usage of glucose by the neurons in satiety center of hypothalamus due to absence of insulin. So the low glucose in these cells leads to stimulation of the feeding center and thereby increased food intake
b. *Polyuria:* Passage of large amounts of urine. As the plasma glucose levels increase, the amount of glucose filtered is also increased. The SGLT transporter in renal tubular cells of PCT gets saturated and is not able to reabsorb glucose from the filtrate and glucose starts appearing in the urine. The glucose when retained in tubule holds back water and other electrolytes in the tubule and results in osmotic diuresis. Other ions like Na^+, K^+ and phosphates are also lost in urine
c. *Polydipsia:* When water is lost excessively, thirst mechanism is stimulated because of cellular dehydration and water intake is increased
d. *Weight loss* is due to loss of calories in the urine and mobilization of other stores like fats and proteins resulting in weight loss
e. *Hyperglycemia* is due to decreased peripheral utilization of glucose by skeletal muscles, adipose tissues and liver. There is also increased glucose output from liver
f. *Glycosuria* is excessive loss of glucose in urine. This happens when the renal threshold (>180 mg/dL) is reached. Glycosuria leads to all the symptoms mentiond above.

Physiological Basis of Treatment of DM

a. *Sulfonylurea derivatives* like Tolbutamide, acetohexamide, glipizide, glyburide are hypoglycemic agents and they decrease blood glucose levels by increasing production of insulin. So they are effective in people with some amount of working β cells. It cannot be used in Type 1 DM. They act by inhibiting ATP-inhibited K^+ channels and decrease K^+ efflux thereby depolarizing the membrane and favours Ca^{2+} influx and release of insulin
b. The other groups of drugs are *biguanides* like Phenformin, Metformin which act in the absence of insulin. They decrease the hepatic output of glucose and thereby decreases blood glucose levels. Metformin can be used in combination with sulfonylureas in treatment for Type 2 DM
c. *Thiazolidinediones* like Triglitazone are hypoglycemic agents which increase the insulin-mediated peripheral utilization of glucose. They act by binding to peroxisome proliferator-activated receptor (PPARγ)
d. *Exercise:* It is a very effective startegy to decrease blood glucose levels in Type 1 and Type 2 DM. Exercise increases glucose entry into skeletal muscle by inserting an insulin independent GLUT 4 glucose transporter in muscle cell membranes. This increases glucose uptake by muscle cells for a prolonged duration after exercise also and therefore regular exercise can increase insulin sensitivity.

2. Describe menstrual cycle in detail and explain the hormonal control involved in various phases. Add a note on pregnancy tests.

Menstrual Cycle

- Menstrual cycle is the female sexual cycle and it happens once in 28–30 days. It is associated with uterine bleeding—menstruation
- It is a preparatory cycle for fertilization and implantation of the fertilized ovum
- Therefore cyclic changes happen in the uterus, ovaries, cervix and vagina

- All these changes are under the control of various hormones
- The hormones regulating menstrual cycle are hypothalamic hormones (GnRH), anterior pituitary hormones (FSH and LH) and ovarian hormones (estrogen and progesterone)
- GnRH from hypothalamus is the key controller of gonadotrophin released from anterior pituitary
- GnRH is secreted in pulsatile fashion and the pulsatility of GnRH is very important in regulating secretions of LH and FSH
- GnRH pulsatility is in turn kept in check by levels of estrogen and progesterone. Just before LH surge, pulsatility of GnRH is increased by high levels of estrogen
- We will be now discussing the hormonal regulation for ovarian changes and endometrial changes seperately.

Regulation of Ovarian Changes

Ovarian changes happen in 3 phases:
- Follicular phase
- Ovulatory phase
- Luteal phase.

Follicular Phase

- This phase starts from day 1 of menstruation to the day of ovulation (usually 14th day)
- Day 1 onwards the FSH and LH levels start increasing. Due to the actions of FSH, 10 - 20 follicles start to grow in size
- The granulosa cells of the follicles acquire FSH receptors and start secreting estrogen. Only one follicle continues to grow and become the dominant follicle and this is the follicle which secretes estrogen maximally. Other follicles become atretic
- The estrogen levels start increasing. Estrogen along with FSH induces LH receptors on granulosa cells and theca cells
- LH acts on theca cells to increase androgen synthesis and this androgen is diverted to granulosa cells for synthesis of estrogen
- Now the rising estrogen levels have a **positive feedback** effect on LH secretion from the anterior pituitary resulting in LH peak or LH surge. LH stimulates granulosa cells to synthesize progesterone
- 9 hours after the LH surge, ovulation happens on the 14th day
- As LH increases, progesterone levels increase and the proteolytic enzyme activity (Plasmin) is enhanced resulting in distension of follicle and the rupture of follicle is stimulated by Prostaglandins and leukotrienes. This results in ovulation.

Luteal Phase

- This phase starts after the ovulation and lasts for 14 days. This time period is a constant one
- Following ovulation the follicle is filled with blood and is called as corpus hemorrhagicum
- Soon after the release of ovum, granulosa and theca cells of the follicle proliferate and become lipid laden and are now yellow in color and are called as luteal cells. Now the follicle is called as—corpus luteum
- Corpus luteum, under the influence of LH, starts secreting progesterone, estrogen and inhibin. High levels of these hormones negatively inhibit the secretion of FSH and LH
- The maintanence of corpus luteum function is by the action of LH
- If ovum is not fertilized, corpus luteum reaches a peak secretion of steroidal hormones by 7 days following ovulation and then begins to undergo degeneration and luteolysis and becomes a scar tissue—corpus albicans
- Now the hormone production of corpus luteum drops and progesterone, estrogen and inhibin levels decrease
- The inhibition over FSH and LH is lifted and there is a rise in FSH levels which induces the next cycle with the development of new set of follicles

Regulation of Changes in the uterine endometrium: The uterine changes are given in 3 phases (refer Figs. 1A to D):
- Proliferative phase
- Secretory phase
- Menstrual phase.

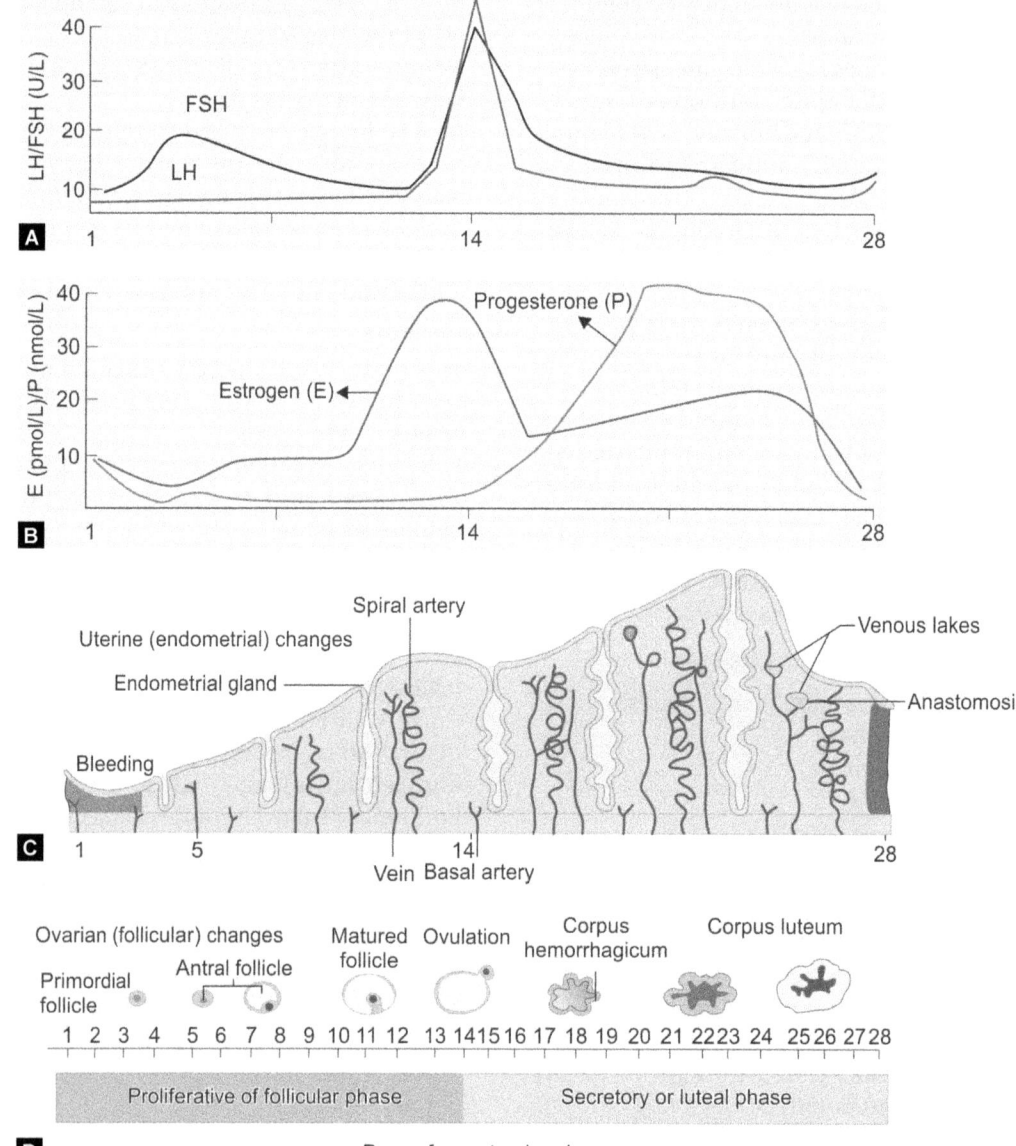

Figs. 1A to D: Menstrual cycle. Hormonal changes, changes in endometrium and changes in ovary.
(*Source:* GK Pal)

Proliferative Phase

- This phase correlates with the follicular phase of ovarian cycle
- Estrogen secreted from the follicle stimulates growth of uterine endometrium and therefore it thickens
- Glands in the endometrium and the blood vessels in endometrium also grows
- This phase is from day 5 till the day of ovulation.

Secretory Phase

- This phase is from the day of ovulation to 25th day of the cycle
- It correlates with the luteal phase in the ovarian cycle
- Progesterone levels are high and they make the endometrium secretory by acting on the glands. Maximum action is 5–7 days after ovulation

- The secretion from the endometrial glands is rich in glycogen and can nourish the fertilized ovum
- The secretory endometrium is favourable for implantation of fertilized ovum
- If fertilization does not happen, corpus luteum starts to regress and the progesterone and estrogen levels decrease
- Withdrawal of hormonal support of the endometrium and release of prostaglandins result in vasoconstriction of the spiral arteries → uterine ischemia happens and endometrial necrosis and shedding of endometrium happens resulting in bleeding.

Menstrual Phase

It starts with the menstrual bleeding with the shedding of outer 2/3rd of endometrium and unfertilized ovum and it continues for 5 days.

Pregnancy Tests

The pregnancy tests are grouped as:
1. **Biological tests:** Injection of urine of pregnant female containing hCG into animals and look for presence of ovulation in female animals and shedding of sperm in male animals
2. **Immunological tests:** Antibodies are produced for hCG and mixed with urine of pregnant female and then with RBC or latex particle coated with hCG. Presence of agglutination indicates negative for pregnancy and absence of agglutination indicates pregnancy
3. **One step immunoassay test (strip test):** The hCG antibody is mixed with a dye and is impregnated on a strip of paper. When the strip comes in contact with the urine containing hCG, a pink-purple band appears, indicating pregnancy
4. **Radiological test: Pregnancy tests 1, 2 and 3 are based on the presence of the hormone hCG present in the urine of pregnant female. It is detected in urine as early as 9 days by radioimmunoassay**
5. **Enzyme-linked immunosorbent assay (ELISA):** It is a quantitative test where even minute levels of hCG can be identified to confirm pregnancy
6. **Radioimmunoassay** can also be done.

---

3. Describe in detail how urine is concentrated in kidneys. Add a note on kidney function tests.

Refer answers to 2004 paper.

Kidney Function Tests

Kidney functions are assessed by methods of renal clearance tests and examination of blood and urine.

Urine Examination

a. *Normal urine volume:* 1.5L/day. Urine output can be decreased in terminal stages of renal failure and glomerulonephritis
b. *Colour:* Pale yellow due to presence of pigments like urochrome and urobilin
c. *Specific gravity of normal urine* (indicates tubular concentrating and diluting ability): Normal value, 1001–1040
   Maximum diluted urine – 1001
   Maximum concentrated urine – 1040
   Water deprivation should result in increase in specific gravity to 1025 and osmolar concentration of urine is increased to 1000 mOsm/L. Failure to concentrate urine indicates abnormal renal function as in acute nephritis. Decrease in specific gravity is seen in renal failure
d. *Urine pH* (indicates tubular capacity to acidify urine): Normal urine pH is 4.5–8
e. *Microscopic examination:* Look for urine sediments
   - Normal constituents are WBCs (1-2), few epithelial cells
   - Abnormal constituents are: RBCs, bacteria, albumin, ketones and granular casts.

Blood Examination

a. Blood urea – 20–40 mg/dL
b. Serum creatinine – 0.6–1.2 mg/dL. Serum creatinine is a good indicator of GFR. Increase in creatinine levels indictaes defects in filtration
c. Serum electrolytes – K^+, Na^+, Ca^{2+}, Mg^{++}, Phosphates, sulfates, serum proteins (in

nephrotic syndrome there is albuminuria leading to decrease in serum albumin)
d. Serum uric acid
e. Serum cholesterol—150-200 mg%. It increases in nephrotic syndrome.

Renal Clearance Tests

- Renal clearance means the volume of plasma getting completely cleared of a substance per minute by the kidneys
- It is calculated if the concentration of the substance in urine and plasma are known and the volume of urine excreted per unit time is also known
- $C_x = U_x \times V / P_x$
- C_x = Clearance of the substance X
- Ux = Urine concentartion of the substance
- V = Urine flow per mnute
- P_x = Plasma concentration of the substance X.

If X is urea then

- U_{urea} = 20mg/mL
- V = 1 mL/min
- P_{urea} = 30 mg/dL
- C_{urea} = 20 × 100/30 = 67 mL/min
- Renal clearance tests can be used to estimate GFR, tubular reabsorption and secretion.

a. GFR is estimated by studying the clearance of inulin or creatinine. Inulin is s fructose polymer and is excreted only by filtration. It is neither secreted nor reabsorbed. It is also not toxic and not metabolised in the body
b. PAH clearance is used to assess tubular secretion capacity and to estimate renal plasma flow
c. Osmotic clearance: Amount of plasma cleared of the osmotically active particals. Normal value - 3 mL/min
d. Phenol sulphonephthalein (PSP) excretion test: The ability to excrete PSP by the kidneys is an indicator of general function of the kidneys. Decrease in PSP excretion (about 70% is excreted in 2 hours) indicates loss of function of nephrons. Increased excretion indicates early renal inflammation.

Other Methods

a. Micropuncture method: Samples of fluid from various tubular sites are taken by micropuncture and compared with reference standards
b. Stop flow technique: Stopping the ureteral flow for 1-2 minutes and then while collecting samples, the first few are from collecting duct, then from DCT, Loop of Henle and the last few are from PCT.
c. Microcryoscopic study: Slices of renal tissues at different depths are studied.
d. Radiographic studies: Plain radiograph abdomen, intravenous pyelography (IVP)
e. Ultrasound examination, radionuclide studies, MRI, PET
f. Renal biopsy.

---

4. Describe a normal ECG recorded from standard limb lead and explain how each wave is produced. Describe ECG changes in abnormal conditions.

Refer answers to 2005 paper.

ECG Changes in Abnormal Conditions

Cardiac Arrhythmias

Sinus rhythm:
In a normal heart, the electrical activity originates and spreads towards the ventricles following which contraction of ventricles happen. This happens rhythmically and the normal heart rate is 70/min and is said to be the sinus rhythm as the impulse originates from the SA node.

During respiration there is alteration in the rhytm, increase in rate during inspiration and decrease in rate in expiration—**sinus arrhythmia**. This is because of fluctuation of parasympathetic output to heart.

Diseases affecting sinus node:
- Sinus bradycardia: Decrease in heart rate but follows sinus rhythm as in sleep
- Sinus tachycardia: Increase in heart rate as in exercise, emotions, fever etc.
- Sick sinus syndrome: Diseases affecting sinus node leading to marked bradycardia, dizziness and syncope.

Conduction Defects (refer Figs. 2A to D)

- Other portions of the conducting system other than the SA node can also generate impulses
- Since the rate of SA node is faster the impulses discharged here are conducted below to the conducting system at a faster rate and is followed by the other tissues
- But in disease conditions if there are blocks in conduction, other parts of conduction system can generate electrical activity and they are said to be *ectopic pacemakers*
- If there is interruption of conduction of impulses from atria to ventricle it is said to be atrioventricular block (AV Block)
- There are three types of AV blocks: First degree block, second degree block and third degree or complete heart block
  a. First degree block: Conduction between atria and ventricle is slowed as prolonged AV Nodal delay and there is no complete interruption of conduction. It is said to be first degree block. Each P wave is followed by a QRS complex, but there is prolongation of PR interval (refer Fig. 2A)
  b. Second degree block: Here not all the atrial impulses are conducted to the ventricles and there may be a ventricular beat following every second or third atrial beat, 2:1 or 3:1 block. This type is said to be **Mobitz type II block** (refer Fig. 2B).
  In another type of incomplete block, there are repeated sequences of beats in which the PR interval lengthens progressively until a ventricular beat is dropped – **Wenckebach phenomenon**. This type is said to be **Mobitz type I** (refer Fig. 2C)
  c. Third degree or complete heart block: Here conduction of impulses from atria to ventricle are completely interrupted and the ventricles beat at a slow rate— idioventricular rhythm. It could be a AV nodal block or infranodal block (refer Fig. 2D).
  The ventricular rate may be lowered to 40-35/min and sometimes there could be a minute of asystole leading to cerebral ischemia and fainting— *Stokes-Adams syndrome*. Causes could be septal MI and damage to His bundle
  d. Bundle branch block: Block of one branch of bundle of His—right or left bundle branch block. Ventricular rate is normal, but QRS complex is prolonged and deformed
  e. Hemiblock or Fascicular block: Block in anterior or posterior fascicle of the left bundle branch. Left anterior hemiblock leads to left axis deviation and left posterior hemiblock causes right axis deviation.

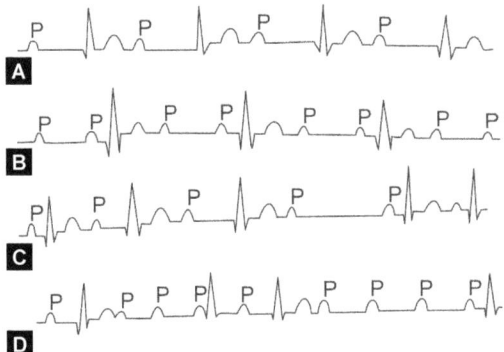

Figs. 2A to D: Conduction defects. (A) First degree block; (B) Second degree heart block, Mobitz type II block; (C) Second degree block, Mobitz Type I; (D) Third degree heart block.
(*Source:* GK Pal)

Arrhythmias

Atrial Arrhythmias

Atrial extrasystole:

- Excitation arises from an individual ectopic foci in atria and spreads to the ventricle
- The P wave of extrasystole is abnormal but the following QRST complex is normal (refer Fig. 3A)
- It is seen in conditions like anxiety, excess intake of tea, coffee, coronary artery disease etc.

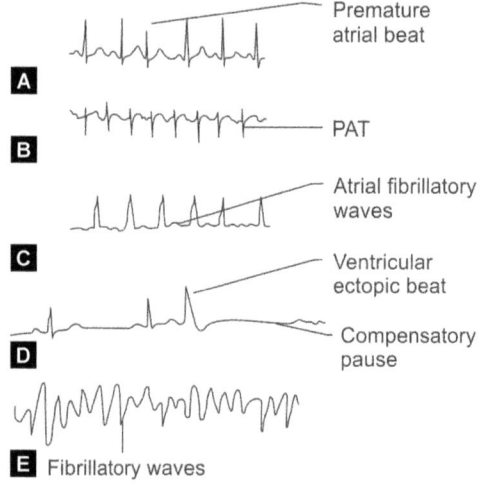

Figs. 3A to E: Atrial and Ventricular arrhythmias.
(PAT: Paroxysmal atrial tachycardia)
(*Source:* GK Pal)

Atrial tachycardia:
- Atrial rates can be upto 220/min (refer Fig. 3B)
- It could be due to an ectopic foci discharging rapidly or due to a reentrant circuit.

Atrial flutter:
- The rate is 200 – 350/min
- It is commonly due to a counter-clockwise circus movement in right atrium. ECG recording shows a sawtooth like flutter waves
- It is usually associated with 2:1 or greater AV block. AV node cannot conduct more than 230 impulses per minute.

Atrial fibrillation:
- Atria rates are 300–500/min (refer Fig. 3C)
- Atria beats completely irregularly and in a disorganised fashion
- Due to AV nodal delay ventricles beat in an irregular rate, 80–160/min. It could be chronic, paroxysmal or genetic
- It happens because of multiple concurrent circulating reentrant excitation waves in both atria
- In atrial tachycardia, flutter and fibrillation the diastolic phase is shortened and so the ventricular filling and cadiac output are reduced and symptoms of heart failue happens.

Ventricular Arrhythmias
Ventricular ectopics:
- These ectopics appear as bizarrely shaped prolonged QRS complexes (refer Fig. 3D)
- If the next succeeding normal SA nodal impulse depolarise the atria the P wave is buried in the QRS complex
- When this reaches the ventricle it is refractory from the ectopic impulse
- Therefore there is a compensatory pause following an ectopic beat.

Paroxysmal ventricular tachycardia:
- These are a series of rapid, regular ventricular depolarisations due to circus movement involving the ventricles
- The QRS morphology is totally deformed as in Torsede des pointes
- Ventricular tachycardia can be differentiated from supraventricular tachycardia by a His bundle electrogram
- Ventricular tachycardia is more serious as it decreases the cardiac output and also can be complicated by ventricular fibrillation.

Ventricular fibrillation:
- This happens due to a very rapid discharge of multiple ectopic foci or a circus movement
- Ventricles contract in a totally irregular and ineffective way. There is improper pumping of blood and if it lasts for few minutes it can be fatal (refer Fig. 3E)
- VF can also be produced in electric shock or by an extrasystole during a critical interval, the 'Vulnerable period'. It coincides in time with the midportion of T wave.

Accelerated AV Conduction

Wolf-Parkinson-White syndrome (WPW syndrome)
- In this condition there is an aberrant bundle connecting the atria and ventricle other than the AV node
- Impulse travels faster in this bundle and excites one ventricle

- The manifestation of this event merges with the normal QRS complex and there is shortening of PR interval and prolonged and slurred QRS complex
- PJ interval is normal.

Lown-Ganong-Levine syndrome:
- In this condition there is aberrant bundle passing from atria to ventricle that bypasses the AV node but enters the intraventricular conducting system distal to the node
- Patients have paroxysmal supraventricular tachycardia
- ECG shows short PR intervals and normal QRS.

ECG Changes in Myocardial Infarction
- When there is decrease in blood supply to myocardium it results in ischemia and if the block continues it leads to myocardial infarction
- In ischemia the ECG change seen is T wave inversion and in infarction there is ST segment elevation in the leads overlying the myocardial wall (refer Fig. 4).

Causes for ST elevation:
- There is rapid repolarisation of the infarcted tissue
- Decrease in RMP of infarcted tissue
- Delayed depolarisation of infarcted cells.

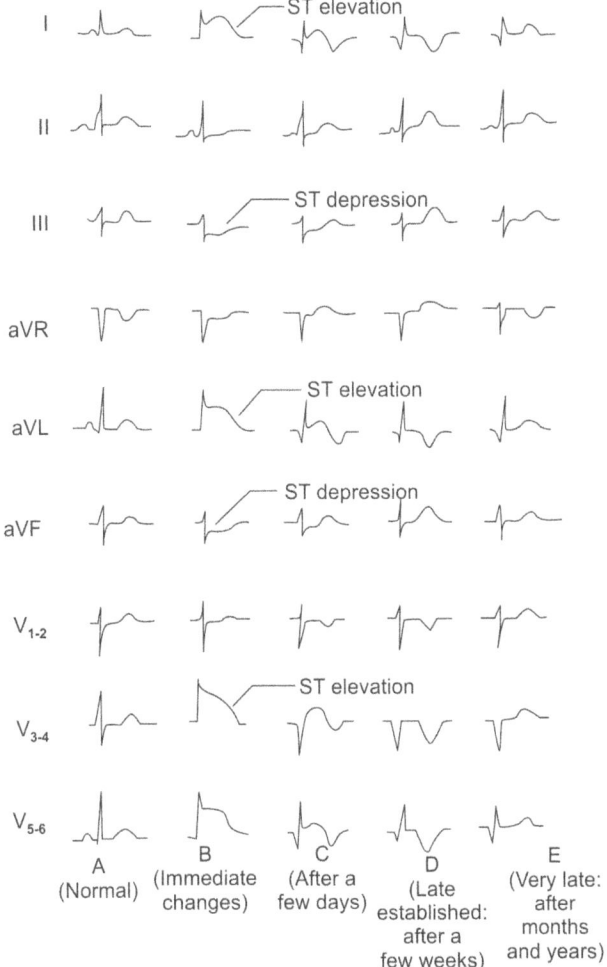

Fig. 4: ECG changes in anterior wall myocardial infarction. ST elevation is seen in leads I, avL and V3 – 6. These leads overlie the anterior wall. There is ST depression in leads opposite to the infarcted area as in Leads III, aVR, aVF.
(Source: GK Pal)

Effect of Electrolyte Imbalance in ECG

Hyperkalemia:
- Plasma K^+ levels ±7 mEq/L – Tall and slender T waves, PR interval and QRS complexes are normal
- As the K^+ levels increase (± 8.5meq/L) there is no evidence of atrial activity, QRS complex is broad and slurred, Tall T waves
- Further increase in K^+ levels leads to ventricular tachycardia and fibrillation

Hypokalemia:
- Plasma K^+ levels ± 3.5 meq/L, PR interval and QRS duration are normal
- ST segment depression is present, a prominent U wave is seen
- Further lowering of K^+ levels (±2.5 meq/L) PR interval is lengthened, ST segment depressed, T wave is inverted, U wave is seen and true QT interval is same.

Hyponatremia: Low voltage electrocardiographic complexes are seen.

Hypercalcemia: Heart relaxes less in diastole and stops in systole – Calcium rigor.

Hypocalcemia: Prolongation of ST segment and consequently QT interval.

---

5. **Describe the connections and functions of basal ganglia in detail. Explain the clinical disorders and physiological basis of management.**

Basal ganglia is a groups of nuclei in the forebrain and upper part of brainstem underlying the cortical mantle (refer Fig. 5).

They are:
1. Caudate nucleus
2. Putamen
3. Globus pallidus
4. Subthalamic nucleus
5. Substantia nigra.

Caudate nucleus + Putamen – **Striatum**
Putamen + Globus pallidus – **Lenticular nucleus**
Globus pallidus – **Internal and External segments**
Substantia nigra – **Pars reticulata and Pars compacta.**

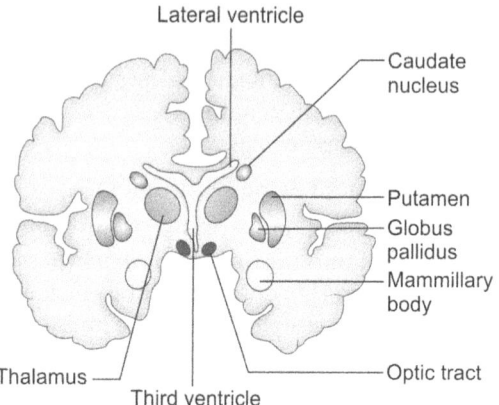

Fig. 5: Basal ganglia.
(*Source:* Sembulingam)

Connections of Basal Ganglia

Afferents (refer Fig. 6)

All afferents enter basal ganglia via striatum. They are from most of the cortex and thalamus. Also receives from Raphe magnus nucleus (RMN) and Pedunculopontine region of brainstem:

1. Corticostriate projections: Originate from many areas of cortex, premotor, SSI and supplementary motor cortex
2. Thalamostriate fibers: Arise from centeromedian nucleus and end on striatum
3. Rapestriatal projection: Serotonergic fibers from raphe nucleus in RF
4. Pedunculostriate projection: Arises from pedunculopontine nucleus of brainstem.

Efferent Connections (refer Fig. 7)

- Output from basal ganglia is through Internal segment (IS) of Globus pallidus and Pars reticulata (PR) of Substantia nigra (SN)
- **From IS of GP:**
    a. Via thalamic fasciculus to venterolateral (VL) and venteroanterior (VA) and centeromedian nuclei of thalamus → Prefrontal and premotor cortex
    b. Via Ansa lenticularis fibers go to subthalamic nucleus, substantia nigra and red nucleus of midbrain and reticular formation of brainstem.
- **From PR of SN to:**
    a. VL and VA nuclei of thalamus
    b. To Pedunculopontine nucleus, habenula and superior colliculus.

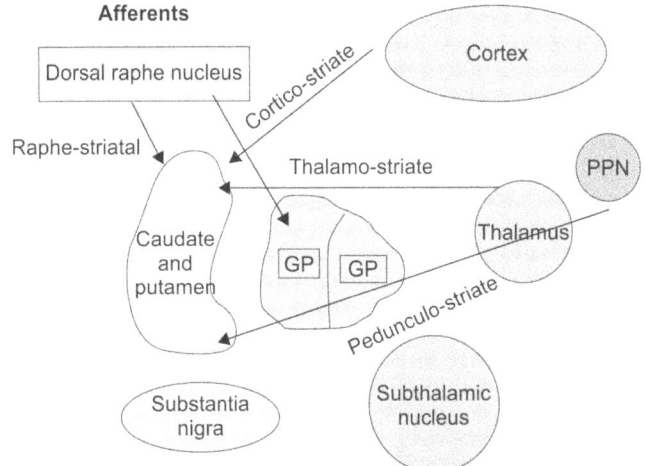

Fig. 6: Afferent connections to basal ganglia.

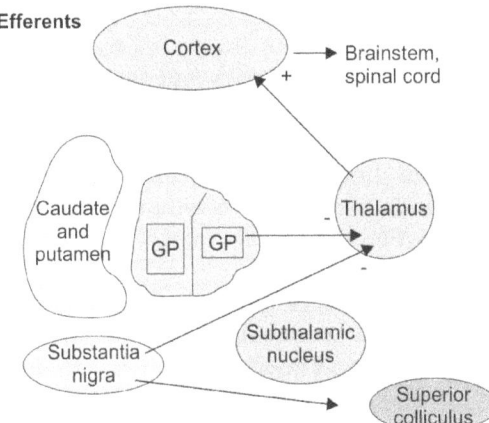

Fig. 7: Efferent connections of basal ganglia.

- Output from IS of GP to thalamus is inhibitory whereas from thalamus to cortex is excitatory
- Efferents to red nucleus → Rubrospinal tract.

Motor Loop:

The connection between basal ganglai and cortex is forming a motor loop.

Various areas of cerebral cortex projects to striatum → Striatum projects to IS of globus pallidus → Thalamic nuclei → back to cortex.

Internuclear connections:

1. Dopaminergic Nigrostriatal system – From SN to striatum
2. GABA-ergic inhibitory projections
   a. Striatum to PR of substantia nigra
   b. Striatum to IS and External segment (ES) of GP
   c. ES of GP to STN.
3. Excitatory glutaminergic projections from STN:
   a. To IS and ES of GP
   b. To PR of SN.

Neural pathways through basal ganglia: Direct and Indirect pathways. Both the pathways modulate the inhibitory output from basal ganglia. Direct pathway facilitates and indirect pathway further inhibits output (refer Fig. 8).

Direct pathway in basal ganglia: Cerebral Cortex → Striatum (Caudate and Putamen) → internal segment (IS) of Globus Pallidus (GP) → Thalamus → Motor cortex.

Cortex excites striatum (Glutamate)
↓
Striatum inhibits IS of GP (GABA)
↓
IS of GP inhibits the inhibition of thalamus via thalamic fasciculus (goes to VA and VL nuclei of thalamus) (GABA)
↓
Impulses are conducted from thalamus to prefrontal and premotor cortex. The final effect is disinhibition.

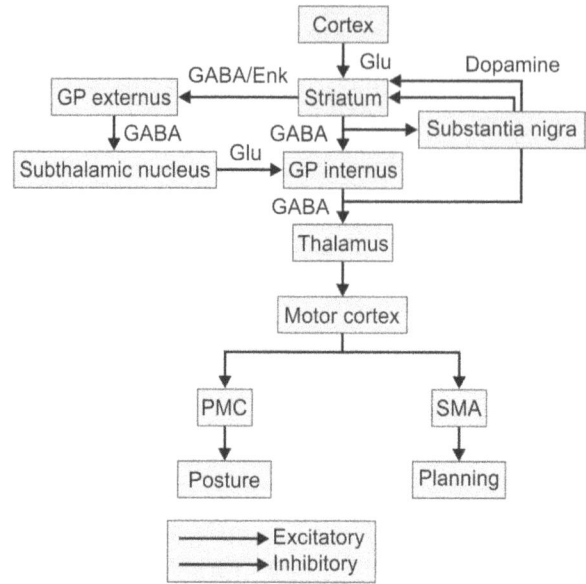

Fig. 8: Direct and indirect pathways in basal ganglia.
(PMC: premotor cortex; SMA: supplementary motor area; Glu: glutamate; GP: globus pallidus; Enk: enkephalin)
(*Source:* GK Pal)

Indirect pathway:

Cortex → Striatum → ES of GP → STN → IS of GP → Thalamus → cortex

- Striatum inhibits ES of GP (GABA)
- Inhibition by ES of GP on STN is removed
- STN activates IS of GP (Glutamate)
- So stimulation of striatum activates IS of GP
- The final effect of this pathway is inhibition of thalamocortical fibers by the IS of GP.

Nigrostriatal projections have important effects on both pathways. Dopaminergic connections of PC to striatum has an excitatory effect on direct pathway and inhibitory effect on indirect pathway

- In health there is a balance between the two pathways
- Alteration of either of them results in imbalance in motor output
- So BG disorders may have both hypo and hyperkinetic movement disorders

Functions of Basal Ganglia

1. Basal ganglia is involved in planning and programming of voluntary movement. The neurons of basal ganglia fire impulses even before the movements starts. Caudate loop is involved in planning of movements (direct pathway through caudate nucleus)
2. Controls muscle tone through inhibition of motor cortex and inhibitory medullary RF. The pathway involved is cortex – striatum – GP – SN- Medullary RF – Spinal cord via reticulospinal tract. In lesion of BG there is hypertonia
3. Controls the limb movements. In diseases of BG unpurposeful limb movements appear
4. Controls automated associative limb movements like swinging of arms while walking. Putamen circuit (direct pathway through putamen nucleus) is involved in control of subconscious movements
5. Timing the movements is also a role of BG
6. BG exerts an inhibitory effect on spinal reflexes which help to regulate posture
7. Somatic movements associated with emotions are controlled by BG
8. Provides muscle tone for skilled movements

9. Functions in motivated behavior
10. Caudate nucleus plays a role in cognition because of its connections with associative cortex. Lesion leads to deficits of performance based learning
11. Because of its connections with RF, GP has a role in arousal mechanism
12. Lesion of head of left caudate nucleus leads to dysarthric aphasia.

Disorders of Basal Ganglia

BG disorders are associated with movement disorders like:
- Hyperkinetic movements:
  1. Rigidity
  2. Chorea
  3. Athetosis
  4. Ballismus
  5. Rest tremors.
- Hypokinetic movements:
  1. Akinesia
  2. Bradykinesia.

Parkinson's Disease

- Also called as Paralysis agitans
- Due to destruction of Nigrostriatal Dopaminergic neurons, to Putamen is mostly affected
- Causes:
  1. Primary or idiopathic
  2. Complication of drugs: Phenothiazines.
- Characterized by:
  1. Hyperkinetic features:
     - Rigidity: Lead-pipe or cogwheel
     - Tremors: Resting tremors, at 6–8 Hz frequency.
  2. Hypokinesia
     - Weakness of movements and lack of initiation of movements—akinesia
     - Bradykinesia.
  3. Lack of automated movements
  4. Mask like face without expression
  5. Festinant or short shuffling gait—patient walks in an attitude like he is going to catch the center of gravity.
- Treatment:
  - Treatment with L-Dopa rather than Dopamine as it cannot cross the Blood brain barrier
  - Bromocryptine, a dopamine agonist can also be used
  - Anticholinergics like atropine, tries to reduce the acetylcholine levels in basal ganglia and regulates the ratio between dopamine and acetylcholine
  - L-deprenyl
  - Dopamine agonists like bromocryptine
  - Transplantation of adrenal medulla in BG
  - Implantation of fetal BG.

Chorea

- Due to disease of the caudate nucleus
- Characterized by rapid, irregular, involuntary movements of short duration
- Seen in Huntington's disease, rheumatic fever in children.

Athetosis

- Due to lesion in lenticular nucleus
- Characterized by continuous, slow, twisting movements. Movements are worm like writhing movements of extremities like the fingers and wrist.

Hemiballism

- It is due to damage to Subthalamic nucleus, due to hemorrhage in it
- Characterized by spontaneous attacks of inco-ordinated movements affecting whole of opposite side of body.

Huntington's Disease

- Genetic disorder inherited as an autosomal dominant disease
- There is damage to GABAergic and cholinergic neurons of striatum
- Loss of GABAergic neurons leads to hyperkinetic movements
- Early sign is a jerky trajectory of the hand when reaching to touch a spot especially towards the end of the target
- Later hyperkinetic choreiform movements appear and incapacitate the patient
- Speech becomes slurred and incomprehensible and later dementia sets in and death happens in 10–15 years
- There is no effective treatment.

Wilson's Disease

- Also called as hepatolenticular degeneration
- It is due to accumulation of copper in brain and liver
- Cirrhosis of liver is seen
- In brain the damage is more in lenticular nucleus especially putamen and symptoms of Parkinsonism is seen.

Kernicterus

Damage to GP following deposition of unconjugated bilirubin.

It is usually seen in hemolytic disease of newborn.

Symptoms are—rigidity, chorea, athetosis, mental defeciency and may lead to death.

---

6. Describe the refractory errors of eye and explain the physiological basis of their corrections.

Myopia – Shortsightedness

In myopia the ciliary muscles are relaxed and the eyeball may be elongated and therefore parallel rays of light from a distant object are brought to focus in front of the retina. It can also be due to increased curvature of the cornea or the lens. It is the most common refractory error. It may be genetic or acquired (refer Fig. 9B).

Correction

It can be corrected by using biconcave lenses. The lens diverges the light rays before they strike the cornea and then they are covereged by the lens in the eye, so that the object is focussed on the retina (refer Fig. 9C). The lens power is given in negative dioptres. Surgical correction like keratoplasty can also be done.

Hypermetropia – Farsightedness

Here the parallel rays of light from a distant object are brought to focus behind the retina. It occurs due to decrease in anteroposterior diameter of the eye or due to decreased curvature of cornea or lens (refer Fig. 9D). It is seen in 80% of the newborn and infants and is corrected as the eye grows in length.

Correction

It can be corrected by using biconvex lenses so that they converge the light rays before they fall on the cornea and therefore the light rays fall on the retina (refer Fig. 9E). The refractory power of the biconvex lens is given in positive dioptres.

Astigmatism

It is a condition where curvature of cornea is not uniform. The curvature in one meridean is different from the other meridian and light rays in that meridian are refracted to a different focus, so that part of the retinal image is blurred. It also happens if the lens curvature is not uniform or if the lens is pushed out of alignment.

It is of two types—regular and irregular astigmatism.

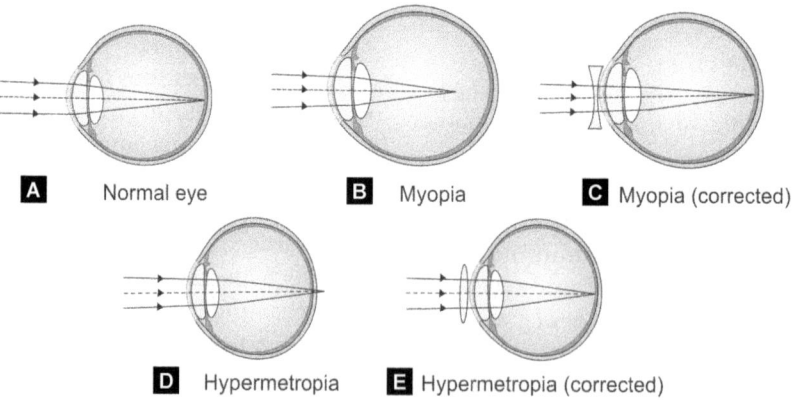

Figs. 9A to E: Refrectory errors of the eye with corrections.
(*Source:* GK Pal)

Regular astigmatism: Here the greatest and least curvatures of cornea are at right angles.

Irregular astigmatism: Curvatures are irregular in different meridians and light rays get refracted irregularly and there is severe blurring of vision.

Correction

Astigmatism in myopia is corrected with cylindrical concave lens and hypermetropia with astigmatism is corrected with cylindrical and convex lens.

Presbyopia

It is commonly seen in aged people above the age of 40 years.

The near point has receded beyond the normal reading distance due to loss of plasticity of lens and denaturation of lens proteins. The loss of plasticity results in loss of accommodation property of the lens. Accommodation of eye is lost and the near point recedes from 9 cm to 83 cm.

Correction

It is corrected using convex lens for near work and upper segment for glasses for far work and it is given as the Bifocal lenses.

7. **Define hemostasis. Explain the steps involved in intrinsic mechanism of clotting. Add a note on hemophilia.**

Refer answers to 2003 paper.

8. **Describe in detail the phases of deglutition.**

Refer answers to 2003 paper.

9. **Classify hypoxia, what are the causes and features of each type? What types respond best to oxygen therapy?**

Refer answers to 2006 paper – Causes, classification, features.

Types of Hypoxia best responding to O_2 Therapy

- O_2 therapy can be either 100% O_2 at normal pressures or hyperbaric oxygen, at high pressure
- O_2 therapy does not benefit all types of hypoxia
- It is useful in all types of hypoxic hypoxia except in conditions of A-V shunt
- It is of limited use in anemic, stagnant and histotoxic hypoxia. In these conditions it can increase only the dissolved O_2 content in blood
- In carbon monoxide poisoning using hyperbaric O_2 is useful as it displaces CO from hemoglobin
- In cyanide poisoning also hyperbaric O_2 therapy is useful.

10. **Draw and label the visual pathway. What are the effects of lesions at various levels of pathways.**

Refer answers to 2004 paper.

II. SHORT NOTES

1. **Blood groups.**

- The blood groups are classified based on the presence of antigens or agglutinogens on the membranes of RBCs
- An individual with a particular antigen on RBC membrane will not possess the corresponding antibody or agglutinin in his plasma
- This forms the basis of blood grouping
- There are more than 30 blood group systems based on the presence of nearly 400 antigens
- The blood group systems are: ABO system, Rh system, MNS, Lutheran, P, Kell, Kidd, Duffy, Lewis etc.
- Most of the antigens are cold antigens and therefore they do not react in body temperature
- The ABO and Rh systems are the major blood group systems as they react in body temeperature and when they react with their corresponding agglutinins they produce major reactions
- Since the above two systems of blood groups are more important it is discussed in detail
- **Karl Landsteiner has framed two laws based on the presence and absence of agglutinogens and agglutinins**
  a. If a particular agglutinogen (antigen) is present on the RBC membrane, the

corresponding agglutinin (antibody) will be absent in the plasma

b. If a particular agglutinogen is absent on the RBC membrane then the corresponding agglutinin will be present in the plasma.

ABO system follows both the laws whereas Rh system follows only the first law.

ABO System

- This blood group system is based on the presence of the antigens A and B or both or none on RBC membrane
- There are 4 types of blood groups—A group, B group, AB group and O groups
- A has two subtypes—A_1 and A_2
- AB has A_1B and A_2B subtypes
- Antigens are present on the RBC membrane and also in secertions like saliva, semen, amniotic fluid and other tissues like salivary glands, testis, pancreas etc.
- These antigens are basically Oligosaccharides and they differ among each other in their terminal sugars
- Agglutinogen A has N-acetylgalactosamine as the terminal sugar and B antigen has Galactose as the terminal sugar and O does not have any terminal sugars
- Antigens start appearing since fetal age of 6 weeks
- Agglutinins of ABO systems are Anti A and Anti B antibodies and they belong to IgM type of antibodies and therefore they do not cross the placenta
- Antibodies are not present since fetal life and they start appearing in the 2nd week of neonatal life and reach a peak level by 10 years of age

The blood types, antigens and antibodies in the ABO system are:

Blood groups	Agglutinogen present	Agglutinin present
A	A	Anti B
B	B	Anti B
AB	A and B	Nil
O	Nil	Anti A and Anti B

Rh System

- Rh system is the 2nd most important blood group system
- There are 6 antigens of this system – C, D, E, c, d and e
- But D antigen on the RBC membrane is the most antigenic
- Therefore individuals with D antigen are Rh positive and its absence is considered to be Rh negative
- 90–95% of Indian population is Rh postive
- Rh system does not follow 2nd law of Landsteiner's, i.e. in an Rh negative individual the Anti D antibody is not present in plasma
- But exposure to D antigens for the first time stimulates the immune system to form Anti D antibodies of an Rh negative person
- These antibodies can later react on D antigens if they are exposed to it in the second attempt.

Importance of Doing Blood Grouping

a. The knowledge of the blood group of an individual helps in compatible blood transfusions in emergency situations of blood loss like surgery, trauma etc.
b. Blood grouping helps us to identify Rh incompatability between mother and fetus and prevetion of hemolytic disease of the newborn
c. The basis of antigens on RBC has given us an understanding about other hemolytic diseases
d. Certain blood group antigens are susceptible to certain diseases like malaria, viral infections and it also provides resistance to certain diseases
e. It is also useful for organ transplantation
f. ABO and Rh blood grouping is useful to settle paternity disputes.

Procedure for Determining the Blood Group

- To determine the blood group of an individual, a suspension of RBC is made by diluting a drop of blood in one mL normal saline
- On a porcelain tile, drops of Antisera A, B and D are put

- To the antisera, a drop of RBC suspension is added and mixed with seperate sticks for each antisera and left aside for 10 minutes
- After 10 minutes, look for agglutination reactions in each of the antisera
- Agglutinated RBCs look like clumps
- If there is agglutination in Antisera A the person's blood group is A and agglutination in Antisera B it is B group and in Anti D the person is Rh positive
- Agglutination is present because of the presence of a particular antigen on RBC membrane and is agglutinated when mixed with its corresponding antisera.

Blood group	Agglutination in Antisera A	Agglutination in Antisera B	Agglutination in Antisera D
A Positive	+	-	+
A negative	+	-	-
B Positive	-	+	+
B Negative	-	+	-
AB Positive	+	+	+
AB Negative	+	+	-
O Positive	-	-	+
O Negative	-	-	-

2. Anticoagulants

Anticoagulants are chemicals which prevent coagulation of blood.

Uses of Anticoagulants

- They are used to prevent clotting of blood in blood bank while storing blood.
- They are mixed with blood when it has to be transported to laboratories for investigations
- They are given as drugs to prevent formation of intravascular clots in persons having the tendency to form clot.

Classification of Anticoagulants

They are classified as in vitro and in vivo anticoagulants.

In vitro Anticoagulants

- EDTA
- Double oxalates
- Trisodium citrate
- Heparin
- ACD, CPD.

In vivo Anticoagulants

- Heparin
- Coumarin derivatives - Warfarin.

Ethylenediamine tetra-acetic acid (EDTA): This is the anticoagulant of choice in the laboratories. It makes Ca^{2+} unavailable for clotting by chelating it. It is used to determine ESR.

Trisodium citrate: This anticoagulant is used for determining clotting disorders and also ESR. This prevents clotting by chelation of Ca^{2+}.

Double oxalate mixture: It is a mixture of Ammonium oxalate and Potassium oxalate. It prevents clotting by forming insoluble calcium oxalate precipitate.

Heparin: A naturally occurring anticoagulant is used as an in vitro and in vivo anticoagulant. It activates Anti-thrombin III.

Sodium flouride is an anticoagulant used in the labs for tests to analyze blood glucose levels.

ACD and CPD: Acid citrate dextrose and citrate phosphate dextrose are the anticoagulants used in the blood bank. Dextrose helps in nourishing the blood cells.

Coumarin derivatives: They act as anticoagulants by inhibiting vitamin K. Vitamin K acts as a cofactor in the synthesis of coagulation factor II, VII, IX and X.

3. Micturition reflex.

Refer answers to 2006 paper.

4. Fat absorption.

Absorption of Fats

- It starts in the duodenum and is completely absorbed by the time the fats reach jejunum
- Absorption of fats is favored by formation of micelles by the bile salts and lecithin
- The lumen of intestine contains water and therefore movement of digested fats is favored only by micelle formation
- Refer 2010 paper for "Micelle formation"

- On reaching enterocytes, fats move out of micelles and enter enterocytes by passive diffusion
- The rate-limiting step in absorption of fats is formation and movement of micelles from the chyme in the lumen to the brush border
- The bile salts forming the micelles, are absorbed in the terminal ileum
- Fate of fats, entering the enterocytes is dependent on their size
- Fats containing 10-12 carbon atoms, easily pass through the basal side of the enterocytes and enter the portal blood vessels as free fatty acids and are transported
- Fatty acids with more than 12 carbon atoms are esterified to triglycerides and the absorbed cholesterol is also esterified and they are coated with protein (β lipoprotein), cholesterol and phospholipids to form **chylomicrons**
- The chylomicrons now exocytose through the basal side of the enterocytes to enter the lymphatics in the villus, the Lacteal
- They are transported in the lymphatics and are drained into the thoracic duct and finally they enter the blood circulation
- Absorption of large chain fatty acids are more in the upper parts of the intestine and some amount of absorption happens in terminal parts also
- In moderate fat intake, nearly 95% of ingested fats are absorbed.

Steatorrhea

- Steatorrhea is malabsorption of fats resulting in excretion of fat in stools
- The indigested fats appear in stools and the stools are fatty, bulky and clay-coloured. This is said to be Steatorrhea
- The fecal fat content is more than 40-50 g/day.
- It happens due to either destruction of exocrine pancreas, lipase deficiency or absence of bicarbonate in pancreatic juice which results in acidic environment in the intestine precipitating the bile salts
- Acids also inhibit pancreatic lipase and therefore patients with gastrin-secreting tumor have steatorrhea
- It is also seen in conditions with defective absorption of bile salts in terminal ileum.

5. Plasma proteins.

Refer answers to 2004 paper.

6. Gastrointestinal hormones.

- GI hormones are classified as Gastrin family and secretin family
- Gastrin family includes Gastrin and Cholecystokinin- Pancreozymin (CCK-PZ)
- Secretin family includes secretin, glucagon, gastric inhibitory peptide (GIP) and vasoactive intestinal peptide (VIP)
- Others include motilin, substance P, gastrin releasing peptide (GRP) and guanylin
- Three important hormones are gastrin, secretin and CCK-PZ.

Gastrin

- Gastrin is secreted by the 'G' cells in gastric antral glands
- Gastrin is a polypeptide and has different forms—G34, G17 and G14
- G17 is the form present in the stomach
- It is also present in the hypothalamus and anterior pituitary.

Regulation of Secretion of Gastrin

- **Stimuli that increase gastrin secretion**
    - **Luminal:**
        1. Peptides and amino acids
        2. Distension
    - **Neural**
        1. Increased vagal discharge via GRP
    - **Blood-borne**
        1. Calcium
        2. Epinephrine
- **Stimuli that inhibit gastrin secretion:**
    - **Luminal**
        1. Acid
    - **Blood-borne**
        1. Secretin, GIP, VIP, glucagon, somatostatin, calcitonin.

Actions of Gastrin
a. Stimulates secretion of HCl and pepsinogen in stomach
b. Has trophic action on gastric mucosa
c. Stimulates gastric motility
d. Contracts gastroesophageal sphincter (GES) and prevents reflux gastritis
e. Stimulates secretion of pancreatic juice
f. Stimulates mass movements of colon
g. Stimulates insulin secretion
h. Causes gastro-colic reflex
i. Stimulates Histamine from enterochromaffin like cells (ECL) cells in GI mucosa.

Cholecystokinin
- Secreted from I cells in upper small intestine (SI)
- It is a Polypeptide hormone
- Many forms – CCK 58, 39, 33, 12, 8, 4
- From SI it is 12 and 8.

Actions of CCK
a. Stimulates release of pancreatic solution rich in enzymes
b. Augments action of secretin to produce alkaline pancreatic juice
c. Causes contraction of gallbladder (GB) and release of bile
d. Inhibits gastric acid secretion
e. Inhibits gastric motility and emptying
f. Stimulates growth of pancreas
g. Enhances intestinal motility and colonic motility
h. Augments contraction of pyloric sphincter
i. Stimulates glucagon secretion
j. In brain it acts to enhance food-intake.

Secretin
- First hormone to be discovered
- Secreted from S cells in upper SI
- Polypeptide hormone.

Functions of Secretin
1. Enhances secretion of HCO_3 rich pancreatic juice
2. Increases alkaline rich bile secretion
3. Augments action of CCK
4. Decreases gastric secretion and motility
5. Contracts pyloric sphincter.

7. Neural regulation of respiration.
- Breathing is an automatic process occurring throughout life without conscious effort
- Respiration is a process which is highly regulated
- Spontaneous respiration is due to rhythmic discharge of neurons from respiratory centers supplying the inspiratory muscles
- This is under cortical (voluntary) and medullary and pontine control (automatic)
- These centers in turn are regulated by alterations in the PCO_2, PO_2 and pH of arterial blood and other non-chemical influences.

Cortical Control or Voluntary Control of Respiration

Impulses from cerebral cortex
↓
Corticospinal tract
↓
Motor neurons supplying the inspiratory muscles

- Impulses also reach the innervation of expiratory muscles
- There is a reciprocal inhibition between the motor neurons supplying the I and E neurons
- There is an exception for this at the start of expiration were the "I" neurons are active
- The inspiratory muscles are active for some time during expiration to brake the elastic recoil of lungs and make expiration smooth.

Automatic Control of Respiration
Impulses from brainstem respiratory centers in pons and medulla → Supplies neurons in intermediolateral horn cells of cervical and thoracic segments → Supplies inspiratory muscles.

Medullary Respiratory Centers
- Dorsal respiratory group of neurons (DRG): Has inspiratory neurons (I neurons)

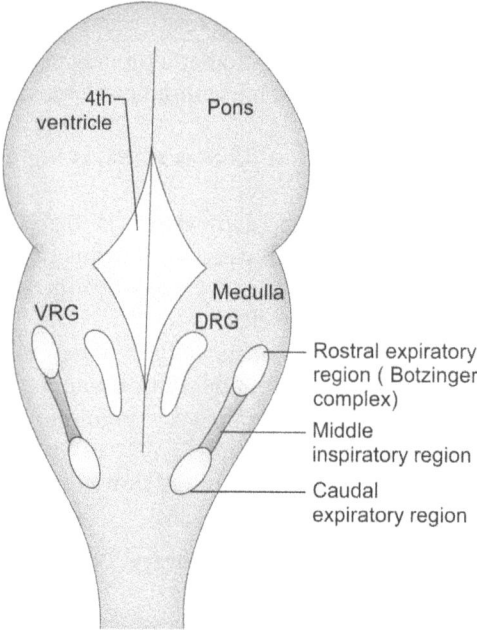

Fig. 10: Respiratory centers in medulla.
(DRG: Dorsal repiratory group of neurons (has only inspiratory neurons); VRG: Ventral respiratory group of neurons (has both inspiratory and expiratory neurons).
(*Source:* GK Pal)

- Ventral respiratory group of neurons (VRG): Has inspiratory (I) and Expiratory (E) neurons (refer Fig. 10)
- Central pattern generator (CPG): Prebotzinger complex (refer Fig. 11).

Dorsal Respiratory Group of Neurons

- Located near nucleus tractus solitarius (NTS)
- Contains only inspiratory neurons
- They project to cell bodies of phrenic nerves in spinal cord
- Its activity is weaker to start with and gradually increases in a ramp fashion for 2 seconds and abrupty stops for 3 seconds
- The ramp signal helps in steady increase in lung volume during inspiration
- Receives input from peripheral chemoreceptors through 9th and 10th cranial nerves.

Ventral Respiratory Group of Neurons

- Located in venterolateral medulla in region of nucleus ambiguus (NA)
- Contains both inspiratory and expiratory group of neurons
- 3 regions—rostral, middle and caudal inspiratory regions
- Middle region—has inspiratory neurons
- Rostral and caudal—has expiratory neurons—supply expiratory muscles
- They are active only during forceful respiration
- I and E neurons reciprocally inhibit each other.

Pacemaker Cells for Respiration

- Located close to DRG and VRG neurons

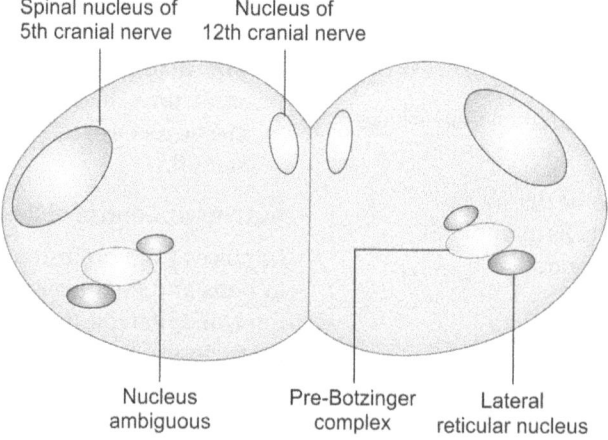

Fig. 11: Location of pacemaker (Pre-Botzinger complex) for rhythm generation in medulla.
(*Source:* GK Pal)

- Present in the Pre-Botzinger complex between Nucleus ambiguus and Lateral reticular nucleus
- They are pace-maker cells and are responsible for generating respiratory rhythm → Rhythmically activate phrenic nerves
- It receives input from higher centers.

Pontine Centers
- There are two centers:
  1. Pneumotaxic center
     - Located in nucleus parabrachialis and Kolliker-Fuse nucleus in the upper part of pons
     - Active during both inspiration and expiration
     - On stimulation, it shortens the duration of inspiration. When its activity is less, the duration of inspiration is longer
     - Its major function is to limit inspiration, by inhibiting apneustic center
     - It co-ordinates switching between inspiration and expiration.
  2. Apneustic center
     - Present in lower part of pons
     - On stimulation → Leads to prolonged inspiratory spasms – Apneusis
     - It sends inputs to DRG to cause a prolonged inspiration
     - It is constantly stimulating DRG
     - But its actions are kept in check by inputs from pneumotaxic center and vagal afferents from airways (refer Fig. 12).

Mechanism of Breathing
- The neurons in DRG discharge steadily and spontaneously in a ramp like fashion for 2–3 seconds
- Muscles of inspiration contract steadily resulting in expansion of the lung and chest wall resulting in inspiration
- As the inspiration happens, the stretch receptors in lungs and airways are stimulated and impulses from here travel through vagus nerve to stop the firing of DRG neurons

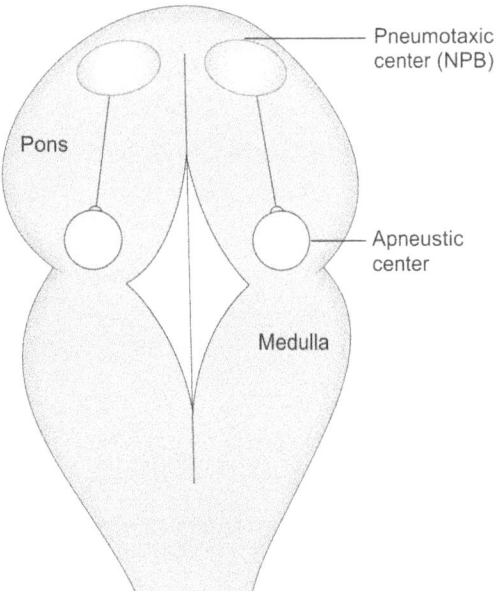

Fig. 12: Respiratory centers in pons, pneumotaxic and apneustic centers.
(*Source:* GK Pal)

- Impulses from pneumotaxic center through inhibition of apneustic center stops the firing of DRG
- Inspiratory muscles relax and the lung and chest wall recoils and induces expiration.
- At the end of expiration the next cycle starts (refer Fig. 13).

Factors Influencing Respiratory Centers
- Afferents from higher centers: Cerebral cortex, Limbic system, Hypothalamus
- Afferents from peripheral receptors: Baroreceptors, chemoreceptors, J receptors, pain receptors, proprioceptors, pulmonary stretch receptors and thermoreceptors
- Reflexes: Hering-Breuer reflex, sneezing reflex, swallowing reflex, cough reflex, speech.

Afferents from Higher Centers
- Cerebral cortex imparts control over the respiratory centers and therefore voluntary hyperventilation and breath holding is possible

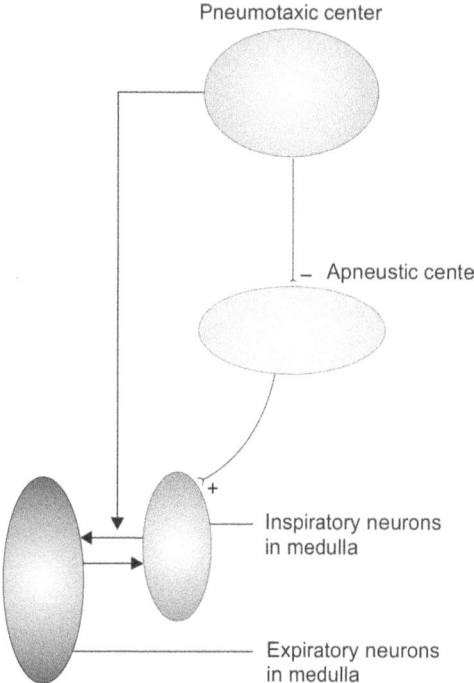

Fig. 13: Interaction of medullary and pontine centers in regulation of respiration.
(*Source:* GK Pal)

- Limbic cortex sends impulses to respiratory centers and therefore the changes in ventilation in relation to emotions can happen
- Hypothalamic connections are responsible for respiratory changes associated with body temperature changes.

Afferent Impulses from Peripheral Receptors

Baroreceptors: They regulate blood pressure through the regulation of vasomotor and cardiac vagal centers. But stimulation of baroreceptors also inhibit respiratory center and causes apnea.

Chemoreceptors: There are peripheral and central chemoreceptors. They monitor the PO_2, PCO_2 and pH levels in the arterial blood. Decrease in arterial PO_2 levels will stimulate peripheral chemoreceptors and they will send impulses to DRG to stimulate respiration. Central chemoreceptors are more sensitive to PCO_2 and H^+ levels and when it increases they stimulate respiration.

'J' receptors: These are endings of unmyelinated C fibers of vagal afferents and are located between the pulmonary capillaries and alveolar walls. They are stimulated in conditions of increase in interstitial fluid between the capillary endothelium and alveolar epithelium as in pulmonary edema, pulmonary congestion, pulmonary embolism etc. On stimulation, it induces apnea followed by tachypnea, bradycardia and hypotension. In physiological conditions these receptors are stimulated while exercising, especially in high altitude.

Proprioceptors: While doing exercise, movements in the muscles and joints stimulate the proprioceptors and impulses from here stimulate respiration by stimulating DRG.

Pulmonary stretch receptors (Hering-Breuer reflex): The pulmonary stretch receptors are located in the smooth muscles of the airways and are stimulated by inflation of lungs.

There are two types of reflexes:
- *Hering-Breur inflation reflex:* It is activated during inspiration. When the inspiration is more and tidal volume is more than 1 L, the reflex is initiated and it sends impulses to the respiratory centers and inhibits inspiration and stimulates expiration. This reflex is more important in infants to control the tidal volume
- *Hering-Breur deflation reflex:* This reflex is activated during expiration and causes arrest of expiration and stimulates inspiration.

Thermoreceptors: Increase in body temperature stimulates these receptors and send impulses to the cerebral cortex which in turn sends impulses to respiratory centers to increase respiration. Respiration helps to lose body temperature.

Reflexes

Sneezing reflex: Stimulation of nasal mucosa by irritant substances results in sneezing. The act of sneezing involves a deep inspiration followed by forceful expiration with opened glottis initially and later gottis opens to allow air to flow through mouth and nose.

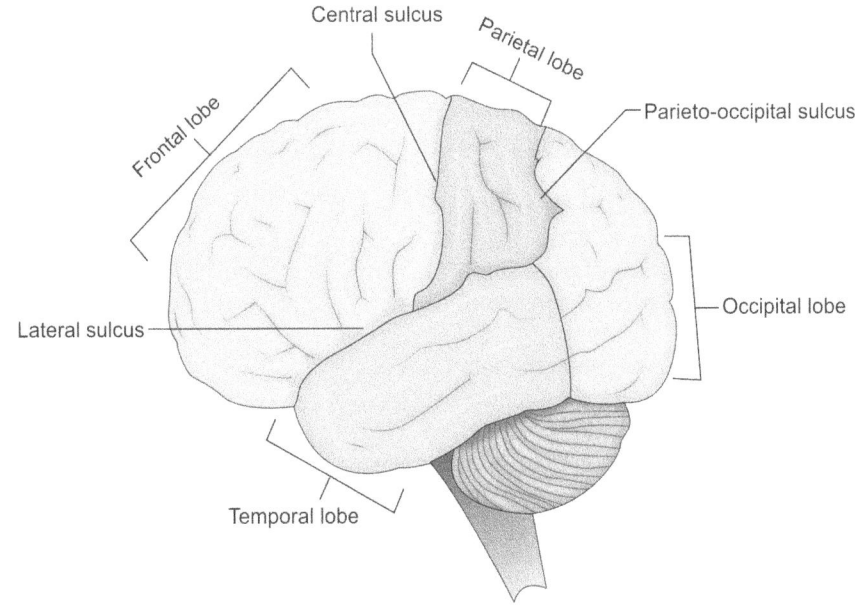

Fig. 14: Parietal lobe.
(*Source:* Sembulingam)

Cough reflex: Stimulation of irritant receptors in the tracheobronchial mucosa leads to deep inspiration followed by forceful expiration against a closed glottis. It is a protective reflex useful for clearing the airway of the irritant substance.

Deglutition reflex: On swallowing there is temporary stoppage of respiration— deglutition apnea. It is a protective reflex which prevents entry of food into the airway.

Vomiting reflex: Apnea happens for a short time during vomiting to prevent aspiration of contents.

8. Hypoxia.
Refer answers to 2006 paper.

9. Excitation-contraction coupling.
Refer answers to 2003, paper.

10. Functions of middle ear.
Refer answers to 2005 paper.

11. Functions of parietal lobe.
Major functions of parietal lobe are somatosensory in nature. It is posterior to the frontal lobe and is posteriorly seperated from occipital lobe by the calcarine fissure and laterally from temporal lobe by the sylvian fissure.

The areas in this lobe are areas 3, 1, 2, 5, 7, SSII, 39 and 43 (refer Fig. 14).

Functions
1. Perception of somatic sensations like touch, pressure, vibration, pain etc.
2. Spatial recognition, two point discrimination and tactile localisation
3. Since taste area is in this lobe, perception of taste is a function
4. Area 39 helps in language and speech
5. Area 5 and 7 help in stereognosis and hand-eye coordiantion
6. Also involved in learning and memory
7. Helpful in recognition of different intensities of stimuli.

12. Functions of thalamus.
- Thalamus functions as a major relay station for most sensory impulses reaching the cortex

- Thalamus acts as a crude center for sense perception like crude touch, pain, crude form of temperature sensation
- It also contributes to motor function by relaying impulses from cerebellum and basal ganglia to motor cortex
- Relays impulse between different areas of cortex
- Contributes to regulation of autonomic activities and maintenance of consciousness
- Due to the intimate connections of thalamus with frontal cortex and hypothalamus it is involved in various emotions
- It is an integrating center for sleep, intralaminar nuclei for NREM sleep and lateral geniculate body for REM sleep
- Concerned with recent memory and emotions due to its involvement in Papez circuit
- Concerned with language
- Important role in genesis of synchronization of EEG waves and alertness of the individual. Induces alertness due to its connections with RAS.

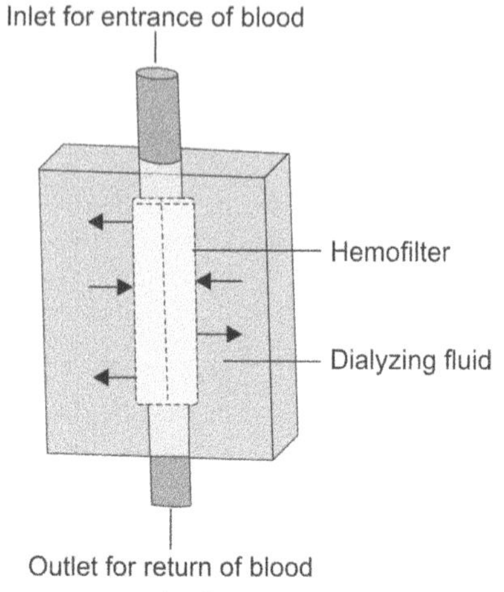

Fig. 15: Basic principle of dialysis. The blood to be dialysed passes through small coiled cellophane tubes which is seperated from the dialyzing fluid in the machine. Solutes diffuse from their higher to lower concentrations between blood and the dialyzing fluid through the semipermeable cellophane membrane.
(*Source:* Sembulingam)

13. Artificial kidney.

- Acute and chronic renal failure is treated with **artificial kidney or dialysis**
- It helps to remove the toxic substances from the body and restores body fluid volume and composition to normal
- There are two types of dialysis—**hemodialysis and peritoneal dialysis**
- Basic principle of dialysis is diffusion of solutes from higher to lower concentration across a semi-permeable membrane
- Blood which is needed to be purified is passed through minute blood channels bounded by a thin semi-permeable membrane (refer Fig. 15)
- The other side of the membrane contains the dialyzing fluid with which exchange of substances happen.

Peritoneal Dialysis

- It can be done by the patient 4 – 5 times/day in his/her place
- The peritoneal membrane is used as the semi-permeable membrane across which movement of substances happen between plasma and the dialyzing fluid
- A catheter is inserted into the peritoneal cavity and is connected to a bag with 2 litres of dialyzing fluid
- There is an outlet tube through which the fluid containing the waste products are removed and measured
- The exchange takes place for 20 minute
- The input and output measurements are made
- This can be done with the patient ambulatory.

Hemodialysis or Artificial Kidney

- Here the blood which has to be purified is passed through a machine
- It is usually done in a hospitalized patient by an expert
- The radial artery of the patient is connected to the machine and at a time 500 mL of blood enters the machine and passes through a coiled cellophane tube which is surrounded by the dialyzing fluid
- The fluid contains less amount of sodium, potassium and more amounts of glucose, bicarbonate and calcium ions
- The fluid is devoid of waste products like urea, uric acid etc and therefore they

move out of the blood into the fluid by the gradient
- This favors removal of excess of unwanted ions and addition of solutes which are necessary
- By this process the wastes are removed and electrolyes are restored in the blood and the purified blood is returned back into the patient's body through a peripheral vein
- The blood is anti-coagulated with heparin when it passes through the machine.

14. Feedback mechanisms.

- Most of the control systems in the body are negative feedback regulations
- There are negative and positive feedback mechanisms.

Negative Feedback Mechanism

- In negative feedback regulation, if a particular activity is increased or decreased, the control system initiates a chain of actions by which the activity returns back to normal
- So the control system has a sensor to sense the change, a control center that receives signals from the sensor and sends command to the effector which will bring about the change.

Examples

Body temperature regulation, regulation of pH, regulation of blood glucose levels, regulation of thyroid hormone secretion.

Blood pressure regulation:

Increase in mean arterial pressure
↓
Sensed by baroreceptors
↓
Impulses are carried by IXth and Xth cranial nerves
↓
Inhibits vasomotor center and stimulates cardiac vagal center
↓
Decreases heart rate and stroke volume
↓
Decreases cardiac output
↓
Decreases mean arterial pressure.

Positive Feedback Mechanism

- In positive feedback regulation the output of the control system is enhanced or amplified so that controlled variable continues to move in the direction of the initial change
- For example: Parturition reflex (refer Fig. 16)
- Positive feedback occurs in only certain instances whereas the negative feedback regulation is the most common one happening in the body.

15. Female contarceptives.
Refer answers to 2004 paper.

16. Nerve action potential.
Refer answers to 2004 paper.

17. Hypothyroidism.

Hypothyroidism due to thyroid gland dysfunction is primary hypothyroidism.
- Hypothyroidism may also occur due to disease in the pituitary gland or in hypothalamus.
- Symptoms of hypothyroidism vary in children and adults.
- In children hypothyroidism due to iodine deficiency—cretinism.

Symptoms

In Newborns

- Respiratory distress syndrome, poor feeding, hoarse cry, umbilical hernia,

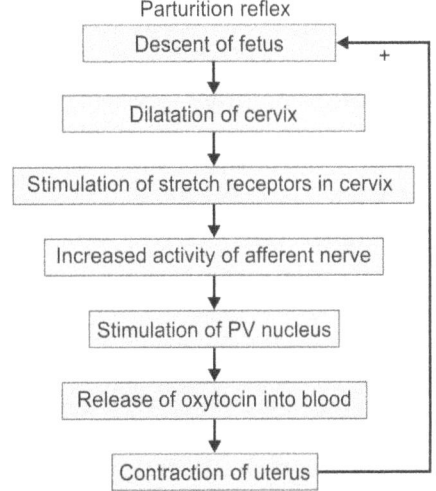

Fig. 16: Parturition reflex (positive feedback regulation).

retarded bone age, no visible symptoms detected, so early thyroid screening and TH replacement is essential to prevent mental retardation.

In Children
- Mental retardation, stunted growth, pot belly, enlarged and protruding tongue, delayed or absent sexual maturity, deaf mutism with rigidity, precocious puberty can also occur.

In Adults: Hypothyroidism in Adults is Myxedema
- ↓ BMR, hypothermia and cold intolerance, Skin is dry and cold.

CNS Symptoms
- They are dull and lethargic, speech and mentation is slow, reflex time is prolonged
- Depression, excess sleep, frank psychosis (myxedema madnesss).

CVS Symptoms
- Bradycardia, ↓ myocardial contractility, cardiac output ↓, hypertension
- Serum cholesterol and TGL levels ↑ leading to atherosclerosis.

Skin
- Non-pitting edema (myxedema)
- Hoarseness of voice, thick skin, thick facial features, enlarged tongue, hair is brittle, thin, coarse and lacks lustre.

GIT Symptoms
- ↓ Appetite and food intake, constipation, BMR and caloric use ↓→ weight gain
- Amenorrhea is present, conception is difficult, stillbirths and abortion are common.

18. B-lymphocytes.
- B lymphocytes mediate humoral immunity
- B lymphocytes are produced in the bone marrow and their maturation also happens in the bone marrow
- Following maturation they reach the lymphoid tissues and reside there till their activation by respective antigens
- Humoral immunity provides protection against extracellular pathogens, takes part in immediate hypersensitivity reactions type I, II and III.

Stages of humoral immunity include:
Refer answers to 2005 paper.

19. Cytoskeleton.
- Maintains structural integrity
- Allows change in cell structure and shape
- Provides motility of cells
- Contains microtubules, intermediate filaments and microfilaments.

Microtubules
- Long hollow tube with 25 nm diameter
- Made of globular protein – tubulin (refer Fig. 17A)
- It has the property of aggregating and disaggregating
- So it is a dynamic structure.

Functions
- Forms cytosolic guide rail for transporting particles within the cell and towards the cell membrane
- It contributes to cell strength and shape

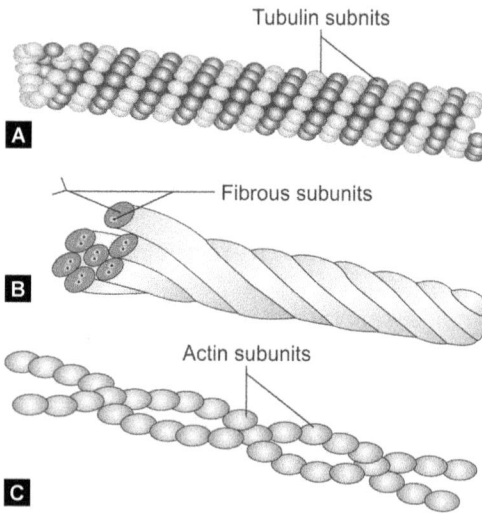

Figs. 17A to C: Cytoskeletal elements. (A) Microtubule; (B) Intermediate filament; (C) Microfilament.
(*Source:* Sembulingam)

- Forms spindle to move chromosome during cell division
- Forms pillar for cilia. Helps in cell motility.

Intermediate Filaments (refer Fig. 17B)
- It has a diameter of 8-14 nm
- Connects the nuclear membrane to cell membrane and membranes of organelles
- Forms supple skeletal network of cell and helps to resist rupture of cell from external pressure
- Their proteins form biomarkers.

Microfilaments (refer Fig. 17C)
- They have a diameter of 7 nm
- Made up of actin
- They are helpful in contractiliy of muscles and platelets
- They are present in microvilli and help in its motility
- Helps in cell motility.

20. Erythropoietin.
- Erythropoietin is a glycoprotein hormone secreted by the interstitial cells in the peritubular capillary bed of the kidneys. It has 165 amino acid residues and 4 oligosaccharide chains
- In adults 85% of it is produced in the kidneys and 15% from the liver. It is also produced in the brain.

Actions of EPO
- The major action of erythropoietin is to increase the erythropoietin-sensitive committed stem cells that are converted to red blood cell precursors and subsequent maturation to RBCs
- It stimulates maturation of RBCs from proerythroblast stage to mature RBC
- It also stimulates synthesis of hemoglobin
- It causes the release of RBCs from bone marrow into circulation
- In the brain it exerts a protective effect against the excitotoxic damage induced by hypoxia
- In uterus and oviducts it mediates estrogen-dependant angiogenesis.

Mechansim of Action
The receptor for EPO belongs to cytokine receptor superfamily. On binding with EPO it stimulates the tyrosine kinase bound to the receptor resulting in activation of a cascade of serine and threonine kinases which results in growth and development of target cells.

Regulation of Secretion
- The stimulus for secretion of EPO is hypoxia. It can also be stimulated by cobalt salts and androgens
- Secretion is also facilitated by alkalosis, catecholamines through β receptors
- Thyroxine and other hormones like growth hormone, ACTH also stimulate secretion of EPO
- Estrogen inhibits secretion of erythropoietin.

21. Calcitonin.
- It is synthesized by the C cells or parafollicular cells in thyroid gland
- It is also neural in origin
- It is polypeptide in nature
- It is secreted in response to increase in serum calcium levels.

Regulation
- Most important stimulus for secretion of calcitonin is rise in plasma calcium levels
- Other stimuli are catecholamines through β receptor, dopamine, gastrin, glucagon and secretin stimulates its secretion.

Actions of Calcitonin
- It lowers circulating calcium and phosphate levels. Calcium is lowered by inhibition of bone resorption. It also inhibits activity of osteoclasts in vitro
- It also increases calcium excretion via urine
- It helps in bone development in young individuals
- It protects against postprandial hypercalcemia
- It protects the bones of mother from excess calcium loss during pregnancy.

22. Functions of blood.

Nutritive function: Carries nutrients like glucose, proteins, vitamins, minerals and fats from GIT to cells.

Respiratory functions: Carries O_2 from lungs to tissues and CO_2 from tissues to lungs.

Excretory functions: Blood transports various metabolic waste products (urea, uric acid, creatinine) to excretory organs for excretion.

Transport function: Various hormones, Enzymes and antibodies are transported in blood.

Protective function: Neutrophils and monocytes phagocytose the micro-organisms, lymphocytes take part in immunity, eosinophils detoxify, disintegrate and remove foreign particles. Platelets prevent loss of blood.

Homeostatic function: Maintains fluid and electrolyte balance. Maintains pH and body temperature.

Storage function: Readymade source of glucose, water, proteins and electrolytes.

23. Korotkov's sound.

- These sounds are heard during recording of arterial blood pressure (BP) by auscultatory method
- This is based on the principle that streamline flow in an artery is silent and turbulent flow creates sounds
- While recording blood pressure by auscultatory method by using a Sphygmomanometer, Riva-rocci cuff is tied in the upper arm overlying the brachial artery
- The cuff is inflated well above the systolic pressure in the artery
- At this point, on auscultation over the artery no sounds are heard as the artery is completely occluded by the inflated cuff
- Now the cuff pressure is gradually released and auscultation is done over the Brachial artery
- At the point at which the cuff pressure is just below the systolic pressure, there is a spurt of blood, flowing through the vessel only during systole
- Since the vessel is still constricted the flow is intermittent and turbulent and it creates an intermittent taping sound
- These sounds are called as Korotkoff's sounds
- As the cuff pressure is lowered further, the sounds become louder, dull, muffled and then disappear as the artery is full open and thereby the flow becomes streamline again.

Krotkoff, sounds are described in 5 phases:
- **Phase 1:** It starts appearing with a tapping sound. It denotes systolic BP. This phase lasts for 10-12 mm Hg fall in BP
- **Phase 2:** Sounds become murmur-like and is for 14-15 mm Hg fall in mercury column.
- **Phase 3:** Sounds become clear, knocking or banging in quality. It is heard for 14-15 mm Hg fall in mercury column
- **Phase 4:** Sounds again become muffled in quality. It is dull and faint. It lasts for 4-5 mm Hg fall in mercury column
- **Phase 5:** No sounds are heard here. It is taken to be the diastolic BP.

24. Heart sounds.

Refer answers to 2006 paper.

25. Timed vital capacity.

- When vital capacity is related to time it is said to be timed vital capacity
- **It is defined as the percentage of vital capacity that is expired in a unit of time**
- It is also called as Forced vital capacity or Forced expiratory volume (FEV) as the person exhales rapidly and forcibly in a unit of time
- FEV1: Volume expelled in the 1st second – 80% of VC
- FEV2: Volume expelled in the 2nd second – 90% of VC
- FEV3: Volume expelled in 3rd second – 100% of VC
- FEV1/FVC ratio is a good indicator to diagnose Obstructive and restrictive pulmonary diseases
- In Obstructive disease FEV1/FVC ratio is decreased

- In restrictive disorders it may be normal or increased.

26. Oxygen dissociation curve.

Refer answers to 2004 paper.

27. Non-respiratory functions of lung.

Non-respiratory Functions

1. **Acts as a reservoir for blood:** The pulmonary vessels are highly compliant and therefore can store blood without much increase in pressure. In cases of imbalance in left ventricular output and systemic venous return, the stored blood in the pulmonary circulation helps to regulate cardiac output
2. **Filters** small emboli, particles in blood, detached cancer cells, fat cells, air emboli in blood
3. **Processes inhaled air:** The atmospheric air which enters the airways are hydrated as it passes through the airways
4. **Olfactory function**
5. **Metabolic function:**
   a. Synthezises and secretes surfactant
   b. Pulmonary capillary endothelial cells secrete angiotensin converting enzyme (ACE) and thereby converts angiotensin I to angiotensin II
   c. Synthezises, stores and secretes substances like prostaglandins, histamine and kallikrein
   d. Partially removes prostaglandin, bradykinin, adenine nucleotides, serotonin, norepinephrine and acetylcholine.
6. **Helps in defense:** With the help of pulmonary alveolar macrophages, IgA, mucus secretion, beating of cilia, cough reflex
7. **Helps in speech**
8. **Helps in absorption** of drugs like anaesthetic gases, aerosols and bronchodilators
9. **Fibrinolytic mechanism** present in the lungs lyses the clot.

28. ECG leads.

ECG is recorded using electrodes. It could be Unipolar electrodes (an active electrode is connected to an indifferent electrode at zero potential) or bipolar electrode (Using two active electrodes). There are also limb leads placed on the limbs and chest leads placed on the precordium.

Bipolar Limb Leads

Bipolar limb leads are the earlier ones and there are three bipolar limb leads—Lead I, II and III. In these leads, when depolarization moves towards a positive electrode it will record a positive deflection and when depolarization moves in the opposite direction it will record a negative deflection. These leads record the potential differences between two limbs. The body fluids are good conductors of current and therefore leads can be placed anywhere in the limbs to record the potential differences (refer Fig. 18).

- Lead I – Electrodes are in left and right arms, with left arm positive
- Lead II – Electrodes are in right arm and left leg and left leg is positive
- Lead III – Electrodes are on left leg and left arm, leg is postive.

Unipolar Limb Leads

There are three unipolar limb leads, those which record the potential difference between an active electrode and an indifferent electrode (by connecting all bipolar electrodes to a common terminal an indifferent electrode is obtained).

They are aVR, aVL and aVF. 'a' stands for augmented lead. It is recorded between one limb and the other two limbs, this increases the size of the potential by 50% without changing the configuration from the unaugmented leads. R stands for right arm, L for left arm and F for left foot.

- aVF reflects the activity of inferior surface of heart
- aVL records the activity of left outer aspect of heart
- aVR records the electrical activity of cavity of ventricles.

Unipolar Leads

There are six unipolar chest leads; V1, V2, V3, V4, V5 and V6 (refer Fig. 19).

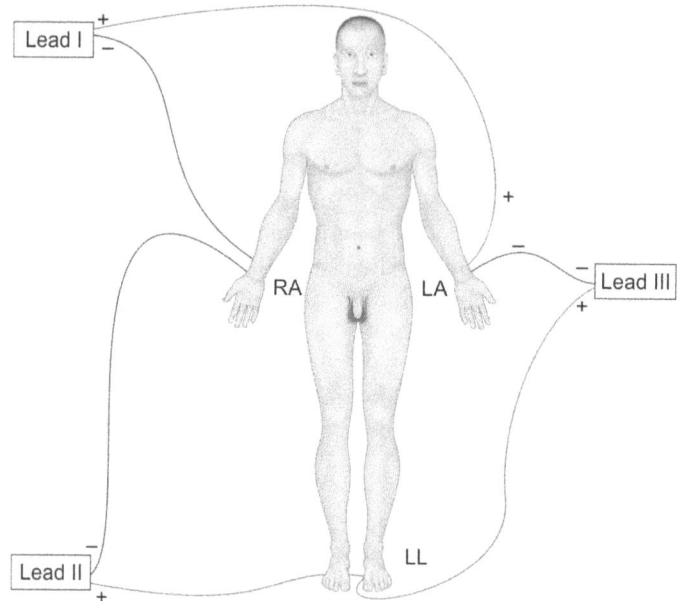

Fig. 18: Position of electrodes for standard limb leads.
(*Source:* Sembulingam)

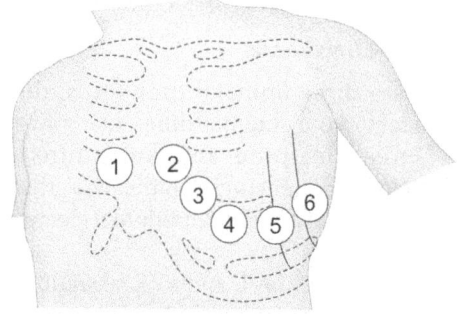

Fig. 19: Position of electrodes for unipolar chest leads.
(*Source:* Sembulingam)

- V1—4th Intercostal space (ICS), right of sternum
- V2—4th ICS left of sternum
- V3—Midway between V2 and V4
- V4—5th left ICS in midclavicular line
- V5—5th left ICS in anterior axillary line
- V6—5th left ICS, in mid axillary line.

V1 and V2 reflect the electrical activity of right ventricle, so QRS deflection is negative.

V3 and V4 record the electrical activities of both the ventricles and interventricular septum. QRS defelection is biphasic.

V5 and V6 record the electrical activities of left ventricle. QRS defelection is positive.

Esophageal Leads

Unipolar leads can be inserted via catheters and can be placed in the esophagus to record potentials in the heart.

29. Baroreceptors.

Refer answers to 2003 paper.

30. Color blindness.

Refer answers to 2005 paper.

31. Parkinsonism.

Refer answers to 2005 paper.

32. Middle ear.

Refer answers to 2005 paper.

MBBS Examination 2008

ANSWER ALL QUESTIONS

I. Essay questions (15 Marks each)

1. Discuss the regulation of serum calcium concentration. What is tetany? How do you treat it?
2. Enumerate the functions of liver and write about jaundice.
3. Name the functional lobes of cerebellum. Describe the connections and functions of neocerebellum. Mention the clinical features of cerebellar disease.
4. Write about the functions of hypothalamus
5. What is menstrual cycle? Explain the ovarian changes taking place in the menstrual cycle.
6. What are different types of salivary glands? Describe the composition, functions and regulation of secretion of saliva.
7. Enumerate the descending tracts of spinal cord. Describe in detail the pyramidal tracts. Mention its functions and effects of lesion at different levels.
8. Define arterial blood pressure. Describe the nervous regulation of arterial blood pressure.

II. Short notes (5 Marks each)

1. Ovulation.
2. Glomerular filtration rate.
3. Physiologic principles of tissue transplantation.
4. Micturition.
5. Movements of small intestine.
6. T lymphocytes.
7. Enzymes of exocrine pancreas.
8. Corpus luteum.
9. Tubular maximum for glucose.
10. Reactions due to incompatible blood transfusion. What is autologous transfusion?
11. Travelling wave theory.
12. Electroencephalogram.
13. Reynold's number.
14. Plasticity of smooth muscle.
15. Decompression sickness.
16. Conditioned reflex.
17. Heart failure.
18. Refractive errors.
19. Differences between three types of muscles.
20. Write the features of acromegaly.
21. Tubuloglomerular feedback.
22. Mechanism of HCl secretion in the stomach.
23. Extrinsic mechanism of coagulation of blood.
24. Write the functions of platelets.
25. Write the actions of parathormone.
26. Cystometrogram.
27. Explain neuroendocrine reflex.
28. Erythroblastosis fetalis.
29. Haemophilia.
30. Surfactant.
31. Chloride shift.
32. Artificial respiration.
33. Taste pathway.
34. Effects of lesion in optic pathway.
35. Brown-Sequard syndrome.
36. Functions of thalamus.
37. Pacemaker potential.
38. Regulation of coronary circulation.
39. Neuromuscular transmission.

III. Short answers (2 Marks each)

1. Functions of eosinophil.
2. Name anticoagulants used in the laboratories.
3. Write differences between adult hemoglobin and fetal hemoglobin.
4. Functions of sertoli cells.
5. Functions of large intestine.
6. Migrating myoelectric complex (MMC).
7. Achalasia cardia.
8. Name the homones of hypothalamus.
9. Write the actions of prolactin.
10. Name second messengers.
11. Define sarcomere. Mention normal length of sarcomere.
12. Myasthenia gravis.
13. Windkessel effect.
14. Phonocardiogram.
15. Haldane effect.
16. VO_2 Max.
17. Babinski sign.
18. Alpha block.
19. Functions of aqueous humor.
20. Rinne's test.

I. ESSAY QUESTIONS

1. **Discuss the regulation of serum calcium concentration. What is tetany? How do you treat it?**

- Normal plasma concentration of calcium is 10 mg/dL (5 meq/L or 2.5 mmol/L). Plasm calcium is in bound form (non-diffusible) and in ionic and complexed form (diffusible)
- 99% of the body calcium is present in the bones. In the bone, calcium pool is of two types—readily exchangable reservoir and a stable pool
- Calcium has various actions in the body; acts as a second messenger, needed for muscle contraction and coagulation of blood
- All these actions are done by ionic calcium. It is very important to regulate the ECF calcium levels as hypocalcemia increases neuromuscular excitability and may lead to tetany
- In tetany the skeletal muscles go in for spasm and laryngospasm may lead to fatal asphyxia. So the calcium levels are needed to be regulated
- There are 3 hormones regulating blood calcium levels.

The hormones involved in calcium homeostasis are:

- Parathormone
- 1, 25 Dihydroxycholecalciferol or calcitriol
- Calcitonin.

Parathormone and calcitriol increase serum calcium levels and calcitonin decreases calcium levels.

Calcium homeostasis is done by these hormones.

Parathormone

- Parathormone is a polypeptide hormone with 84 amino acids secreted by the chief cells of the parathyroid gland.
- The main actions of parathyroid hormone (PTH) are to increase blood calcium levels and decrease Phosphate levels.

Effect on Bones

- It increases activity of both osteoclasts and osteoblasts
- But the osteoclastic activity is the major effect resulting in resorption of bone and release of calcium and phosphates into the extracellular fluid (ECF)
- PTH stimulates the differentiation of precursors into osteoclasts, increases their numbers and size. The products of resorption are present in blood and are excreted in urine
- PTH increases calcium resorption from the bones in 2 phases—rapid phase and slow phase
- **Osteolytic activity:** PTH causes demineralization of bone and there is transport of calcium from the bone fluid into the osteocytes and from there to the osteoblasts through gap junctions. Osteoblasts

pump calcium into surrounding matrix and then into ECF. This process is termed osteocytic osteolysis
- **Action on osteoclasts:** This effect comes into action after a few days of exposure to PTH. The number and activity of osteoclasts are increased. Osteoclasts increase bone resorption and thereby increases calcium and phophate levels in the blood. Also levels of hydroxyproline and hydroxylysine are increased
- **Action on osteoblasts:** At low doses PTH increases osteoblastic activity but in high doses it inhibits action of osteoblasts.

Action on Kidneys
- There are 3 major actions on the kidneys:
  1. Increased reabsorption of calcium in the thick ascending limb of loop of Henle and distal convoluted tubule (DCT). 25–30% of the filtered Ca^{2+} is reabsorbed in the DCT and Loop of Henle by the action of PTH. 65% of filtered Ca^{2+} is reabsorbed in the proximal convoluted tubule (PCT)
  2. Decreases reabsorption of phosphate in the kidneys by its action on the PCT and induces phosphaturia. Serum phosphate levels are lowered by the action of PTH
  3. Stimulates the formation of 1, 25 Dihydroxycholecalciferol (calcitriol) by the kidneys. PTH stimulates the 1α Hydroxylation of 25 hydroxycholecalciferol to form the active form of vitamin D3. Calcitriol in turn increases reabsorption of calcium from gastrointestinal tract (GIT) and kidneys.

Calcitriol
Calcitriol is the active form of vitamin D_3 and is also called as 1, 25 Dihydroxycholecalciferol.

Actions of Calcitriol
- **Action on GIT:** It increases absorption of calcium from the GIT by increasing its permeability of brush border of the enetrocytes. It also increases synthesis of Calbindin, a calcium binding protein in enterocytes
- **Actions on bones:** It induces bone resorption and mineralization. In presence of PTH, calcitriol induces bone resorption
- **Action on kidneys:** It increases reabsorption of calcium and phosphates from the renal tubules
- **Other actions:** Increases calcium transport into skeletal muscles and bones, stimulation and differentiation of immune cells, it regulates growth and induces formation of growth factors.

Regulation of Synthesis of Calcitriol
- **Plasma calcium levels:** Increase in plasma calcium levels decreases Parathormone secretion which in turn decreases synthesis of calcitriol. Decrease in blood calcium levels increases PTH levels and calcitriol synthesis increases
- **Plasma phosphate levels:** Phosphate levels regulate synthesis of calcitriol by negatively inhibiting the enzyme 1, α hydroxylase
- **Levels of Calcitriol:** The calcitriol has a direct negative feedback effect on its synthesis. It also acts on the parathyroid gland and inhibits synthesis of PTH
- **Other factors** like prolactin, estrogen, growth hormone, human chorionic somatomammotrophin and calcitonin stimulate synthesis and Thyroid hormone excess and acidosis decrease synthesis.

Calcitonin
Refer August 2007 paper.

Tetany
- Tetany is neuro-muscular hyperexcitability due to hypocalcemia
- The decrease in calcium ions in plasma results in reduction in the amount of depolarization needed to excite the nerves.

The signs and symptoms are:
a. *Carpopedal spasm:* There is flexion at metacarpophalangeal joints, extension at interphalangeal joints and opposition of thumb. In the legs the toes are plantarflexed and feet are drawn up

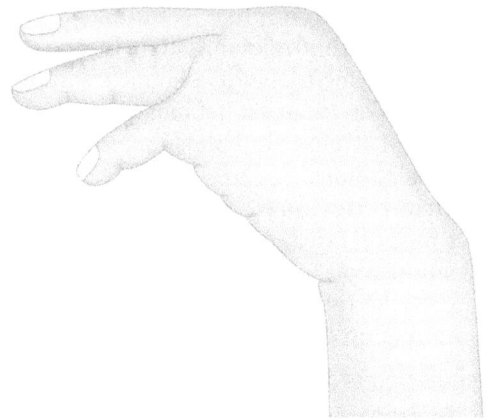

Fig. 1: Trousseau's sign.
(*Source:* GK Pal)

b. *Trousseau's sign:* It is seen in latent tetany. On inflation of the sphygmomanometer cuff to the arm and occlusion of blood vessels results in appearance of the carpal spasm (refer Fig. 1)
c. *Chvostek's sign:* On tapping the facial nerve at the angle of the jaw there is twitching of facial muscles
d. *Laryngeal stridor:* Spasm of laryngeal muscles results in constriction of larynx and it may result in asphyxia
e. *Paraesthesia:* Tingling sensation in peripheral parts of limbs

Tetany is treated with infusion of ionized calcium and parathormone replacement.

2. Enumerate the functions of liver and write about jaundice.

Liver has various functions in the body, especially in metabolism and excretion.
The functions of liver are:
a. Storage function: Liver stores protein, glycogen, Vitamins A, D and B12 and iron
b. Synthesis function: Liver synthesises albumin, clotting factors (I, II, V, VII, IX and X), lipids, bile salts, cholesterol, heparin and enzymes like serum glutamic oxaloacetic transaminase (SGOT), serum glutamic pyruvic transaminase (SGPT) etc.
c. Metabolic functions: Liver takes part in metabolism of carbohydrates, proteins, lipids and vitamins.
   Carbohydrate metabolism: It takes part in glycogenolysis, glycogenesis and gluconeogenesis.
   Protein metabolism: Synthesizes many proteins like albumin. It also converts ammonia to urea. It is the site of synthesis of urea.
   Lipid metabolism: Synthesis of triglycerides from free fatty acids and glycerol, formation of ketones following lipolysis and synthesis of lipoproteins (HDL, LDL)
d. Secretory function: Liver secretes bile acids and bile salts in bile
e. Excretory function – Liver excretes heavy metals like lead and arsenic. Bile pigments and some hormones are excreted in bile following its metabolism in liver. Cholesterol is also excreted
f. Detoxification functions: Many drugs are detoxified in the liver. Certain unwanted substances are conjugated with glucuronic acid and are made water soluble and excreted in urine
g. Defense function: Kupffer cells lining the sinusoids remove the pathogens ingested with food
h. It is also the site of formation of RBCs in fetal life and also a site of destruction of RBCs
i. Along with skin and kidneys liver is also a site of synthesis of 1, 25 Dihydroxycholecalciferol.

Jaundice

Jaundice is yellowish discoloration of skin, sclera and other body fluids. There is deposition of bilirubin in the tissues and tissue fluids. This happens when serum bilirubin level exceeds 2 mg/dL. Normal serum bilirubin level is 0.2-0.8 mg/dL.

Before understanding pathophysiology of jaundice we need to know about the formation of biliruin from hemoglobin.

Fate of Hemoglobin
Refer answers to 2006 paper.

Types of Jaundice
Jaundice can be due to either excess formation of bilirubin as in hemolytic anemia or due to improper excretion of bile.

Based on the above two reasons there are three types of jaundice:
- Prehepatic jaundice or hemolytic jaundice
- Hepatic jaundice
- Obstructive jaundice.

Hemolytic Jaundice
- In conditions where there is excessive lysis of RBCs as in spherocytosis, sickle cell anemia etc., there is formation of excess of bilirubin
- Since there is excessive release of bilirubin nomal liver is not able to conjugate the bilirubin
- Serum unconjugated bilirubin (Bilirubin + Albumin) levels are high. So no bilirubin is present in urine (Acholuric jaundice)
- The amount of bilirubin delivered to intestines is high and therefore there is increase in formation of stercobilinogen in intestine
- Feces appears dark in color. Urine urobilinogen levels are also high
- Van den Bergh reaction is indirectly positive.

Hepatic Jaundice
- It usually happens due to infective or toxic damage to the liver
- Liver is unable to effectively conjugate bilirubin. Whatever conjugated bilirubin present is also not able to be excreted by the damaged liver cells
- So both conjugated and unconjugated bilirubin levels are increased in serum
- As conjugated bilirubin levels are high it is excreted in urine and therefore urine bilirubin levels are high and urine appears yellow in color
- Bile excreted in intestine is decreased so stercobilin levels in feces are decreased. Urine urobilin levels are also decreased
- Since there is liver damage albumin synthesis is less and there is decrease in albumin to globulin (A/G) ratio
- Serum alkaline phosphatase levels are increased
- Van den Bergh test reaction is biphasic.

Obstructive Jaundice
- There is obstruction in the flow of bile from the liver as in biliary calculi or tumor
- Conjugated bilirubin levels rise in serum
- Since there is no bile entering the intestine there is no stercobilinogen in the feces and stools are clay colored
- Urobilinogen is also not formed and there is no urinary urobilinogen
- The conjugated bilirubin levels rise in serum and since it is water soluble there is excretion in the urine and urine is deep yellow in color
- A/G ratio may be normal but later decreases due to liver damage
- Van den Bergh test is directly positive
- Serum alkaline phosphatase level is markedly increased as it is not excreted in bile.

Physiological Jaundice
- It is seen in new borns and so also called as Neonatal jaundice
- It is seen within 2–5 days after birth and disappears by 1–2 weeks.
  It is due to:
  - Excessive destruction of RBCs after birth resulting in high serum bilirubin levels
  - It is also due to hepatic immaturity: In fetal life, bilirubin is removed from circulation by the placenta. After birth the liver is immature to handle the load of bilirubin in the first 10 days. So serum bilirubin rises till 7–10 days after that it starts to decrease as the liver takes up the conjugating function
  - It is usually more common in preterm infants and low birth weight babies
  - This condition is treated with phototherapy. Here the babies are

exposed to white light. This converts bilirubin to lumirubin which is water soluble and can be easily excreted in urine.

3. Name the functional lobes of cerebellum. Describe the connections and functions of neocerebellum. Mention the clinical features of cerebellar disease.

Refer answers to 2006 paper – Functional lobes, connections and functions of cerebellum.

Clinical Features of Cerebellar Lesions

- Patients with cerebellar lesion do not show much abnormalities when they are at rest
- The symptoms are well established when they move
- There is **no paralysis or sensory defects**
- The effect of lesion is manifested on the same side of lesion
- There is marked incoordination of movements—ataxia
- This is due to errors in rate, range, force and direction of movement
- There is hypotonia
- There is loss of equilibrium.

Ataxia is expressed as:

- Instability during walking which is expressed as **drunken gait or wide-based gait**
- There are also defects in skilled movements like **scanning of speech**
- **Past pointing or dysmetria:** Attempting to touch an object with one finger results in overshooting to one side or the other. This is followed by correction of the overshoot which results in overshooting to the other side
- Therefore the finger oscillates back and forth resulting in **intention tremors**
- It is called so as it is seen when the person attempts to do an action
- The person with cerebellar lesion is unable to brake a movement or stop a movement. For example in a normal person flexion of the forearm against resistance is kept in check when the resistance is suddenly released. But in a person with cerebellar lesion the patient is unable to brake the movement and the forarm flies backward in an arc—**rebound phenomenon**
- They also show the feature of **adiadochokinesia**—inability to do rapid alternating opposite movements such as repeated supination and pronation of the hands
- They show **decomposition of movement:** The movements are dissected into individual components and carried out in each joint at a time
- Defects in flocculonodular lobe (vestibulocerebellum) results in **vertigo, nystagmus and motion sickness**.

4. Write about the functions of hypothalamus.

- It is a small part located inferior to thalamus, composed of dozen nuclei (refer Fig. 2)
- It is divided into four major areas
  a. **Preoptic region:** Medial and lateral preoptic nucleus
  b. **Supraoptic region:** Supraoptic, suprachiasmatic, paraventricular and anterior nuclei
  c. **Tuberal region:** Venteromedial, dorsomedial, arcuate, lateral and posterior nuclei
  d. **Mamillary region:** Medial and lateral mammillary nuclei, pre and supra mammillary nuclei.

Connections

There are afferent and efferent connections to and from hypothalamus.

Afferents are from limbic system, brainstem, thalamus, retina, basal ganglia and cortex.

From Limbic System

a. Medial forebrain bundle: This is the major connecting system of hypothalamus with other areas. It connects piriform cortex and amygdala with lateral hypothalamus. It also extends to tegmentum of midbrain and end on raphe nuclei here. They are related to emotions and olfaction.
b. Fornix: Largest fiber system and connects hippocampus with mamillary body.

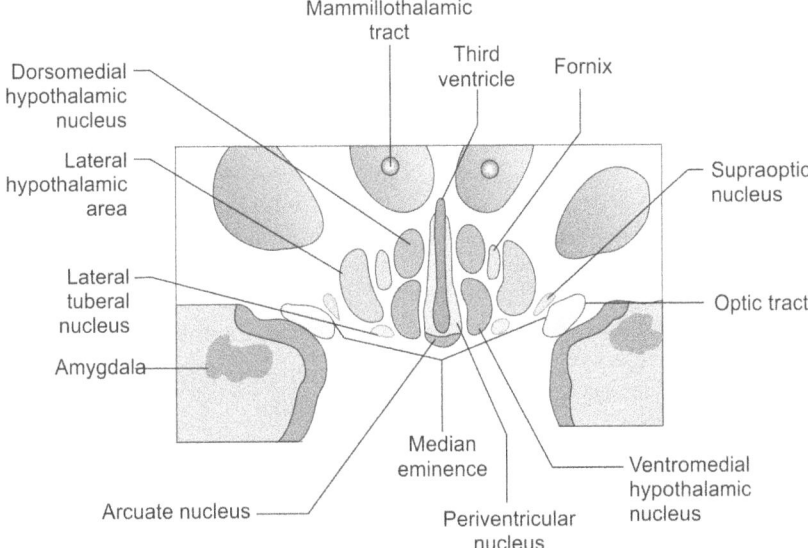

Fig. 2: Nuclei in hypothalamus.
(*Source:* Sembulingam)

c. Stria terminalis: Connects amygdala with preoptic area and anterior nucleus of thalamus.
d. Medial hypothalamic tract: Connects hippocampus with arcuate nucleus.

Afferents from Brainstem

a. Mamillotegmental tract: Connects tegmentum with mamillary body
b. Dorsal longitudinal fasciculus arises from periaqueductal grey and ends on dorsal and caudal areas of hypothalamus.
c. Noradrenergic fibers project from locus ceruleus to dorsal hypothalamus
d. Serotonergic fibers project from raphe nucleus to hypothalamus, amygdala and cortex.

From Other Areas

a. Retinohypothalamic tract: Connects optic nerve with suprachiasmatic nucleus and is involved in regulation of circadian rhythm.
b. Thalamohypothalamic tract: Connects midline and dorsomedial nucleus to various areas of hypothalamus.
c. Pallidohypothalamic tract: Connects globus pallidus to hypothalamus.
d. Corticohypothalamic fibers: Connects various areas of cerebral cortex to hypothalamus.

Efferents

Efferents to limbic system:
a. Stria terminalis: Connects venteromedial nucleus with amygdaloid nucleus
b. Ventral pathway: Connects lateral hypothalamus with lateral nucleus
c. Medial forebrain bundle: Connects lateral hypothalamus with septal nucleus and then project to hippocampus.
d. Posterior longitudinal fasiculus connects autonomic center in hypothalmus with autonomic areas in brainstem and spinal cord.
e. Mamillothalamic tract: It is a part of Papez circuit. It connects mamillary body to anterior thalamic nucleus and ends on cingulate gyrus.
f. Mamillotegmental tract arises from mamillary body and ends on tegmental reticular nuclei in midbrain.
g. Hypothalamohypophyseal tract: Connects supraoptic and paraventricular nuclei to posterior pituitary.

h. Hypothalamic connections with infundibulum. Fibers arise from various nuclei of hypothalamus and ends on median eminence.

Functions

a. Regulation of food intake
b. Regulation of body temperature
c. Regulation of thirst
d. Regulation of anterior pituitary hormones
e. Regulation of posterior pituitary hormones
f. Regulation of sleep wake cycle
g. Control of autonomic nervous system
h. Control of reproduction
i. Control of emotions
j. Control of circadian rhythm
k. Role in stress
l. Role in visceral and somatic function
m. Role in reward and punishment.

Regulation of Food Intake

- There are 2 groups of neurons involved in food intake:
  1. Venteromedial (VM) nucleus (satiety center)
  2. Lateral nucleus (feeding center).
- Feeding center stimulates appetite and increases food intake and satiety center inhibits feeding center and brings satiety.

Hypotheses Regulating Food Intake

These are the hypothesis regulating food-intake:

1. **Glucostatic hypothesis:** Activity of satiety center is regulated by glucose utilization of the neurons. When the glucose utilization is low their activity is less and vice versa. When satiety center activity is less the feeding center's activity is unchecked and the person feels hungry. When utilization is high, the glucostats activity is unchecked and there is inhibition of feeding center and the person feels satiated. Hypoglycemia is an appetite stimulant and the decrease in plasma glucose decreases the utilization of glucose by the cells
2. **Lipostatic hypothesis:** This hypothesis is based on the fact that the adipose tissues send humoral signals like Leptin, a hormone secreted by adipose tissue. When fat depots are more, the leptin levels increase and it decreases food intake and increases energy output
3. **Gut-peptide theory:** After food intake, there are hormones released from the GIT which act on the hypothalamus and thereby inhibits food intake
4. **Thermostatic theory:** Food intake is increased in cold weather and decreased in warm weather.

Hormones and neurotensin (NT) Regulating Food Intake

- Hormones increasing food intake:
  a. Neuropeptide Y
  b. Orexins
  c. Ghrelin
  d. Melanin-concentrating hormone (MCH)
  e. Agouti related peptide (AGRP)
  f. Galanin
  g. Growth hormone-releasing hormone (GHRH)
- Hormones decreasing food intake:
  a. Estrogen
  b. Dopamine
  c. Alpha-melanocyte-stimulating hormone (α-MSH)
  d. Cocaine- and amphetamine-regulated transcript (CART)
  e. Corticotrophin releasing hormone (CRH)
  f. Gut hormones
  g. Cholecystokinin
  h. Leptin.

Temperature Regulation

- Humans need to maintain body temperature at 37°C
- Preoptic region of anterior hypothalamus has a role in regulation of body temperature in warmth. When body temperature goes above set point it stimulates heat dissipating mechanisms like vasodilation and sweating
- Posterior hypothalamus acts in cool temperature and involved in heat conserving mechanisms like vasoconstriction, piloerection and sympathetic stimulation.

Regulation of Thirst
- Thirst center is located in the hypothalamus
- It is located in the lateral hypothalamus
- It is stimulated by osmoreceptors in increase in tonicity of body fluids
- A decrease in extracellular fluid (ECF) volume also stimulates thirst center.

Regulation of ECF Volume
Achieved by regulation of antidiuretic hormone (ADH), aldosterone and thirst mechanism.

Regulation of Endocrine Functions
- Hypothalamus controls anterior pituitary and through anterior pituitary it regulates secretion of other endocrine glands
- It secretes posterior pituitary hormones
- Hypothalamus is considered to be the master of Endocrine orchestra
- It is a part of the brain and therefore is the link between neural and endocrine systems.

Control of Reproduction
- Hypothalamus releases gonadotropin-releasing hormone (GnRH) which regulates the release of follicle stimulating hormone (FSH) and luteinizing hormone (LH) from anterior pituitary gland
- They in turn control reproductive function in males and females
- They regulate spermatogenesis, development of accessory sex organs in males and menstrual cycle and secondary sexual characteristics in females
- Also the sexual behaviour are influenced by hypothalamus (preoptic and anterior hypothalamus).

Regulation of Sleep Wake Cycle
- Hypothalamus regulates sleep wake cycle
- There are 2 sleep centers:
  1. Diencephalic sleep zone
  2. Basal forebrain sleep zone.
- Stimulation of these areas at the frequency of 8 Hz induces slow wave sleep.

Control of Autonomic Nervous System (ANS)
- Hypothalamus controls and integrates the activities of ANS
- Through ANS it is a major regulator of visceral activities
- Stimulation of posterior hypothalamus results in increase in HR, BP, pupillary dilatation, piloerection (sympathetic system stimulated)
- Stimulation of anterior hypothalamus results in decreased HR, increased HCl secretion, urination etc (parasympathetic system stimulated).

Regulation of Emotional and Behavioral Patterns
- With the limbic system (LS) it participates in the expressions of emotions
- The Papez circuit (Fig. 3) is responsible for emotions.

Regulation of Circadian Rhythm
- The suprachiasmatic nucleus establishes patterns of awakening and sleep that occur on a circadian (daily) schedule
- This is mediated through Retino-hypothalamic tract
- **Examples:**
  a. Cortisol secretion
  b. Body temperature
  c. Adrenocorticotropic hormone (ACTH) secretion
  d. Melatonin secretion
  e. Sleep-wakefulness.

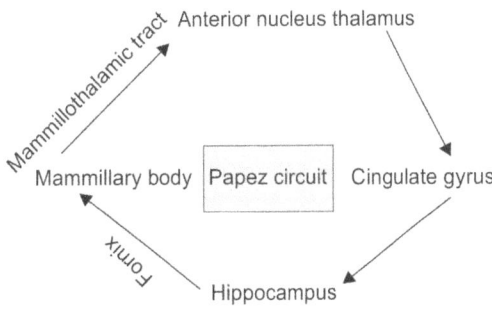

Fig. 3: Papez circuit.

Regulation of Reward and Punishment Areas:
- Hypothalamus along with LS and Cortex integrate and bring about smooth responses for reward and punishment
- VM nucleus is associated with reward and posterior and lateral nuclei of hypothalamus with punishment.

5. What is menstrual cycle? Explain the ovarian changes taking place in the menstrual cycle.

Refer answers to 2006 paper.

6. What are different types of salivary glands? Describe the composition, functions and regulation of secretion of saliva.

- There are major and minor salivary glands
- They can be classifed as mucous and serous salivary glands based on the type of secretory cells in the salivary acini (refer Fig. 4)
- There are 3 pairs of major salivary glands situated in the oral cavity—parotid, sublingual and sub-mandibular salivary glands
- Parotid glands are purely serous in nature and they secrete watery saliva
- Sublingual gland is a mucous gland secretes thick viscous saliva
- Submandibular glands are mixed glands; they have both serous and mucous types of secretory cells lining the acini

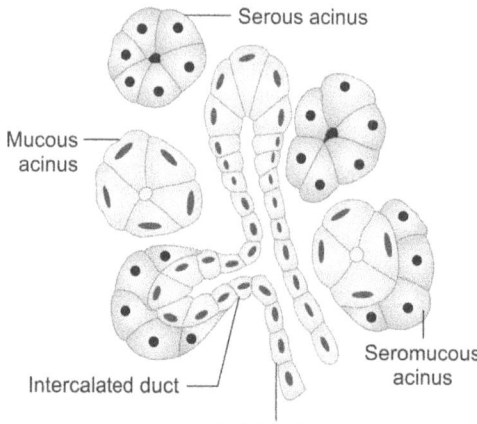

Fig. 4: Histology of salivary gland showing the duct system and acini with mucous and serous cells.
(*Source:* GK Pal)

- Minor salivary glands are present in the mucosa of oral cavity, buccal mucosa etc.

Composition, Functions and Regulation of Secretion of Saliva

Refer answers to 2003 paper.

7. Enumerate the descending tracts of spinal cord. Describe in detail the pyramidal tracts. Mention its functions and effects of lesion at different levels.

Refer answers to 2006 paper.

8. Define arterial blood pressure. Describe the nervous regulation of arterial blood pressure.

Refer answers to 2006 paper.

II. SHORT NOTES

1. Ovulation.
- In a female with a 28 days cycle, ovulation occurs on the 14th day
- Just before ovulation, outer wall of the follicle swells and a small protrusion, the stigma is seen
- After a few minutes a fluid starts oozing out followed by the release of ovum along with the corona radiata around it.

Hormonal Changes
- 2 days before ovulation, estrogen levels increase and there is a positive feedback regulation of estrogen on LH secretion
- LH levels reach 6-10 times the normal value and peaks 10-12 hours before ovulation
- High LH levels are essential for the final growth, maturation and ovulation
- LH acts on the granulosa cells to increase progesterone secretion.

Causes:
- Theca externa cells to release proteolytic enzymes from lysosomes, which will dissolve the follicular capsule and degeneration of stigma
- Blood vessels grow rapidly into the follicle and prostaglandins are secreted into the follicle
- Both these events cause the follicle to swell and break the stigma and release the ovum.

Indicators of Ovulation

a. **Rise of basal body temperature**: There is a rise in 0.5°C in basal body temperature after ovulation. The rise is due to the thermogenic effect of progesterone which is secreted by corpus luteum. It is recorded first thing in the morning, orally, before getting up from bed, before eating or drinking anything
b. **Mittleschmertz**: After ovulation, bleeding into the ruptured follicle happens, some amount of blood is also spilt into the abdominal cavity close to the ovary and results in fleeting abdominal pain
c. **Spinnbarkeit**: During proliferative phase, under the influence of estrogen, cervical mucus is very thin and at the time of ovulation it is the thinnest and a drop of mucus between the thumb and index finger can be stretched to 10 cm, this is Spinnbarkeit
d. Sometimes following ovulation **mid-cycle** spotting can also be present
e. **Fern test**: At the time of ovulation, under the effect of estrogen, the cervical mucous is thin and when spread on a slide and viewed under the microscope gives a fern shape. In the luteal phase when progesterone is present this fern pattern is absent
f. **Demonstration of LH peak**: LH suge is seen just before ovulation and therefore regular estimation of LH levels can give us an idea about ovulation
g. Laparoscopic examination
h. Ultrasound scanning of pelvis.

2. Glomerular filtration rate.

Refer answers to 2003 and 2005 papers.

3. Physiologic principles of tissue transplantation.

Tissues or organs are transplanted when there is damage to an organ as in liver failure or kidney failure. Most commonly transplanted tissues are cornea, kidneys, skin, bone and liver. The organs after transplantation may function normally for a short period after which it may be necrosed and damaged due to rejection of the tissue by the donor. It happens because of a mounting immune response, especially the cellular immunity is responsible for graft rejection.

The rejection happens because of mismatch of the MHC antigen between the donor and recepient.

Various types of transplants:

a. Autograft: Tissue of the same person is transplanted from one part of the body to another part, e.g. skin transplant
b. Isograft: Transplant of tissue between identical twins. The transplanted tissue is never rejected.
c. Allograft: Transplantation of tissue/organ between individuals of same species but not identical twins, e.g. kidney transplant
d. Xenograft: Transplantation of tissues between different species. Animals to humans transplantation. It is rejected faster.

Physiological basis of Prevention of Transplant Rejection

The goal of treatment is to prevent rejection of transplanted tissue without getting the patient to suffer from massive infection or cancer.

a. Destruction of T lymphocytes and other rapidly dividing cells by using the drug such as azothioprine, a purine metabolite. The adverse effect of using this drug is the patient becomes susceptible to infections and cancer
b. Administration of glucocorticoids inhibits cytotoxic T cell proliferation by inhibiting production of IL-2
c. Treatment with cyclosporine or tacrolimus prevents transcription of IL-2 gene by preventing the dephosphorylation of NF-AT, a transcription factor. These drugs inhibit all the T cell mediated responses and they can also cause kidney damage
d. There are new drugs being developed to stop the second co-stimulation that is needed for normal activation of T lymphocytes.

4. Micturition.

Refer answers to 2006 paper.

5. Movements of small intestine.

Refer answers to 2004 paper.

6. T Lymphocytes.

Lymphocytes are produced in the bone marrow and some of them are transported to thymus gland. There they are processed to become T lymphocytes and are transported to lymphoid tissues and reside there till activation by antigens. These cells take part in cell mediated immunity. They are of 3 types.

Types of T Cells

There are 3 main types of T cells: Helper T cells (CD4 cells), Cytotoxic T cells (CD8 cells) and Memory T cells.

- *Helper T cells:* Helper T cells or CD4 cells recognise the antigen presented along with MHC II and Cytotoxic or CD8 cells recognise the antigens presented with MHC I. After co-stimulation of Helper T cells, they secrete many cytokines. The most important cytokine is IL-2 which is needed for all the immune responses and is the major stimulator for T cell proliferation. IL-2 is also the co-stimulator for resting Helper T cells and Cytotoxic T cells. It also enhances activation and proliferation of B cells and Natural killer cells
- *Cytotoxic T cells:* The T cells that express CD8 develop into Cytotoxic T cells. They recognise foreign antigens expressed along with MHC I on the membranes of body cells infected by viruses, tumor cells and cells of tissue transplant. But to get activated into a killer cell it needs co-stimulation by IL-2 produced by Helper cells. Therefore for maximal activation of Cytotoxic T cells it needs antigen presentation with MHC I and II
- *Memory T cells:* The T cells for a specific antigen which remain in the lymph organ after the immune response is over are termed as Memory T cells. If the same pathogen is encountered for the second time, these cells get activated and they initiate a swift and fast immune response. The second response is faster and vigorous

and the pathogen is eliminated even before any symptom develops.

Elimination of the Pathogens

The killing of the pathogen is done by the cytotoxic T cells.

a. The activated CD8 cells synthesize and secrete proteins called "Perforins" which are inserted into the membrane of the pathogen. The perforins are water channels which allow influx of water and thereby swelling of the microbe and cause its lysis
b. Release of Lymphotoxins by activated T cells. These cytokines destroy the microbes
c. Cytotoxic T cells secrete interferons which will favour the phagocytic activity of the neutrophils and macrophages by promoting opsonisation.

7. Enzymes of exocrine pancreas.

Pancreatic juice contains enzymes for digestion of lipids, proteins and carbohydrates.

Digestion of Lipids

a. Pancreatic lipase is the major fat digesting enzyme. It digests triglycerides into monoglycerides and fatty acids
b. Colipase: It exposes the active sites of pancreatic lipase and facilitates its lipolytic action
c. Phopholipase A2: It acts on phospholipids and converts it to fatty acids and lysophospholipids
d. Cholesterol ester hydrolase acts on cholesterol esters and splits it into cholesterol and fatty acids.

Digestion of Proteins

Proteolytic enzymes are secreted in the inactive forms—trypsingen, chymotrypsinogen.
Proelastase and procarboxypeptidase A and B.

a. Trypsinogen on secretion into duodenum is activated to trypsin by the enzyme enterokinase in the Intestine.
Trypsinogen → Trypsin, happens in presence of intestinal enzyme, enterokinase
b. Chymotrypsinogen → Chymotrypsin, in presence of trypsin

c. Proelastase and Procarboxylase → Elastase and carboxylase, in presence of trypsin
d. Trypsin and Chymorypsin act on proteins and polypeptides and cleaves the peptide bonds in basic and aromatic aminoacids
e. Elastase acts on elastin and some other proteins
f. Carboxypeptidases also act on proteins and polypeptides
g. Nucleases split ribose and deoxyribose nucleotides
h. Collagenase digests collagen

Digestion of Carbohydrates

Pancreatic α amylase: It is secreted in active form and just like salivary amylase it hydrolyzes glycogen, starch and other complex carbohydrates to form disaccharides.

8. Corpus luteum.

- On the 14th day of the menstrual cycle after the release of ovum from the Graafian follicle the inside of the follicle is filled with blood—*corpus haemorrhagicum*
- The granulosa and the thecal cells of the follicle proliferate and the clotted blood is replaced with yellowish lipid rich luteal cells forming the *corpus luteum*. Following this starts the luteal phase of menstrual cycle. The luteal cells start secreting estrogen and progesterone
- If pregnancy occurs, the corpus luteum persists and continues to produce progesterone which is essential for the survival of the fetus. Its function is maintained by human chorionic gonadotrophin (hCG) secreted from trophoblasts
- If fertilization has not occurred the corpus luteum regresses and degenerates 4 days before the next menstrual cycle. Gradually it is replaced by a scar tissue—*Corpus albicans*.

Functions of Corpus Luteum

a. Corpus luteum secretes estrogen and progesterone during the luteal phase of menstrual cycle

b. The progesterone secreted from the corpus luteum prepares the endometrium for the implantation of the fertilized ovum
c. On fertilization of the ovum, the corpus luteum continues to secrete progesterone till the placenta takes over the function of secreting progesterone.

9. Tubular maximum for glucose.

Transport maximum or tubular maximum (Tm) is the maximum amount of the solute that can be actively transported (reabsorbed or secreted) per minute by the renal tubules.

Tm is the level of the substance in tubular fluid at which the carrier protein, transporting the substance, gets saturated and beyond this level, the substances are no more reabsorbed or secreted and starts appearing in the urine.

Therefore the amount of substance transported depends on the amount of the solute present in the tubular fluid upto the Tm for the solute.

Therefore Tm is the amount of substance delivered to the tubule per minute and is given as the **tubular load**.

Tubular load is the quantity of a solute filtered by the glomerulus and presented to the tubule.

Tm depends on plasma concentration of the solute and the rate of filtration of the substance, so it is given as **Tm = Plasma concentration X GFR.**

Tubular Maximum for Glucose

The transporter in the epithelial cells of PCT used for reabsorption of glucose, on reaching its Tm, glucose is no more reabsorbed and it starts appearing in the urine.

Tm for glucose in males is 375mg/min and 300 mg/min in females.

Therefore the glucose transporter can transport glucose from tubular fluid into plasma up to plasma glucose levels of 300 mg% (300 mg/100 mL × 125 mL/min).

But glucose starts appearing in urine if a plasma concentration reaches 200 mg/dL. This is because of differences in the Tm of the tubules of various nephrons for reabsorption of glucose.

Tm is applicable only for substances which are actively transported and not for substances which are passively transported.

Substances having a Tm are—glucose, amino acids, uric acid, pulmonary arterial hypertension (PAH) etc.

Substances which do not have a Tm are— Na^+, HCO_3^-

Renal threshold is the concentration of a solute in plasma at or above which the substance starts appearing in the urine.

10. Reactions due to incompatible blood transfusion. What is autologous transfusion?

Due to Mismatched Transfusion

- Happens immediately → Agglutination of RBCs → Hemolysis - Acute hemolytic transfusion reactions. Usually happens in ABO incompatibility
- **Complications are:**
  - Shivering and fever
  - Hemoglobinemia and hemoglobinuria
  - Jaundice: Excessive lysis leads to hemolytic jaundice
  - Acute renal failure: Due to the hemoglobin released by hemolysis may block the renal tubules, release of toxic compounds from lysed RBCs and due to circulatory shock
  - Clumped RBCs block vessels of vital organs leading to stroke, myocardial infarction etc.
  - Hyperkalemia: K^+ is released from RBCs.

Autologous Blood Transfusion

- It is transfusion of one's own blood. It is usually done before elective surgeries. 1000–1500 mL of blood can be withdrawn in a period of 3 months and is stored in blood bank
- The patient is under iron treatment during the time period of withdrawal of blood
- The same blood is transfused during the time of surgery
- The hemoglobin level of the subject should be more than 12g/dL to withdraw blood
- It has come into use in fear of transmission of AIDS by heterologous transfusion
- It is also useful since it can prevent transfusion reactions.

11. Traveling wave theory.

- Traveling wave theory was proposed by George Von Bekesy in 1941
- The sound waves travel through the external ear and hit the tympanic membrane and this creates a movement of the stapes attached to oval window
- Movement of stapes sets up a travelling wave in the perilymph of scala vestibuli
- This travelling wave induces a vibration in the cochlea and the basilar membrane
- The wave causes distortion in basilar membrane
- As the wave travels the basilar membrane from the base to apex of cochlea it reaches a maximum amplitude at a particular point depending upon the frequency of the sound wave
- Sounds of lower frequency create waves which attain maximum amplitude closer to the apex of cochlea
- High frequency sounds create waves which attain maximum amplitude near the base of cochlea
- Thus the brain understands the frequencey of sounds based on the impulses arising from various points of the basilar membrane.

12. Electroencephalogram.

Refer answers to 2006 paper.

13. Reynold's number.

- The blood flow in a straight vessel is laminar or streamline. The velocity of blood flow in the center of the stream is greatest and lowest immediately below the vessel wall
- Laminar flow occurs at velocities up to a level called as the **critical velocity**
- At or above this velocity, the flow becomes turbulent

- Laminar flow is silent but turbulent flow creates sounds
- The probability of turbulence is also related to diameter of vessel and viscosity of blood
- **This is given as the Reynold's number (Re)**
  Re = ρDV/η
  ρ = Density of fluid
  D = Diameter of tube
  V = Velocity of flow
  η = Viscosity of fluid
- Higher the value of Re greater is the turbulence
- When D is in cm, V is in cm/s^{-1}, η is in poises, flow is not turbulent if Re is < 2000. When Re > 3000 there is always turbulent flow.

14. Plasticity of smooth muscle.

- Plasticity is a property of smooth muscles
- There is no proper length-tension relationship for the smooth muscles and there is no resting length assigned to it
- If a piece of visceral smooth muscle is stretched there is a great increase in tension initially. But if the muscle is held at the same length for some time the tension gradually decreases and even falls below the level exerted before the muscle was stretched
- This property is well explained in the bladder wall muscle in humans
- As the bladder gets filled initially there is a small rise in tension and then it wears off
- This continues till the physiological capacity is reached and then the bladder wall contracts forcefully
- Smooth muscle therefore behaves like a viscous mass rather than a rigid structure. This property is said to be plasticity.

15. Decompression sickness.

Refer answers to 2005 paper.

16. Conditioned reflex.

Refer answers to 2003 paper (Associative learning, short note).

17. Heart failure.

Heart failure is inability of heart to pump out blood efficiently and therefore tissue perfusion is compromised.

There are classifications of heart failure:

- *Right heart failure:* In this type of failure there is congestion of blood in the atria and large veins and that leads to edema, hepatomegaly and rised JVP
- *Left heart failure:* There is back logging of blood in the pulmonary circulation and it leads to pulmonary edema causing dyspnoea and orthopnea. There can be failure of both ventricles also which may be due to disease of the myocardium
- *High output failure:* Here there is relative decrease in cardiac output rather than absolute decrease as in a large A-V fistula, thyrotoxicosis, severe anemia, thiamine deficiency. Here the output is inadequate to the needs of the tissues
- *Low output failure:* Cardiac output is in its lower limit at rest and in conditions of demand it is further depressed as in myocardial infarction, pericarditis etc.
- *Systolic failure:* In this condition stroke volume is reduced because of weak ventricular contractions as in ventricular hypertrophy following long term hypertension. Initially the hypertrophy is compensatory and eventually the heart fails. Initially the cardiac output is decreased only during exercise and normal at rest but as the failure progresses output is decreased even at rest. Ejection fraction decreases and end systolic volume increases
- *Diastolic failure:* Here the elasticity of the heart muscle is decreased and thereby the ventricular filling is decreased and so output is decreased
- *Backward failure:* Behind the failed ventricles there is backlogging of blood increasing the atrial and venous pressures. Symptoms are – left side failure – Pulmonary congestion and pulmonary edema, resulting in dyspnea and decreased oxygenation of blood. Right side—increased peripheral venous pressure, resulting in fluid transudation from capillaries leading to edema
- *Forward failure:* In left side leads to inadequate cardiac output and decreased

perfusion to muscles especially during exercise. There is activation of renin-angiotensin-aldosterone system and there is water retention and edema.

Symptoms

- Decreased cardiac output as in forward failure leads to weakness, fatigue, exercise intolerance, hypotension etc.
- Backward failure presents with symptoms of dependent edema like ankle or sacral edema, hepatomegaly, raised JVP (right heart failure) and dyspnea, orthopnea, paroxysmal dyspnea (left heart failure)
- Orthopnea: Dyspnea on lying supine. Usually on lying supine there is pooling of blood in lungs added to the already congested lungs. This can be relieved by sitting up or raising the head end
- Paroxysmal nocturnal dyspnea: Sudden left heart failure leads to inability to cope up with the right heart output. This leads to pulmonary congestion and pulmonary edema resulting in sudden dyspnea awakening from sleep
- Weakness, fatigue and exercise intolerance
- Ankle and sacral edema
- Hepatomegaly
- Ascites
- Raised JVP.

Treatment

- Treatment aims at improving cardiac contractility and decreasing the load on heart. Also the symptoms are treated
- Salt-restricted diet decreases volume expansion
- Digitalis derivative, digoxin increases intracellular calcium in cardiac myocytes and increase cardiac contractility. They also slow the ventricular rate in patients with atrial fibrillation
- Angiotensin converting enzyme inhibitors (ACE inhibitors) are used to inhibit formation of Angiotensin II. Also Angiotensin receptor blockers are used. The above two drugs inhibit aldosterone production and thereby decreases blood pressure and decrease the afterload against which the ventricle has to pump
- Aldosterone receptor blockers can also be used
- Diuretics are given to decrease the fluid overload
- β adrenergic blockers have shown to decrease the mortality and morbidity in heart failure
- Nitrates and hydralazine reduce the venous tone and increase venous capacity sa that venous return is decreased.

18. Refractive errors.

Refer answers to 2004 paper.

19. Differences between three types of muscles.

S. No.	Characteristics	Skeletal muscle	Cardiac muscle	Smooth muscle
1.	Location	Attached to bones	In the heart	Two types: 1. Single unit- walls of hollow viscera 2. Multi-unit – Ciliary muscles and iris etc
2.	Structure	Well developed cross-striations	Cross-striations +	No cross-striations
3.	Sarcoplasmic reticulum	Well developed	Well developed, more than in skeletal muscle	Poorly developed
4.	Size and shape	50–500 µm, Cylindrical, multi-nucleate	15 µm, short, cylindrical, branching and single nucleus	2–10 µm, elongated, single nucleus, spindle shape
5.	Physiological structure	Non-syncytial	Functionally syncytial	Multi-unit—Non-syncitial Single unit—syncitial

Contd...

Contd...

S. No.	Characteristics	Skeletal muscle	Cardiac muscle	Smooth muscle
6.	Sarcotubular system	Present, T-tubule at AI junction	Present, T-tubule at Z line	Present but not so characteristic
7.	Nucleus	Multiple	Single	Single
8.	Regulatory protein	Troponin	Troponin	Calmodulin
9.	Ca^{++} for contraction	From SR	ECF (Less) and SR	ECF (More) and SR
10.	Nerve supply	Somatic nerves	Autonomic nerves	Autonomic nerves
11.	RMP	–90 mV	–90 mV	–55 mV
12.	Absolute refractory period	1–3 ms	180–200 ms	Not defined
13.	Fatigue	Possible	Not present	Possible but difficult to demonstrate
14.	Control and rhythmicity	No automaticity and rhythmicity. Contracts only on nerve stimulation	Due to presence of pace-maker automaticity and rhythmicity present	Pace-maker cells present so automaticity and rhythmicity present
15.	Gap junction	Absent	Present	Present only in single unit type

20. Write the features of acromegaly.

Refer answers to 2005 paper.

21. Tubuloglomerular feedback.

- Tubuloglomerular (TG) feedback is an autoregulatory mechanism in the kidneys to regulate the renal blood flow (RBF) and thereby glomerular filtration rate (GFR) (refer Fig. 5)
- This feedback mechanism is dependant on the NaCl content in tubular fluid
- NaCl content in the tubular fluid is sensed by Macula densa cells and signals are sent to the afferent arterioles to regulate RBF and GFR

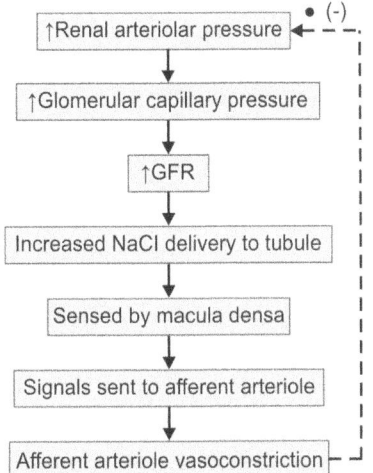

Fig. 5: Tubuloglomerular feedback.

- Increased renal arterial pressure increases glomerular capillary pressure and thereby increases filtration
- Increased GFR leads to increased NaCl content in the tubular fluid. This is sensed by macula densa cells and they send signals to cause vasoconstriction of afferent arterioles and thereby decreases RBF and GFR and NaCl content is brought back to normal
- If NaCl content is less, it is sensed by the macula densa cells and signals are sent to afferent arterioles resulting in vasodilation followed by increased RBF and GFR
- The chemicals mediating this feedback may be thromboxane A_2 or adenosine for vasoconstriction and nitric oxide (NO) for vasodilation and they are released by the macula densa cells

22. Mechanism of HCl secretion in the stomach.

Refer answers to 2005 paper.

23. Extrinsic mechanism of coagulation of blood.

Refer answers to 2005 paper.

24. Write the functions of platelets.

Refer answers to 2004 paper.

25. Write the actions of parathormone.

Refer first essay in this paper.

26. Cystometrogram.
Refer answers to 2005 paper.

27. Explain neuroendocrine reflex.
Refer answers to 2004 paper.

28. Erythroblastosis Fetalis.
Refer answers to 2003 paper.

29. Hemophilia.
- Hemophilia is a bleeding disorder usually seen in the males. In majority of cases there is deficiency of Factor VIII. This is said to be Classical Hemophilia or **Hemophilia A**
- It is an X-linked recessive disease. Therefore the males are affected and females are carriers of the disease
- There are soft tissue hematomas and hemarthrosis which may happen repeatedly resulting in crippling arthropathy
- Usually there are no spontaneous hemorrhages but there is excessive bleeding after even a mild injury as in tooth extraction
- Condition is characterized by prolonged clotting time (normal CT = 3–8 minutes) and normal bleeding time. Activated partial thromboplastin time (APTT) is prolonged
- Treatment is done by fresh blood transfusion. Factor VIII can also be prepared fom fresh frozen plasma and injected
- Christmas disease or **Hemophilia B** is due to deficiency of factor IX. It is also a sex-linked recessive disease. Symptoms are similar to Hemophilia A. Diagnosis is done by the assay of Factor IX
- **Hemophilia C** is due to deficiency of Factor XI. It affects both males and females.

30. Surfactant.
- It is a protein-lipid complex secreted by the Type II alveolar epithelial cells lining the alveoli (refer Fig. 6)
- Surfactant is a mixture of Dipalmitoyl phosphatidylcholine (DPPC), other lipids and proteins - SP-A, SP-B, SP-C and SP-D
- It acts as a detergent to reduce the surface tension of the fluid lining the alveoli and prevent its collapse during expiration

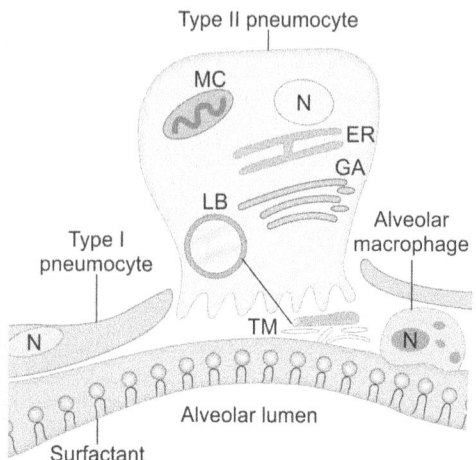

Fig. 6: Arrangement of surfactant molecules in alveolar lumen.
(MC: mitochondria; N: nucleus; ER: endoplasmic reticulum; GA: golgi apparatus; LB: lamellar bodies; TM: tubular myelin)
(*Source:* GK Pal)

- The phopholipids have hydrophobic tails and a hydrophilic head. They arrange themselves with the tails facing the alveolar lumen and intersperse between water molecules
- So during inspiration as the alveoli enlarge the surfactant molecules move apart and surface tension of water increases and during expiration they come closer and the suface tension is lowered
- Surfactant is important at birth. After birth the infant tries to breathe and makes inspiratory movements and the lungs expand after which the lung tends to recoil and the presence of surfactant prevents the collapse of the alveoli
- Surfactant defeciency results in alveolar collapse, which results in Infant respiratory distress syndrome (IRDS)
- Maturation of surfactant in the lungs is enhanced by glucocorticoids. During term the fetal and maternal cortisol increases and favours matuartion of surfactant.

Other functions of surfactant
- Stabilizes the lung alveoli
- It also decreases the effect of surface tension, which if not countered will increase the pulmonary capillary

hydrostatic pressure and thereby fluid accumulation in the alveolus. So surfactant prevents pulmonary edema
- As it prevents alveolar collapse, it decreases the work of breathing
- They help in immunity.

Regulation of Secretion of Surfactant
- It is regulated by hormones: Glucocorticoids, insulin and thyroxine promote secretion of surfactant.

Factors which affect surfactant secretion:
- High O_2 content affects surfactant secretion as in O_2 therapy in patients undergoing cardiac surgery using pump oxygenator
- Occlusion of pulmonary bronchus or pulmonary artery
- Long term inhalation of 100% O_2
- Cigarette smoking.

31. Chloride Shift.
Refer answers to 2005 paper.

32. Artificial respiration.
Refer answers to 2004 paper.

33. Taste pathway.
Refer answers to 2005 paper.

34. Effects of lesion in optic pathway.
Refer answers to 2004 paper.

35. Brown-Sequard syndrome.
Hemi-section of spinal cord is called Brown-sequard syndrome. It involves lesion of one lateral half of spinal cord.

Following injury to the spinal cord there are there following stages:
1. Stage of spinal shock
2. Stage of reflex activity
3. Stage of reflex failure

Immediately after the lesion there is complete loss of function below the level of lesion. This happens because of sudden removal of impulses from higher centers.

The symptoms of Brown-Sequard are seen in the second stage. Symptoms are explained as the features above the level of lesion, at the level and below the level of lesion, on the same side and opposite side of lesion.

	Sensory		Motor	
	Same side	Opposite side	Same side	Opposite side
Above the level of lesion	Small area of hyperasthesia	Normal	Normal	Normal
At the level of lesion	Complete loss of sensation (anaesthesia)	Not affected	Lower motor neuron type of paralysis	Not affected
Below the level of lesion	**Damage to Dorsal column fibers:** Loss of Fine touch, tactile localisation, two point discrimination, vibration sense, stereognosis and position sense	**Damage to lateral and anterior spinothalamic tract:** Loss of pain, temperature and crude touch sensations. All other sensations are intact	Upper motor neuron type of paralysis as the inhibition from higher centers are removed. Temporary loss of vasomotor tone	Not usually affected

36. Functions of thalamus.
Refer answers to 2007 paper.

37. Pacemaker potential.
Refer answers to 2005 paper.

38. Regulation of coronary circulation.
Refer answers to 2005 paper.

39. Neuromuscular transmission.
It is the junction between the motor neuron and the muscle fiber it supplies.

Structure of NMJ
- The NMJ is formed by the axon terminal of the motor neuron
- On approaching the muscle fiber, the axon loses its myelin sheath and divides into many branches and the nerve terminals bulge to form the terminal buttons which approaches the muscle fiber at its center
- NMJ has a presynaptic membrane, synaptic cleft and postsynaptic membrane (refer Fig. 7).

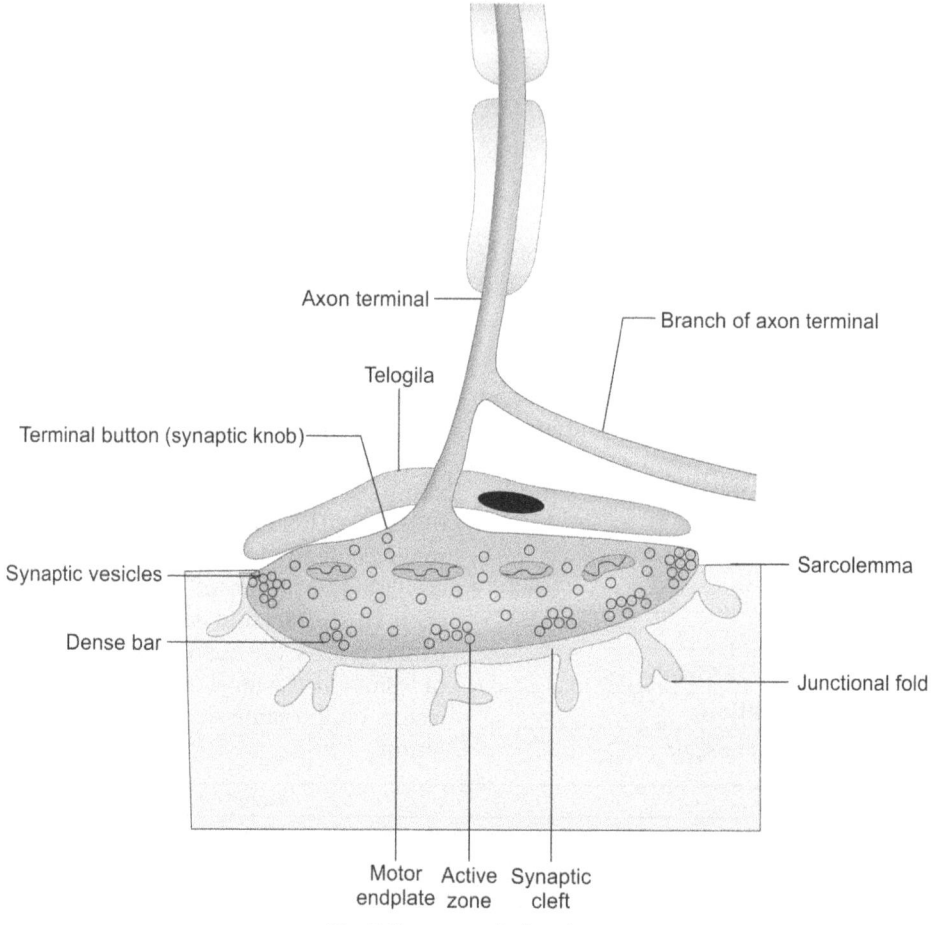

Fig. 7: Neuromuscular junction.
(*Source:* GK Pal)

Presynaptic Terminal
- It is the membrane of the terminal button of the axon
- It has many ACh vesicles and mitochondria within the membrane
- The membrane is studded with many Voltage-gated Ca^{2+} channels.

Synaptic Cleft
- It is a space of 50–100 nm width between the presynaptic and postsynaptic membranes
- It has ECF in it and acetylcholinesterase enzyme is also present in it.

Postsynaptic Membrane
- It is the muscle membrane in contact with the nerve terminal and it is thrown into many folds – Junctional folds and is thickened and deepened – Synaptic trough
- The muscle membrane here is called as the motor end plate
- It contains the Nicotinic acetylcholine receptors.

Impulse Transmission in NMJ

Stimulation of nerve fiber
↓
AP generated in nerve fiber
↓
Conduction of AP in nerve fiber
↓
Impulse reaches nerve terminal
↓

Voltage-gated Ca^{2+} channels in nerve terminal open
↓
Ca^{2+} influx into presynaptic membrane
↓
Exocytosis of ACh vesicles and ACh is released into synaptic cleft
↓
ACh moves across the cleft and binds to Nicotinic ACh receptors in muscle membrane
↓
The receptor is a Non-specific cation channel which opens on binding with ACh
↓
Influx of Na$^+$ ions into postsynaptic membrane
↓
Local depolarization of muscle membrane – End plate potential (EPP)
↓
Generation of action potential in the neighboring muscle membrane by the EPP

Drugs Acting on NMJ

Blockers of NMJ

- *Curare:* It binds with the ACh receptors and prevents binding of ACh to their receptors. This blocks the neuromuscular transmission
- *Bungarotoxin:* This is acquired from snake venom. It also prevents impulse transmission by binding the ACh receptors
- *Succinylcholine:* They act just like ACh and make the muscle membrane depolarized. But the choline esterase does not have any effect on these substances and therefore the muscle is continuously depolarized and cannot be stimulated again
- *Botulinum toxin:* They are derived from the bacteria *Clostridium tetani* and it prevents release of ACh vesicles from terminal buttons.

Stimulators of NMJ

- *Drugs having ACh like action:* Drugs like Carbachol, Nicotine, etc act on Ach receptors like ACh but cannot be removed or slowly removed by ACh esterase. This makes the muscle to have repeated depolarizations resulting in muscle spasm
- *Drugs that inhibit Choline esterase:* Drugs like Neostigmine, Physostigmine, diisopropyl flurophospahte (DFP) stimulate the NMJ by inactivating cholinesterase. This results in continuous activation of ACh on receptors and repeated muscle spasm. It takes weeks together for removal of ACh and therefore it has a fatal poisoning effect.

Diseases Affecting NMJ

Myasthenia Gravis

- It is an autoimmune disease
- Antibodies are formed against the Nicotinic ACh receptors in NMJ
- There is weakness, fatigue and the muscles become weak with use and therefore symptoms worsen towards the evening
- Antibodies not only combine with ACh receptors, they also flatten the postsynaptic membrane and cause endocytosis of ACh into presynaptic membrane
- Because of these effects, the muscle response to stimulation gradually decreases
- Symptoms improve after rest and are better on getting up in the morning
- The extraocular and facial muscles are the first to be affected and ptosis and diplopia are present.

Treatment:

- Acetylcholine esterase (AChE) inhibitors – ACh E inhibitors increase the amount of ACh in the NMJ and they can displace the antibodies and improve functions
- Thymectomy: Decreases the immune response by inhibiting T cell activation
- Immunosuppressants
- Plasmapheresis.

Eaton-Lambert Syndrome

- It is also an autoimmune disease
- Antibodies are formed against voltage gated Ca^{2+} channels in the presynaptic membrane

- Here the symptoms of muscle weakness improve with repeated stimulation, as Ca^{2+} levels increase with each stimulus.

III. SHORT ANSWERS

1. Functions of eosinophil.

- **Antiallergic function:** The granules of eosinophils release chemicals like histaminase, leukotriene C4 and Aryl sulphatase. These chemicals neutralize the effects of histamine and other mediators of allergic reaction and thereby bring down the effects of allergy
- They also **prevent degranulation** of mast cells
- Eosinophils are abundant in the mucosa of respiratory tract, mucosa of GIT and urinary tract and **provide mucosal immunity**
- Eosinophils are **weakly phagocytic**, they ingest and destroy antigen-antibody complexes and reduce the effects of immune reactions
- They are also **anti-parasitic** in nature. Eosinophils attach to large parasites like schistosomiasis and release the granules containing major basic protein and other hydrolytic enzymes which are larvicidal in nature and destroy the parasites.

2. Name anticoagulants used in the laboratories.

- **Ethylenediamine tetra-acetic acid (EDTA):** This is the anticoagulant of choice in the laboratories. It makes Ca^{2+} unavailable for clotting by chelating it. It is used to determine ESR
- **Trisodium citrate:** This anticoagulant is used for determining clotting disorders and also ESR. This prevents clotting by chelation of Ca^{2+}
- Double **oxalate mixture:** It is a mixture of ammonium oxalate and potassium oxalate. It prevents clotting by forming insoluble calcium oxalate precipitate
- **Heparin:** A naturally occuring anticoagulant is used as an invitro and invivo anticoagulant. It activates anti-thrombin III
- **Sodium flouride** is an anticoagulant used in the labs for tests to analyze blood glucose levels.

3. Write differences between adult hemoglobin and fetal hemoglobin.

- **Adult hemoglobin (HbA)** has 2 alpha chains and 2 beta chains making up the globin part of hemoglobin. It starts appearing in the RBCs by 5th month of extrauterine life. Affnity of Hb to oxygen is normal
- **Fetal hemoglobin (HbF)** has 2 alpha chains and 2 gamma chains making up the globin part of Hb. 80% of Hb in the fetus at the time of birth is HbF. Disappears by 5th month of age. It has greater affinity for oxygen and it shifts the O_2 – Hb dissociation curve to the left. High affinity is due to its poor binding capacity with 2, 3, DPG. It is also resistant to action of alkalis. Life span is 1-2 weeks.

4. Functions of sertoli cells.

- They play a major role in the maturation of spermatozoa. Spermatids mature into spermatozoa in the deep folds of cytoplasm in the Sertoli cells
- They provide nutrition to the developing spermatozoa and help in spermeation
- They take part in the formation of blood-testis barrier which selectively allows certain substances to enter seminiferous tubule
- They phagocytose damaged germ cells
- They secrete seminal fluid
- Sertoli cells produce substances like:
  - Mullerian inhibiting substance (MIS): Causes regression of Mullerian duct and promotes development of structures from the Wolffian duct
  - Inhibin: Inhibits FSH secretion
  - Activin
  - Androgen binding protein (ABP): This helps to maintain a high concentration of androgens in the seminiferous tubule which is essential for spermatogenesis
  - Estrogen is produced from androgen in the presence of aromatase which is present in the Sertoli cells.

5. Functions of large intestine.

- It acts as a **reservoir** for undigested food material and they are stored here till they are expelled as feces
- **Absorption:** The most important components absorbed in the Colon are water and electrolytes. The large absorptive capacity of colon can be used to instill certain drugs like anesthetics, analgesics etc through the colon
- **Formation of feces:** The undigested residue of the food substances are made into formed fecal matter in the colon
- **Colonic bacteria:** Colon has large numbers of beneficial bacteria which helps to form many useful substances like vitamin K, B complex vitamins and folic acid
- **Short-chain fatty acids** are also synthesized in the large intestine by action of intestinal bacteria on complex carbohydrates, resistant starch and other dietary fibers
- Goblet cells in the mucosa of large intestine produce large volume of **Mucus** which helps in smooth passage of feces
- Alkaline nature (pH 8) of large intestinal secretion **neutralizes acids** formed by bacteria on feces
- Undigested cellulose, hemicellulose and some fats are digested by the colonic bacteria
- Heavy metals like lead, mercury etc are excreted through feces.

6. Migrating myoelectric complex.

- Migrating myoelectric complexes (MMCs) are the type of movements seen in the GIT during the interdigestive period. These movements are initiated in the stomach and they migrate to the distal ileum. Each cycle of the MMCs have 3 phases
- Phase I: It start as a quiescent phase
- Phase II: The next phase has irregular electrical and mechanical activity
- Phase III: The phase with a regular burst of activity
- These waves occur at an interval of 90 minutes and they travel at the rate of 5 cm/min. They are accompanied by increased secretion of gastric juice, bile and pancreatic juices
- MMCs are said to clear the lumen of the stomach and intestines and prepare it for receiving the next meal
- They are stimulated by the GI hormone Motilin secreted from the stomach, small and large intestines
- These waves come to a halt immediately following intake of food after which peristalsis starts.

7. Achalasia cardia.

- It is a condition in which the resting tone of the lower esophageal sphincter (LES) is increased and there is improper relaxation of the sphincter on food intake and food does not reach the stomach
- Food starts accumulating in the proximal esophagus and it starts getting distended
- This is because of the defect in the myentric plexus at the LES. There could also be a mismatch of the release of neurotransmitters at the LES
- Acetylcholine released by parasympathetic nerves, makes the sphincter tonic. Nitric oxide and VIP relax the sphincter
- Achalasia cardia could be due to increase in the Acetylcholine released by the nerves supplying the LES and a decrease in the levels of Nitric oxide or VIP. This makes the sphincter to become tonic
- It can be treated by injecting botulinum toxin which inhibits the release of acetylcholine. Pneumatic dilatation of the sphincter can also be done
- Myotomy is also done to relax the sphincter

8. Name the homones of hypothalamus.

- The hypothalamus is both an endocrine organ as well as a neural structure. It is said to be the master of endocrine orchestra
- Hypothalamus releases many releasing and inhibiting hormones which regulate the anterior pituitary hormones and also secretes the posterior pituitary hormones.

Anterior Pituitary Regulating Hormones

1. Growth hormone releasing hormone (GRH)

2. Growth hormone inhibiting hormone (GIH) or somatostatin
3. Prolactin inhibiting hormone (PIH - Dopamine)
4. Thyrotrophin releasing hormone (TRH)
5. Corticotrophin releasing hormone (CRH)
6. Gonadotrophin releasing hormone (GnRH).

Posterior pituitary hormones secreted by hypothalamus are:

1. Anti-diuretic hormone or arginine vasopressin
2. Oxytocin.

9. Write the actions of prolactin.

- Prolactin is a peptide hormone with 199 amino acids secreted from the anterior pituitary gland
- It acts on the breast of pregnant females and stimulate milk secretion
- During pregnancy, estrogen and progesterone helps in the ductal and lobular devlopment of the breast
- After delivery of the fetus, Prolactin acts on the hormones-primed breast and stimulates synthesis of milk and its secretion
- Prolactin also inhibits GnRh secretion and its action
- It also inhibits the effects of LH and FSH at the level of ovary and thereby prevents ovulation in the nursing mother. Therefore it acts as an effective contraceptive tool after child birth
- Role of prolactin in males is not clear but in large quantities they induce impotence.

10. Name second messengers.

- Cyclic AMP—cAMP
- Cyclic GMP—cGMP
- Inositol triphosphate—IP_3
- Diacylglycerol—DAG
- Ionic calcium—Ca^{2+}.

11. Define sarcomere. Mention normal length of sarcomere.

Refer answers to 2006 paper.

12. Myasthenia gravis.

Refer answers to 2005 paper.

13. Windkessel effect.

- The distal portion of aorta and large arteries contain large amount of elastin in the tunica media of the vessel wall
- During systole when the blood is pumped into the vessels they distend with blood and are stretched because of the large amount of elastin present in the vessel wall
- Following systole the stretched vessel walls recoil and convert the blood flow into a continuous one
- This recoiling effect also contributes to the diastolic BP
- This is said to be the **Windkessel effect** and the large arteries and aorta are the **Windkessel vessels** (refer Fig. 8).

14. Phonocardiogram.

This is an instrument used to record heart sounds. The sounds are picked by a microphone, amplified and fed to a recorder

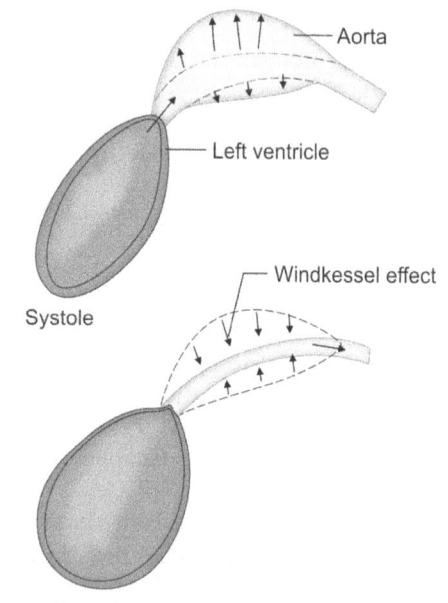

Fig. 8: Windkessel effect in aorta in systolic and diastolic phase of cardiac cycle.
(*Source:* GK Pal)

and can be heard with a loud speaker. The recording is said to be the phonocardiograph.

Phonocardiograph

- The first heart sound is heard as "LUBB", is low pitched and frequency is less than 50/sec. Duration is 0.14-0.17 secs. The phonocardiographic recording shows 7-13 waves and the sound coincides with carotid pulse, R wave of ECG and 'C' wave of JVP. It is due to closure of AV valves
- Second heart sound: It is heard as "DUP". It is high pitched, >50 Hz in frequency, duration is shorter; 0.1-0.14 sec. Phonocardiographic recording shows 4-6 waves. It coincides with T wave of ECG. It is due to closure of semilunar valves
- Third heart sound: It is heard normally in small children and adults with thin chest wall. Phonocardiographic recording shows 1-4 waves. Duration is less than 0.1 secs. It is due to rapid filling phase of ventricular diastole
- Fourth heart sound: It is a low pitched sound and inaudible in adults. It can be recorded by phonocardiogram and shows 1-2 waves. It is due to atrial systole or second rapid filling phase. It is audible in heart failure and myocardial infarction.

15. Haldane effect.

- The effect of PO_2 or oxyhemoglobin saturation on CO_2 content is known as **haldane effect**
- The relationship between PO_2 and CO_2 content is inverse
- When blood passes through pulmonary capillaries, O_2 diffuses into blood, binds to hemoglobin and forms Oxy-Hb
- Oxygenation of Hb shifts the CO_2 dissociation curve to the right and Hb gives out CO_2
- So in the lungs, loading of O_2 helps in unloading of CO_2
- In the tissues, low PO_2 increases the capacity of Hb for carrying CO_2.

16. VO_2 max.

- The normal O_2 consumption in an adult is 250 mL/min
- During exercise the amount of O_2 consumption increases by 15-20 times
- The maximum amount of O_2 that can be consumed by a normal adult is called Maximum O_2 consumption or VO_2max
- The normal VO_2max in adults is 3 L/min
- It varies between athelets and non-athelets
- It is an indicator of an individual's capacity of aerobic exercise.

17. Babinski sign.

- It is an abnormal plantar reflex
- On eliciting a plantar reflex, the normal response is adduction and plantar flexion of all the toes
- In Babinski sign, there is dorsiflexion of big toe and fanning out of all the other toes
- It is a normal response in infants below 2 years of age as the myelination of pyramidal tract is not complete till this age
- In adults if this response is seen it is due to lesion of pyramidal tract.

18. Alpha block.

- Alpha waves in EEG, occurs at a frequency of 8-13 per second. Amplitude is 50-100 µV
- These waves are present in all normal individuals when they are awake and resting with closed eyes
- It disappears entirely during sleep
- It is found in the parieto-occipital region
- *Alpha block:* Alpha rhythm disappears on opening the eyes and is replaced by faster and low amplitude waves resembling the beta waves (refer Fig. 9)
- It is also called as desynchronization.

19. Functions of aqueous humor.

- Contributes to refractive power of eye
- Maintains shape of eye and intraocular pressure
- Provides nutrition to cornea and lens.

20. Rinne's test.

- It is a tuning fork test used to identify the type of deafness

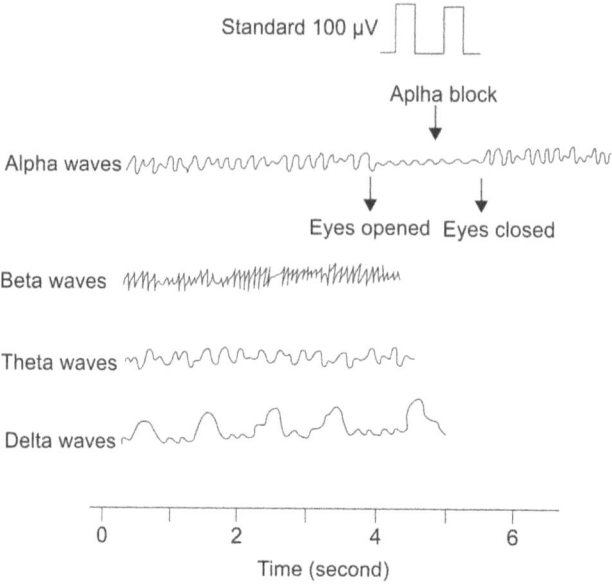

Fig. 9: EEG waves with alpha block.
(*Source:* Sembulingam)

- This test is based on the principle that air conduction is better than bone conduction.

Method

- Base of the vibrating tuninig fork is placed in the mastoid process behind the ear till the subject no longer hears the sound, then the vibrating blade is held in air next to the ear

- In normal condition the subject hears vibration in air after bone conduction has stopped (air conduction is better than bone conduction)
- In conduction deafness, vibration in air is not heard after bone conduction is over as there is no conduction of sound through external and middle ear.

MBBS Examination 2009

ANSWER ALL QUESTIONS

I. Essay questions (15 Marks each)

1. Describe in detail the synthesis and functions of thyroid hormones. Add a note on hypothyroidism.
2. Describe the composition, functions and regulation of secretion of gastric juice.
3. Name the functional divisions of the cerebellum. Describe the structure, connections, and functions of cerebellum. Mention two signs of cerebellar lesions.
4. Define cardiac cycle. Describe in detail with the help of a diagram the mechanical changes during cardiac cycle. Add a note on heart sounds
5. Enumerate the nuclei of hypothalamus. Explain the connections and functions of hypothalamus.
6. Explain the countercurrent mechanism in the concentration of urine. Add a note on diuresis.
7. Enumerate the ascending tracts in the spinal cord. Describe the pathway for pain in detail. Add a note on referred pain.
8. Describe the neural regulation of respiration. Add a note on periodic breathing.

II. Short notes (5 Marks each)

1. Composition of semen and its uses as a diagnostic tool.
2. Functions of juxtaglomerular apparatus.
3. Explain components and functions of bile.
4. Explain the stages of development of erythrocytes.
5. Describe the metabolic actions of cortisol.
6. Describe briefly the formation and functions of corpus luteum.
7. Describe the formation and circulation of lymph.
8. Enumerate the hormones secreted by anterior pituitary gland. Describe the actions of growth hormone.
9. Classify the fluid compartments of body giving their normal values, mention two methods to determine ECF.
10. Describe the formation and functions of immunoglobulins.
11. Neuromuscular junction.
12. Compare REM and NREM sleep.
13. Triple response.
14. Describe formation, circulation and functions of cerebrospinal fluid (CSF).
15. Functions of vestibular apparatus.
16. Explain 'dark adaptation'.
17. Organ of Corti.
18. Describe decompression sickness.
19. Describe chemical control of respiration.
20. What is myasthenia gravis? Describe the biological basis of its treatment.
21. Micturition reflex.
22. Gastric emptying.
23. Indicators of ovulation.
24. Myxedema.
25. Enterohepatic circulation of bile.
26. Conn's syndrome.
27. Functions of glucocorticoids.
28. Significance of Rh group.
29. Transport mechanisms across cell membrane.

30. Albumin: Globulin ratio.
31. Compliance.
32. Brown-Sequard syndrome.
33. Blood brain barrier (BBB).
34. Surfactant.
35. Chronaxie and rheobase.
36. Pupillary light reflexes.
37. Pace maker potential.
38. Atrial natriuretic peptide.
39. Draw the optic pathway. Depict the lesions at various levels.
40. Peculiarities of pulmonary circulation.

III. Short answers (2 Marks each)

1. Briefly describe the process of deglutition.
2. Heparin.
3. Name two indications of exchange transfusion.
4. Purpura.
5. Plasma cells.
6. Functions of plasma proteins.
7. Phagocytosis.
8. Physiological basis of pregnancy diagnosing tests.
9. Role of oxytocin in female reproduction.
10. List the important functions of saliva.
11. Explain the basic defect in astigmatism and its correction.
12. Draw a labelled diagram of arterial pulse and explain.
13. Draw a labelled diagram of pathways for taste.
14. Rigor mortis.
15. Phantom limb.
16. Oxygen debt.
17. What is Bohr's effect? What is its physiologic significance?
18. Draw a normal ECG and label it.
19. Refractory period.
20. Define terms: Chronaxie, rheobase and utilization time.
21. Actions of insulin.
22. Estrogen functions.
23. Aldosterone escape.
24. Functions of saliva.
25. Significance of erythrocyte sedimentation rate.
26. Functions of corpus luteum.
27. Blood–testis barrier.
28. GAP junctions.
29. Glomerular filtration rate.
30. Dietary fibre.
31. Wernicke's aphasia.
32. Acetylcholine.
33. Parkinson's disease:
34. Rapid–eye movement sleep.
35. Anti–G suit.
36. Clinical significance of electro-encephalogram.
37. Chloride shift.
38. Jugular venous pulse.
39. Contents of middle ear.
40. Functions of placenta.

I. ESSAY QUESTIONS

1. **Describe in detail the synthesis and functions of thyroid hormones. Add a note on hypothyroidism.**

Hormones Synthesized from Thyroid Gland are:

- From follicular cells: Thyroxine (T4) and triiodothyronine (T3)
- From parafollicular cells: Calcitonin.

Synthesis of Thyroid Hormone

- Synthesis takes place in the follicular cells and the hormone is stored in follicular lumen as colloid (refer Fig. 1)
- Thyroid hormones are iodothyronines, formed by coupling of iodinated tyrosine molecules by ether linkages.

Following are the steps in synthesis of thyroid hormones:

a. Iodide trapping
b. Thyroglobulin synthesis
c. Oxidation of iodide
d. Organification
e. Coupling
f. Storage
g. Release

Iodide Trapping

- Iodide is transported from the blood in thyroid capillaries to the follicular

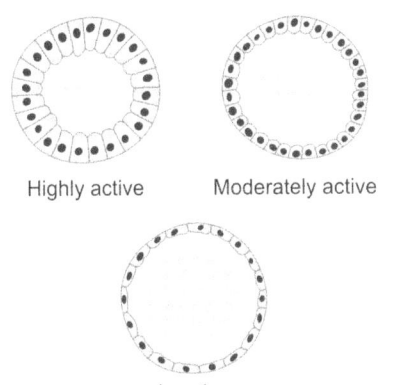

Fig. 1: Thyroid follicle: Active follicle, Moderately active follicle and inactive follicle with colloid content. Inactive follicle is lined by flattened epithelial cells and the colloid content is more. In an active follicle the cells are columnar and colloid content is less.
(*Source:* GK Pal)

cell through sodium-iodide symporter (NIS)
- NIS transports I⁻ against electrochemical gradient
- TSH stimulates I⁻ trapping and concentration in the gland
- Iodide immediately moves towards the apical membrane of the follicular cell.

Thyroglobulin Synthesis
- As iodide is being trapped, thyroglobulin is also synthesized in the endoplasmic reticulum of follicular cells and transferred to colloid
- TG is a glycoprotein. Has 131 tyrosine amino acids.

Oxidation of Iodide
- Iodide on reaching the colloid - apical membrane interface is oxidized to iodine
- This reaction is catalysed by Thyroid peroxidase enzyme (TPO) present in the colloid-membrane interface
- $2I^- + H_2O_2 \rightarrow I_2 + 2\,HO^-$

Organification
- The tyrosine molecules of thyroglobulin get iodinated in the colloid to form iodotyrosines
- This is organification and is catalyzed by TPO (refer Fig. 2)
- It forms either Mono-iodotyrosine (MIT) or Di-iodotyrosine (DIT) depending on the number of iodine attached to tyrosines.

Coupling Reaction
Two DIT molecules couple to form tetraiodotyrosine (T_4) or thyroxine.
OR
One molecule of MIT and DIT couple to form triiodothyronine (T_3)
OR
One molecule of DIT and MIT couple to form reverse T_3 (RT_3), an inactive component formed in the follicular cells.

This is coupling reaction and is catalyzed by TPO (refer Fig. 3).

Storage
- TG after iodination is stored in the colloid until release

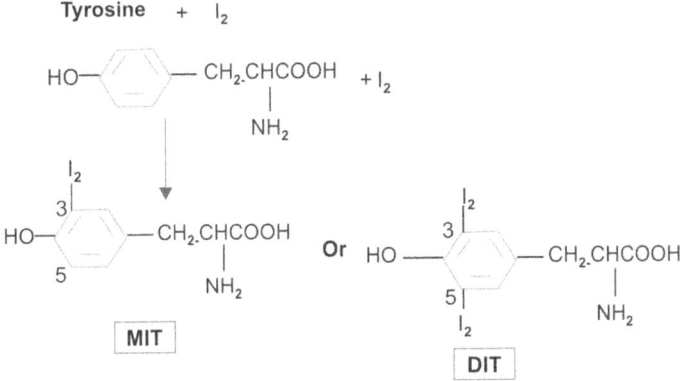

Fig. 2: Organification reaction—I_2 molecule is bound to tyrosine molecules. If it is bound in one position (3) then MIT (Monoiodotyrosine is formed). If I_2 is bound in two positions (3 and 5) it is DIT (Diiodotyrosine).

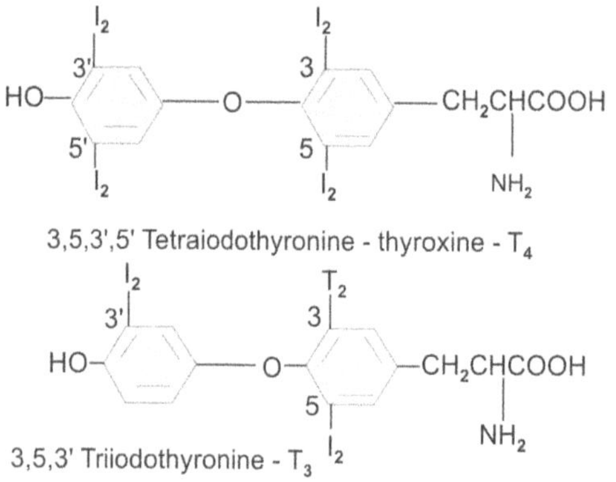

3,5,3',5' Tetraiodothyronine - thyroxine - T_4

3,5,3' Triiodothyronine - T_3

Fig. 3: Coupling reaction. Two MITs couple to form T_4 (throxine) and one MIT and one DIT binds T_3 (triiodothyronine) is formed.

- In each molecule of thyroglobulin (TG): MIT-7, DIT-6, T_4- 2, T_3- 0.2 molecules are present
- The gland is capable of storing secretions needed for 100 days.

Release of the hormone:

- On stimulation by TSH, colloid droplets (with TG and T_3 and T_4) are endocytosed through the protein Megalin into the cell
- The droplet gets attached to a lysozome and forms a phagosome (refer Fig. 4)
- Proteolytic enzymes of the phagosome break the peptide bonds between thyroid hormone (TH) and TG
- This releases T_3, T_4, MIT and DIT
- Released thyroid hormones enter into the capillaries by diffusion
- MIT and DIT are deiodinated by the enzyme, thyroid deiodinases, which are selective for iodotyrosines and not for iodothyronines
- Small amounts of TG are also released.

Functions of Thyroid Hormone

Refer answers to 2004 paper.

Hypothyroidism

Refer answers to 2007 paper.

2. **Describe the composition, functions and regulation of secretion of gastric juice.**

Refer answers to 2005 paper.

3. **Name the functional divisions of the cerebellum. Describe the structure, connections, and functions of cerebellum. Mention two signs of cerebellar lesions.**

Refer answers to 2006 paper.

Signs of Cerebellar Lesions

1. No paralysis
2. No sensory deficits
3. Deep reflexes not affected much except for pendular knee jerk.
4. Hypotonia
5. All movements are characterized by ataxia

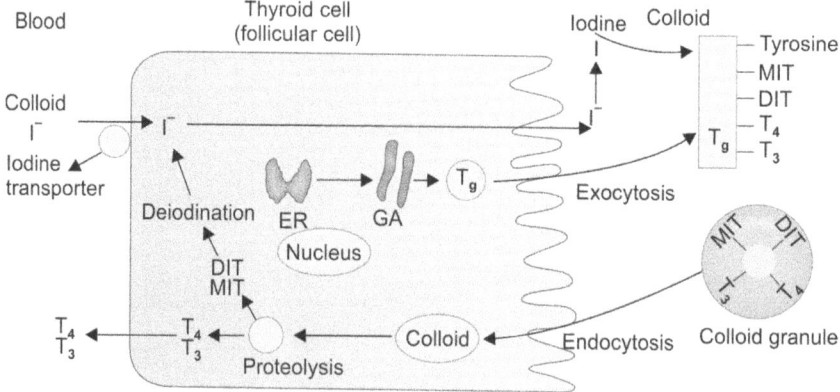

Fig. 4: Synthesis of thyroid hormone in follicular cell.
(*Source:* GK Pal)

6. **Ataxia:** Defect in co-ordination due to errors in the rate, range, force and direction of movement.

It manifests as:
- Drunken gait
- Scanning speech
- Dysmetria
- Intention tremor
- Rebound phenomenon: Pendular knee jerk
- Disdiadochokinesia
- Decomposition of movements
- Nystagmus.

4. **Define cardiac cycle. Describe in detail with the help of a diagram the mechanical changes during cardiac cycle. Add a note on heart sounds.**

Cardiac Cycle

Refer answers to 2005 paper.

Heart Sounds

Refer answers to 2006 paper.

5. **Enumerate the nuclei of hypothalamus. Explain the connections and functions of Hypothalamus.**

Hypothalamus has many numbers of nuclei and they are grouped as anterior, middle, posterior and lateral groups.

They are:
- Anterior group: Preoptic, supraoptic and paraventricular nuclei
- Middle group: Arcuate, venteromedial, dorsomedial and tuberal nuclei
- Posterior group: Supramamillary, mamillary and posterior hypothalamic nuclei
- Lateral group: Lateral preoptic area and lateral hypothalamic nuclei.

Connections and Functions

Refer answers to 2008 paper.

6. **Explain the countercurrent mechanism in the concentration of urine. Add a note on diuresis.**

Refer answers to 2004 paper.

Diuresis

Diuresis refers to increased urinary output. There are two types of diuresis—water diuresis and osmotic diuresis

1. **Water diuresis** refers to increase in urine output after excess intake of water following which there is inhibition of antidiuretic hormone (ADH) secretion and and no water reabsorption occurs at distal convoluted tubule (DCT) and collecting duct (CD), so there is excess urinary output. Output may be as high as 20L/day. Urine is highly diluted and osmolality is <30 mOsm/kg H_2O
2. **Osmotic diuresis** is increased urinary output due to presence of osmotically active substances in the urine, e.g. glucose in urine. These substances stay back in the tubule as they are not reabsorbed at the proximal convoluted tubule (PCT) and they also retain water with them. Output may be more than 20L/day, osmolality >300 mOsm/kg H_2O.

7. **Enumerate the ascending tracts in the spinal cord. Describe the pathway for pain in detail. Add a note on referred pain.**

The ascending tracts in the spinal cord are:
i. Dorsal column: Fasciculus gracilis and Fasiculus cuneatus
ii. Spinothalamic tracts: Lateral and anterior Spinothalamic tracts
iii. Spinocerebellar tracts: Dorsal and ventral spinocerebellar tracts
iv. Spinotectal tract
v. Spino-olivary tract
vi. Spinovestibular tract
vii. Spinoreticular tract.

Pain Pathway

- Pain sensation is carried by the lateral spinothalamic tract (LSTT)
- There are two types of pain—fast pain and slow pain
- So the LSTT has fibers for fast pain and for slow pain. There are separate pathways for fast and slow pain (refer Fig. 5).

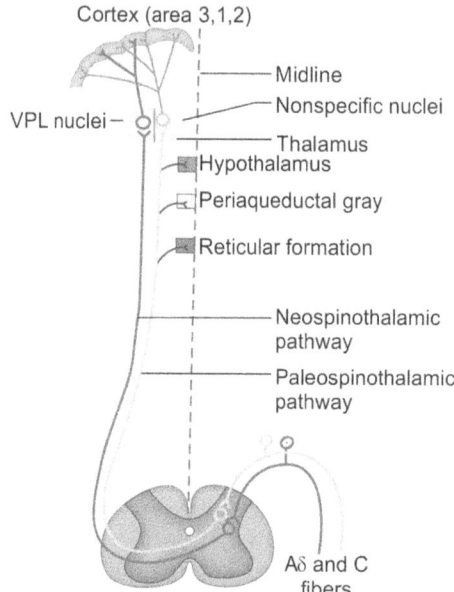

Fig. 5: Neospinothalamic and paleospinothalamic tracts.
(VPLN: venteral posterolateral nucleus of thalamus)
(*Source:* GK Pal)

Fast Pain

- Fast pain is sensed by the free nerve endings of Aδ fibers
- The pain sensation from periphery is carried through the Aδ fibers
- Their cell bodies are present in the dorsal root ganglion
- The fibers on entering spinal cord terminate on cells in laminae I and V of the dorsal grey horn
- These are the second order neurons. Neurotransmitter released here is glutamate
- Second order neurons cross to the opposite side and ascend up as **neospinothalamic tract** in the anterolateral column of spinal cord
- Neospinothalamic tract reaches thalamus and ends on the ventral posterolateral nucleus of the thalamus (VPLN)
- The tract on its way to thalamus gives a few branches to periaqueductal grey (PAG) in midbrain
- The third order neurons start from thalamus and reach somatosensory area I
- This pathway is concerned with localisation and interpretation of pain.

Slow Pain

- Slow pain is sensed by the free nerve endings of unmyelinated C fibers
- Slow pain is carried by the same fibers to spinal cord and they terminate in the laminae II and III of dorsal grey horn
- This is the first order neuron. The neurotransmitter released here is **Substance P**
- The second order neuron arises from laminae I and V and the fibers cross to the opposite side and ascends up as **paleospinothalamic tract**
- It ascends up along with neospinothalamic tract in the anterolateral column of spinal cord
- This tract gives many fibers to PAG, reticular formation and tectum
- It then ends in the non-specific nucleus of thalamus
- Third order neuron arises from here and is projected to entire cerebral cortex
- This pathway is concerned with alertness, arousal and perception of pain rather than localisation of pain.

Referred Pain

Refer answers to 2006 paper.

8. Describe the neural regulation of respiration. Add a note on periodic breathing.

Neural Regulation of Respiration

Refer answers to 2007 paper.

Periodic Breathing

Periodic breathing means respiratory activity alternating with apnea.

Cheyne-Stokes Respiration

Refer answers to 2005 paper.

Biot's Breathing

- Has one or more large tidal volumes separated by apnea (refer Fig. 6)
- It is seen in irregular intervals
- It is seen only in pathological conditions
- Present in diseases ↑ intracranial tension – Tumors, Meningitis, pontine hemorrhage, Central medullary lesions.

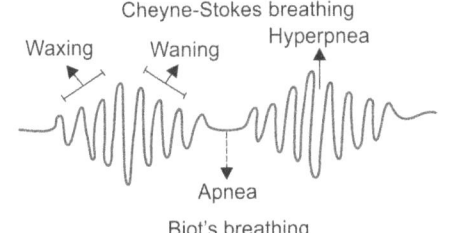
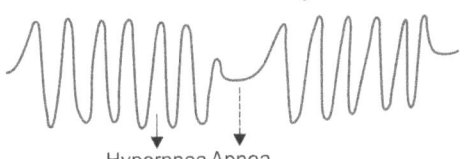

Fig. 6: Periodic breathing; Cheyne-Stokes breathing and Biot's breathing.
(*Source:* Sembulingam)

II. SHORT NOTES

1. Composition of semen and its uses as a diagnostic tool.

- Semen is a white colored secretion ejected from the male urethra during sexual intercourse
- It contains sperm and other secretions from seminal vesicles, prostate, urethral glands and Cowper's glands
- The average volume in each ejaculation is 2.5–3.5 mL
- The volume decreases after repeated ejacultion
- There are 100 million sperms per mL of semen.

Composition of Semen

- pH—7.35–7.5
- Specific gravity—1.028
- Sperm count—100 million/mL, <20% abnormal forms

Other Components

From Seminal Vesicles

- Phosphorylcholine
- Ergothionine
- Ascorbic acid
- Flavins
- Prostaglandins.

From Prostate

- Spermine
- Citric acid
- Cholesterol, phospholipids
- Fibrinolysin, Fibrinogenase
- Zinc
- Acid phosphatase
- Phosphate
- Bicarbonate
- Hyaluronidase
- 60% of the sperms should show normal motility within 3 hours after collection
- Abnormal sperms should not be more than 30–35%.

Semen analysis is used for:

- Assessing male fertility
- It reflects the normal funtions of testis and accessory sex organs
- For investigation of infertility cases
- To find out the effectiveness of vasectomy
- For medico-legal cases like—rape, adultery etc.

2. Functions of juxtaglomerular apparatus.

- Juxtaglomerular (JG) apparatus is a combination of tubular cells and vascular cells
- It is located near the glomerulus where the afferent arteriole enters and efferent arteriole leaves the glomerulus (Fig. 7).

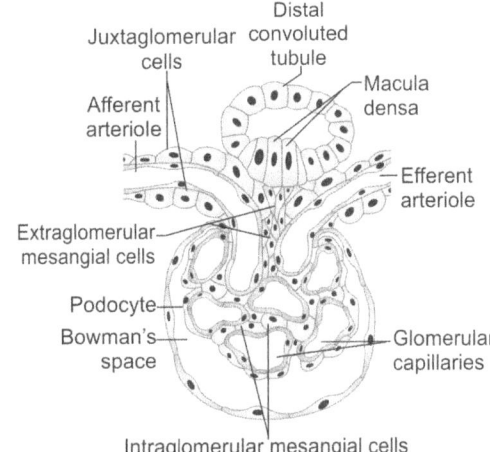

Fig. 7: Juxtaglomerular apparatus. It includes Juxtaglomerular cells, Macula densa and Lacis cells.
(*Source:* GK Pal)

It is made up of the following components:
a. Juxtaglomerular cells
b. Macula densa cells
c. Lacis cells.

Juxtaglomerular Cells

- These are myoepithelial cells lining the afferent arteriole just befor it enters the glomerulus
- These cells are rich in endoplasmic reticulum and they secrete the hormone renin
- They act as baroreceptors and they sense the change in the renal arterial pressure and respond to the pressure gradient between the afferent arteriole and the interstitium
- When the renal arterial pressure drops JG cells release renin
- These cells also sense the ECF volume and respond to hypovolemia by secreting renin
- They are also supplied by sympathetic nerves and when the stimulation is there it releases renin
- Renin activates Renin-Angiotensin-Aldosterone system and thereby regulates ECV volume and pressure (refer Fig. 8).

Macula Densa Cells

- They are present in the renal tubules at the junction of thick ascending limb of loop of Henle and the distal convoluted tubule
- These cells are modified; they are more columnar and densely packed
- They are in close contact with the mesangial cells and the JG cells
- They act as chemoreceptors and they sense the NaCl content in the tubular fluid
- They act through tubuloglomerular feedback (Ref. Aug 2008 answers) and regulate the renal blood flow and GFR.

Mesangial Cells or Lacis Cells

- These are present in between the afferent and efferent arterioles and are in close contact with the JG cells and Macula densa cells
- They are contractile in nature and therefore they regulate GFR
- They also secrete some amount of renin.

3. Explain components and functions of bile.

- Bile is secreted by the hepatocytes and the ductal cells
- Bile salts are secreted into the bile from the hepatocytes and other components like bile pigments are added to it from blood

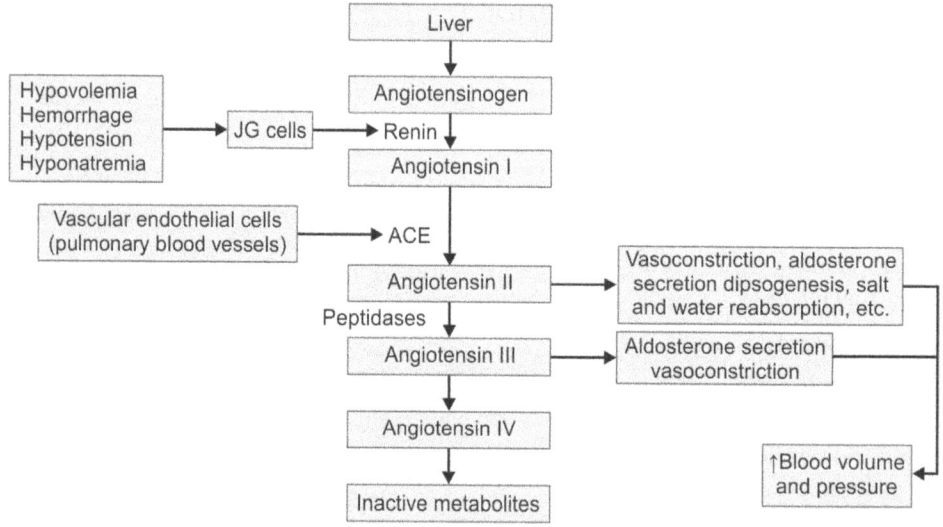

Fig. 8: Renin-angiotensin pathway.
(*Source*: GK Pal)

- Ductal cells add HCO_3^- to bile and make it an alkaline secretion.

Composition of Bile

- pH—7.8-8.6
- Colour—light golden yellow
- Water—97%
- Solids—3%.

Organic Substances

- Bile salts
- Bile pigments
- Cholesterol
- Fatty acids
- Fats
- Lecithin
- Mucin.

Inorganic Salts

- Cations - Na^+, K^+, Ca^{2+} and Mg^{2+}
- Anions - HCO_3^-, Cl^-, SO_4^{2-} and PO_4^{3-}.

Functions of Bile

a. *Digestive function:* Bile salts emulsify the fats and helps in digestion of fats. By emulsification, bile salts break down large fat globules into smaller molecules thereby increasing the surface area on which lipase can act and digest fats
b. *Absorption of fats and fat-soluble vitamins:* The fats are surrounded by the amphipathic bile salts and form the micelles which help in transporting the fats to the brush border of the small intestine and helps in its absorption
c. *Excretory function:* Bile pigments, the breakdown products of hemoglobin are the most important substances excreted in bile. Heavy metals like copper and iron are also excreted. Toxins are also excreted in bile. Bile salts lost in the bile helps in excreting fats
d. *Laxative function:* Bile salts when they remain in the GIT they hold back water and they increase the motility of GIT
e. *Regulation of pH in GIT:* High HCO_3 content in the bile helps in neutralizing the acid entering the small intestine
f. *Prevents gall stone formation:* Bile salts keep the cholesterol and lecithin in solution and thereby prevents formation of cholesterol stones in the gall bladder
g. Mucin present in the bile lubricates the chyme in the intestine
h. *Choleretic function:* Bile salts in the bile increases secretion of more bile from the liver.

4. **Explain the stages of development of erythrocytes.**

Refer answers to 2006 paper.

5. **Describe the metabolic actions of cortisol.**

Refer answers to 2006 paper.

6. **Describe briefly the formation and functions of corpus luteum.**

Refer answers to 2008 paper.

7. **Describe the formation and circulation of lymph.**

- Lymph is present in the lymphatic channels
- Across the capillaries, plasma is getting filtered into the interstitium at the arteriolar end and reabsorption of fluid happens at the venular end into the blood vessels
- But not all the fluid is reabsorbed at the venular end and some fluid is lost from plasma in each cycle of circulation
- This left out fluid is reabsorbed into the lymphatic vessels from the interstitium and finally they drain into the veins, thereby restoring the normal plasma volume
- From glands, substances like fats, proteins and organic and inorganic substances from degrading cells also enter the interstitium and then into the lymph.

Circulation of Lymph

Tissue fluid from interstitium
↓
Forms lymph and enters lymphatic capillaries
↓

Lymph capillaries merge with other capillaries
↓
Lymph capillaries drain into Lymphatic afferents
↓
Lymph enetrs lymph nodes
↓
Lymph leaves through lymphatic efferents
↓
Merge with other vessels and drain forms lymphatic trunk
↓
Drains into collecting duct (right lymphatic duct and thoracic duct)
↓
Drains into subclavian vein at the junction with internal jugular vein

8. Enumerate the hormones secreted by anterior pituitary gland. Describe the actions of growth hormone.

Anterior pituitary hormones are the following:

1. Growth hormone (GH)
2. Prolactin (PL)
3. Thyroid stimulating hormone (TSH)
4. Adrenocorticotrophin (ACTH)
5. Gonadotrophins: Follicle stimulating hormone (FSH) and leuteinizing hormone (LH)

Actions of Growth Hormone

Refer answers to 2003 paper.

9. Classify the fluid compartments of body giving their normal values, mention two methods to determine ECF.

Total body water is classified in two compartments:
- Extracellular space – Extracellular fluid – 14 L (20% of body weight)
- Intracellular space – Intracellular fluid – 28 L (40% of body weight).

Extracellular fluid is distributed as:

- Interstitial fluid—fluid present in between cells
- Intravascular—plasma
- Transcellular fluid—CSF, ocular fluid, peritoneal and pleural fluids, synovial fluid, GIT secretion
- Lymph—flows in the lymphatic channels.

Determination of ECF Volume

- ECF volume is measured by the indicator dilution technique
- Substances used to measure ECF volume should remain only in the ECF. The substances used are inulin, mannitol, sucrose and thiocyanate.
- ECF volume forms 20% of the body weight of an individual and therefore it can be calculated approximately if the body weight is known. For example, in a male of 70 kG the ECF volume will be 14 L.

Indicator Dilution Technique

- A known volume of the substance is injected into the blood. After some time when the substance has uniformly distributed in the space, a sample of blood is taken and the concentration of substance in the blood is estimated and ECF volume is calculated using this formula:

ECF Volume

$$= \frac{\text{Amount of substance injected} - \text{Amount excreted}}{\text{Average concentration of the substance}}$$

$$= \frac{150\,\text{mg} - 10\,\text{mg}}{0.01\,\text{mg/mL}}$$

$$= 14000\,\text{mL}$$

10. Describe the formation and functions of immunoglobulins.

- Matured B lymphocytes are located in the lymph nodes in a dormant form
- When an antigen enters blood, it is phagocytosed by the macrophages present in lymph nodes
- The macrophage processes the antigen and presents it to B cells which have the receptor for that antigen. It is also presented to T cells and Helper T cells are produced
- T Helper cells are also essential for activation of B cells
- The B cells get transformed into Plasmablasts, precursors for plasma cells

and they start dividing many times to form the clone of Plasma cells
- Plasma cells start producing immunoglobulins at a rate of 2000 molecules per second by each plasma cell
- Following that, plasma cells rupture and release Immunoglobulins into the lymph and are carried to blood.

Functions of Immunoglobuins

Immunoglobulins attack the antigens in two ways:
- Direct attack on the antigens
- Complement activation and thereby inactivation of antigens.

Direct inactivation of antigens is by:
i. Agglutination of antigens, by binding to antibodies making them a large clump which favors phagocytosis by the phagocytes
ii. Precipitation of antigen-antibody complexes
iii. Antibodies cover the antigen and neutralize it
iv. Directly attacks the membrane of the pathogen and lyses it.

Activation of complement system and thereby destroying the antigens:
i. Opsonization and phagocytosis of antigens by neutrophils and macrophages
ii. Lysis of antigens by forming a lytic complex which gets inserted on the pathogen and destroying it
iii. Agglutination of antigens
iv. Neutralization of antigen by complement proteins
v. Chemotaxis
vi. By activation of basophils and mast cells.

11. Neuromuscular junction.
Refer answers to 2008 paper.

12. Compare REM and NREM sleep.
See Figure 9.

13. Triple response.
Refer answers to 2006 paper.

14. Describe formation, circulation and functions of cerebrospinal fluid (CSF).
- CSF is a colorless fluid that protects the brain and spinal cord (SC)
- It also carries nutrients and oxygen from blood to brain
- It circulates in the cavities of brain (ventricles) and SC and also in the subarachnoid space.

Formation of CSF
- CSF is formed from the choroid plexus in the walls of all the ventricles
- Rate of formation is 0.35 mL/min or 20 mL/hr or 500 mL/D
- Normal volume of CSF at any time is 70–150 mL
- Formation is by passive diffusion, Active transport and facilitated diffusion
- There are 2 steps—ultrafiltration and active secretion
- The choroid plexus are network of capillaries which are covered by ependymal cells of the ventricles
- These cells form CSF from blood by filtration and secretion

	NREM sleep	REM sleep
Timing in sleep cycle	Occurs first	Occurs after NREM sleep
Duration in normal adults	75% of total sleep	25% of sleep
Autonomic symptoms	Sympathetic inhibition (low BP, HR, respiration)	Sympathetic excitation (high BP, HR)
Eye ball movement	No movement	Rapid eye movement occurs
Dreams	Dreams are not memorized	Dreams well memorized
Muscle tone	Is inhibited	Profoundly decreased
Type of sleep	Enters into deep sleep	Sleep lightens
EEG waves	Slow-wave, high amplitude	High frequency, low voltage
Mechanism	Inhibition of reticular activating system (RAS)	Activation of pontine reticular formation

Fig. 9: Differences between rapid eye movement (REM) and non-rapid eye movement (NREM) sleep.

- The cells are joined by tight junctions to prevent leakage between the cells.

Circulation of CSF

- CSF is formed in lateral ventricles and pass to the third ventricle through interventricular foramen or Foramen of Monro (refer Fig. 10)
- More CSF is formed in third ventricle and flows through cerebral aqueduct to the fourth ventricle
- Then CSF enters the subarachnoid space through three openings in the roof of fourth ventricle—a median aperture of Magendie and two lateral apertures of Luschka
- CSF then circulates in the central canal and subarachnoid space of brain and spinal cord.

Drainage of CSF

- CSF is gradually reabsorbed into the blood through the **Arachnoid villi** into the *superior sagittal sinus*
- 20% is reabsorbed through spinal veins
- CSF is absorbed at the same rate at which it is formed
- So the CSF pressure is always constant
- It is around 8 mm Hg or 110 mm H_2O.

Functions of CSF

- CSF offers mechanical protection by acting as a shock absorber
- CSF offers the optimum chemical environment for accurate neuronal signaling
- CSF acts as a circulating medium for exchange of nutrients and waste products between the blood and nervous tissue
- Continuous formation and drainage removes metabolic wastes from brain
- Acts as lymph in brain
- Provides nutrition
- Reduces the weight of brain.

15. Functions of vestibular apparatus.

- Vestibular apparatus helps in regulating posture either due to effect of gravity or rotation
- The afferents from this organ (through vestibulo-spinal tract) helps to adapt the position of trunk and limbs to that of head. Thus enabling the erect posure of head and normal position of body
- Vestibulospinal tract helps to regulate tone in antigravity muscles
- The vestibular apparatus supports the head during movement, orientation of head in space and reflexes (tonic labyrinthine and righting reflexes)
- Vestibular apparatus relay to thalamus and cortex and helps in conscious awareness of position and acceleration of body
- Information from here is relayed to cranial nerves 3, 4 and 6 and helps in visual fixation during rotation—vestibulo-ocular reflex
- Vestibular apparatus also has a predictive function and thereby prevents from fall.

Vestibulo-ocular Reflex (VOR)

- When head rotates, eyes move in the opposite direction to head movement
- VOR helps to fix vision on the same object in spite of head movement
- Speed of the eye movement equals that of the head movement
- Allows objects to remain in focus during head movements.

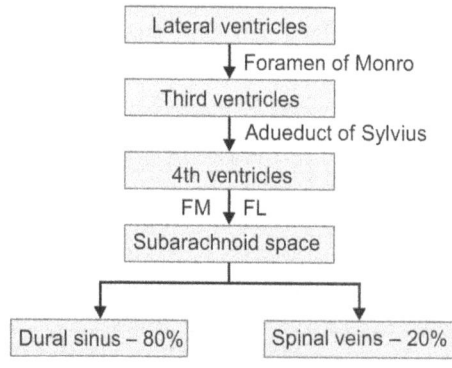

Fig. 10: Formation, circulation and drainage of CSF. CSF is formed from choroid plexuses in lateral, 3rd and 4th ventricles. (FM: foramen Magendie; FL: foramen Luschka)

16. Explain 'dark adaptation'.

Refer answers to 2005 paper.

17. Organ of Corti.

- The organ of Corti is the organ of hearing and is present in the inner ear in cochlea (refer Fig. 11)
- It is placed on the Basilar membrane and contains the receptors for hearing—hair cells
- The organ of Corti consists of the hair cells, supporting cells, tunnel of Corti, basilar membrane, tectorial membrane and reticular lamina
- There are two groups of hair cells—the inner hair cells and outer hair cells seated on the basilar membrane seperated by the rods of Corti
- There is a tringular space between the rods—the tunnel of Corti.

Hair Cells

- The inner hair cells are 3500 in number and are arranged in a single row along the entire length of cochlea
- There are 20, 000 outer hair cells and are arranged in 3 rows
- At the bases of the hair cells are the nerve endings which later become the cochlear divison of vestibulo-cochlear nerve
- The apical ends of the hair cells contain the cilia that pass through reticular lamina
- The cilia of outer hair cells are embedded in the thin gelatinous tectorial membrane
- The hairs of the inner hair cells do not touch the membrane

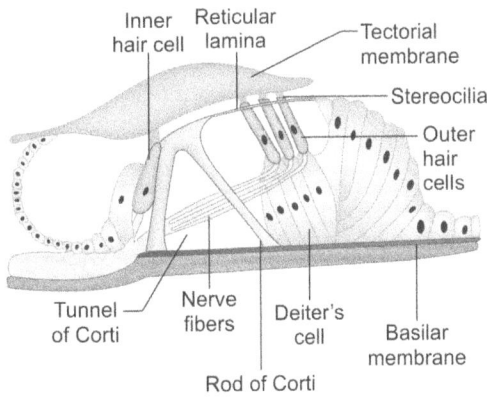

Fig. 11: Organ of Corti with hair cells.
(*Source:* GK Pal)

- When the sound waves reach the organ of Corti it acts as the transducer to convert sound waves into action potentials which travel through the cochlear nerve to reach the auditory area in the cortex.

18. Describe decompression sickness.
Refer answers to 2006 paper.

19. Describe chemical control of respiration.
Refer answers to 2005 paper.

20. What is myasthenia gravis? Describe the biological basis of its treatment.
Refer answers for 2005 paper.

21. Micturition reflex.
Refer answers to 2006 paper.

22. Gastric emptying.

- Gastric emptying is a slow process in which food from stomach is gradually emptied into the duodenum and jejunum
- **There are 3 mechanisms in gastric emptying:**
  a. **Peristaltic contractions:** These are ring like contractions starting in the body of stomach and gradually push the contents towards the antrum. The waves in the proximal part are weak and as it reaches the antrum the waves become stronger and dig into the chyme. So adequate mixing and breaking down of food particles happen in the antrum
  b. **Contractions of antrum:** Antral contractions are very strong and they help in proper mixing of gastric juice with food contents. Not only mixing of food and gastric juice happens but also the force of contraction forces the food towards the pylorus. But the Pyloric sphincter ahead is strongly contracted (refer Fig. 12)
  c. **Retropulsion:** Forceful contraction of antrum and closure of pyloric sphincter pushes the food back into the proximal part of the antrum and this continues for few times. The retropulsion helps in mixing and grinding the food particles. The Pyloric sphincter opens partially allowing small quantities of

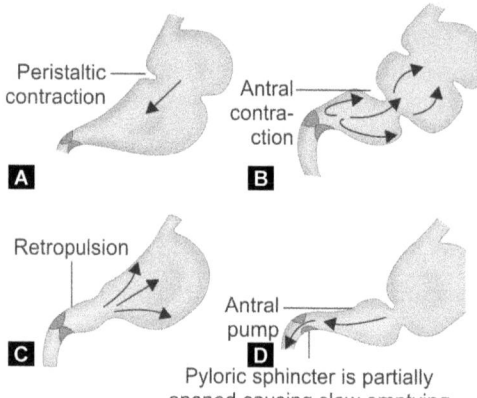

Figs. 12A to D: Gastric emptying; In A, B and C the Pyloric sphincter is closed. The contractions in antrum digest the food and is converted to chyme. (C) There is forward movement of chyme and as the sphincter is closed there is retropulsion of chyme which further breaks food particles. (D) Sphincter is partially open allowing small amounts of chyme to be emptied.
(*Source:* GK Pal)

chyme at a time to be squirted into the duodenum.

Regulation of Gastric Emptying

Regulation is done by neural and humoral mechanisms. Factors which affect emptying are—pH of contents in duodenum, osmotic pressure, products of fat and protein digestion.

a. **Low pH:** Acidic content in the duodenum are sensed by receptors in the duodenum and gastric emptying is delayed by Secretin released from small intestines
b. **Osmolality of contents:** If the osmolality of the contents entering the duodenum is high it is sensed by osmoreceptors here and hormones are released which inhibit gastric emptying
c. **Products of digestion of fat:** Presence of digested fats and fatty acids are sensed by the duodenum and CCK is released which causes delay in gastric emptying
d. **Products of protein digestion:** Protein products like peptides and amino acids in duodenum cause release of gastrin which in turn causes antral contraction and closure of pyloric sphincter resulting in delaying the gatsric emptying
e. **Volume and type of meal:** When volume of meal is more there is delayed emptying. Watery meal hastens the emptying. Carbohydrate emptying is faster and fat emptying is the slowest
f. **Stretch of duodenum:** When duodenal wall is streched it induces enterogastric reflex which inhibits gastric emptying
g. **Neural factors:** Vagus stimulation promotes emptying and sympathetic stimulation delays emptying.

23. Indicators of ovulation.

Refer answers to 2008 paper.

24. Myxedema.

Refer answers to 2005 paper.

25. Enterohepatic circulation of bile.

- Bile acids and salts present in the bile on entering the inetstine are absorbed from the terminal part of the ileum and re-enter the portal vein to be secreted back into the bile from hepatocytes (refer Fig. 13)
- This process repeats many times—enterohepatic circulation
- The conjugated bile salts are absorbed and recirculated in the above manner
- Also, bile salts are unconjugated and some of it is also absorbed
- Colonic bacteria act on free bile acids and are converted to secondary bile acids and a part of it is also absorbed back into the portal vein
- 95% of secreted bile salts are absorbed by the enterohepatic circulation and only 200–500 mg/day are excreted.

Significance of Enterohepatic Circulation

- Only the amount of bile salts which are excreted, are synthesized and replaced daily, to maintain the pool of bile salts in the body which are essential for digestion and absorption of fats
- The total amount of bile salts is 2–4 g
- This amount is circulated daily many times to digest and absorb fats in the diet taken.

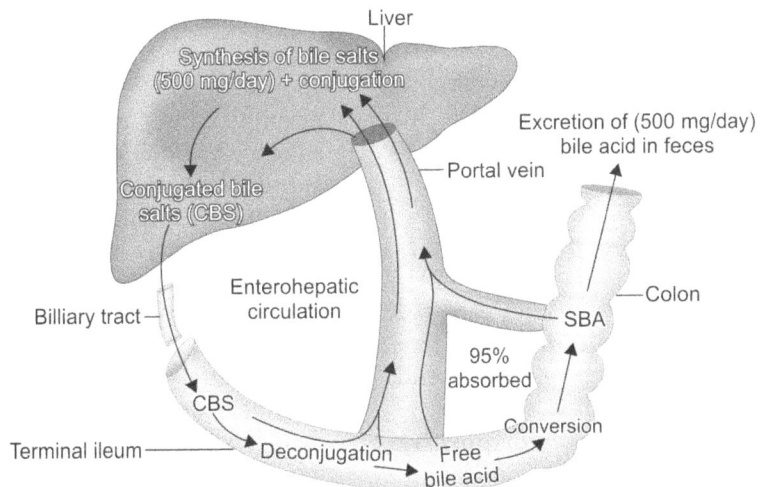

Fig. 13: Enterohepatic circulation. It is the circulation of bile salts following its synthesis from liver in bile and its secretion into duodenum and its reabsorption in terminal ileum and recirculation through portal veins.
(SBA: secondary bile acids)
(*Source:* GK Pal)

26. Conn's syndrome.

- Hyperaldosteronism can be primary or secondary
- **Primary hyperaldosteronism is Conn's syndrome**
- The cause of excess secretion of aldosterone could be due to an adenoma in the adrenal cortex, adrenal hyperplasia or carcinoma of adrenal gland
- Conn's syndrome is due to a tumor in the adrenal cortex, in the zona glomerulosa layer
- Actions of aldosterone are Na^+ reabsorption in the kidneys along with Cl^- and water reabsorption and K^+ and H^+ secretion in exchange for Na^+ reabsorption
- So in hyperaldosteronism the symptoms are due to Na^+ retention and K^+ and H^+ depletion
- Patient presents with hypertension which is due to salt and water retention without edema
- Hypokalemia leads to muscle weakness
- Loss of H^+ leads to alkalosis
- Tetany can be present due to alkalosis induced hypocalcemia
- They also present with polyuria due to impairment of concentrating ability of kidneys
- Due to salt and water retention and increase in ECF volume, renin levels are low
- Edema is absent inspite of water retention due to aldosterone escape phenomenon
- In **secondary hyperaldosteronism** the high levels of aldosterone are due to increased renin secretion secondary to other diseases like cirrhosis of liver, heart failure and nephrosis.

27. Functions of glucocorticoids.

Refer answers to 2004 paper.

28. Significance of Rh group.

- Rh system is the second most important blood group systems in the body. It was discovered in the Rhesus monkey in 1940
- There are 6 antigens in this system, C, D, E and c, d and e
- D antigen is higly antigenic and therefore individuals with D antigen on their RBC membrane are Rh Positive and persons without D antigen are Rh negative

- Rh antigen is inherited as a dominant gene
- Therefore Rh positive may be homozygous with DD or heterozygous with Dd. Rh negative is homozygous with dd
- The antibody in Rh system is Anti D antibody
- There are no naturally occuring antibodies here as in the ABO system
- But if an Rh negative person receives Rh positive blood his immune system recognizes the Rh antigen as foreign and starts producing antibodies
- So in first encounter of Rh positive blood there is not much complication. On the next exposure, massive antigen antibody reactions happen resulting in agglutination and hemolysis
- Therefore the Rh system does not follow the 2nd law of Landsteiner's which states that "If a particular antigen is absent on the RBC membrane the corresponding antibody will be present in the plasma"
- The **most significant aspect** of Rh incompatibility is the mismatch of Rh factor between the mother and the fetus
- If the mother is Rh negative and she conceives an Rh positive fetus, at the time of delivery of the fetus, during the placental seperation, a small amount of Rh positive blood leaks into mother's circulation
- As the first baby is already born, it is not affected
- The mother's immune system starts producing Anti D antibodies
- If she conceives the next time and that fetus is also Rh positive, the antibodies in the maternal circulation which belongs to IgG type crosses the placenta and attacks the fetal RBCs
- There is agglutination and hemolysis of fetal RBCs
- In the subsequent similar pregnancies the damage to the fetus is severe
- The child presents with the symptoms of Hemolytic disease of the newborn or Erythroblastosis fetalis.

The symptoms are:
- Anemia: Due to hemolysis the child has anemia
- Edema: The child has generalized edema—hydrops fetalis
- Jaundice: Hemolysis releases bilirubin and results in jaundice
- Kernicterus: The high bilirubin levels in the neonates damages the basal ganglia. In adults the blood brain barrier prevents the entry of bilirubin into the brain. But in infants blood brain barrier is not fully developed, so, the bilirubin easily damages the basal ganglia resulting in motor defects
- Erythroblasts appear in the circulation: Excessive hemolysis induces erythropoiesis and erythroblasts (the precursors) start appearing in the circulation.

Treatment:
- If the hemolysis is mild, no treatment is needed
- In severe conditions treatment can be given as intrauterine transfusions or after birth, exchange transfusion can be given along with phototherapy.

Prevention:
- After the delivery of the Rh positive fetus by the Rh negative mother, the mother is immunized with Anti D antibodies
- These antibodies neutralize the antigens which have entered the mother's circulation and prevent formation of further antibodies.

29. Transport mechanisms across cell membrane.

The cell membrane, being a semi-permeable one, does not allow all substances to pass through it.

It is easier for lipids and lipid-soluble sustances to pass through the bilipid layer.

Water and water soluble substances need channels/carriers to be transported across the membrane.

Substances on either sides of the membrane differ in their concentrations also, therefore they either move along the gradients or against the gradients.

So transport across the cell membrane is classified as:
- Active transport
- Passive transport
- Vesicle-mediated transport (refer Fig. 14).

Passive Transport
Here the movement of substances is along the concentration or electrical gradient and there is no energy expenditure.

Types:
1. Simple diffusion
2. Facilitated diffusion
3. Osmosis
4. Filtration
5. Bulk flow
6. Solvent drag.

Simple Diffusion
- **Lipid soluble** substances diffuse by dissolving in the membrane and diffuse to either side of membrane—O_2, N_2, steroids etc.
- **Water soluble** substances move through water filled channel proteins
- No energy expenditure
- Moves substances along concentration gradient (refer Fig. 15A).

Diffusion through Channels
- Channels are water-filled pores (refer Figs 15B and C)
- This allows water soluble substances to move across the membrane
- The channels have selective permeability
- They may be gated or Non-gated
- Gates could be either change in—voltage, binding ligands or stretch (Mechanical).

Factors Affecting Net Diffusion
A. Cell membrane permeability
   - Thickness of membrane—inversely proportional
   - Lipid solubility—directly proportional
   - Distribution of protein channels in membrane
   - Temperature—directly proportional
   - Size of molecule—inversely proportional

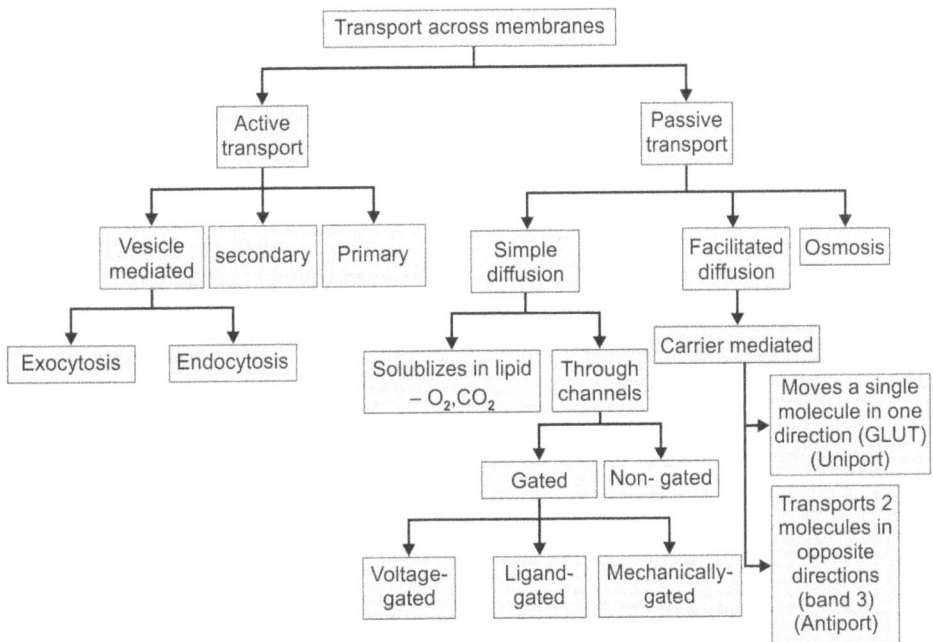

Fig. 14: Classification of transport across cell membrane.

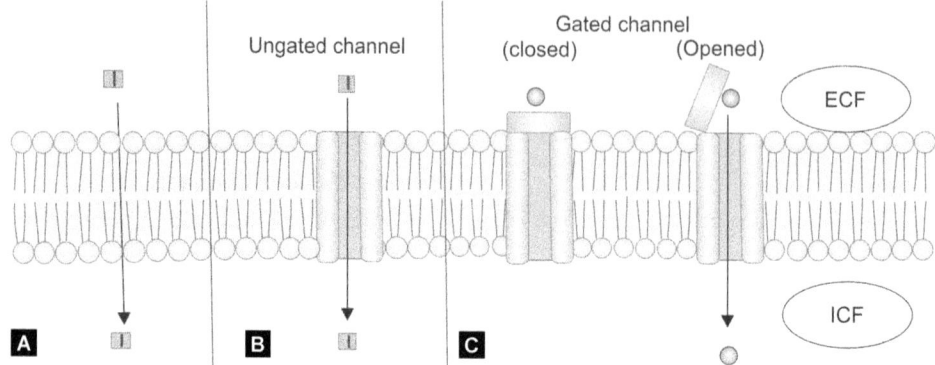

Figs. 15A to C: (A) Simple diffusion through lipid membrane; (B) Simple diffusion through non-gated channels; (C) Diffusion through Gated channels.
(*Source:* Sembulingam)

- Area of membrane—directly proportional.
B. Concentration gradient—directly proportional
C. Electrical gradient
D. Pressure gradient—directly proportional.

Facilitated Diffusion
- Large water soluble substances (e.g. glucose) are carried by a protein which changes configuration on binding
- This change in configuration shifts the molecule in or out (refer Fig. 16)
- Carrier is highly selective and specific
- Types:
  - Uniport
  - Symport
  - Antiport.

- Characteristics
  - Specificity
  - Saturation
  - Competition.

Osmosis
Diffusion of water or other solvent molecules through a semi-permeable membrane (i.e. membrane impermeable to solute and not to solvent) from a solution containing lower concentration of solutes to the solution containing higher concentration of solutes—**osmosis**.

Filtration and Bulk Flow
Filtration or movement of water and solutes through the capillary wall are examples of filtration.

If filtration involves movement of greater volume of water it is called bulk flow.

Solvent Drag
During bulk flow if sovents are carried along – Solvent drag.

Active Transport
- It is also carrier mediated
- Moves substances uphill against concentration gradient
- So associated with energy expenditure. Energy is derived from ATP, either directly or indirectly
- Types:
  - Primary active transport
  - Secondary active transport.

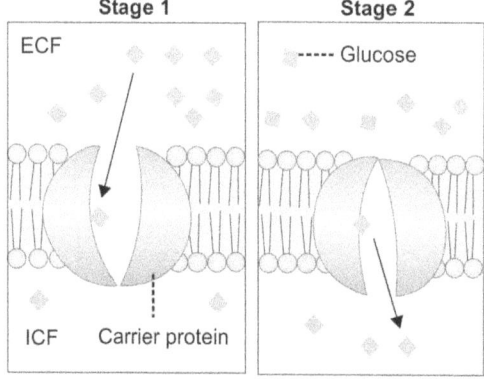

Fig. 16: Facilitated diffusion. A uniport transporting Glucose molecules.
(*Source:* Sembulingam)

Primary Active Transport

Here substances are moved uphill across the cell membrane with the help of pumps. It involves energy expenditure which is directly derived from break down of ATP.

Ex.
- Na^+- K^+ Pump
- H^+ -K^+ Pump
- Ca^{++} ATPase

Na^+- K^+ Pump

Sodium Potassium ATPase is a ubiquitous pump. It pumps out 3 Na^+ molecules from the cell in exchange for 2 K^+ molecules into the cell. Na^+ concentration is more in the ECF and K^+ concentration is more in the ICF (refer Fig. 17). So both the ions are pumped against their concentration gradients out and in of the cell respectively. The pump is present in all the cells to maintain the cell volume and to maintain the membrane potential.

Secondary Active Transport

In the secondary active transport the substances are moved against the concentration gradient with the help of energy derived indirectly from the ATP. Na^+- K^+ Pump, when it pumps out Na^+ from the cell, creates a concentration gradient for Na^+ into the cell. This gradient for Na^+ is utilised for movement of other ions across the cell membrane. So the transporters of secondary active transport moves Na^+ in exchange (sodium counter-transporter) or along (sodium cotransporter) with another molecule (both organic and inorganic substances) (refer Fig. 18).

Ex.
- Na^+-Glucose symport
- Na^+ – Amino acid symport
- Na^+ – H^+ exchanger
- Na^+ – Ca^{++} exchanger.

Vesicle-mediated Transport

- Large polar molecules – like protein hormones in endocrine glands are transported across the cell as membrane wrapped vesicles

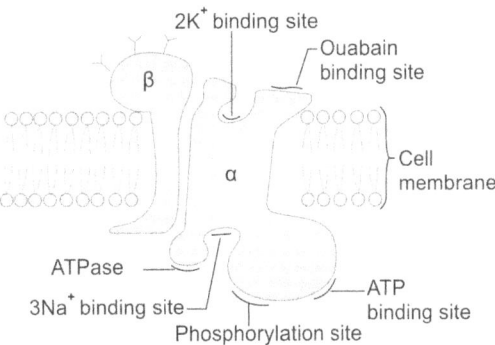

Fig. 17: Sodium-potassium pump; Primary active transporter.
(Source: GK Pal)

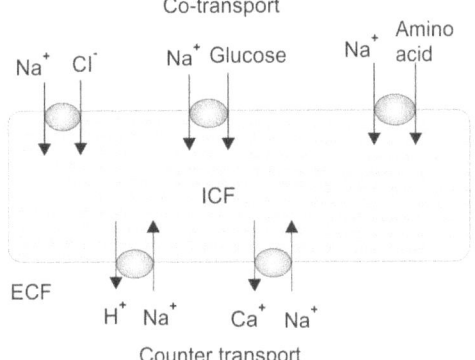

Fig. 18: Secondary active transporters; Na^+-Glucose symporter, Na^+- Aminoacid symport, Na^+-H^+ exchanger, Na^+- Ca^{2+} Exchanger.
(Source: Sembulingam)

- Types:
  - Endocytosis
  - Exocytosis.

Endocytosis

It is the process by which substances are internalized within the cell (refer Fig. 19). There are 3 types:
- Phagocytosis
- Pinocytosis
- Receptor mediated endocytosis.

Phagocytosis: Engulfing of solid substances (cell eating) as that of micro-organisms by the neutrophils.

Pinocytosis: Engulfing the liquid components (cell drinking).

Receptor-mediated endocytosis: Here the substances to be internalized get attached to a

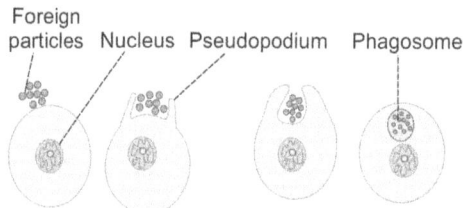

Fig. 19: Process of endocytosis.
(*Source:* Sembulingam)

receptor protein present on the cell membrane and the whole complex is engulfed.

Exocytosis

It is the process by which substance are extruded from the cell. It is the reversal of endocytosis. The substances to be extruded are in the vesicle which moves towards the cell membrane and gets attached to the membrane and is later pinched out of the cell.

30. Albumin: Globulin ratio.

- Albumin is synthesized in the liver and globulin is synthesized by the reticulo-endothelial system
- Normal value of albumin is 3–5 g/dL, average is 4.8 g/dL
- Normal value of globulin is 2–3 g/dL and average is 2.3 g/dL
- So the normal Albumin: Globulin ratio is 1.7:1
- In liver disorders albumin synthesis is decreased resulting in low serum albumin levels and an increase in serum globulin level as it is synthesized in R-E system. This is called as compensatory increase. It results in reversal of A:G ratio
- Thymol turbidity test is done to find out the reversal of A:G ratio
- Marked turbidity is seen in liver insufficiency. This is due to increase in γ-globulin levels.

31. Compliance.

Refer answers to 2003 paper.

32. Brown-Sequard syndrome.

Refer answers to 2008 paper.

33. Blood brain barrier (BBB).

- It is a barrier formed between the brain capillaries and brain matter

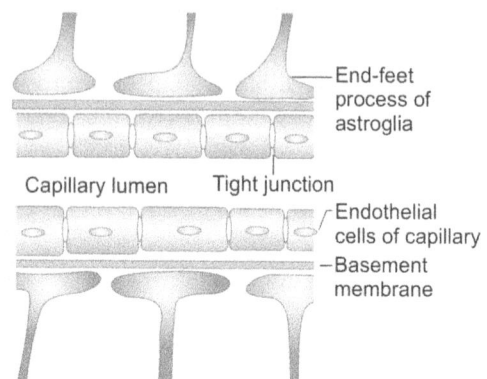

Fig. 20: Blood brain barrier formed by feet of astrocytes, tight junctions of endothelial cells.
(*Source:* GK Pal)

- The barrier is formed by tight junctions (TJ) between capillary endothelial cells and TJ between the epithelial cells lining the choroid plexus
- It is also surrounded by the feet of astrocytes which cover the capillary wall (refer Fig. 20)
- BBB prevents the entry of proteins into brain and allows slow movement of smaller molecules
- Though passive diffusion is very limted, there are vesicle-mediated transports and other carrier-mediated and active transport mechanisms in cerebral capillaries
- Lipid-soluble substances like CO_2, O_2 and steroids penetrate brain with ease
- Water also moves across easily
- Glucose which is the major source of energy and enters through the glucose transporter GLUT 1
- There are other transporters like Na^+-K^+-$2Cl^-$ transporter.

Circumventricular Organs (CVO)

- Some of the areas of the brain do not have a BBB
- They are called as the circumventricular organs. Posterior pituitary is also present out of the BBB
- It includes small structures in the brainstem: Median eminence of the hypothalamus, area postrema, Organum vasculosum of the lamina terminalis (OVLT) and subfornical organ (SFO)

- These structures have fenestrated capillaries whose permeability is high and therefore are said to be outside the BBB
- These organs contain receptors for many peptides and chemicals and they function as chemoreceptor zones in the brain.

For example:

a. Area postrema triggers vomiting when exposed to certain chemicals in plasma
b. Angiotensin II acts on SFO and induces thirst
c. OVLT is the site of osmoreceptor controlling vasopressin secretion
d. Circulating IL-1 induces fever by acting on CVO.

Functions of BBB

a. It maintains the constancy of environment of the neurons in the CNS
b. It maintains the concentrations of K^+, Ca^{2+}, Mg^{2+} and H^+ in the fluid bathing the neurons for their normal functioning
c. Protects the brain from exogenous and endogenous toxins in blood
d. Prevents the escape of neurotransmitters from brain.

Clinical Aspects

a. The knowledge about BBB and the drugs that penetrate it is important for treatment of neurological diseases, as in Parkinsonism, the low dopamine level is treated by giving the precursor L-dopa (which crosses BBB) rather than dopamine which cannot cross the BBB
b. BBB breaks in areas of infections and injury
c. It is also broken by marked increase in BP and IV injection of hypertonic fluids
d. In case of brain tumors, there are new vessels formed which lack the BBB and therefore radioisotopes can be injected to make the tumor identifiable.

34. Surfactant.
Refer answers to 2008 paper.

35. Chronaxie and rheobase.
Refer answers to 2004 paper (Short Note 4).

36. Pupillary light reflexes.

- The effect of light on the eye induces changes in the pupils—pupillary light reflexes
- They are direct and indirect light reflexes
- Changes are found in the diameter of pupils.

Direct Light Reflex

Here when light rays are shone on one eye, there is constriction of pupil of the same eye.

Indirect Light Reflex

When light is shone on one eye there is constriction of pupil in the same eye and also in the other eye.

Pathway for Light Reflex

- The pathway for direct light reflex is—from the retina impulses pass through the optic nerve, optic chiasma, optic tract
- Some fibers from optic tract reach the pretectal nucleus in the midbrain
- The fibers from pretectal nucleus reach the 3rd cranial nerve nuclei bilaterally
- From here fibers reach the ciliary ganglion on both sides
- Fibers from ciliary ganglion, short ciliary nerves supply the sphincter pupillae of both eyes
- For both, direct and indirect reflexes, pathways are the same
- Crossing over of fibers happen at the optic chiasma and at the pretectal nucleus
- In neurosyphilis there is lesion in the pretectal nucleus and therfore pupillary light reflexes are lost and accommodation reflex is present. this is called as **Argyll Robertson pupil**

Light rays fall on retina
↓
Impulses travel through Optic nerve
↓
Optic chiasma
↓
Optic tract
↓
Pretectal nucleus (Bilateral)

↓
Edinger-Westphal Nucleus (Bilateral)
↓
Ciliary ganglion (Bilateral)
↓
Short ciliary nerve (Bilateral)
↓
Constriction of pupil (Bilateral)

37. Pacemaker potential.

Refer answers to 2005 paper.

38. Atrial natriuretic peptide.

It is a hormone secreted from the right atrium. It is polypeptide in nature with 28 AA. It is secreted in response to atrial stretch as in increased central venous pressure (CVP).

Factors Regulating Secretion of ANP

- Increase in ECF volume as in IV fluid infusion
- Conditions like immersion in water up to the neck which increases CVP.

Actions of ANP

- Increases excretion of sodium in urine by increasing GFR by causing dilatation of afferent and efferent arterioles
- Inhibits reabsorption of Na^+ in the tubules
- Lowers blood pressure by causing vasodilatation in arterioles and by causing extravasation of fluid from capillaries
- It also inhibits release of renin from the Juxta glomerular cells.

39. Draw the optic pathway. Depict the lesions at various levels.

Refer answers to 2004 paper.

40. Peculiarities of pulmonary circulation.

- It is a low pressure and low resistance system (MAP – 15 mm Hg)
- Pulmonary arteries have less amount of smooth muscles → more compliant → can accommodate more blood
- Pulmonary arterioles are also thin-walled and have lesser amounts of smooth muscles
- Pulmonary capillaries are arranged in a network around the alveolus so that blood flows in a thin sheet through them.
- The capillary walls are thin and can be collapsed by ↑ alveolar pressure
- In reponse to hypoxia, the pulmonary arterioles go for vasoconstriction whereas in systemic vessels, hypoxia induces vasodilatation and thereby increases blood flow
- Hypoxia happens when the alveoli are ill-ventilated and therefore vasoconstriction in the supplying vessels diverts the blood to the vessels supplying the neighbouring well-ventilated alveoli
- Blood flow in pulmonary capillaries is decided by the pulmonary—arterial and venous and alveolar pressures
- Pulmonary vascular resistance falls as the pulmonary arterial pressure increases as in ↑ Cardiac output because of:
  i. Recruitment of capillaries
  ii. Capillary distension.

III. SHORT ANSWERS

1. Briefly describe the process of deglutition.

Refer answers to 2003 paper.

2. Heparin.

- Heparin is a naturally occuring anti-coagulant present in the granules of basophil and mast cells
- It is a highly conjugated polysaccharide
- By itself it doesn't have an anticoagulant property
- It combines with anti-thrombin III and increases its anti-coagulant activity
- Antithrombin III, in presence of Heparin removes thrombin from circulation and thereby prevents coagulation
- Antithrombin III and heparin combination removes other activated clotting factors like Factors XII, XI, X and IX.

3. Name two indications of exchange transfusion.

- Exchange transfusion is a technique in which the blood of a person is gradually removed in small volumes by inserting a catheter in the veins and replacing with

another blood sample or plasma into the vein in equal small volumes
- It is indicated in Haemolytic disease of newborn due to Rh incompatability and Hyperbilirubinemia, ABO hemolytic disease.

4. Purpura.

- Platelets have a major function of sealing the vascular injuries
- When the platelets come in contact with the injured vessels or exposed collagen they get activated and change their shape
- Platelets have receptors for collagen and thereby adhere to the exposed collagen in the vessel wall
- Activated platelets release ADP and Thromboxane A2. This attracts more platelets and they form a platelet plug and seal the injured vessel
- This sealing mechanism is important to seal minute ruptures in small vessels
- Such minor ruptures happen many times in a day
- Platelets fuse with the endothelium of vessels and heal the injury
- In case of decrease in platelet count, these minute hemorrhages are not sealed and blood clots beneath the skin which later appear as purple spots—purpura.

Causes of Purpura

i. Idiopathic thrombocytopenic purpura
ii. Thrombasthenia
iii. Allergic purpura
iv. Drug induced
v. Splenomegaly.

5. Plasma cells.

- Preformed B lymphocytes are stored in the lymph tissues
- B Lymphocytes mature in the lymph nodes
- Each type of B cells is capable of forming only one type of antibodies for which it is specialized for
- When the specific antigen enters the blood stream it is carried to the lymph tissues and is phagocytosed by the macrophage present there and is presented to the B cells and T lymphocytes
- Once the B cell specific for the antigen is activated it starts dividing many times and similar clone of B cells are produced
- Helper T cells are also activated which helps in final maturation of B cells
- The B cells get differentiated into plasmablasts
- Plasmablasts are precursors for plasma cells
- Plasma cells start producing immunoglobulins specific for the antigens at a rate of 2000 molecules per second per plasma cell
- As the antibodies are formed the cell size increases and finally bursts and releases the immunoglobulins into the lymph and then into the circulation.

6. Functions of plasma proteins.

Albumin, globulin and fibrinogen are the plasma proteins.

Functions

a. Fibrinogen helps in blood coagulation
b. Albumin helps in maintaining colloidal oncotic pressure which is around 25–30 mm Hg. Oncotic pressure is related inversely to molecular shape, size and directly proportional to concentration of molecules. Therefore 80% of oncotic pressure is contributed by albumin
c. Maintains acid-base balance in blood. Plasma proteins act as buffers and they are amphoteric in nature. Therefore they buffer both acids and base and maintain pH at 7.4
d. Maintains the viscosity of blood: Since 80% of the total plasma proteins is contributed by albumin they regulate the viscosity of blood
e. Diastolic blood pressure is regulated by peripheral resistance which in turn is regulated by viscosity of blood and therefore plasma proteins regulate BP
f. Immunoglobulins provide immunity
g. Transport function: Plasma proteins combine with the following substances and transport them—hormones, drugs, metals, bilirubin etc.

7. Phagocytosis.
Refer answers to 2005 paper.

8. Physiological basis of pregnancy diagnosing tests.
- The pregnancy tests are grouped as:
  1. ***Biological tests:*** Injection of urine of pregnant female containing hCG into animals and look for presence of ovulation in female animals and shedding of sperm in male animals
  2. ***Immunological tests:*** Antibodies are produced for hCG and mixed with urine of pregnant female and then RBC or latex particle coated with hCG. Presence of agglutination indicates negative for pregnancy and absence of agglutination indicates pregnancy
  3. ***Radiological test***
- Pregnancy tests 1 and 2 are based on the presence of the hormone hCG present in the urine of pregnant female. It is detected in urine as early as 9 days by radioimmunoassay.

9. Role of oxytocin in female reproduction.
a. Oxytocin acts on myoepithelial cells in the ducts of breast after delivery of fetus—milk let down
b. It also acts on uterine muscles—uterine contraction and aids in delivery of fetus
c. It also acts on non-pregnant uterus—helps in sperm transport.

10. List the important functions of saliva.
Refer answers to 2003 paper.

11. Explain the basic defect in astigmatism and its correction.
- It is a condition where curvature of cornea is not uniform
- The curvature in one meridian is different from the other meridian and light rays in that meridian are refracted to a different focus, so that part of the retinal image is blurred
- It also happens if the lens curvature is not uniform or if the lens is pushed out of alignment
- It can be corrected using cylindrical lens.

12. Draw a labelled diagram of arterial pulse and explain.
- The blood forced into the aorta during systole not only moves the blood forward but also sets up a pressure wave that travels along the arteries (refer Fig. 21)
- The pressure wave expands the arterial walls as it travels and the expansion is palpable as the pulse
- The arterial tracing shows two waves and one notch
- The upstroke is the percussion wave (p wave) and it is due to the ejection of blood in systole
- The downstroke is the dicrotic wave (d wave) and is due to rebound of blood against the closed aortic valve
- The dicrotic notch (n) is due to the closure of the aortic valve.

13. Draw a labelled diagram of pathways for taste.
Refer answers to 2005 paper.

14. Rigor mortis.
- It is the stiffening of muscle after the death of an individual
- This is due to lack of ATP after death
- The depletion of ATP in muscle cells results in failure of detachment of myosin head from actin
- The cross-bridges remain attached to the actin molecule and the muscle remains in a contracted state or rigidity

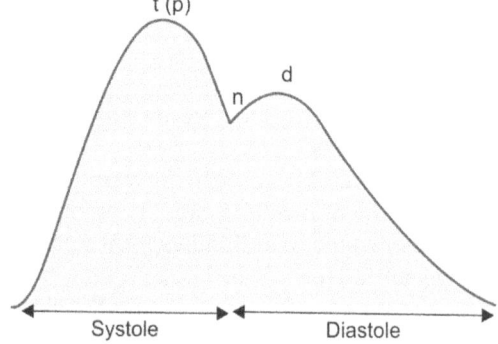

Fig. 21: Arterial pulse tracing from a peripheral artery. 't' is the tidal wave, 'd' dicrotic wave, 'n' is dicrotic notch.
(*Source:* GK Pal)

- It appears by 3-6 hrs after death and is complete by 12 hours
- It disappears after 40-60 hours due to disintegration and myolysis
- It helps to identify the time of death.

15. Phantom limb.

- Phantom limb phenomenon is a condition where the subject feels pain or itch in an amputated limb that does not exist
- It is explained by the law of projection
- **Law of projection:** This codes the location of stimulus
- Along the pathway anywhere from the receptor to brain, wherever stimulated, the conscious sensation is referred to the location of receptor
- Irrespective of application site of stimulus along the pathway the sensation is felt at the site of receptor
- So in phantom limb, irritation of the cut end of nerve terminals from an amputated limb results in feeling of pain or itch in the absent limb
- It can also be due to cortical plasticity.

16. Oxygen debt.

- During exercise there is increase in O_2 consumption to supply the need of O_2 for the exercising muscles
- But even after the stoppage of exercise there is continuous increase in ventilation
- This extra O_2 consumed after exercise is used to remove the lactate accumulation, to replenish the ATP and phosphocreatine stores which were depleted and to replace the O_2 that has been removed from the myoglobin
- The amount of extra O_2 consumed depends on the extra demand of energy consumed during exercise which has exceeded the capacity of aerobic energy synthesis
- This is said to be the O_2 debt
- This can be calculated by finding the O_2 consumption after exercise till the basal consumption is reached.

17. What is Bohr's effect? What is its physiologic significance?

- Decrease in O_2 affinity of hemoglobin when pH of blood falls is called the Bohr effect.
- This signifies that deoxyhemoglobin has more affinity for H^+ than Oxyhemoglobin
- It happens at the tissue level
- In the tissue level, CO_2 release is more and this increases pCO_2 in blood which shifts the Oxygen-Hb dissociation curve to the right (decreases Hb affinity for O_2) and releases O_2
- The unsaturation of hemoglobin at the tissue level is due to decrease in PO_2 but an extra 1-2% of unsaturation is due to the rise in PCO_2 and thereby shift of curve to right (Bohr Effect)

18. Draw a normal ECG and label it.

See Figure 22.

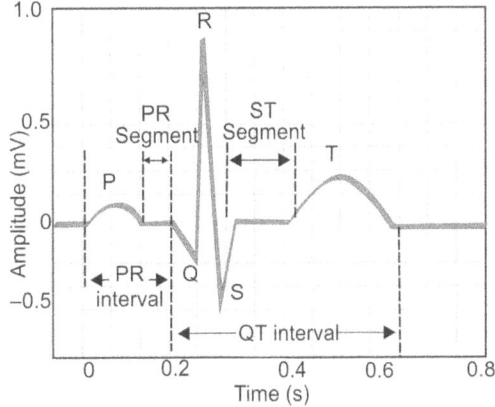

Fig. 22: Normal ECG in Lead II with waves, segements and intervals.
(*Source:* GK Pal)

19. Refractory period.

- Refractory period is the time period in which when a second stimulus is given, the membrane is unresponsive to the second stimulus
- The total refractory period has; the relative and absolute refractory periods
- Absolute refractory period: It is the period during the action potential (AP) when a second stimulus of any strength and duration when given does not produce another AP. In a nerve AP it corresponds to start of firing level to 1/3rd of repolarization is complete. It is because the voltage-gated sodium channels after getting inactivated at the peak has to go back to resting state to be opened again

- Relative refractory period: It is defined as the period after ARP after which application of a suprathreshold stimulus can produce an AP. In nerve AP it is after the end of ARP to the start of After-depolarization. The cause for RRP is that the stronger stimulus spreads to larger area of membrane to open up larger numbers of voltage-gated sodium channels resulting in AP.

20. Define terms: chronaxie, rheobase and utilization time.

Refer answers to 2004 paper (Short note 4).

21. Actions of insulin.

Metabolic Actions

- Insulin is needed for the carbohydrate, lipid and protein metabolisms. It is the hormone of abundance.
- It is essential for the utilzation of glucose by muscle, adipocytes, leukocytes etc.

Effect on Carbohydrate Metabolism

- It increases peripheral uptake of glucose by muscles and adipose tissue by inserting the glucose transporter GLUT 4 on their cell membrane
- It also enhances glucose utilization by stimulating glycolysis in muscle and liver and glycogenesis in the liver and muscle.
- It decreases glucose production by inhibiting gluconeogenesis and glycogenolysis.

Effect on Lipid Metabolism

Effects on liver:

- In liver, insulin favors storage of glucose as glycogen and when it reaches a level glucose is converted to fat in the liver
- It favors synthesis of cholesterol from acetyl-CoA
- It is anti-ketogenic, decreases entry of FFA into liver and favours ketone body utilization by peripheral tissues.

Effects on Adipose Tissue

- Favors deposition of fat in adipose tissue by stimulating lipoprotein lipase in capillary of adipose tissue
- In adipose tissue it inhibits hormone-sensitive lipase (HSL) and thereby supresses lipolysis

- **In muscle**, it inhibits lipolysis of triglycerides
- Insulin is needed for the utilization of LDL and VLDL and therefore their levels are elevated in diabetes mellitus.

Effects on Protein Metabolism

- It is an anabolic hormone
- It stimulates transport of amino acids into the cells
- It stimulates translation of mRNA and results in protein synthesis
- In liver, gluconeogenesis is inhibited and amino acids are used for protein synthesis
- Insulin inhibits protein metabolism

Effects on Ion Transport

- It increases transport of K^+, PO_4^{3-}, Mg^{2+} into skeletal muscles and also K^+ and PO_4^{3-} into the liver and renal tubules.
- It is an important hormone to decrease serum K^+ levels after food intake.

Effect on Growth and Development

- Anabolic action of insulin favors growth
- It is therefore needed for normal growth of the individual
- Children with insulin deficiency tend to have reduced muscle mass, bone mass and retarded growth.

22. Estrogen functions.

- Estrogen stimulates proliferation of endometrium in 1st half of menstrual cycle
- It feeds back to regulate LH secretion, positively in the 1st half and negatively in the 2nd half of menstrual cycle
- It makes the cervical mucus thin and watery, thereby permitting entry of sperm into female reproductive tract
- It increases size of ovaries and facilitates growth of follicle
- Induces changes in Fallopian tube and increases its motility. Increases the size of internal and external genitalia
- It increases the excitability of uterine myometrium and therefore peaks at the time of parturition
- Responsible for female behavior and development of secondary sexual characteristics
- Develops the ducts of mammary gland

- Lowers plasma cholesterol and rises HDL levels
- Causes fusion of epiphysis and stops the linear growth, both in males and females
- Has properties of retaining salt and water and responsible for pre-menstrual bloating sensation
- Prevents osteoporosis by inhibiting osteoclastic activity by inhibiting IL-1, 6 and TNF-α and stimulating TGFβ
- Inhibits the formation of Acne
- Makes the skin soft and vascular.

23. Aldosterone escape.

The actions of aldosterone are:
- Reabsorption of Na⁺ and Cl⁻ from collecting duct which is followed by water reabsorption
- It also causes secretion of K⁺ from collecting duct.

Aldosterone escape:
- When there is hyperaldosteronism, there is increased reabsorption of salt and water from the renal tubules
- This results in increased ECF volume followed by increase in blood pressure
- But this does not continue indefinitely
- When ECF volume has increased 10-15% above the normal, there is pressure diuresis and it limits further rise in ECF volume
- This phenomenon is called as **aldosterone escape**
- It is because of secretion of atrial natriuretic peptide (ANP) from the right atrium in response to increase in ECF volume → excretion of water and salt from the body. Therefore hyperaldosteronism is not associated with edema.

24. Functions of saliva.

Refer answers to 2003 paper.

25. Significance of erythrocyte sedimentation rate.

- ESR is increased in many diseases and therefore does not have any diagnostic value
- The normal value is 3-7 mm/hr in males and 5-9 mm/hr in females
- It is elevated in chronic inflammatory conditions
- It is used to assess the prognosis of a disease when the patient is getting treated.

26. Functions of corpus luteum.

Refer Answers to 2008 paper.

27. Blood-testis barrier.

Blood-testis barrier is formed by the bases of neighboring Sertoli cells close to the basal lamina of seminiferous tubule in testis.

The functions of the barrier are:
a. Prevents passage of large proteins from moving from interstitium to the tubular lumen or adluminal compartment
b. The fluid in the lumen of seminiferous tubule is rich in androgen, estrogen, glutamic and aspartic acids and maintenence of this composition is essential for spermatogenesis and it is maintained by the barrier
c. It protects the germ cells from noxious agents in circulation
d. Prevents entry of germ cell division products into the circulation and thereby prevents formation of autoimmune response
e. Maintains an osmotic gradient for movement of fluid into tubular lumen.

28. GAP junctions.

This is a type of intercellular connection.

There are intercellular connections for:
a. Holding the cells together and to the basement membrane
b. For communication between cells
- **Gap junctions** are the type of intercellular connections which allow passage of molecules and impulses between adjacent cells (refer Fig. 23)
- The junction is made up of channels from lateral aspects of the neighboring cells
- Each half of the channel from each cell is surrounded by 6 subunits of proteins—connexins
- The intercellular space is reduced here to 2-3 nm
- Gap junctions are present in the cardiac myocytes and they allow rapid spread of

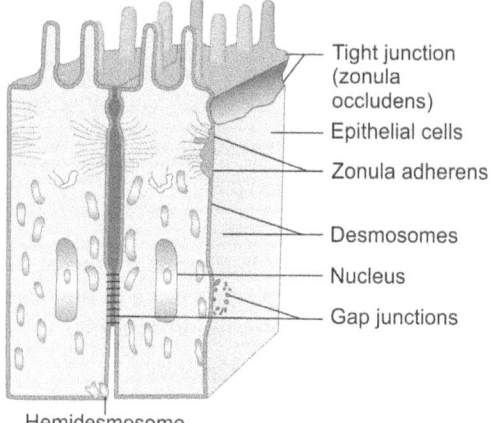

Fig. 23: Intercellular connections.
(*Source:* GK Pal)

action potentials from one cell to the other one.

29. Glomerular filtration rate.

GFR is defined as the rate at which the filtrate is formed in all the nephrons of both the kidneys per unit of time. The normal values are: 125 mL/min, 90–140 mL/min or 180L/day.

Factors affecting filtration are:

- Filtration co-efficient which is a product of permeability of filtration membrane and the surface area across which filtration happens
- Glomerular capillary hydrostatic pressure—directly proportional to GFR
- Glomerular oncotic pressure—inversely proportional to GFR
- Bowman's space hydrosatic pressure—inversely proportional to GFR
- Renal blood flow
- Afferent and efferent arteriolar resistance
- Sympathetic stimulation.

Measurement of GFR:

- It is done by measuring renal clearence of inulin and creatinine.

30. Dietary fiber.

- Dietary fibers include cellulose, hemicellulose, lignin etc.
- These substances when ingested are not digested due to lack of microorganisms for digesting them
- So they pass out without getting digested.

Functions of dietary fibers are:

- The undigested fibers when they are present in the colon they tend to hold water and increase the bulk of feaces and therefore can be **used for treating constipation**
- It **decreases the rate of absorption** of nutrients form intestines and thereby prevents sudden increase in blood glucose levels after food intake. Due to slow absorption of carbohydrates, insulin demand is also decreased. So it can be used as a **supplementary treatment in diabetes mellitus**
- It **decreases blood cholesterol levels** by excreting bile salts. Bile salts get trapped in the fiber and is excreted. The rate of formation of bile salts are increased and cholesterol is used for it. So it is used for **controlling hypercholesteremia**, obesity etc.
- It **prevents colon cancer** by diluting the carcinogens and minimizing their contact with the colon.

31. Wernicke's aphasia.

- Lesion in the sensory speech area - Wernicke's area (Area 22) (refer Fig. 24)
- It can happen due to blockage of vessels supplying the area or due to injury
- Also called as fluent aphasia
- Here the person is able to hear spoken words or identify written words
- But cannot comprehend spoken or written words
- Motor speech is intact. So speech is not disturbed. Person speaks excessively
- There is impairment of reply to written words as they are not able to comprehend written words also.

32. Acetylcholine.

- It is an acetyl ester of choline
- It is synthesized from choline and acetate
- Choline is an amine and is taken into the cholinergic neurons via transporters and also synthesized in the neurons
- Acetate is activated by coenzyme A

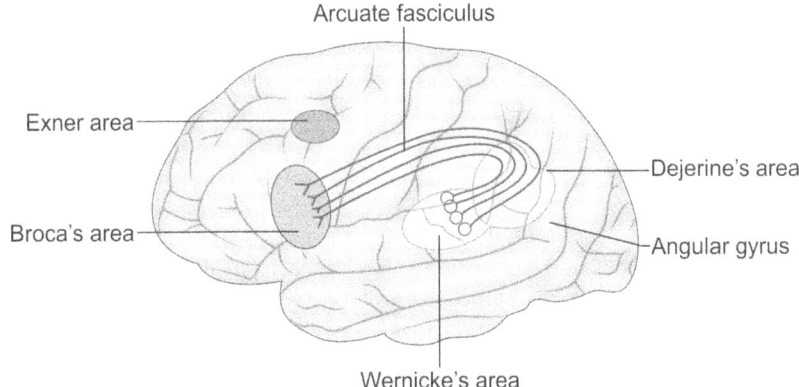

Fig. 24: Speech areas in the cerebral cortex.
(*Source:* GK Pal)

- The enzyme Choline acetyl transferase catalyzes the reaction between acetate and choline to form acetylcholine
- It happens in the nerve endings and following this acetylcholine (ACh) is stored inside the secretory vesicles
- ACh is released from—somatic motor nerve terminals in the neuromuscular junction (NMJ), postganglionic parasympathetic nerve terminals, preganglionic nerve terminals of sympathetic and parasympathetic nerves and in the CNS
- ACh receptors: There are two types of receptors:
  - Muscarinic receptors: Stimulated by muscarine. It is present on the smooth muscles and glands. They are blocked by the drug atropine. Muscarinic receptors are metabotropic and there are 5 subtypes—M1, M2, M3, M4 and M5
  - Nicotinic receptors: They are ionotropic receptors. These receptors are stimulated by nicotine and are present in the NMJ and the postganglionic neurons. There are two subtypes. These two types are blocked by different drugs. These receptors are made up of 5 subunits which surround a central pore and acts as a cation channel.
- **There are both muscarinic and nicotinic receptors present in the brain in large amounts.**

Removal of ACh:
- After the action of ACh is over it should be removed from the site of action to induce repolarization. It is by hydrolysis of ACh to choline and acetate by the enzyme Acetylcholinesterase. The enzyme is present in the synaptic cleft in large amounts.

33. Parkinson's disease.
Refer answers to 2005 paper.

34. Rapid–eye movement sleep.
- Sleep is said to be a state of altered consciousness or partial unconsciousness from which a person can be aroused
- Sleep deprivation results in impaired attention, learning and performance
- Sleep has two components—non-rapid eye movement (NREM) and rapid eye movement (REM) sleep.

REM Sleep
- In a period of sleep of 7–8 hrs, REM and NREM sleep phases alternate
- REM sleep occurs 3–5 times during the sleep period alternating with NREM sleep
- Initial episode of REM sleep will be lasting for 10–20 minutes. Then with each episode, it prolongs and the final episode is for 50 minutes
- In adults REM sleep totals for about 90 – 120 minutes. With increasing age, period of REM sleep decreases

- 50% of an infants' sleep is REM sleep. 35% for 2 year old infant and 25% for adults
- REM sleep is thought to be important for maturation of brain in infants. This has been identified by the high percentage of REM sleep in infants.

Physiological Changes in REM Sleep

- Most of the dreaming occurs in REM sleep. These dreams can be remembered
- Eyes move rapidly back and forth under the eyelid
- Neuronal activities are higher—brain blood flow and O_2 use is high
- EEG recordings are similar to that of an active and awake person
- Excepting the motor neurons governing respiration and eye, impulses in most of them are inhibited
- Inhibition of motor neurons results in loss of muscle tone and even some time paralysis
- Parasympathetic activity increases and sympathetic activity decreases → decrease in HR and BP
- Periodically sympathetic activity is also increased
- Bruxism, erection of penis and twitching of facial muscles are seen in REM sleep.

Control of REM Sleep

- NREM and REM sleep are mediated by different parts of the brain
- REM sleep: Neurons in pons and mid brain.

35. Anti-G suit.

- Effect of gravity on circulatory system is multiplied during acceleration or deceleration
- The gravitational force acting on the body during acceleration is expressed in 'g' units
- 1 'g' is force of gravity on the body on earth's surface
- Positive 'g' is force acting on long axis of the body from head to foot and blood is thrown into the lower parts of the body
- Negative 'g' is the forces acting in the opposite direction
- In positive 'g', arterial pressure in the head is reduced but as the intracranial and venous pressures are also reduced there is not much compensation of cerebral blood flow
- But when the force exceeds 5 'g' there is failure of vision and 'black out' happens. It can be prevented by using the antigravity 'g' suit.
- It is a double-walled pressure suit containing water or compressed air
- It compresses on the abdomen and legs with a force proportionate to the positive 'g'
- This decreases venous pooling and enhances venous return.

36. Clinical significance of electroencephalogram.

- Used to study normal functions of brain
- To study the changes in brain activity during sleep
- To diagnose various brain disorders like epilepsy, tumors, sites of trauma, degenerative diseases.

37. Chloride shift.

Refer answers to 2005 paper.

38. Jugular venous pulse.

JVP tracing is recorded from internal jugular vein. It reflects the pressure changes in the right atrium as there are no valves in this vein and therefore any pressure change in right atrium is reflected to this vein.

The JVP tracing has three positive waves and two negative waves (refer Fig. 25).

They are:

- 'a' wave—due to atrial contraction

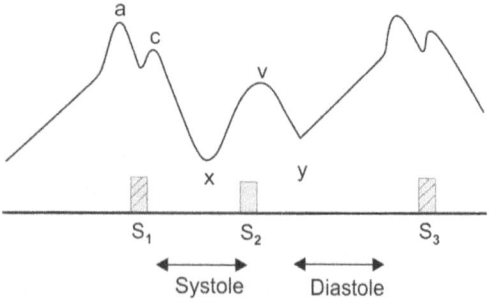

Fig. 25: Jugular venous pulse; a, c and v are positive waves, x and y are negative waves.
(*Source:* GK Pal)

- 'c' wave—due to bulging of tricuspid valve into right atrium during onset of ventricular systole
- 'v'—due to atrial filling
- 'x' descent—fall in atrial pressure due to its relaxation
- 'y' descent—due to emptying of blood from right atrium to right ventricle.

Conditions Altering JVP

- **Increased JVP:**
  - Right heart failure
  - Superior vena caval obstruction
  - Congestive cardiac failure
  - Constrictive pericarditis.
- **Prominent 'a' wave:**
  - Pulmonary stenosis
  - Pulmonary hypertension
  - Tricuspid stenosis.
- **Canon wave or giant 'a' wave:** Right atrium contracts with closed tricuspid valve
  - Complete heart block.

39. Contents of middle ear.

Refer answers to 2005 paper.

40. Functions of placenta.

I. Hormone secretion
II. Transport of substance between mother and child
III. Protection of fetus.

Placental Transport

- Placental transport occurs through—simple diffusion, active transport and endocytosis
- Gases, water and electrolytes cross the placenta by diffusion
- Amino acids are transported by carrier mediated secondary active transport
- Glucose is transported by carrier mediated facilitated diffusion.

Hormonal Functions of Placenta

- Placenta secretes:
  - Human chorionic gonadotrophin (hCG)
  - Human chorionic somatomammotrophin (hCS)
  - Progesterone
  - Estrogen
  - Corticotrophin releasing hormone (CRH)
  - Gonadotrophin releasing hormone (GnRH)
  - Prolactin.

MBBS Examination 2010

ANSWER ALL QUESTIONS

I. Essay questions (15 Marks each)

1. Describe the enteric and colonic movements. Discuss the role of the enteric nervous system. Add a note on defecation.
2. How did Hans Selye, group the adrenocortical hormones? Elucidate their physiological functions.
3. What are the types of muscular exercise? Discuss the various physiological changes occurring during and after exercise.
4. Elucidate how pressure vibrations in the air are perceived as sound.
5. Name the different blood group systems. Mention the importance of blood groups. Explain the procedure for determining the blood group of an individual. Give the basis and principles of treatment of erythroblastosis fetalis.
6. Name any four hormones producing hyperglycemia. Explain the actions of the chief hypoglycemic hormone on liver, skeletal muscle and adipose tissue. Briefly explain GTT. Add a note on diabetes mellitus and physiological basis of its treatment.
7. Discuss the short-term and long-term regulation of arterial blood pressure. Add a note on neurogenic hypertension.
8. With the help of a diagram, describe the auditory pathway. Add a note on conduction deafness.

II. Short notes (5 Marks each)

1. Cells in fibrous tissue, their functions.
2. Functional categorization of plasma proteins.
3. Starling forces and edema.
4. Digestive proteases.
5. Transporters of amino acids in gut and kidneys.
6. Counter current in juxtamedullary nephrons.
7. Abnormalities of micturition.
8. Actions of parathormone.
9. Neurohumoral reflexes.
10. Immunological test for pregnancy.
11. Kirchhoff's law and Einthoven's law.
12. Excitation contraction coupling in cardiac muscle.
13. Triple response in skin.
14. Physiological dead space.
15. Dysbarism.
16. Causes of muscle tone.
17. Function of paleostriatum.
18. Climbing, mossy and parallel fibres.
19. Control of appetite.
20. Induction of sleep.
21. Describe the phases of gastric juice secretion.
22. Micelle formation.
23. Describe cystometrogram.
24. Functions of Sertoli cells.
25. Functions of placenta.
26. Plasma proteins.
27. Hepatic and gallbladder bile.
28. Deglutition.
29. Differences between cretinism and dwarfism.
30. Explain the hormonal regulation of menstrual cycle.
31. Theories of hearing.
32. Anterior spinothalamic tract.

33. Postural reflexes.
34. Aqueous humor.
35. Taste pathway.
36. Cerebral circulation.
37. Color vision.
38. CO_2 transport.
39. Chemoreceptors.
40. Endothelins.

III. Short answers (2 Marks each)

1. Measurement of total body water.
2. Lipids in cell membrane.
3. Remodelling of bone tissue.
4. Landsteiner's laws.
5. Fibrinolysis.
6. Lingual lipase.
7. Limiting pH of urine.
8. Leptin.
9. Mullerian regression factor.
10. Composition of semen.
11. Tracing of arterial pulse.
12. Reynold's number.
13. Preload and afterload in the heart.
14. Sneezing reflex.
15. Denervation hypersensitivity.
16. Reciprocal inhibition.
17. Consolidation of memory.
18. Formation of cerebrospinal fluid.
19. Gustatory receptors.
20. Dark adaptation.
21. Phagocytosis.
22. Role of sweat glands in thermoregulation.
23. 'B' lymphocytes in immunity.
24. ESR and its clinical significance.
25. Fetoplacental unit.
26. Actions of relaxin and inhibins.
27. Endogenous pyrogens.
28. Defecation reflex.
29. PAH clearance.
30. Brown fat tissue.
31. Broca's area.
32. Spinal animal.
33. Scuba diving.
34. Cardiac Index.
35. Bohr's effect.
36. Inverse stretch reflex.
37. Respiratory distress syndrome.
38. Thalamic syndrome.
39. Unipolar limb leads.
40. Astigmatism.

I. ESSAY QUESTIONS

1. Describe the enteric and colonic movements. Discuss the role of the enteric nervous system. Add a note on defecation.

Movements of the Small Intestines

Refer answers to 2004 paper.

Movements of the Large Intestine

1. Haustral contractions
2. Peristalsis
3. Mass movement.

Haustral Contractions

- This is similar to the segmentation contraction of the small intestines
- Here the circular muscles contract and form a ring like contractions and the taenia coli contract and make the neighboring area to relax
- This type of contractions helps to mix the contents of the colon and exposes the content to absorptive surface for absorption.

Peristalsis

Similar to small intestines peristalsis helps in moving the contents forward

Mass Movements

- This is a type of peristalsis occuring only in the colon
- It occurs 3 to 4 times a day, usually after the meals and lasts for 3 minutes
- Here, one whole segment of the colon contracts tonically and pushes the contents into the next segment
- They also push the fecal matter into the rectum distending it
- The distension initiates defeacation reflex
- Mass movements are stimulated by - Distension of rectum, gastro-colic reflex and stimulation of parasympathetic nerves.

Functions of Large Intestinal Movements

- Excretion of feces
- Effective absorption of water and electrolytes.

Defecation Reflex

- Defecation is the process of expulsion of faecal matter from the rectum
- It is a reflex response and is also under voluntary control (refer Fig. 1)
- The center for this reflex is the S3 segement of spinal cord which is inturn influenced by higher centers
- Parasympathetic nerves stimulate defecation.

Sphincters of the Anus

- There are internal and external anal sphincters
- Internal sphincter is thickened smooth muscles of the anus and external sphincter is made of skeletal muscles and therefore under voluntary control

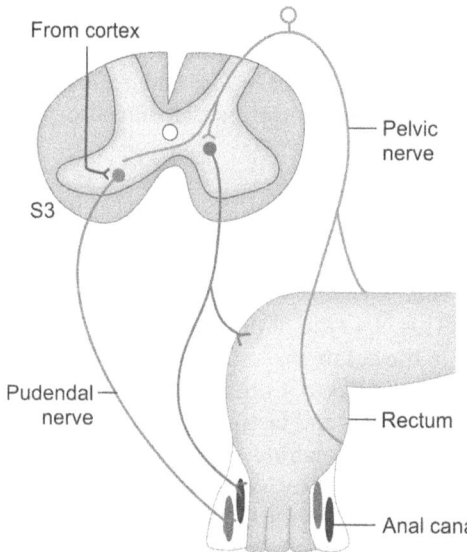

Fig. 1: Defecation reflex. Sensory fibers (Pink lines) Sense stretch of rectal wall due to its filling is sent to sacral segment S3 by pelvic nerves and efferents (Green lines) come through pelvic nerves to rectum and internal anal sphincter. In voluntary defecation, External sphincter is inhibited through pudendal nerve.
(*Source:* GK Pal)

- The internal sphincter is supplied by sympathetic and parasympathetic nerves and external sphincter is supplied by somatic motor nerves – Pudendal nerve.

Reflex

- The reflex is initiated as the rectum is distended and as the distension happens, there is increase in intrarectal pressure. The urge to defaecate is stimulated when the pressure rises to 18 mm Hg
- **Receptors:** The stretch receptors located on the rectal walls sense the stretch of rectum due to its distension with fecal matter
- **Afferents:** The pelvic nerves from the rectal wall carry the information to S3 spinal segment
- **Center for integration:** S3 spinal segment
- **Efferents:** From S3 segments efferents come out through pelvic nerves and reach the internal sphincter and via pudendal nerves reach the external sphincter
- As the rectal pressure increases, the pelvic nerve to internal sphincter is inhibited and the sphincter relaxes
- But as the pressure rises the pudendal nerve impulses are increased and the tonic external sphincter is made to contract strongly.

Higher center control is from the cortex and it controls the spinal cord via corticospinal tracts.

Distension of rectum with feces
↓
Transmission of impulses through pelvic nerves to S3 segment
↓
Parasymapthetic nerve stimulation
↓
Further intense peristaltic contraction of rectum
↓
Further rise in intra-rectal pressure
↓
On reaching a pressure >55 mm Hg
↓

Further relaxation of internal and external sphincters
↓
Voluntary control based on favorability of situation either causes defecation to occur or not

- If situations are **not favorable** the external sphincter becomes more tonically contracted due to impulses from higher centers through pudendal nerves and after some time the internal sphincters also close and the rectum relaxes and accommodates the feces
- If situations are **favorable** the internal and external sphincters relax and the anterior abdominal wall muscles contract and the muscles of rectum contract forcibly to expel the feces.

Role of Enteric Nervous System in Intestinal Motility

- GIT is innervated by autonomic nerves and the enteric nervous sytem
- Sympathetic nerves arise from prevertebral and paravertebral ganglia. It is usually inhibitory to GIT and inhibits motor activity and secretions
- Parasympathetic (PS) supply is by the vagus nerve and is stimulatory to the GIT. It increases motility and secretions. But PS nerves inhibit the sphincters and thereby relax it and favours emptying.

Enteric Nervous System

- This is the intrinsic nervous system of the GIT; it includes neurons and nerve fibers
- There are two plexuses – Submucosal or Meissner's plexus and Myentric or Auerbach's plexus. Meissner's plexus regulates secretory functions of GIT and Myentric plexus regulates motility of GIT
- Submucosal plexus lies between submucosal and circular muscle layer and myentric plexus is between circular and longitudinal muscle layers of the wall of GIT (refer Fig. 2)
- They are connected with the extrinsic nerves and function as interneurons
- These neurons can regulate GI motility and their actions can be modified by the extrinsic nerves
- The sympathetic and parasympathetic nerves project to both the plexuses
- The vagus nerve which is cholinergic terminates on intrinsic nerve plexuses and stimulates secretion and motility
- Sympathetic nerves which are noradrenergic they terminate on the intrinsic neurons and thereby inhibits secretions and motility.

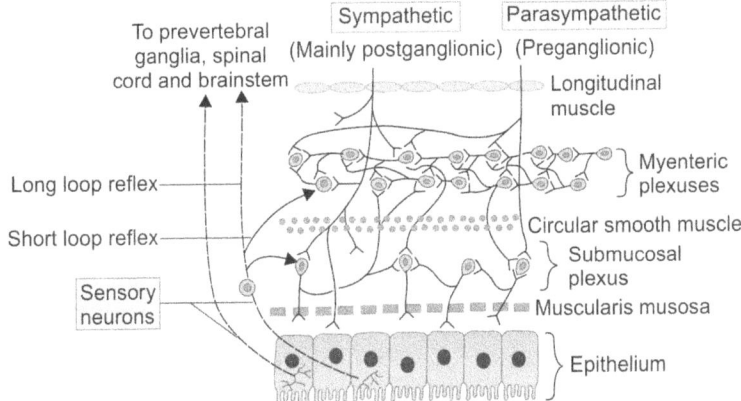

Fig. 2: Enteric nervous system; submucosal plexus is present between mucosa and circular muscle layers. Myentric plexus is present between circular and longutidanal layers.
(*Source:* GK Pal)

2. How did Hans Selye, group the adrenocortical hormones? Elucidate their physiological functions.

Hans Selye grouped the adrenocortical hormones based on their chemical structure and number of carbons – 21, 19 and 18 carbon structures. C 21 steroids are Glucocorticoids and mineralocorticoids. C19 steroids are adrenal sex steroids.

Physiological Functions of Glucocorticoids

Refer answers to 2004 paper.

Actions of Mineralocorticoids

Mineralocorticoid, as the name implies acts on reabsorption of Sodium and secretion of Potassium ions by acting on the nephrons. Aldosterone acts on the Principle (P) cells in the collecting ducts.

Reabsorption of Na⁺

- Aldosterone acts on P cells and inserts EnaC (Epithelial sodium channels) on the luminal side of P cells and stimulates reabsorption of Na⁺ ions
- It also stimulates the Na⁺-K⁺ ATPase on basolateral side and creates a gradient for Na⁺ reabsorption.

Secretion of K⁺ and H⁺

- K⁺ secertion happens in exchange for Na⁺ reabsorption. K⁺ and H⁺ compete with each other for secretion in exchange for Na⁺ reabsorption
- K⁺ and H⁺ secertion is also affected by the acid-base levels in the body
- Reabsorption of Na⁺ is associated with reabsorption of water and therefore aldosterone regulates ECF volume and thereby blood pressure.

Actions of Adrenal Androgens

- Adrenal androgens are—dehydroepiandrosterone and androstenedione
- They are anabolic in nature and promote protein synthesis
- They induce masculanizing effect when the levels are excess
- They induce pubic and axillary hair growth in females at time of puberty—**adrenarche**
- The adrenal androgens induce growth.
- They are the source of estrogens in post-menopausal women.

3. What are the types of muscular exercise? Discuss the various physiological changes occurring during and after exercise.

Types of exercises are based on the types of muscle contraction. They are classified as isotonic and isometric exercises.

Isometric Exercise

- In this type of exercise, the muscle length remains the same and the force generated is increased
- Since no shortening of muscle happens there is no work being done
- Examples are—pushing against the wall and holding the weight as in weight lifting.

Isotonic Exercise

- In this type of exercise there is shortening of muscle fiber and therefore external work is done
- Here tension in the muscle remains the same and length of the muscle shortens
- Examples are—walking, running, jogging etc.

Physiological Changes During Exercise

- Exercise is a type of stress to the body and therefore there are many physiological changes happening in the body to face this stress
- The changes are happening to provide additional amount of energy needed for the exercising muscle and to remove waste metabolites put out by the working muscles
- So bodily changes happen at the level of O_2 uptake, cardiovascular changes, respiratory changes and changes in the muscles and other tissues.

O_2 Uptake

- Normal O_2 uptake at rest is 250 mL/min. It can increase to 3L/min during exercise

- So it is given as the maximum amount of O_2 consumed by an individual during exercise or VO_2max
- VO_2max is the product of maximal cardiac output and maximal O_2 extraction by the tissues
- VO_2max improves with training. In a sedantary individual it is around 3L/min and in athelets it is upto 5L/min
- There is a linear increase in O_2 uptake in the initial phases of exercise and it reaches the VO_2max. But as the severity of exercise increases and as the VO_2max is reached, there is no further increse in O_2 uptake
- So the excess energy requirement is dealt by utilisation of anerobic glycolytic pathway of metabolism and also break down of creatinine phosphate for energy
- This results in production of lactic acid and the blood pH decreases resulting in hyperventilation. This further limits the production of lactic acid
- Increase in O_2 uptake continues to be increased even after termination of exercise and the extra O_2 consumed, is used to repay the O_2 debt
- This O_2 debt is used to remove the lactic acid, replenish ATP stores and phosphoryl creatine and the O_2 store in myoglobin.

Changes in the Respiratory System

- Changes happening in RS during exercise is to supply the extra amount of O_2 needed by the muscles and to remove the extra CO_2 put out by the working muscles
- Hyperventilation during exercise helps to achieve this demand and also to maintain pO_2 and pCO_2 at normal levels in arterial blood.

Increased Ventilation During Exercise

- Increase in ventilation matches the energy requirement of working muscles
- Increase in ventilation is by increasing the depth and rate of respiration
- Normal rate of respiration is 12–18 cycles /min and the depth of respiration is assessed by the tidal volume and it is 500ml at rest. So the minute ventilation is around 6L/min
- During exercise, tidal volume and rate increases, initially both are increased and once TV reaches its saturation, further increase is by increasing the rate of respiration. It can be increased to 80 – 100 L/min
- The **pattern of increase in ventilation** is by an abrupt increase in the beginning followed by a small pause then a gradual increase and after stopping the exercise there is an abrupt decrease in ventilation followed by a gradual decline to baseline level
- The initial abrupt increase is due to psychic stimuli from the cortex followed by neural stimuli arising from the proprioceptors in muscles, joints and tendons
- The gradual increase in ventilation is due to the chemical changes happening in the PO_2, PCO_2 levels and pH in arterial blood
- Arterial PO_2 and PCO_2 levels remain the same, even in severe exercise, but the stimulation of chemoreceptors happen because of increase in sensitivity of the chemorecptors for the normal fluctuations in the levels of PO_2 and PCO_2
- The other important mechanism by which ventilation increases is due to increase in body temperature
- Increase in plasma K^+ levels in blood following its release from the exercising muscles, also stimulates respiration.

Increase in O_2 Uptake

O_2 uptake increases following exercise from 250 mL/min to 4000 mL/min.

This is happening because of:

a. **Increased blood flow to lungs** as the cardiac output increases, due to increase in heart rate and stroke volume
b. **Increase in PO_2 gradient** between the alveolus and pulmonary arterial blood. Exercising muscles extract more O_2 from arterial blood and therefore the venous blood reaching the pulmonary artery has low PO_2. This increases the gradient for O_2 movement
c. **Increase in diffusion capacity** of the respiratory membrane. Most of the

pulmonary capillaries remain closed in resting states. During exercise these capillaries also open up and therefore the surface area across which exchange happens increases.

Changes in the Cardiovascular System

Changes in the CVS happen to supply the extra O_2 needed by the exercising muscles.

This happens by:

- Increase in heart rate, increase in cardiac output, increase in blood flow to skeletal muscles, decreased blood flow to other organs
- The cardiovascular change during exercise depends on the type of exercise being performed.

Isometric Exercise

There is a prompt increase in heart rate (HR) on the start of exercise.

Causes for increase in HR

- HR rises even before starting the exercise due to psychic stimuli
- The increase is mainly due to decreased vagal tone and increase in sympathetic discharge to the heart
- Impulses from joints and muscles increase HR and rise in body temperature also increases HR
- Release of catecholamines from adrenal medulla also increases HR
- The maximum increase in HR is a good indicator of fitness and it is based on the basal heart rate
- The target heart rate achieved during exercise in the adults is 195/min and in children it is 200/min and above. With advancing age it declines.

Changes in BP

- There is an increase in systolic and diastolic blood pressure following isometric exercise
- Systolic pressure increases due to increase in HR
- Diastolic pressure increases due to compression of the blood vessels by the contracting muscles
- There is not much change in stroke volume
- Blood flow to the steadily contracting muscle is decreased.

Isotonic Exercise

There is increase in HR and the causes are the same as the above.

Changes in BP

- Systolic BP rises moderately
- Diastolic BP remains same or decreases as the peripheral resistance decreases
- Peripheral resistance decreases due to vasodilatation
- Vasodilatation is due the vasodilator metabolites ($\uparrow PCO_2$, $\downarrow PO_2$, Lactate, adenosine etc) produced by the working muscle
- Stroke volume is increased.

Changes in Cardiac Output

- Cardiac output (CO) increases to supply the extra demand faced by the body
- It decides the O_2 delivery to the tissues and rise in cardiac output is the rate limiting step for O_2 extraction
- CO increases from 5L/min at rest to 25L/min during exercise
- CO increase is due to both, increase in HR and Stroke volume
- Increase in stroke volume is due to - Increase in myocardial contractility following sympathetic stimulation and increase in EDV due to activation of skeletal muscle pump, thaoracic pump and abdominal pump.

Skeletal Muscle Blood Flow

The blood flow to the exercising muscles increases 30 times from the baseline value. At rest the muscle blood flow is 2-4 mL/100 g/min.

The causes for increase in muscle blood flow:

- The increase happens even before start of exercise due to a neural mechanism. It involves the sympathetic cholinergic system
- This is followed by the local mechanisms. As the exercise progresses the working

muscle put out vasodilator metabolites—$\downarrow PO_2$, $\uparrow PCO_2$, $\uparrow K^+$, lactate etc. These chemicals dilate the blood vessels
- The heat generated by the contracting muscles increases the blood flow by dilating the vessels.

O2 extraction by the muscles is also increased as the metabolites and increased body temperature and 2, 3, DPG levels shift the O_2-Hb dissociation curve to the right and thereby liberates O_2 to the muscles.

Redistribution of Blood Flow

- As the blood flow to exercising muscles increase, there is a compromise in blood flow to certain organs and increased blood flow to other organs
- So the redistribution also contributes to the increase in skeletal muscle flow along with the increased cardiac output.

Redistribution

- Blood flow to the visceral organs is decreased
- Blood flow to skin is also decreased initially but as the exercise progresses, the rise in body temperature causes vasodilataion and increased blood flow to skin helps in losing the body heat
- Cerebral blood flow is maintained
- Coronary blood flow increases by neural and local mechanisms
- Blood flow to adipose tissues increase to mobilize fatty acids.

---

4. Elucidate how pressure vibrations in the air are perceived as sound.

Sound waves are produced by vibrating objects. Each wave consists of an alternating compression and rarefaction of the molecules in the media it travels.

Mechanism of Hearing is Discussed Under the Following Headings

- Properties of sound waves
- Conduction of sound waves
- Transduction of sound energy
- Transmission of impulses to brain
- Perception of sounds.

Poperties of Sound Waves

Pitch of Sound

- It is the frequency of sound and is given as number of waves per second. The unit is in Hertz (Hz)
- Human ear can respond to 20–20,000 Hz, but is sensitive within the range of 1000–3000 Hz
- The pitch of an average male voice is 125 Hz and a female voice is 250 Hz
- Human ear auditory apparatus can distinguish about 2000 pitches.

Intensity of Sound

- Intensity or loudness of sound is the amplitude of the sound wave
- The unit is in decibels
- A decibel is 1/10 of a bel and is the least change in intensity which can be detected.
- Decibel is a log scale. 0 decibel is the minimum audible sound.

Pure Tone

Single frequency sound is called the pure tone.

Conduction of Sound Waves

Sound waves travel in the air medium and enter the external ear, travel through the middle ear and reach the inner ear.

Conduction in External Ear

- External ear consists of the pinna and the external auditory meatus
- Pinna collects the sound waves and passes it to the external auditory meatus. It helps in identifying the source of sound
- The external auditory meatus funnels the sound towards the tympanic membrane at a high pressure
- When the sound waves strike the tympanic membrane it vibrates according to the frequency of the sound and stops promptly when the sound disappears. It is critically dampened.

Conduction in Middle Ear

- Middle ear has the 3 ossicles—malleus, incus and stapes
- The manubrium of malleus is attached to the umbo of tympanic membrane

- Head of malleus articulates with body of incus
- Long process of incus articulates with head of stapes
- The footplate of stapes is attached to oval window
- As the sound waves hit the tympanic membrane, it vibrates and the vibration is transmitted to the ossicles and they vibrate as a single unit (refer Fig. 3)
- The sound waves have been travelling in the air media and when they reach the inner ear it is transmitted to a fluid medium. This results in loss of sound energy by 30 dB
- This is prevented by the **impedence matching** mechanism in the middle ear
- Impedence matching is done by the differences in surface area of the tympanic membrane and the membrane covering the oval window
- Tympanic membrane surface area is much greater than the surface area of membrane covering the oval window. This helps in concentrating sound in a smaller area and thus amplifying it
- Lever action of the ossicles also amplifies the sound. There is an overall increase in sound pressure by 28 folds.

Conduction in the Inner Ear

- The movement of the stapes vibrates the membrane covering the oval window
- This creates a spreading wave in the perilymph in scala vestibuli of the cochlea
- The wave is transmitted directly to perilymph in scla tympani
- As the wave moves up the cochlea it reaches a maximum height and then drops off
- The point in cochlea where it reaches a maximum height is dependent on the frequency of the sound detected
- High pitched waves reach a maximum near the base of cochlea and the low frequency waves reach a maximum near the apex
- The waves in the scala vestibuli cause the basilar membrane to vibrate
- The movement of the basilar membrane makes the organ of corti to move up and down

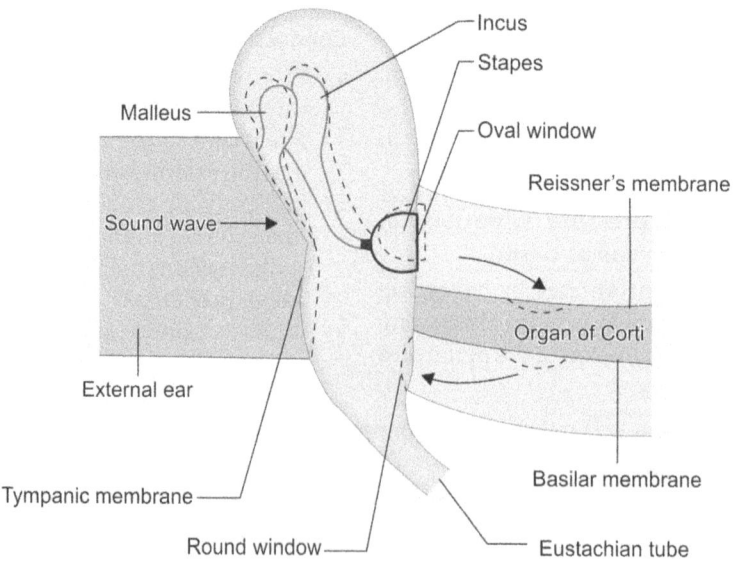

Fig. 3: Conduction of sound waves in the external, middle ear and internal ear. Dashed lines indicate the movement of structures following transmission of sound waves in the ear.
(*Source:* GK Pal)

- The tops of hair cells in organ of corti are held rigid by the reticular lamina and the hairs of outer hair cells are embedded in the tectorial membrane
- When the stapes moves due to sound transmission both membranes move in the same direction but they are hinged on different axes and this causes bending of the hairs
- The hairs of inner hair cells are not attached to tectorial membrane
- But it can be moved or bent by the fluid moving between the tectorial membrane and the hair cells.

Transduction of Sound Energy

- The hairs in the hair cells are arranged with taller hair in one end and smaller hairs in descending order
- The largest hair is the kinocilium and the smaller ones are the stereocilia
- When the smaller hairs bend towards the larger hairs there is depolarisation of the hair cells and when the movement is in the opposite direction there is hyperpolarisation of the cells (refer Fig. 4)
- When the movement of basilar membrane moves the organ of corti upwards and this causes lateral bending of stereocilia which results in depolarisation
- This is due to opening of K^+ channels in the hair cells due to the pull provided by the tip link protein
- K^+ in the endolymph of scala media, the compartment in which the organ of Corti is placed, enters through the channel and depolarises the hair cells
- This result in release of the neurotransmitter, glutamate which stimulates the nerve fibers in the bases of hair cells and these nerves together form the cochlear branch of vestibulo-cochlear nerve
- Now the electrical impulse travels through the VIII cranial nerve to the higher centers
- These afferents arise from inner hair cells.

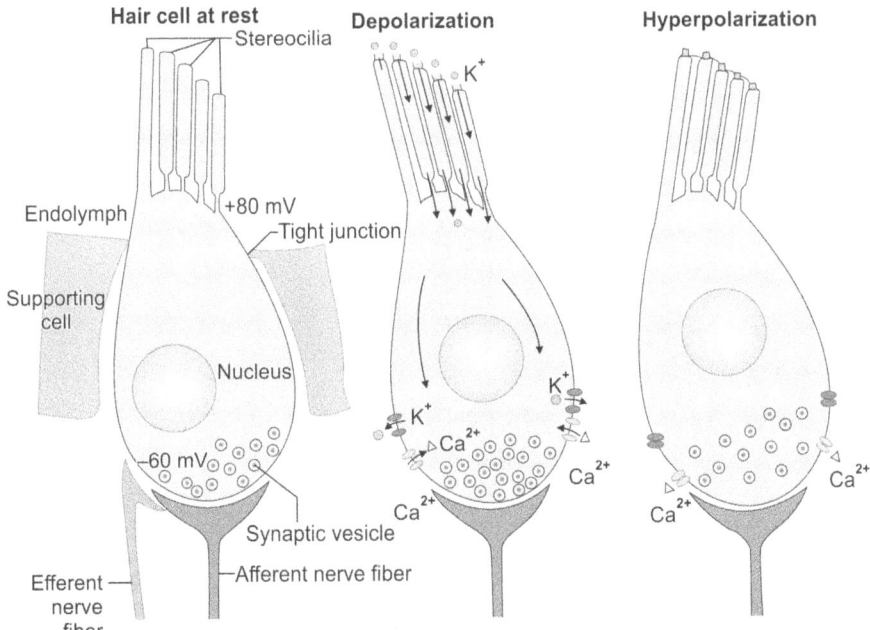

Fig. 4: Transduction of sound waves in the cochlear hair cells. Pressure waves move the basilar membrane; thereby hairs of the hair cells are bent. If the smaller hairs are bent towards kinocilium there is depolarisation of the cell and stimulation of nerves in the bases of the cells. If hairs are bent in the opposite direction it results in inhibition of impulse transmission. (*Source:* GK Pal)

Transmission of Impulses

The action potentials generated in the cochlear division of VIII cranial nerve travels in the following pathway (Fig. 5).

Organ of Corti
↓
Bipolar cells of spiral ganglion
↓
Cochlear nuclei (dorsal and ventral) in brainstem
↓
Superior olivary nuclei of both sides
↓
Lateral lemniscus (both sides)
↓
Inferior colliculus (both sides)
↓
Medial geniculate body in thalamus (both sides)
↓
Primary auditory cortex (Area 41) (both sides)
↓
Auditory association areas (Areas 42, 22) (both sides)

Perception of Sound and Encoding of Sound Signals

Encoding of sound signals are discussed under:

- Coding of pitch of sound
- Coding of intensity of sound
- Localization of sound.

Coding of Pitch of Sound

Discrimination of pitch (sound frequency) is done at the level of organ of Corti and in the auditory cortex.

Organ of Corti:

The pitch discrimination in the organ of Corti is explained by the place theory and the Volley theory.

Place theory:

- This theory holds good to explain in perception of pitches between 2000 and 20,000 Hz
- The waves generated by higher frequency sounds reach a maximum height in perilymph in the scala vestibuli near the oval window or close to the base of

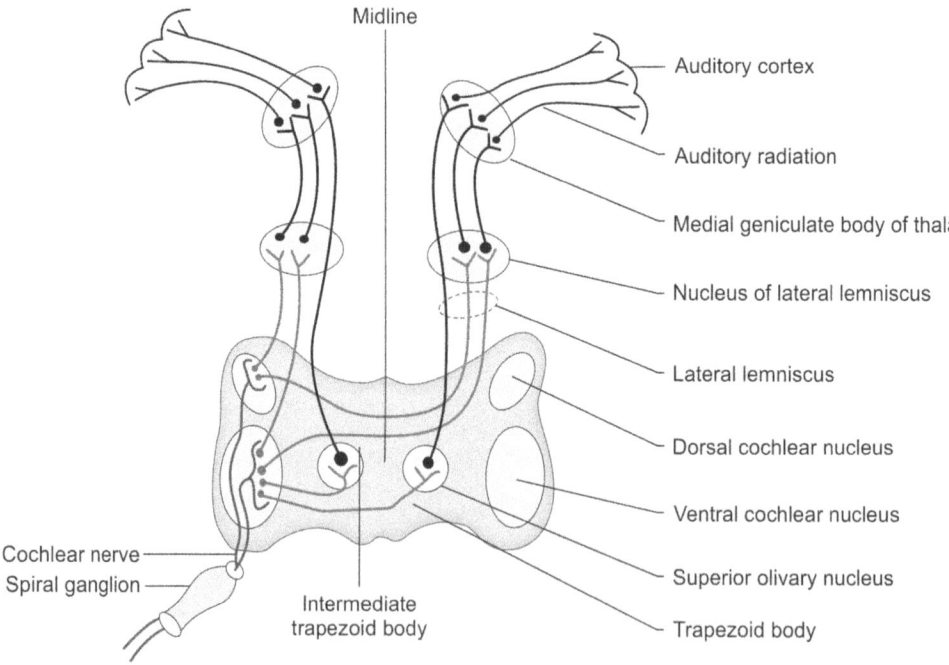

Fig. 5: Auditory pathway from right cochlea. There is bilateral route through brainstem and bilateral cortical representation.
(*Source:* Sembulingam)

the cochlea. This vibrates the basilar membrane of this region to a maximum and the hair cells present here are stimulated and send impulses through nerves arising from their bases (refer Fig. 6)
- Lower frequency sounds produce waves which reach a maximum height close to the heloctrema or apex of cochlea
- Therefore different hair cells respond to different frequencies of sound based on their location in the basilar membrane
- There are 30,000 fibers in the cochlear nerve and each gets stimulated by a particular frequency of sound.

Frequency theory or Volley principle:
- This theory explains the coding of frequency of sound below 2000 Hz
- According to this theory same numbers of impulses are transmitted through the cochlear nerves as that of the frequency of sound waves
- The other factors affecting pitch are the loudness of sound and duration of exposure.

Auditory area:
- In the auditory cortex there is a point to point representation of the basilar membrane
- So different sound frequencies reach different points in the cortex and they are decoded as different frequency sounds.

Coding of Sound Intensity
- It occurs at the level of cochlear nerve
- The intensity of sound is coded by the frequency of impulses travelling through the nerve

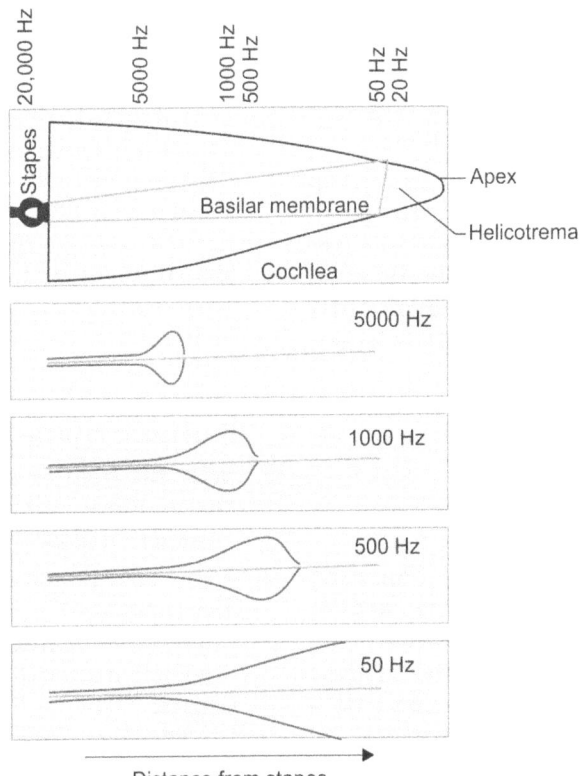

Fig. 6: Pitch discrimnation based on Place theory. Sound waves of various frequencies displace basilar membrane of organ of Corti at different sites; High frequency sound close to base of cochlea and low frequency waves close to the apex.
(*Source:* GK Pal)

- There is also increase in stimulation of number of nerve fibers
- As the intesity of sound increases the area of basilar membrane getting stimulated and the numbers of hair cells getting stimulated and thereby number of nerves getting stimulated are also increased.

Localization of Sound

- Sound localization is possible by the human ear even if the source of sound is seperated by 1°
- Localization of sound is a function of neurons above the level of brainstem
- It is possible because of the time lag in entry of sound between the two ears
- The other factor is the difference in intensity of sound in both the ears. Sound is louder in the side of the ear close to the source
- Pinna helps in collecting the sound and thereby helps in localization
- Superior olivary nucleus, inferior colliculi and the auditory cortex play a major role in localizing sound by latency difference as well as intensity difference. They have specialized neurons for these functions.

5. **Name the different blood group systems. Mention the importance of blood groups. Explain the procedure for determining the blood group of an individual. Give the basis and principles of treatment of erythroblastosis fetalis.**

Blood Groups

Refer answers to 2007 paper.

Erythroblastosis Fetalis

Refer answers to 2006 paper.

6. **Name any four hormones producing hyperglycemia. Explain the actions of the chief hypoglycemic hormone on liver, skeletal muscle and adipose tissue. Briefly explain GTT. Add a note on diabetes mellitus and physiological basis of its treatment.**

Hormones Producing Hyperglycemia

- Adrenaline
- Glucocorticoids
- Thyroxine
- Growth hormone.

The chief hypoglycemic hormone is insulin.

Actions of Insulin

Refer answers in 2007 paper.

7. **Discuss the short-term and long-term regulation of arterial blood pressure. Add a note on neurogenic hypertension.**

Short-term Regulation and Long-term Regulation of BP

Refer answers to 2006 paper.

Neurogenic Hypertension

- These are done experimentally to demonstrate the role of baroreceptors in regulating blood pressure
- Bilateral clamping of the carotid arteries proximal to carotid sinuses results in increase in BP
- Similar changes are seen when the carotid sinus nerves (IXth cranial nerve) on each side are cut
- The rise is not too high as the aortic sinuses are still functioning
- If the vagus nerve from the aortic sinus is also cut it results in rapid rise in BP even upto 300/200 mm Hg
- Similar results are seen when the nucleus tractus solitarius (NTS) in medulla is bilaterally damaged. This can even be fatal
- These forms of hypertension are said to be neurogenic hypertension.

8. **With the help of a diagram, describe the auditory pathway. Add a note on conduction deafness.**

Refer answer to question number 4 and Figure 5 of this paper.

Conductive deafness: Impaired sound transmission in external or middle ear.
- Causes:
    i. Plugging of external auditory canal by wax or foreign body
    ii. Destruction of ossicles
    iii. Thickening of ear drum
    iv. Perforation of tympanic membrane
    v. Rigidity of attachment of stapes

vi. Otitis media
vii. Eustachian tube obstruction.

Tests for Hearing

Watch test: Watch is brought close to the ear and the patient is noted to tell when he/she is able to hear the ticking sound. Compare the distance at which it is heard with that of the examiner.

Tuning Fork Tests

- These tests are done with tuning forks of 256 and 512 Hz
- They are used to distinguish between conduction and sensorineural deafness.

a. **Rinne's test:**
   - **Principle:** Air conduction is better than bone conduction
   - Here bone conduction is compared with air conduction
   - Base of the vibrating tuning fork is placed on the mastoid process on one side and the patient is asked to raise his hand when the sound disappears (sound is heard because the vibrations are transmitted via bone and are perceived as sound)
   - Then the vibrating fork is brought close to the auditory meatus and if he is still able to hear the sound then, AC is better than BC and it is Rinne's positive

   Observations:
   - In normal subjects, Rinne's test is positive (AC>BC)
   - In conductive deafness it is negative (BC>AC)
   - In neural deafness both are negative.

b. **Weber's test:**
   - Here the base of the vibrating tuning fork is placed on the glabella or the vertex
   - The subject normally hears equally on both sides
   - In conductive deafness, the sound is heard well in the defective side as the masking sounds are not heard
   - In neural deafness it is heard well on the normal side.

c. **Schwabach's test:**
   - The bone conduction of the subject is compared with the bone conduction of the examiner (presuming that the examiner's bone conduction is normal)
   - Base of the vibrating tuning fork is placed on a mastoid process and the subject is asked to say when he ceases to hear the sound
   - Then the examiner places it on his mastoid process
   - In normal condition both the subject and the examiner hears the sound for same duration
   - In conductive deafness, the subject hears for longer period as the masking effect is not there
   - In neural deafness the examiner hears it for longer duration.

Audiometry

- Here the audiometer is used to perform the test. Here pure tones of various frequencies are given and the subject's hearing ability is tested. It is done to detect conductive deafness. Air conduction is tested by using ear phones to hear sounds and for bone conduction a vibrator is placed on mastoid process. The subject is made to sit in a sound-proof room. Sounds of various frequencies are given and the minimum threshold for each frequency is plotted as a graph for each ear and the loss of hearing for individual frequencies can be identified.

II. SHORT NOTES

1. **Cells in fibrous tissue, their functions.**
- Fibrous tissue is a connective tissue. It contains large amount of collagen fibers, few cells and large matrix
- The fibers may be arranged regularly or in irregular pattern
- Irregular arrangement is seen in areas where there is stress and strain from all directions as that in the skin
- Regular arrangements are seen in the tendons and ligaments
- It contains the cells—fibroblasts
- Fibroblast is an immature connective tissue cell which has the capacity to produce any type of connective tissue

- It is motile and can undergo mitosis
- It lays down almost all of the fibers found in the connective tissue.

2. Functional categorization of plasma proteins.

- Normal plasma concentration is—6 to 8 g/100 mL
- Plasma proteins are categorized as Albumin (55%), Globulin (38%) and Fibrinogen (7%)
- They are classified based on their electrophoretic pattern.

Albumin

- Their levels are 4.8 g/dL
- Molecular weight is the least and is 69000
- They are synthesized in the liver
- They regulate plasma colloidal oncotic pressure
- It helps in transport of bilirubin, hormones, ions, fatty acids, metals etc.
- It also helps in regulating acid base balance.

Globulin

- Normal level is 2-3 g/dL
- Their molecular weight is 90000–156000
- There are—α, β and γ globulins with subtypes for each one
- There are different forms of globulins—glycoprotein, lipoprotein, transferrin, haptoglobins, ceruloplasmin and Immunoglobulins
- They act as transport proteins as in transferrin transports iron, ceruloplasmin copper, lipoproteins lipids etc.
- The immunoglobulins provide immunity
- The normal Albumin: Globulin ratio is 1.5–2.5:1 ratio.

Fibrinogen

- Normal value is 0.3 g/dL
- Their molecular weight is 500,000
- It has the highest molecular weight
- It helps in coagulation of blood and provides viscosity of blood
- There are other plasma proteins like prealbumin, prothrombin etc.
- There are nearly 100s of plasma proteins
- All the above proteins are amphoteric in nature since they have both the NH_2 and COOH groups, they act as buffers for both acids and bases.

3. Starling forces and edema.

- Filtration and absorption across the capillary wall happens due to the balance of forces acting across the wall
- The forces are—capillary hydrostatic pressure, capillary oncotic pressure, interstitial hydrostatic pressure and interstitial osmotic pressure
- These forces are called as the Starling's Forces (refer Fig. 7)
- According to the Starling's hypothesis the filtartion/absorption occurs as a result of net effect of all the above pressures.

Effective filtration pressure is given as:

$$K(P_c + \pi_i) - (P_i + \pi_c)$$

- K = Filtration co-efficient (permeability of capillary and surface area of filtration membrane)
- P_c = Hydrostatic pressure in the capillaries
- P_i = Hydrostatic pressure in interstitium
- π_c = Capillary oncotic pressure
- π_i = Interstitial osmotic pressure
- P_c is 37 mm Hg at the arteriolar end of the capillary and is 17 mm Hg at the venous end of the capillary
- Capillary oncotic pressure is 25 mm Hg
- These two forces are opposing to each other
- Hydrostatic forces push the fluid out of the capillaries and oncotic pressure (exerted by plasma proteins) draws the fluid into the capillaries
- At the arteriolar end, the hydrostatic pressure exceeds oncotic pressure and filtration happens here
- At the venous end, the oncotic pressure exceeds the hydrostatic pressure and therefore absorption of fluids and metabolites happen here
- The other two forces, the interstitial hydrostatic and osmotic pressures oppose each other. The interstitial hydrostatic pressure varies in different organs

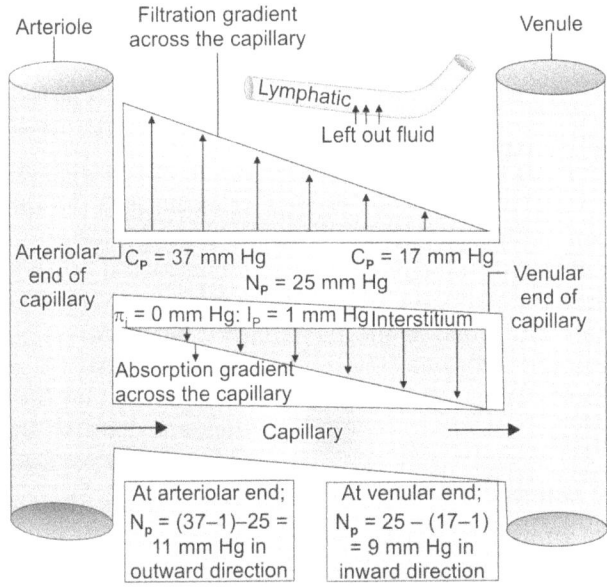

Fig. 7: Role of Starling's forces on filtration along the capillaries.
(C_p: Capillary hydrostatic pressure; π_p: Capillary osmotic pressure or oncotic pressure;
I_p: Interstitial hydrostatic pressure; π_i: Osmotic pressure in interstitium; N_p: Net filtration pressure)
(Source: GK Pal)

- In most subcutaneous tissues it is −2 mm Hg and it is positive in liver and kidneys and 6 mm Hg in the brain
- Pi, opposes the filtration of fluid from the capillaries, whereas the osmotic pressure in interstitium favors filtration
- But the presence of proteins in interstitium is almost negative and therefore πi is equal to 0
- Since the interstitial pressure differs in various organs the filtration and absorption differs in the organs
- In the glomerulus the hydrostatic pressure is high throughout the capillaries and so filtration happens all along and fluid moves into the capillaries all along the intestines.

Edema

It is the accumulation of abnormally large volumes of fluid in the interstitium.

Causes for Edema

a. **Incresed filtration pressure:**
   - Arteriolar dilation
   - Venous constriction
   - Increased venous pressure: Heart failure, venous obstruction, effect of gravity, increased ECF volume.
b. **Decreased osmotic gradient across vessel wall:**
   - Decreased plasma protein level
   - Accumulation of osmotically active substances like the metabolites in interstitium.
c. **Increased capillary permeability:**
   - By chemicals like histamine, kinins and substance P.
d. **Lymphatic obstruction**
   - **Lymph** is the fluid present in the lymphatic ducts
   - Normally across the capillaries, fluid efflux (in arteriolar end) is more than the fluid influx (in venous end)
   - The extra fluid which stays back in the interstitium cannot afford to be lost from circulation
   - This volume is returned back to the circulation through the lymphatic ducts which empty through the thoracic duct into the internal jugular vein

- The normal lymph flow is 2–4L/day
- If there is obstruction for the drainage of this fluid it retains in the interstitium and results in edema
- But the fluid is rich in proteins and long term retention leads to inflammation and fibrosis
- This leads to non-pitting edema
- Example for this type of edema is filariasis, where the parasites block the lymphatics and this result in accummulation of fluid especially in legs and scrotum—elephantiasis.

4. Digestive proteases.

Protein Digestion in Stomach

- The digestion of protein starts in the stomach by the action of the proteolytic enzyme—pepsin
- Pepsin is secreted in the inactive form, the pepsinogen and is activated by the low pH in the gastric lumen due to the presence of HCl
- There are two types of pepsinogens – Pepsinogen I secreted from fundus and body of stomach and Pepsinogen II from pylorus
- *Pepsins* hydrolyze the bonds between aromatic amino acids like phenylalanine and tyrosine and the second amino acids to form polypeptides of diverse nature.

Protein Digestion in Proximal Part of Small Intestione by Pancreatic Juice

- *Trypsin, chymotrypsin and elastases* act on the interior peptide bonds in the peptide molecules—they are called as *endopeptidases*
- The above enzymes are synthesized in the inactive forms like trypsinogen, chymotrypsinogen and proelastases
- The trypsinogen is activated by the intestinal enzyme Enterokinase. Activated trypsin further activates trypsinogen and all the other proteolytic enzymes
- *Carboxypeptidases A and B* hydrolyze the amino acids in the carboxyl and amino ends of polypeptides—so called as *exopeptidases*.

Protein Digestion by Intestinal Proteases in Later Part of Small Intestine

- Some of the digested amino acids are released into the intestinal lumen. But some peptides are further digested by the intestinal brush border peptidases—*aminopeptidases, carboxypeptidases, enteropeptidases and dipeptidases*
- Some undigested di and tripeptidases are transported into the enterocytes where they are digested into amino acids by *intracellular peptidases*.

5. Transporters of amino acids in gut and kidneys.

Transport of Amino Acids in the Gut

- Amino acid transport across the intestinal wall is essential for absorption of amino acids
- There are 7 transportes for amino acid absorption and 5 of them are Na^+ dependent and are similar to Na^+- glucose symport
- 2 of the above ones also require Cl^- as co-transport
- Out of the 7 transporters, 2 are Na^+ independent transporters
- Transport of di and tripeptides are through H^+ dependant rather than Na^+ dependant transporters
- The absorbed amino acids enter the enterocytes and are transported along the basolateral side of the cells through 5 transport systems and 3 of them are Na^+ dependant and 2 are not Na^+ dependant
- Most of the proteins are absorbed from the duodenum and jejunum
- 50% of absorbed protein is from food intake, 25% from digestive juices and 25% from the denuded enterocytes.

Transport of Amino Acids in the Kidneys

- Amino acids are transported in the renal tubules with the help of Na^+- amino acid symport

- This happens only in the proximal convoluted tubule (PCT)
- 100% of Glucose and amino acids are reabsorbed in the PCT by the secondary active transporter Na^+-glucose and Na^+-amino acid co-transporters in the luminal side of the epithelial cells
- From the basolateral surface these organic substance diffuse across the membrane and enter the interstitium.

6. Countercurrent in juxtamedullary nephrons.

Refer answers to 2004 question paper (Essay 1).

7. Abnormalities of micturition.

- The urinary bladder wall is made up of detrusor muscle and there are two sphincters—internal and external sphincters
- Internal sphincter is made of smooth muscle and external sphincter is made of skeletal muscles
- The bladder wall and internal sphincter is supplied by sympathetic and parasympathetic nerves and external sphincter is supplied by somatic motor nerve—pudendal nerve
- The bladder dysfunction usually arises from neural defects at different levels.

The types of bladder dysfunctions are:

a. Deafferentation of bladder: Damage to only afferents from bladder
b. Denervation of bladder: Damage to both afferents and efferents to bladder
c. Defects in spinal cord transection: Due to interruption of pathways from higher center controls to bladder.

a. **Deafferentation of bladder:**
   - Here there could be disease of the afferents from the bladder either due to diseases like Tabes dorsalis or transection of dorsal nerve root of sacral segment
   - The reflex contractions of the bladder are abolished and the bladder becomes distended, thin-walled and hypotonic
   - But some minute intrinsic contractions of the wall are still present.

b. **Denervation of bladder:**
   - The afferents and efferents may be damaged due to tumors of cauda equina or filum terminale
   - The bladder is distended and flaccid initially
   - But later the muscle gets active and acquires contraction waves which expels urine in the from of dribbling
   - Repeated contractions make the bladder wall hypertrophic and shrunken
   - The reason for hyperactivity may be due to denervation hypersensitivity.

c. **Defects of spinal cord transection:** The symptoms due to transection of spinal cord are given under three subheadings
   - Stage of spinal shock, Stage of recovery and stage of failure
   - In the stage of spinal shock the bladder is thin and distended and the reflexes are abolished. The bladder gets distended and above the limit there is overflow dribbling of urine (overflow dribbling)
   - After the spinal shock is relievd, the spinal reflexes without higher control comes into action. So as the bladder gets filled the reflex is initiated and urine is emptied
   - Patients can be trained to empty the bladder at intervals by mass reflex
   - The bladder may not be emptied completely resulting in repeated infections of the bladder and hypertrophy of bladder wall happens resulting in shrunken bladder. This further reduces the capacity of the bladder—spastic neurogenic bladder.

8. Actions of parathormone.

- Parathormone is secreted by the chief cells in the parathyroid glands
- It is a polypeptide hormone with 84 amino acid chains
- It is the most important hormone to increase the blood calcium levels.

Refer 2008 answers.

9. Neurohumoral reflexes.

Refer answers to 2004 paper.

10. Immunological test for pregnancy.

- Presence of hCG in the urine or blood of the pregnant female is the basis for pregnancy tests. Immunological tests are based on the antigenic property of hCG. It can be done using Latex particles coated with hCG (Latex agglutination test) or RBCs of sheep blood coated with hCG (hemagglutination test)
- Antisera for hCG is commercially available.

I. Hemagglutination Test

a. If the female is not pregnant: The urine sample of the female is taken and mixed with hCG antisera, since there are no antigens the antibodies are still present and now if either the hCG coated latex particles or sheep RBCs are added there will be agglutination of latex/RBCs. So presence of agglutination indicates absence of pregnancy

b. If the female is pregnant: The urine sample of pregnant female is mixed with hCG antisera, the antigens are neutralized by antibodies, now if the latex particles/Sheep RBCs are added there will be no agglutination since the antibodies are used up by the antigens.

II. One Step Immunoassay Test (Strip Test)

The hCG antibody is mixed with a dye and is impregnated on a strip of paper. When the strip comes in contact with the urine containing hCG, a pink-purple band appears, indicating pregnancy.

III. Enzyme-linked Immunosorbent Assay (ELISA)

It is a quantitative test where even minute levels of hCG can be identified to confirm pregnancy.

IV. Radioimmunoassay can also be done.

11. Kirchhoff's law and Einthoven's law.

- Einthoven's triangle is an imaginery triangle drawn around the heart (refer Fig. 8)
- It is formed by the two arms and the left leg forming the apices of the triangle with the heart in the middle

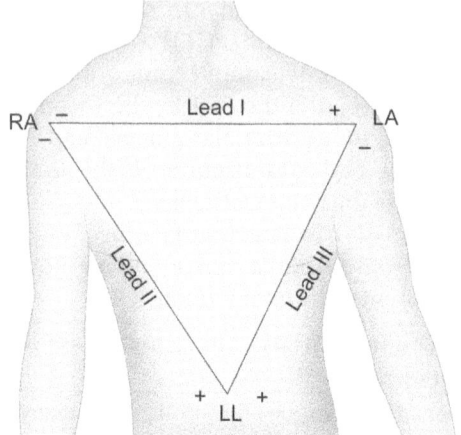

Fig. 8: Einthoven's triangle with placement of Bipolar limb leads.
(RA: right arm; LA: left arm; LL: left leg)
(*Source:* GK Pal)

- The two apices at the upper part of the triangle represent the points at which the arms connect electrically with the fluid around the heart
- The lower part of the apex is formed by the left leg connecting with body fluids.

There are three bipolar limb leads placed in the 3 apices of this triangle.

- **Lead I:** The negative terminal of the electrode is connected to the right arm and the positive terminal is connected to the left arm
- **Lead II:** To record limb lead II, the negative terminal of the electrocardiograph is connected to the right arm and the positive terminal to left leg
- **Lead III:** To record limb lead III, the negative terminal is connected to the left arm and the left leg is connected to the positive terminal.

Eintoven's law states that if the electric potentials in any two of the three bipolar limb leads are known at any instance, the potetial in the third lead can be known by summing the potentials in the first two leads.

For example:

- Momentarily if the right arm is −0.2 mV (negative) with respect to the average potential in the body and the left arm is +0.3 mV (Positive)

- The left leg is +1 mV (Positive)
- Therefore Lead I records a positive potential of +0.5 mV, because this is the difference between −0.2 mV in right arm and +0.3 mV in left arm. Similarly Lead III records a positive potential of +0.7 mV and it can be calculated that Lead II will record +1.2 mV positive potential. These are the instantaneous potential differences in the limbs
- Therefore the potential of any wave or complex in Lead II of ECG is equal to the sum of potentials in Leads I and III while recorded at any instant [Voltage in Lead I + Lead III = Voltage in lead II; (+0.5) + (+0.7) = +1.2 mV)]
- So using Einthoven's law, amplitude of QRS complex can be calculated in any bipolar limb lead either by summing up or subtracting the amplitude in other two leads
- QRS amplitude in Lead II = Lead I + Lead III and amplitude of QRS in Lead III = II − I
- Einthoven's law is the modification of Kirchhoff's law of voltage.

Kirchhoff's Law

- According to Kirchoff's voltage law the algebric sum of the voltage rise in a closed circuit is equal to the algebric sum of voltage drop.
- Kirchoff's current law states that the algebric sum of forces flowing to and from a single point in a network is zero.

12. Excitation contraction coupling in cardiac muscle.

- It is the link between the excitation (arrival of action potential) of the ventricular muscle and the contraction of the muscle
- As in skeletal muscles, E-C coupling happens due to release of Ca^{2+} from the sarcoplasmic reticulum (SR). Excitation ends with release of Ca^{2+} and contraction begins with release of Ca^{2+}
- When an impulse arrives in the ventricular muscle following excitation of - SA node, excitation of subsequent tissues happen in the following pattern → AV node → His bundle → bundle branches → Purkinje fibers → ventricular AP is generated
- Ventricular action potential is of longer duration when compared to the skeletal muscle AP. It has a plateau phase where there is opening of Voltage-gated Long lasting Ca^{2+} channels in the sarcolemma (L-type Ca^{2+} channels). This results in Ca^{2+} influx
- The small amount of Ca^{2+} influx is needed for the release of Ca^{2+} from SR
- So in cardiac muscle, the Ca^{2+} release from SR is a Calcium-induced Ca^{2+} release mechanism (CICR)
- L-type Ca channel is also called as the Dihydropyridine receptor (DHPR) as it binds to Dihydropyridine class of anti-hypertensive drugs
- T tubule, SR and sarcolemma form a junction and the junctional part of SR has the Ryanodine receptor (RYR) which is the Ca^{2+} release channel from SR
- Following the calcium released from SR, the cytosolic Ca^{2+} increases and the Ca^{2+} binds to Troponin C
- This results in confirmational changes in the Troponin/Tropomyosin complex
- Tropomyosin moves into the groove of actin filament and exposes myosin binding sites on the actin filament
- Myosin head binds to actin and brings about muscle contraction.

13. Triple response in skin.

Refer answers to 2009 paper.

14. Physiological dead space.

- Dead space is the space in the airways in which the volume of air present does not take part in gaseous exchange
- There are 3 types of dead spaces—anatomical dead space, alveolar dead space and physiological or total dead space
  1. **Anatomical dead space** is the conducting zone of the respiratory pathway in which the gaseous exchange does not take place and the volume of air is said to be the dead space air
  2. **Alveolar dead space** is the alveoli which do not have blood supply and the volume of air in these alveoli do

not take part in gas exchange and is considered to be wasted ventilation
3. **Physiological dead space** is the sum of the above two dead spaces
- Since in normal conditions there are no alveolar dead spaces, physiological dead space is equal to anatomical dead space
- In a normal adult, of the 500 mL of tidal volume inhaled, 150 mL remains in the anatomical dead space, which is also the physiological dead space.

Measurement of Physiological Dead Space

It is by using the Bohr's equation or Single breath CO_2 technique:

Bohr's equation is used to measure Physiological dead space by measuring the CO_2 levels in the alveolar and arterial blood and the tidal volume.

CO_2 gas is used as it is very less in inspired air and all the CO_2 in expired air is got from the alveoli.

Bohr's Equation

Bohr's equation states that expired air volume is equal to alveolar air volume and inspired air volume in dead space.

Determination of PCO_2 in expired air, alveolar air, inspired air and tidal volume can be used to find out physiological dead space. Since the inspired air has negligible amount of CO_2 all of it should have come from a functional alveolus.

$P_{ECO_2} \times V_T = P_{aCO_2} \times (V_T - V_D) + P_{ICO_2} \times V_D$
$(V_T - V_D) \times P_{aCO_2} + P_{ICO_2} \times V_D = P_{ECO_2} \times V_T$

Since inspired CO_2 is negligible, $P_{ICO_2} \times V_D = 0$, So:

$V_T - V_D = P_{ECO_2} \times V_T / P_{aCO_2}$
$V_D = V_T - [P_{ECO_2} \times V_T / P_{aCO_2}]$
V_T = Tidal volume
V_D = Physiological dead space
$P_{ECO_2} = CO_2$ in expired air
$P_{ICO_2} = CO_2$ in inspired air
$P_{aCO_2} = CO_2$ in alveolar air
If P_{ECO_2} = 28 mm Hg
P_{aCO_2} = 40 mm Hg
V_T = 500 mL
Then,
V_D = 150 mL.

15. Dysbarism.

Refer answers to 2005 paper.

16. Causes of muscle tone.

- Muscle tone is the partially contracted state of the muscle at rest. It is the resistance offered by the muscle to stretching
- All muscles exhibit a tone but it is more pronounced in the anti-gravity muscles. Therefore it helps in maintaining body posture and equilibrium
- Muscle tone is due to stretch reflex which is integrated at the level of spinal cord.

Stretch Reflex

Refer answers to 2005 paper.

Role of Higher Centers on Stretch Reflex and Therefore the Muscle Tone

- Muscle tone depends on the integrity of stretch reflex
- Stretch reflex is under the regulation of spinal cord
- But higher centers are also involved in control of stretch reflex and thereby muscle tone
- The higher centers controlling stretch reflex are cerebral cortex, basal ganglia, brainstem and cerebellum.

Role Cerebral Cortex

- Cerebral cortex is inhibitory to muscle tone through an indirect pathway. Through basal ganglia it stimulates the inhibitory center in the medullary reticular formation
- Basal ganglia acts through inhibitory medullary reticular formation (refer Fig. 9).

Role of Brainstem

- In the brainstem there is a large facilitatory area in the pontine reticular formation and an inhibitory center in the medullary reticular formation
- The inhibitory area is under the control of cerebral cortex, basal ganglia and the cerebellum
- So there is a large inhibitory control over the muscle tone from higher centers than the facilitatory area

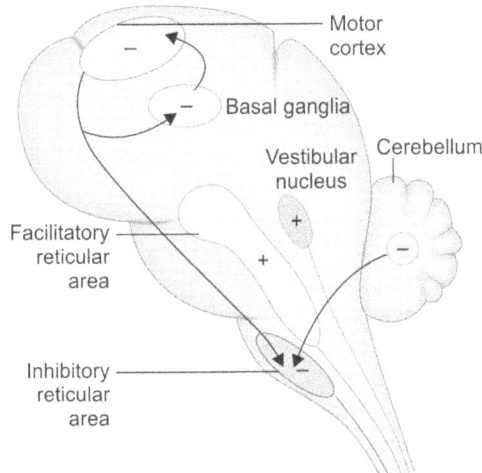

Fig. 9: Higher control of muscle tone. Inhibitory areas—cerebral cortex, basal ganglia, cerebellum and inhibitory medullary reticular area. Facilitatory area—pontine facilitatory reticular formation.
(*Source:* GK Pal)

- These centers regulate the muscle tone by acting on the γ motor neurons
- Cerebellum also has a facilitatory role on the muscle tone. Role of cerebellum is complicated. But in humans cerebellar lesions induces hypotonia
- Vestibular nuclei in the brainstem also facilitate the muscle tone but they act through alpha motor neurons rather than the gamma motor neurons.

17. Function of paleostriatum.

- Globus pallidus (GP) is called as the plaeostriatum. It is an important part of basal ganglia. It has connections with striatum and subthalamic nucleus of the basal ganglia
- It is made of two parts: The internal segment and external segment
- In a direct pathway: The afferents to basal ganglia enter through the striatum and efferents from here go out through the internal segment of globus pallidus. The efferents from here go to thalamus and then to the cortex (refer Fig. 10)
- In the indirect pathway afferents of basal ganglia enter the striatum and through external segment of GP and subthalamic nuclei they stimulate the internal segment of GP which is the final output pathway
- Its important function is to regulate voluntary movement and makes it precise. The interconnection between subthalamic nuclei and GP helps to maintain movements in a smooth and appropriate manner
- GP provides appropriate muscle tone for performance of skilled activity.

18. Climbing, mossy and parallel fibres.

- These are nerve fibers in relation to cerebellum

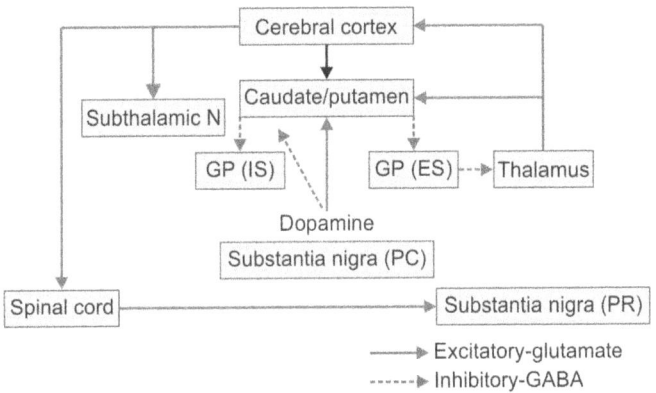

Fig. 10: Connections of nuclei of basal ganglia.
(GP (IS): globus pallidus internal segment; GP (ES): globus pallidus external segment, substantia nigra; PC: pars compacta; PR: pars reticulata)

- Climbing and Mossy fibers are the afferents to cerebellum
- Parallel fibers are axons of the granular cells in the cerebellar cortex (refer Fig. 11).

Climbing Fibers

- Climbing fibers consists of olivocerebellar tract which arises from inferior olivary nucleus in the medulla
- Inferior olivary nucleus receives proprioceptive inputs from all over the body and output signals from cerebral cortex
- These fibers enter through the cerebellum through the inferior cerebellar peduncle of opposite side
- It supplies to the cerebellar cortex and the deep nuclei
- They are stimulatory to the deep nuclei and the Purkinje cells
- The neurotransmitter released is glutamate.

Mossy Fibers

Mossy fibers are also afferents to the cerebellum. It consists of:
- Vestibulocerebellar tract: Vestibular impulses from labyrinths and vestibular nuclei
- Dorsal spinocerebellar tract: Proprioceptive and exteroceptive inputs from all over the body
- Ventral spinocerebellar tract: Proprioceptive and exteroceptive inputs from all over the body
- Cuneocerebellar tract: Proprioceptive impulses from head and neck
- Pontocerebellar tract: Impulses from motor and other cerebral cortex via pontine nucleus
- Tectocerebellar tract: Auditory and visual impulses from inferior and superior colliculi
- They enter the cerebellum through the cerebellar peduncles
- They end on granular cells and golgi cells in the granular layer
- They are stimulatory to these cells and they also end on the deep nuclei.

Parallel Fibers

- The axons of the granular cells in the deep granular cell layer reach the outermost molecular layer of the cerebellar cortex and branch into two divdsions
- It resembles the alphabet 'T'. These fibers are called as the parallel fibers
- The parallel fibers end on Purkinje cells in the middle purkinje layer, basket cells, stellate cells and golgi cells axons in the outer molecular layer
- They are excitatory to all these cells
- So mossy fibers excite granule cells, granule cells excite Purkinje cells, basket cells, stellate cells and golgi cells
- The basket cells and stellate cells in turn inhibit the Purkinje cells—feedforward inhibition
- The axons of granule cells excite the golgi cells and the golgi cells negatively inhibit the granule cells—feedback inhibition.

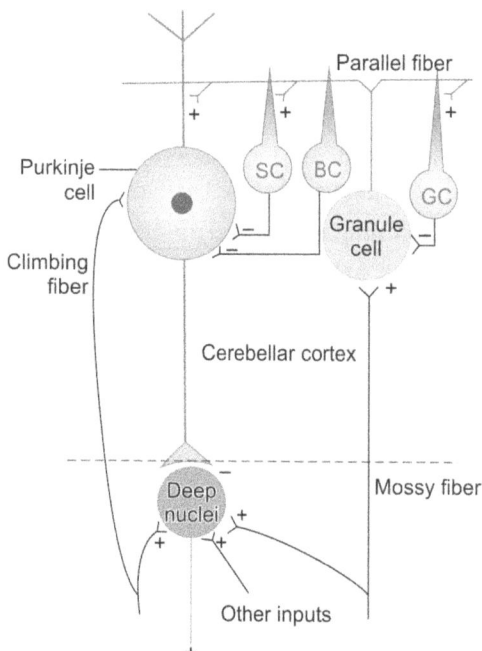

Fig. 11: Climbing, Mossy and Parallel fibers. Climbing and Mossy fibers are afferents to cerebellum and they are excitatory and end on deep nuclei (Both), Purkinje cells and Granule cells respectively. Parallel fibers are axons of Granule cells.
(SC: Stellate cells; BC: Basket cells; GC: Golgi cells)
(*Source:* GK Pal)

19. Control of appetite.
Refer answers to 2003 paper.

20. Induction of sleep.
- Sleep is said to be a state of altered consciousness or partial unconsciousness from which a person can be aroused
- Sleep deprivation results in impaired attention, learning and performance
- Sleep has two components—non-rapid eye movement (NREM) and rapid eye movement (REM) sleep
- NREM sleep has four stages, each with different EEG activities
- EEG patterns in sleep appear in cyclic fashion.

Control of Sleep

Neural Control
- **NREM sleep:**
  - Diencephalic zone: Posterior hypothalamus (HT), intralaminar and anterior nucleus of thalamus.
  - Medullary zone: Reticular formation (RF) at the level of nucleus tractus solitarius (NTS)
  - Basal forebrain zone: Preoptic area of HT and Diagonal band of Broca
- **REM sleep:** Neurons in pons and mid brain. REM sleep is triggered by pontine reticular formation

Chemical Control of Sleep
Evidences show the presence of sleep inducing chemicals in the brain.
- **NREM sleep:**
  - Serotonin induces awakefulness and its antagonists induce sleep
  - Catecholamines prevent sleep
  - Adenosine induces sleep
  - Coffee (caffeine) and Tea (theophylline) bind to and block adenosine receptors and are able to maintain wakefulness.
- **REM sleep:**
  - Acetylcholine induces REM sleep.

Other Controls
- **Afferent control:** Repeated, monotonous low frequency stimulation of mechanoreceptors (at or less than 10 Hz) are their afferents induce sleep by stimulating the above mentioned sleep areas in the brain
- **Circadian control:** Suprachiasmatic nuclei via Retinohypothalamic pathway. NREM or slow wave sleep is under circadian control.

21. Describe the phases of gastric juice secretion.
Refer answers to 2005 paper.

22. Micelle formation.
- Bile salts are secreted into the bile by hepatocytes and they are formed from bile acids
- Bile salts have various functions
- The detergent action of bile salts emulsifies the fats and aids in its digestion
- They decrease the surface tension and along with phospholipids they emulsify fat which is important for its digestion and absorption in the small intestine
- Bile salts are able to form the "micelles" because of their amphipathic nature
- They have both hydrophilic and hydrophobic domains
- One side of the bile salt is hydrophobic and the other side has polar bonds and therefore is hydrophilic
- They form the cylindrical disc like micelles with the hydrophilic domain facing outside and the hydrophobic portion facing inside
- In the micelles, the lipids are collected in the center, cholesterol lies in the hydrophobic center and amphipathic phospholipids and monoglycerides arranged in such a way that their hydrophilic heads are facing outside and hydrophobic tails facing inside
- This typical arrangement of the lipids helps to keep them in solution and for transporting them to the brush border of enterocytes for absorption
- Micelles now move down their concentration gradient through the unstirred layer to the brush border of the mucosal cells
- The lipids now move out of the micelles and the saturated aqueous solution of

lipids comes in contact with the brush border for absorption
- Critical micelle concentration is a value above which all bile salts added to a solution form micelles.

23. Describe cystometrogram.
Refer answers for 2005 paper.

24. Functions of sertoli cells.
Refer answers for 2008 paper.

25. Functions of placenta.

Functions of Placenta

a. Synthesis of hormones (Endocrine function of placenta)
b. Transport of substances across the placenta between the mother and fetus
c. Protection of fetus.

Hormones Synthesized by Placenta

a. Human chorionic gonadotropin (hCG)
b. Human chorionic somatomammotropin (hCS)
c. Placental progesterone
d. Placental estrogen
e. Relaxin.

Human Chorionic Gonadotropin (hCG)

- It is synthesized by syncytiotrophoblasts of placenta
- It is a glycoprotein with α and β subunits
- It starts appearing in the blood of the mother by 6 days after fertilization and reaches apeak by 10–12 weeks
- Clinically, presence of hCG in urine of a female is "the indicator" of pregnancy
- It stimulates the corpus luteum to secrete progesterone till the placenta is fully formed
- hCG helps in sexual differentiation of male fetus
- It induces hyperemesis in the first trimester.

Human Chorionic Somatomammotropin (hCS)

- It is also secreted from the syncytiotrophoblast of placenta
- Its secretion starts by 5th week of pregnancy and reaches a peak towards term
- It is similar to growth hormone and has growth promoting actions, so called as "Maternal growth hormone of pregnancy"
- It stimulates lipolysis, N_2, K^+ and Ca^{2+} retention and decreases glucose utilization by the mother so that the substrates are diverted to the fetus
- Amount of hCS secreted is equal to size of placenta and therefore level of hCS indicates placental viability.

Placental Progesterone

- In the early weeks of pregnancy, progesterone is produced by corpus luteum and later the function is taken over by placenta
- It is produced by co-ordination between the mother and the fetus—the fetoplacental unit
- It makes the endometrium secreetory and thereby nourishes the fertilized ovum
- It keeps the myometrium of the pregnant uterus quiescent which is essential for the survival of the fetus
- It acts on the alveolar system of the maternal breast and facilitates development of maternal breast
- It has an immunosuppressive role in protecting the fetus.

Placental Estrogen

- The major estrogen in pregnancy is estriol
- It stimulates development of the ductular system of the maternal breast
- The levels of estrogen rises during pregnancy but on nearing term estrogen: progesterone ratio rises and estrogen makes the myometrium excitable
- On decrease of levels of estrogen after delivery of fetus, prolactin stimulates milk secretion from the breast.

Relaxin

- Its level in the early pregnancy is high to relax the uterine wall to favour implantation of fetus
- In later weeks it causes relaxation of pubic symphysis and pelvic ligaments to facilitate delivery of fetus.

Other hormones secreted are: CRH, β endorphin, α-MSH, GnRH, inhibin, prolactin etc.

Transport Functions of Placenta

- **Transport of nutrients:** Placenta transports nutrients from the mother to the fetus. The nutrients transported are glucose, fats, amino acids and Ca^{2+}, inorganic phosphates, K^+, Na^+
- **Transports of waste products** from the fetus to the mother: Substances transported are urea, uric acid and creatinine
- **Transport of gases:** Dissolved O_2 is transported from maternal side of placenta to the fetus along the pressure gradient. Fetus receives its O_2 from maternal venous sinuses and therefore is living in an hypoxic environment. But the fetal Hb with 2α and 2γ chains has higher affinity for O_2. CO_2 is also eliminated from fetal circulation into maternal blood by diffusion across the placenta
- **Transport of antibodies:** Maternal antibodies are transferred to the fetus and are responsible for innate immunity.

Protection of Fetus

- It acts as a barrier for prevention of transport of toxic substances from the mother to fetus
- Progesterone produced by placenta helps to maintain pregnancy.

26. Plasma proteins.
Refer answers to 2004 paper.

27. Hepatic and gallbladder bile.

- Bile is synthesized from the hepatocytes and secreted into biliary ductular system
- Hepatocytes form bile, by adding substances which are absorbed from the circulation like bilirubin and also adds bile salts which are synthesized from hepatocytes
- When bile passes through the ducts, its ionic contents get modifed and is high in HCO_3^- content. This is said to be the hepatic bile
- It is highly alkaline in nature. Bile formed in the inter-digestive period is stored in gallbladder
- Gallbladder mucosa is highly folded and has absorptive capacity and therefore it absorbs water and electrolytes and alters the composition of bile.

The bile in gallbladder is:
- Thicker, more viscous and darker in color
- Water content is decreased
- Organic and inorganic constituents are concentrated
- Cl^- and HCO_3^- are decreased and Ca^{2+} and K^+ is increased.
- pH of gallbladder bile is decreased from 8–8.6 to 7–7.6.

Differences between Hepatic Bile and Gallbladder Bile

Properties and features	Hepatic bile	GB bile
pH	8 to 8.6	7 to 7.6
Color	Golden yellow	Black
Consistency	Watery	More viscous
Water	97.5%	87.5%
Solids	2.5%	12.5%
Organic substances		
Bile salts	1.1g/dL	8 g/dL
Bile pigments	0.2g/dL	1g/dL
Cholesterol	0.1g/dL	0.5g/dL
Fatty acids	0.15g/dL	0.5g/dL
Fat	0.1g/dL	0g/dL
Lecithin	0.1g/dL	0.8g/dL
Mucin	Absent	Present
Inorganic substances	0.7g/dL	8.7g/dL

28. Deglutition.
Refer answers to 2003 paper.

29. Differences between cretinism and dwarfism.

Features	Dwarfism	Cretinism
Causes	Defeciency of growth hormone in childhood	Defeciency of thyroid hormone in infancy
Height	Short statured	Short statured
Prportionate growth retardation	yes	yes
Mental development	Normal	Mental retardation is present
Face	Immature facies	Idiotic face

Contd...

Contd...

Features	Dwarfism	Cretinism
Sexual maturity	May or may not be absent	Delayed sexual maturity
Organo-megaly	Absent	Present, resulting in pot belly, enlarged tongue.

30. Explain the hormonal regulation of menstrual cycle.

Refer answers to 2007 paper.

31. Theories of hearing.

a. **Rutherford telephone theory:**
   - According to this theory the ear acts like a telephone and transmits the same number of impulses as that of the frequency of sound
   - For example if the sound is of 6000 Hz frequency, the auditory nerve transmits 6000 impulses
   - But it is not acceptable, as the nerves cannot transmit at this high frequency
   - But lower frquency sounds, less than 2000 Hz/sec can produce a volley of similar number of impulses.

b. **Place theory:**
   - According to this theory, sound waves of different frequencies stimulate the basilar membrane of organ of Corti in different areas (places)
   - Sound waves of higher frequency stimulate the structures near the base of the cochlea and low frequency waves stimulate the structures near the apex.

c. **Resonance volley theory:**
   - This theory combines both the above theories and it proposes that the volley theory is acceptable for low frequency sounds below 2000 Hz and higher frequency sounds are encoded by the place at which the organ of Corti and basilar membrane are stimulated.

- This is the most accepted theory.

32. Anterior spinothalamic tract.

- It is an ascending tract
- It is a part of the anterolateral system
- It carries the sensation of crude touch
- The first order neurons are present in the dorsal root ganglion. They are of pseudounipolar type of neurons
- The central axons of these neurons terminate on second order neurons located in the laminae III, IV and V
- Second order neurons fibers from these laminae cross to the opposite side and occupy the anterior white column
- It ascends in the anterior white column of spinal cord and enters medulla
- It joins with lateral spinothalamic tract and ascends up as spinal lemniscus
- The second order neurons terminate in the ventroposterolateral nucleus (VPLN) in thalamus
- From the VPLN of thalamus, the third order neurons ascend up to terminate in the opposite somatosensory area I (Area 3, 1, 2) and somatosensory area II (refer Fig. 12).

33. Postural reflexes.

- These reflexes help to regulate the body posture and equilibrium. They also help to adjust the body posture during voluntary movement
- They are integrated at various levels in the CNS
- They are classified as segmental, phasic and tonic reflexes.

Local and Segmental Reflexes

Stretch Reflex

Refer answers to 2005 paper.

Positive Supporting Reaction

- Placing the finger on the sole of the foot or giving a pressure sensation, results in contraction of both the protagonists and antagonists of the ankle and transforms the limb into a rigid pillar and as the finger is withdrawn the limb follows the finger. It is also called as the magnetic reaction or positive supporting reaction
- Stimulus for this reflex is touch and pressure sensations from the skin of the sole and impulses from the proprioceptors of leg

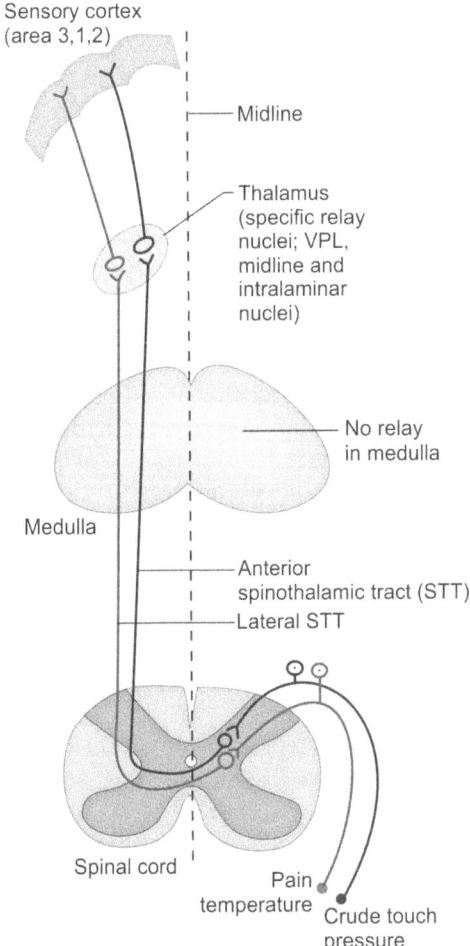

Fig. 12: Anterior and lateral spinothalamic tracts.
(*Source:* GK Pal)

- This reflex helps to maintain the foot in the intermediate position between dorsiflexion and plantar flexion so that erect standing position is possible.

Negative Supporting Reaction

It is the opposite of positive supporting reflex and it results in disappearence of the positive reaction. It is stimulated by impulses coming from the extensors of the limbs. It helps in limb movements for other actions other than standing.

Crossed-extensor Reflex

- This is an example of segmental static reflex. It is a bilateral reflex where stimulus applied in one limb causes response in both the limbs
- A strong stimulus like pain in one limb causes withdrawal or flexion of that limb and at the same time extension of the opposite limb. This helps the animal to stabilize while responding to pain stimulus
- This reflex is also useful while walking. The flexors on one side are active while walking and the extensors are inhibited and the opposite happens in the other limb.

Static or Tonic Reflexes

- These are sustained contraction of muscles to maintain posture and provide background posture while moving
- They involve groups of muscles responding to stimulus arising from one side of the body
- When there is a change in position of head, muscles of the body contract to maintain erect posture.

They are of two types:

a. Tonic neck reflexes
b. Tonic labyrinthine reflexes.

a. **Tonic neck reflexes:**
   - These reflexes are present due to the change in position of neck in relation to body position
   - The reflexes are studied in experimental animals with transections at various levels to know the centers for their integration
   - To study these reflexes the transection is done at the superior border of pons
   - The **stimulus** is turning of the head in relation to body
   - **Receptors** are neck proprioceptors
   - **Center** is in medulla
   - **Response** is change in pattern of extensor contraction.

Neck reflexes in different positions of head of the animal:

1. When head is turned down or ventroflexed, there is flexion of forelimbs and extension of hind limbs. It is like the animal is looking into a hole in the ground

2. When the head is extended or dorsiflexed the forelimbs are extended and hind limbs are flexed. It is like the animal looking over an obstacle
3. When the head is turned to one side the limbs on that side (jaw limbs) become rigid and extended while the contralateral limbs are less so.
   b. **Tonic labyrinthine reflexes:**
      - **Stimulus** is gravity
      - **Receptors** are otolithic organs
      - **Center** is Medulla
      - **Response** is contraction of limb extensor muscles.

Tonic Labyrinthine Reflex in Different Body Positions

- When the animal is in supine position the tone is maximum in antigravity muscles
- When the animal is in prone position the tone is minimum in antigravity muscles
- When the body is in lateral position, the rigidity is less.

These reflexes help to redistribute muscle tone in the limbs to prevent loss of balance when the body is in inclined posture.

Phasic Reflexes

- Phasic or dynamic reflexes help to make rapid adjustments in the posture and are short-term and produce transient changes
- They are also called as righting reflexes
- They help to keep the head upright and in alignment with the body
- These reflexes are integrated in the nuclei of midbrain
- Righting reflexes are demonstrated in experimental animals when the transection is done at the upper border of midbrain.

The reflexes are:

a. *Labyrinthine righting reflexes:* When the animal is held by its body and tipped from side to side, the animal holds the head erect in response to stimulus (gravity) from the otolithic organ (receptors)
b. *Neck righting reflex:*
   - It acts on neck muscles and corrects the position of head to that of the body
   - It happens when the body is in the lateral position and head is erect
   - **The stimulus** is stretch of neck muscles
   - **Receptor** is muscle spindle in neck muscles
   - **Center** is midbrain
   - **Response** is the body gets gradually righted, starting from righting of thorax, shoulders, abdomen and pelvis.
c. *Body on head righting reflex:*
   - It happens when the body is laid on the side and even if the otolithic organs are destroyed the pressure effect of the body initiates righting of the head
   - **Stimulus** is pressure on side of body
   - **Receptor** is exteroceptors
   - **Center** is midbrain
   - **Response** is righting of head.
d. *Body on body righting reflexes:*
   - This happens when the head is prevented from righting, therefore the impulses from the body surface can right the body
   - **Stimulus** is pressure on side of the body
   - **Receptors** are exteroceptors
   - **Center** is midbrain
   - **Response** is righting of body even if body is prevented from righting.
e. *Optical righting reflexes:*
   - Even in the absence of stimuli from labyrinth or body stimulation there can be righting of head due to visual or optical cues. But this needs an intact cerebral cortex. In intact humans, this reflex helps to maintain the head in stable position despite the movements of the body
   - **Stimulus**—visual cues
   - **Receptors**—eyes
   - **Center**—cerebral cortex
   - **Response**—righting of head.
f. **Limb righting reflexes:**
   Placing reaction:
   - It is integrated in cerebral cortex
   - When the snout of a suspended blindfolded animal touches a surface it immediately places both the forepaws on the surface. Exteroceptors are reponsible for the placing reaction

- If a blind-folded animal is suspended in air with one foot touching the surface it can place the foot firmly on the supporting surface. Labyrinthine and exteroceptors are responsible for the placing reaction
- If an animal is thrown into air it can land firmly with four limbs. It is due to visual, labyrinthine and exteroceptor cues. These reflexes help the animal to be prepared to land on a supporting surface.

Hopping reaction:
- When a standing animal is pushed laterally, hopping movements help to support the body and rights the posture
- **Stimulus** is lateral displacement of the body
- **Receptors** are muscle spindles
- **Center** is cerebral cortex
- **Response** is hopping, maintains limb in position to support body.

34. Aqueous humor.
Refer answers to 2006 paper.

35. Taste pathway.
Refer answers to 2005 paper.

36. Cerebral circulation.

Features of Cerebral Blood Flow

- Cerebral blood flow (CBF) is by 2 vertebral and 2 internal carotid arteries
- Venous drainage is by the deep veins and dural venous sinuses
- The cerebral vessels are supplied by sympathetic, parasympathetic and sensory nerves
- CBF—750 mL/min or 54 mL/100g/min. It is 14% of total Cardiac output
- O_2 uptake by the human brain is 3.5 mL/100 of brain/min or 49 mL/min of whole of brain
- CBF is measured by Kety's method, Radioactive methods, PET scan, fMRI scan and by using flow meters
- Cerebral tissues are highly sensitive to hypoxia. If no blood flow for 15 – 30s → unconsciousness, for > 5 min → Brain death
- Structures in brainstem are more resistant to hypoxia than cerebral cortex
- Glucose is the main fuel for brain and prolonged hypoglycemia → Cerebral dysfunction
- Endothelial cells in the cerebral blood vessels are continuous in nature and along with choroid epithelium forms the blood-brain-barrier
- Few regions of the brain do not have this barrier—circumventricular organs.

Regulation of Cerebral Blood Flow

- **The factors which affect the cerebral blood flow are:**
  - Perfusion pressure
  - Intracranial pressure
  - Diameter of blood vessels
  - Resistance or viscosity of blood.
- **The regulation of cerebral blood flow is discussed under:**
  i. Intracranial pressure—major regulator
  ii. Metabolic autoregulation (arterial pCO_2 and pO_2 levels)
  iii. Myogenic autoregulation (65-140 mm Hg MAP)
  iv. Neural regulation—not much of a role for the sympathetics here.
- **Intracranial pressure:**
  - ICP regulates cerebral blood flow by the following mechanisms
  - Monro-Kellie doctrine: According to this phenomenon, at any given time, the contents within the cranial cavity is a constant. It includes the brain tissue, blood and CSF. So if anyone component increases it is at the expense of the other two
  - For example if there is an increase in cerebral venous pressure there is a similar increase in ICP and these two decrease the blood flowing through the arteries.

Cushing's Reflex

- This reflex comes into action when the ICP rises as in brain tumors or intracranial bleeding.

Increased ICP
↓
Compression on cerebral arteries
↓
Decreased blood flow to brain
↓
Hypoxia and hypercapnia in vasomotor center (VMC)
↓
Stimulation of VMC
↓
Increase in heart rate and stroke volume
↓
Increase in cardiac output
↓
Increase in BP
↓
Stimulation of baroreceptors
↓
Bradycardia

So in increased ICP there is increase in BP and decrease in heart rate.

Metabolic Autoregulation

- The metabolic factors which regulate the cerebral blood flow are ↑pCO_2, ↓pO_2, H^+ and adenosine in arterial blood. They cause vasodilatation of cerebral blood vessels
- H^+ cannot cross the blood brain barrier, but CO_2 which easily crosses the blood brain barrier is converted to H_2CO_3 and then to H^+ and HCO_3^-. H^+ then induces vasodilatation
- Hypoxia results in formation of adenosine which also causes vasodilatation.

Myogenic Autoregulation

- Due to the myogenic autoregulation the cerebral blood flow remains a constant between the blood pressures of 60-140 mm Hg.

Neural Regulation

- The cerebral vessels are supplied by sympathetic noradrenergic fibers and parasympathetic fibers
- The sympathetic fibers come into action when there is a marked increase in blood pressure
- This causes vasoconstriction and thereby prevents the rupture of blood vessels and haemorrhage and stroke and also rupture of blood brain barrier.

Measurement of Cerebral Blood Flow

- *Kety method:* This method uses the Fick's principle. Here the person is made to breathe a mixture of Nitrous oxide and air for 10 minutes and samples are taken from artery and vein and blood flow to brain is calculated using Fick's principle and cerebral blood flow is calculated as:
  = N_2O taken up by brain tissue per min/ A-V difference of N_2O
- *Using radioactive substances* like radioactive xenon: Clearance curve of the radioactive isotope is used to measure blood flow to the organ or a region of brain
- *Positron emission tomography (PET):* Used to measure regional blood flow
- *Magnetic resonance imaging (MRI):* Local O_2 utilization and thereby cerebral blood flow can be measured
- Flow meters can be used.

37. Color vision.

Refer answers to 2005 paper.

38. CO_2 transport.

CO_2 is transported in 4 forms:
i. As dissolved form in plasma
ii. As carbamino-compound-combination with plasma proteins
iii. As bicarbonate
iv. As carbamino-hemoglobin-combination with hemoglobin.

As dissolved form:

- CO_2 in dissolved form in plasma is proportional to the partial pressure of CO_2
- It has 20 times more solubility than O_2 in blood

- Some amount of CO_2 combines with plasma proteins to form carbamino-protein complex.

As bicarbonate:
- The major form by which CO_2 is transported is as bicarbonate. Nearly 70% is transported as HCO_3^-
- As the CO_2 enters the blood it saturates the plasma and quickly diffuses into the RBCs
- In the RBC the enzyme carbonic anhydrase catalyzes the reaction of CO_2 combining with water to form H_2CO_3
- $H_2CO_3 \rightarrow H^+ + HCO_3^-$
- As the HCO_3^- levels increase within the RBC, it starts leaving the RBC in exchange for Cl^-
- This exchange happens through the Band 3 protein which is an anion exchanger. It is present on the membrane of RBC
- This is called as the "Chloride shift" or "Hamburger shift" (refer Fig. 13)
- So in the venous blood the RBCs have more osmotically active particles which causes water retention in the RBC and increases its size
- Therefore hematocrit of venous blood is 3% more than the arterial blood
- The H^+ is buffered by hemoglobin within the RBC
- As Hb binds with H^+ the Oxy-Hb curve shifts to the right and O_2 is released to the tissues
- As the venous blood reaches the lungs the reverse process of all the above happens and CO_2 is released and blown out
- High O_2 levels in the lungs helps in unloading of CO_2.

As carbamino compound:
- CO_2 in RBC binds to hemoglobin to form carbamino hemoglobin
- About 23% of CO_2 is transported in this form.

39. Chemoreceptors.
Refer answers to 2005 paper.

40. Endothelins.
- Endothelial cells secrete many chemicals which regulate vascular tone
- There are vasodilators as well as vasoconstrictors secreted by the endothelial cells
- Endothelin is a potent vasoconstrictor secreted by the endothelial cells
- There are Endothelins 1, 2 and 3
- The endothelins are partially secreted into the lumen and most of it move towards the smooth muscles and act on it in a paracrine fashion and induces vasoconstriction
- Endothelins act through two types of receptors – ET_A receptor and ET_B receptors
- Endothelin 1 acts on ET_A receptor and mediates vasoconstriction in many tissues
- ET_B receptor mediates action of all three endothelins.

Functions of Endothelins
- They regulate vascular tone
- It also acts on the kidneys and brain
- Endothelin 2 is present in the kidneys and intestines

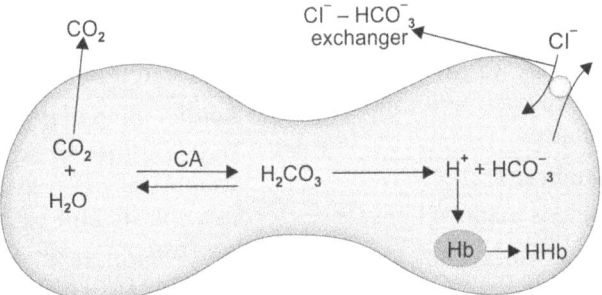

Fig. 13: Chloride shift.
(*Source:* GK Pal)

- Endothelin 3 is present in blood, brain kidneys and GIT
- In brain they regulate transport across BBB
- In kidneys they act on the mesangial cells and decreases GFR
- Endothelins are needed for the migration of cells of myentric plexuses to the distal colon and in its absence the fetus suffers from congenital megacolon
- At birth it is needed for the closure of ductus arteriosus
- It plays a role in pathophysiology of myocardial infarction and congestive heart failure.

III. SHORT ANSWERS

1. Measurement of total body water.

- Total body water can be measured by the indicator dilution principle
- It is measured by injecting a substance which stays in the particular compartment which we want to measure and then calculating the volume of fluid in which the injected test substance is distributed.

It can be calculated by the formula:
- $C = A/V$ i.e, $V = A/C$,
- A = Amount of substance injected
- V = The volume in which the substance is distributed
- C = The final concentration attained
- Total body water can be measured using the above principle and the substances used are – Deutrium Oxide (D_2O), Tritium oxide (^3H_2O) and Aminopyrine
- Total body water in lean body mass is 71–72 mL/100 g of tissue and fat is free of water. The TBW to body weight varies with the amount of fat present and therefore TBW is less in females.

2. Lipids in cell membrane.

- The cell membrane is made of lipids and proteins
- It is semi-permeable in nature
- By semipermeable, we mean that the membrane allows certain substances (lipid soluble substances) to move freely across and others need carrier proteins (water soluble substances) to move across
- The membrane lipids are usually phospholipids such as phosphatidylethanolamine, phosphatidylserine, phosphatidylcholine, sphingomyelin etc. (refer Fig. 14)
- Phospholipids are amphipathic in nature and are made of a hydrophilic head and two hydrophobic tails. In the membrane, they arrange themselves in such a way that the hydrophilic portions face the water compartments – The ECF and ICF and the hydrophobic tails face each other making the membrane a bilipid layer (refer Fig. 15)
- Cholesterol is incorporated in the hydrophilic portion of the membrane to reinforce lipid permeability
- The phospholipids are allowed to move freely in their own layer and the fluidity of the membrane is dependant on the cholesterol-phospholipid ratio.

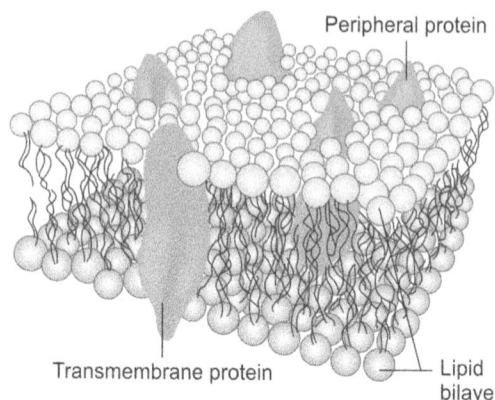

Fig. 14: Phospholipid bilayer. Arrangement of lipid bilayer in cell membrane. The membrane has proteins embedded in it. Proteins are of two types—transmembrane and Peripheral proteins.
(*Source:* GK Pal)

3. Remodelling of bone tissue.

- There are three types of cells in the bones— osteoblasts, osteoclasts and osteocytes
- Osteoblasts and osteocytes are derived from osteoprogenitor cells and osteoclasts belong to monocyte—macrophage family
- Osteoblasts lay down collagen I and are able to form new bone

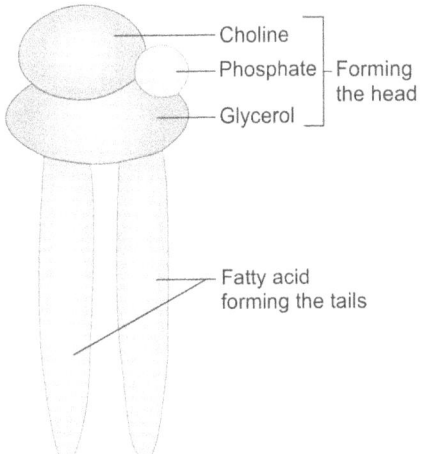

Fig. 15: Structure of a single phospholipid. It has a hydrophilic head and two hydrophobic tails. Because of this amphipathic nature they assemble to form the lipid bilayer. (*Source:* GK Pal)

- Osteoclasts are responsible for resorption of bone and they erode the bone
- The osteclasts resorb the bone followed by osteoblasts laying the new bone. They form together the remodelling units and they remodel the bone in small areas
- The bone remodelling continues throughout life and bone is resorbed and continuously re-laid
- First step in remodelling of bone is arrival of osteoclasts to the site and they attach to the bone through adhesion molecules— the integrins, and a tight seal is formed between the osteoclast and the bone below
- Proton pumps in the endosomes of osteclasts move towards the site of attachment and release acids and acidify the area and a pH of 4.0 is reached
- Acidic pH dissolves the hydroxyapatite and acid proteases secreted by the cell breaks down collagen and forms a shallow depression in the bone
- Products of digestion are endocytosed and they move into the interstitium
- Next the osteoblasts reach the area and start laying down new bone
- This whole cycle takes 100 days. 5% of a bone is remodelled by 2 million remodelling units at any one time.

4. Landsteiner's laws.

- Karl Landsteiner identified the blood group antigens and classified the ABO blood group systems in 1901
- He classified blood groups, based on the presence of antigens or agglutinogens on the RBC membranes
- The major blood group systems are the ABO and Rh systems
- There are other minor blood group systems – Lutheran, Kell, Kid MN systems etc.
- Landsteiner framed 2 laws based on the presence of agglutinogens on RBC membranes and Agglutinins or the corresponding antibodies in plasma of the individual.

Landsteiner's Laws

a. If a paricular agglutinogen is present on the RBC membrane in an individual, the corresponding agglutinin will be absent in plasma
b. If a particular agglutinogen is absent in the RBC membrane the corresponding agglutinin will be present in plasma.

ABO blood group system follows both the laws:

Blood groups	Agglutinigen (RBC membrane)	Agglutinin (Plasma)
A	A	Anti B
B	B	Anti A
AB	AB	No agglutinin
O	No agglutinogen	Anti A and anti B

- Rh system follows only the first law and not the second law
- If the person is Rh positive, RBC membrane expresses the antigen D and there is no anti D antibody in plasma
- But if the individual is Rh negative he does not express D antigen and he also does not have the Anti D antibody
- But once he is exposed to D antigen (as in accidental transfusion of Rh positive blood or the Rh negative mother getting exposed to Rh postive fetal blood during parturition) his immune system produces anti D antibodies which can destroy the RBCs on later exposure.

5. Fibrinolysis.

- Tendency to form clot in an injured vessel is at the same time balanced by anticlotting or fibrinolytic pathways in the vessel to keep the lumen of blood vessel patent
- Fibrinolytic system involves an important protease enzyme plasmin which is present in an inactive form as plasminogen in plasma
- On activation, plasmin lyses the fibrin and fibrinogen to produce fibrin degradation products (FDP) which inturn inhibits thrombin
- Plasminogen is activated by thrombin, and there are plasminogen activators – the tissue type plasminogen activator (t-PA) and urokinase-type plasminogen activator (u-PA) (refer Fig. 16)
- Plasminogen receptors are also located on the endothelial cells and binding to the receptor, plasminogen is activated and prevents clot formation in intact vessels
- There are also tissue plasminogen inhibitors in plasma which are regulated by Protein C and its co-factor Protein S.

6. Lingual lipase.

- Saliva contains the lipolytic enzyme, lingual lipase
- It is secreted by Ebner's glands on the tongue
- It initiates triglyceride digestion
- It is active in the stomach and it digests as much as 30% of the dietary triglycerides
- It yields fatty acids plus 1, 2 diacylglycerols
- Major digestion of lipids starts only in the intestines by the action of pancreatic lipase
- Stomach also secetes gastric lipase but the action is inhibited by low pH in the stomach.

7. Limiting pH of urine.

- Kidneys play a major role in excreting H^+ in the urine and thereby regulate acid-base balance in the body
- H^+ secretion happens in various segments of the tubule by different mechanisms
- As the H^+ are secreted in the renal tubules they are buffered by different types of buffers, in the PCT it is by HCO_3^- buffer and in the distal segments it is by the HPO_4^- and NH_4 buffers
- If not for the buffers, the H^+ secreted drops the pH of urine quickly and further secretion of H^+ is halted
- The maximal H^+ gradient against which the transport mechanisms can secerete H^+ in humans corresponds to a urine pH of about 4.5 (1000 times concentration of H^+ in plasma)—this is the **limiting pH**, beyond which H^+ secretion is halted.

8. Leptin.

- Leptin is a protein hormone of 167 amino acids secreted by the fat cells
- Leptin means "Thin" in Greek.

Actions of leptin in food intake:

- It acts on the hypothalamus to decrease the food intake and increase energy expenditure
- It decreases the activity of Neuropeptide Y, an appetite stimulating agent acting on the feeding center of hypothalamus and increases the activity of pro-opiomelanocortin (POMC) secreting neurons, which decreases appetite
- Animals and humans with defective genes for leptin end up in obesity and diabetes

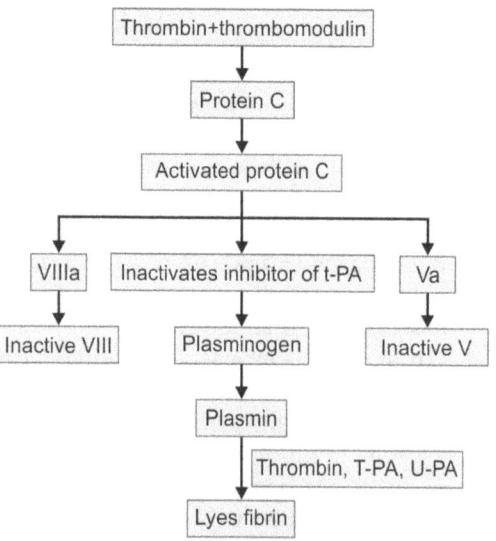

Fig. 16: Fibrinolytic system and its regulation.

- The defect is either due to absence of leptin or defective leptin receptors
- The Leptin receptors are present in the hypothalamic neurons.

Other actions of leptin:
- Leptin when infused into cerebral ventricles causes bone loss
- Leptin also has effects in inducing puberty
- It also acts on brown adipose tissue and induces peripheral increase in energy expenditure.

9. Mullerian regression factor.
- By 7 weeks of age, the embryo has both male and female primordial genital ducts
- In a female fetus, the mullerian duct develops into female internal genitalia—uterus, fallopain tubes
- In a normal male, the Wolffian ducts develop into epididymis and vas deferens
- Similarly the external genitalia are bipotential till the age of 8 weeks
- The presence of functional testis stimulates development of male internal and external genitalia
- Mullerian inhibiting substance (MIS) / Mullerian regression factor, secreted by the Sertoli cell causes the regression of Mullerian ducts
- It is a 536 amino acid homodimer belonging to transforming growth factor beta (TGF-β) superfamily of growth factors
- It acts unilaterally to cause regression of the duct on that side
- Therefore in the male fetus, MIS induces regeression of mullerian ducts and the testosterone induces growth of Wolffian duct related structures and dihydrotestosterone, a metabolite of testosterone induces formation of male external genitalia and secondary sexual characteristics
- MIS reaches a mean value of 48 ng/mL in plasma by 1 to 2 years in boys
- It starts decreasing after that
- In adults it induces maturation of germ cells in both the sexes and causes descent of testis in males.

10. Composition of semen.
Refer answers to 2009 paper.

11. Tracing of arterial pulse.
Refer answers to 2009 paper.

12. Reynold's number.
Refer answers to 2008 paper.

13. Preload and afterload in the heart.
- **Load** is the force exerted on the muscle by an object
- **Tension** is the force of contracting muscle on an object
- Both act on each other.

Preload is the force exerted by an object before the muscle starts to contract. This is the extent to which the muscle is stretched before contraction. As the muscle is stretched the muscle length increases and proportionately the force of contraction increases.

This is based on the Frank-Starling's law:
It states that within the physiological limits, the force of contraction is directly proportional to the initial length of the muscle.

Preload or the initial muscle length is decided by the **End Diastolic Volume (EDV)**. EDV is decided by **Venous return**.

Venous return is decided by:
i. Skeletal muscle pump
ii. Thoracic pump
iii. Abdominal pump
iv. Cardiac pump – Vis A Tergo (Force from behind), Vis A Fronte (Force from front)
v. Total blood volume
vi. Capacity of venous system
vii. Body position

Afterload is the load against which the muscle contracts and in the heart it is the force against which the heart muscle shortens/contracts. It is decided by Peripheral resistance.

Peripheral resistance is decided by:
1. Vessel diameter
2. Viscosity of blood

Cardiac output α 1/Afterload (Anrep effect)

14. Sneezing reflex.
- Sneezing is due to irritation of the nasal epithelium

- It is initiated by stimulation of pain fibers in the trigeminal nerves
- It begins with a deep inspiration followed by forced expiration against a open glottis
- Air is forceful outflow of air at a velocity of 965 km/hr
- This helps in removing the irritants and thereby keeps the airway clean.

15. Denervation hypersensitivity.

- When a nerve is cut and allowed to degenerate the structure supplied by it and close to the cut end shows hypersensitivity or supersensitivity to the neurotransmitter released by that nerve. It is called as denervation hypersensitivity
- It is seen in skeletal and smooth muscles. If the motor nerve to a skeletal muscle is cut and allowed to degenerate the muscle becomes extremely sensitive to acetylcholine
- Denervated exocrine glands except sweat glands also become hypersensitive
- Postganglionic sympathetic nerves to the iris when is cut and norepinephrine is injected intravenously the denervated pupils dilate widely and a minimal response is seen in the normal side
- The causes for the denervation hypersensitivity are:
  - Deficiency of a chemical messenger results in upregulation of its receptors
  - Following the release there is lack of reuptake of the neurotransmitter.

16. Reciprocal inhibition.
Refer answers to 2005 paper.

17. Consolidation of memory.
Refer answers to 2004 paper.

18. Formation of cerebrospinal fluid.
Refer answers to 2009 paper.

19. Gustatory receptors.

- Taste receptors are located in the taste buds
- There are nearly 10,000 taste buds in a young adult and declines with age
- Taste buds are present on the tongue and also in soft palate, pharynx and epiglottis
- Taste buds are present on the papillae of the tongue
- Papillae are elevations on the tongue.

There are three types of papillae:

- Vallate papilla—has 100–300 taste buds
- Fungiform papilla—has 5 taste buds
- Foliate papilla—do not have taste buds
- Filiform papilla—contains tactile receptors and no taste buds
- Cells in taste buds are of 3 types:
  - Type 1 and 2—supporting cells
  - Type 3 cells—receptor epithelial cells and has microvilli projecting (refer Fig. 17).
- They are replaced constantly in 10 days
- Taste receptors are elongate, bipolar shaped and extend from the opening of taste bud to its base
- Through the pore the cilia or hairs project into the oral cavity and come in contact with saliva
- Tastants when dissolved in saliva stimulate the plasma membrane of the taste hairs
- Taste hairs are the site of transduction
- The receptor potential stimulates release of neurotransmitter to trigger nerve impulse in first order neuron
- Each bud is innervated by 50 nerves at bases of receptor cells.

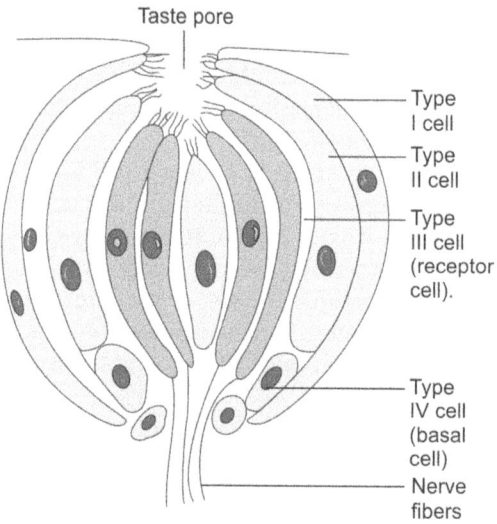

Fig. 17: Taste bud.
(*Source:* Sembulingam)

20. Dark adaptation.
Refer answers to 2005 paper.

21. Phagocytosis.
Refer answers to 2005 paper.

22. Role of sweat glands in thermoregulation.
- The human skin contains 2–3 million sweat glands and there are two types of sweat glands—eccrine and apocrine sweat glands
- **Eccrine glands** are present throughout the body especially on the soles, palm, face and all other parts
- These are the glands taking part in the temperature regulation
- They are coiled tubular glands from which the duct emerges and opens into the skin. These glands are supplied by sympathetic cholinergic nerves
- They are stimulated by hot environmental temperature and their secretion rate is proportional to the temperature
- Sweating is one of the major processes of heat loss
- Vaporization of 1 g of water removes about 0.6 kcal of heat. Sweat glands approximately remove 30 mL of fluid/minute to 1600 mL/hr (as in severe exercise), vaporization of sweat can remove heat at the rate of 30–900 kcal/h
- Vapourization of sweat depends on the humidity in the environment
- Humid environment makes us feel hotter than a dry environment. This is due to decreased evaporation of sweat in humidity.

23. 'B' lymphocytes in immunity.
Refer answers to 2007 paper.

24. ESR and its clinical significance.
It is the rate at which the RBCs settle down/sediment when the blood is anticoagulated and allowed to stand in a long narrow tube for some time. It is expressed as millimeter/hour.

Factors which affect ESR
- Number of RBCs: Increase in number of RBCs decreases ESR and decrease in number raises the ESR
- Increase in size of RBCs increase ESR
- Rouleaux formation: Increased rouleaux forming tendency increases ESR. Fibrinogen and globulin in plasma as in inflammation will increase rouleaux and increase in ESR.

Clinical Significance
- Normal value of ESR is 3–7 mm/hr in males and 5–9 mm/hr in females by Westegren's method
- It is elevated in chronic inflammatory conditions
- It is of no diagnostic value but it gives an idea about the progress of the patient under treatment and therefore is of prognostic value.

25. Fetoplacental unit.
- Placenta produces steroidal hormones; estrogen and progesterone with the interaction of the fetal adrenals
- Placenta forms pregnenolone and progesterone from cholesterol
- Some of this pregnenolone enters the fetal circulation and along with the pregnenolone from fetal liver, forms the substrate for formation of dehydroepiandrosterone (DHEA) and 16-OH DHEAS in fetal adrenals (refer Fig. 18)
- DHEAS and 16-OHDHEAS are transported back to the placenta where DHEAS forms estradiol and 16 OHDHEAS forms estriol
- Estriol is the major estrogen and since its formation requires fetal adrenals, urinary excretion of estriol by mother is a good indicator of well-being of fetus.

26. Actions of relaxin and inhibins.

Relaxin
- It is a polypeptide hormone produced by corpus luteum, placenta, uterus and mammary glands in females and in prostate of males
- In pregancy, it relaxes the pubic symphysis and pelvic joints
- It softens and dilates the cervix and facilitates delivery of fetus
- It also inhibits uterine contraction

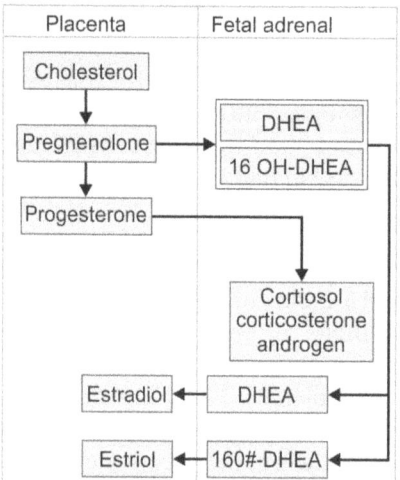

Fig. 18: Fetoplacental unit. Placenta and fetal adrenals, together synthesise progesterone and estrogen.
(*Source:* GK Pal)

- It stimulates growth of mammary glands
- In men, it is present in the semen and helps in sperm motility
- It also aids in sperm penetration of the ovum.

Inhibin

- Inhibin is secreted both in the males and females
- Inhibins are present in extracts of testicular fluids and antral fluids of the ovaries
- Inhibins are formed by 3 glycosylated subunits—glycosylated α subunit and 2 non-glycosylated β subunits, $β_A$ and $β_B$
- They either form hetrodimers or homodimers with α and β subunits
- They inhibit FSH secretion by acting on anterior pituitary
- Heterodimers are inhibins and homodimers are called activins.

27. Endogenous pyrogens.

- Endogenous pyrogens are substances produced by monocytes, macrophages and Kupffer cells by action of endotoxins from bacteria and are capable of producing fever
- Cytokines like IL-1β, IL-6, β-IFN, γ-IFN and TNF-α can individually induce fever.

They induce fever by the following mechanism:

- For inducing fever, the cytokines have to act on thermoregulatory center in hypothalamus
- Cytokines are polypeptides and therefore they cannot penetrate the blood brain barrier
- But they act on Organum Vasculosam of Lamina Terminalis (OVLT), one of the circumventricular organs
- This will activate the preoptic area of hypothalamus
- Prostaglandins are released in the hypothalamus which induces fever
- PGE_2 is one of the prostaglandins which induce fever.

28. Defecation reflex.

Refer answers to 2010 paper.

29. PAH clearance.

Clearance is defined as the quantity of blood or plasma cleared of a particular substance per unit of time. It is the amount of substance excreted by the kidney within a minute.

Clearance = mg of substance excreted per minute/mg of substance per mL of plasma or serum

It is given as $C = U \times V/P$

U = Concentration of substance in urine
P = Concentration of substance in plasma or serum
V = Volume of urine excreted per minute.

Clearance of different substances is used to measure various functions of the nephrons.

Clearance of a substance (Inulin) which is completely filtered but neither reabsorbed nor secreted is used to measure GFR.

Para-aminohippuric acid (PAH) is removed by filtration and secretion but not by reabsorption. Therefore it is used to measure tubular secretory capacity and also renal plasma flow.

PAH clearance to assess secretory capacity of renal tubules:

- PAH is secreted across the renal epithelial cells by means of carrier protein which is a transport maximum (T_m) limited process

- T_m of PAH is 80 mg/min. When plasma PAH levels are low the clearance of PAH is by filtration and secretion
- If Plasma PAH level is high and T_m of PAH is reached then the clearance of PAH is only through filtration and the constant amount of PAH secreted becomes a smaller quantity of total PAH excreted
- Since T_m of PAH is nearly constant, clearance of PAH is used to study the secretory capacity of tubules.

PAH Clearance used to Measure Renal Plasma Flow (RPF)

- Since PAH is completely removed from arterial blood by filtration and secretion, its clearence is a good indicator of RPF.

Methodology

- PAH is infused continuously at low doses to maintain the plasma concentration of PAH
- RPF is calculated by = $U_{PAH} V/P_{a(PAH)} - P_{v(PAH)}$
  U_{PAH} = Urinary concentration of PAH
  V = Volume of urine excreted per minute
  $P_{a(PAH)}$ = PAH concentration in arterial blood
  $P_{v(PAH)}$ = PAH concentration in venous blood
- At low concentrations, T_m is not reached and all the PAH is removed from arterial blood and nothing returns by venous blood ($P_{v(PAH)}$) so it is absent in renal vein and the equation is therefore written as:
  $$RPF = U_{PAH} V/P_{a(PAH)}$$
- Since the above equation is equal to PAH clearance (C_{PAH}):
  $$RPF = C_{PAH}$$
- About 10% of the plasma flowing to kidneys circulates to non-excretory areas of kidneys and therefore the RPF is given as **Effective RPF (ERPF)**:
  $$ERPF = C_{PAH}$$
- Normally urine concentration of PAH (U_{PAH}) is 14 mg/mL, urine flow rate (V) is 0.9 mL/min, Concentration of plasma PAH (P_{PAH}) = 0.02 mg/mL.
- Therefore:
  ERPF = 14 × 0.9/0.02 = 630 mL/min
- From this value RPF is calculated by:
  ERPF/0.9 = 630/0.9 = 700 mL/min.

30. Brown fat tissue.

- Brown fat is a specialized type of lipid and is a small component of total body fat
- It is usually present abundantly in infants and in adults it is present only in specific locations like between the scapulae, in the nape of neck, surrounding large vessels of thorax and abdomen
- In contrast to white fat, in these fat cells there are multiple fat droplets and are supplied by sympathetic nerves
- In white fat, the cells have a single large fat droplet and only its vessels are supplied by nerves
- Brown fat cells have large numbers of mitochondria
- In these mitochondria, along with the usual proton conductance for ATP production there is a second proton conductance through an uncoupling protein (UCP1)
- There is uncoupling of metabolism and generation of ATP and more heat is also generated
- There are also UCP 2 and 3 proteins
- On sympathetic stimulation, nor-epinephrine released from nerve terminals will act on the β_3 receptors, which are specific for brown fat and they induces lipolysis
- Increased fatty acid oxidation will increase heat production
- Brown fat acts this way in cold-adapted animals and humans and increases heat production
- There is increased sympathetic stimulation to brown fat after food intake and thereby it increases heat production along with the specific dynamic action (SDA) which usually follows food intake.

31. Broca's area.

- It is the motor speech area (Area 44) and is located in the foot of the Primary motor cortex (Area 4) (refer Fig. 19)
- In spoken speech, impulses from the ear are transmitted to the primary auditory area (Area 42) in the temporal lobe

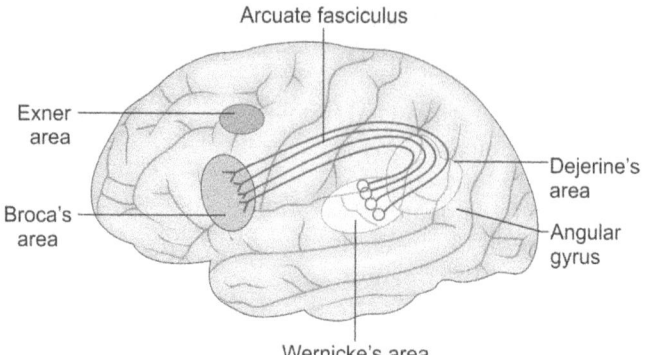

Fig. 19: Speech areas in cerebral cortex.
(*Source:* GK Pal)

- From here the impulse reaches the auditory association areas and then to the sensory speech area – Wernicke's area (Area 22). Here comprehension of speech happens
- From the Wernicke's area impulses are transmitted to the Broca's area
- It regulates the functions of the muscles of the lips, tongue, pharynx and larynx and it helps in vocalisation of the reply
- In lesion of Broca's area there is normal comprehension of speech but there is poverty of speech
- This type aphasia is called as Non-fluent aphasia.

32. Spinal animal.

- Spinal animal is an experimental procedure in which the control of brain on spinal cord is removed by transection below the medulla and ideally below C5 level
- Transection at this level maintains normal respiration.
  Following the transection the animal shows three phases:
  I. Stage of spinal shock
  II. Stage of recovery
  III. Stage of failure.
- This type of experimental procedure is done to study the various reflexes integrated in the spinal cord level.

33. SCUBA diving.

SCUBA is self-contained underwater breathing apparatus.

The type used for commercial purpose is open-circuit demand system.
It contains the following parts:
- One or more tanks of compressed air or breathing mixtures
- A first stage reducing valve to reduce the high pressure in tank to low pressure
- An inhalation demand valve to create a small negative pressure for inhalation of air
- An exhalation valve to breathe out air into the sea
- A mask and a tube with dead space.

Operation of Scuba

- During inhalation, the first step is operation of the first stage reducing valve to reduce the pressure of air from the tank and delivers air at a pressure minimally above the surrounding water pressure
- Inspiration creates a negative pressure on the diaphragm of the demand valve and opens it to allow air to enter the mask and then to lungs
- By this method only the amount needed enters the mask
- Then the expiration follows and the air is breathed out into the sea.

34. Cardiac Index.

- Cardiac output per minute per square meter of body surface area is cardiac index
- Cardiac index = Cardiac output at rest / Body surface area
- 5L/min / 1.7m^2 = 3L/min/mm^2

- Normal average value = 3.2 L/min/mm^2
- Cardiac index is used to standardize cardiac output for the different body surface areas.

35. Bohr's effect.

- The decrease in affinity of hemoglobin for oxygen when the pH of blood falls is called the Bohr effect
- It is due to the fact that deoxygenated hemoglobin binds H$^+$ more actively than oxyhemoglobin
- It usually happens at the tissue level, when CO_2 is released by the tissues into circulation and it increases generation of H$^+$ and decreases blood pH
- So Bohr's effect is partially due to fall in pH and increase in pCO_2
- It shifts the O_2-Hb dissociation curve to the right.

36. Inverse stretch reflex.

- When a muscle is stretched, the muscle spindle is stimulated and results in muscle contraction
- This happens only upto a particular level of stretch
- If the tension in the muscle is increased beyond a level, the muscle relaxes
- Relaxation of muscle in relation to strong stretch is called the inverse stretch reflex or autogenic inhibition
- Receptor for this reflex is Golgi tendon organ
- It is present in the tendons of muscles
- It is stimulated when the extrafusal fibers contract and thereby stretches the GTO in the tendon
- The afferents from here are carried by the Ib fibers
- They end on interneurons in spinal cord and through them inhibit the motor neurons supplying the same muscles and produces IPSP in them. This causes relaxation of the same muscle (refer Fig. 20)
- This reflex helps in regulation of tension developed in the muscle.

37. Respiratory distress syndrome.

- Respiratory distress syndrome is seen in both infants and adults. In infants it is called as Infant respiratory distress syndrome (IRDS) and in adults—adult respiratory distress syndrome (ARDS)
- In infants it is also called as hyaline membrane disease. It is due to deficiency of surfactant.

IRDS

- When the fetus is in utero, the lungs stay collapsed. After birth, the fetus gasps and makes several inspiratory efforts by which the lungs expand
- During expiration, the surface tension of the fluid lining the alveoli tends to collapse the lungs but this is prevented by the surfactant which reduces the surface tension of the fluid
- In infants born premature, the surfactant is not formed and it results in collapse of alveoli in many areas
- This is called as atelectasis
- There is also pulmonary edema which decreases the gaseous exchange in the lungs
- **Treatment:** IRDS can be treated with synthetically available surfactant and surfactant prepared from bovine preparation. Positive end expiratory pressure can also be applied
- **Prevention:** If preterm delivery is suspected glucocorticoid hormones can be administered to the mother to hasten the maturation of surfactant in fetus.

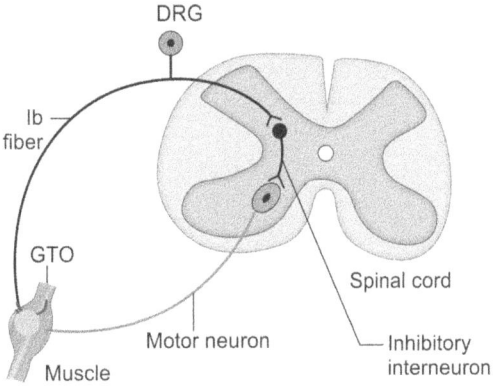

Fig. 20: Inverse stretch reflex.
(DRG: Dorsal root ganglia; GTO: Golgi tendon organ)
(*Source:* GK Pal)

ARDS

- It is seen in adults who have undergone cardiac surgeries with pump oxygenators and interruption of pulmonary circulation
- It is also seen in occlusion of main bronchus, occlusion of pulmonary artery or long term inhalation of 100% O_2.

38. Thalamic syndrome.

- Thrombosis of the artery supplying thalamus leads to dysfunction of thalamus
- Signs and symptoms:
  1. Alteration of various sense perception
  2. Emotional disturbances
  3. Ataxia, weakness and tremor.
- Loss of sensations:
  1. Most of the sensations relay in thalamus and therefore in thalamic syndrome there is loss of sensations in contralateral side of body
  2. Loss of tactile localization, tactile discrimination and stereognosis
  3. Loss of kinesthetic sensations → thalamic phantom limb, ameliognosia, sensory ataxia
  4. Hyper-reactivity to pain.
- Damage to motor system:
  5. Hypotonia
  6. Choreoathetosis
  7. Thalamic hand: Moderate flexion of the wrist with hyperextension of fingers.
- Disturbances in sleep-wakefulness cycle.

39. Unipolar limb leads.

- Unipolar limb leads are the leads placed in the left arm (VL), left foot (VF) and right arm (VR)
- Here one lead acts as the active electrode and is connected to the positive terminal
- It is placed on any one of the above limbs
- The other electrode is an indifferent electrode which is at zero potential and is connected to the negative terminal of the electrocardiograph. (Indifferent electrode is got by connecting 3 electrodes placed on the left arm, left leg and right arm and all are connected to a common terminal through resistance, the indifferent electrode stays at zero potential)
- Normally, the unipolar limb leads are augmented leads and therefore they are given as aVL, aVR and aVF. In augmented leads the recorded potential is increased in amplitude by 50%.

40. Astigmatism.

Refer answers to 2004 paper.

MBBS Examination 2011

ANSWER ALL QUESTIONS

I. Essay questions (15 Marks each)
1. Write in detail the electron microscopic structure of skeletal muscle and the molecular mechanism of muscular contraction.
2. Discuss the composition, mechanism and regulation of gastric secretion.
3. Define cardiac output. Discuss the factors regulating the cardiac output. Add a note on Fick's principle.
4. Trace the visual pathway and the effects of lesion at various points in the pathway.
5. Define GFR. Explain briefly about mechanism of factors regulating GFR.
6. Define Haemostasis. Describe briefly about the mechanism of clotting. Add a note on hemophilia.
7. Name the functional Division of Cerebellum. Describe the structure, connections and functions of cerebellum. Mention any two signs of cerebellar lesion.
8. Describe the structure and function of the conducting system of the heart. List the properties of cardiac muscle.

II. Short notes (5 Marks each)
1. Neuromuscular junction.
2. Regulation of salivary secretion.
3. Functions of pancreatic juice.
4. Erythropoiesis.
5. Micturition reflex.
6. Spermatogenesis.
7. Glucagon.
8. Fetoplacental unit.
9. Secondary active transport.
10. Fibrinolytic system.
11. Normal ECG in Lead II.
12. Regulation of coronary blood flow.
13. Compliance of lung.
14. Carbon dioxide transport.
15. Dysbarism.
16. Functions of thalamus.
17. REM sleep.
18. Decerebrate rigidity.
19. Taste pathway.
20. Theories of hearing.
21. Resting membrane potential.
22. Negative feedback mechanism with example.
23. Pathophysiology of diabetes mellitus.
24. Small intestinal movements.
25. Neuroendocrinal reflex.
26. Functions of placenta.
27. Describe the phases of gastric juice secretion.
28. Hormonal regulation of menstrual cycle.
29. Dwarf.
30. Composition and functions of saliva.
31. Non-respiratory functions of lung.
32. What is FRC? How will you measure FRC and its clinical Importance?
33. Artificial respiration.
34. Referred pain and its theories.
35. Special features of coronary circulation.
36. Color vision.
37. Taste pathway.
38. Explain dark adaptation.
39. What is myasthenia gravis? Explain the biological basis of it's treatment.
40. Brown-Sequared syndrome.

III. Short answers (2 Marks each)
1. Milieu interior.
2. Functions of large intestine.

3. Steatorrhea.
4. Dietary fiber.
5. Multi-unit smooth muscle.
6. Sarcomere.
7. Cytokines.
8. Autoimmune disease.
9. Na^+-k^+ pump.
10. EMG.
11. State Frank-Starling law of the heart.
12. List short-term regulation of blood pressure.
13. Intrapleural pressure.
14. State dead space and its normal value.
15. Define histotoxic hypoxia with an example.
16. What is Bell-Magendie law?
17. Four functions of reticular activating system.
18. Functions of prefrontal lobe.
19. What is endochochlear potential?
20. Delta waves in EEG.
21. Four functions of plasma protein.
22. Helper cells.
23. Kernicterus.
24. Secondary active transport.
25. Rigor mortis.
26. Name the second messengers.
27. Name the hormones involved for the growth.
28. What is Turner's syndrome—three features?
29. APUD cells of its secretion.
30. Law of intestine.
31. Double Bhor effect.
32. Aldosterone escape.
33. What are different types of water absorption?
34. What is Houssay animal?
35. Name the hormones involved in calcium homeostasis, and the main organs that will act.
36. Draw the diagram of alveocapillary membrane and write the thickness of it.
37. What is scuba?
38. Who discovered J receptors? What is its physiological significance?
39. What are otolith organs?
40. What is alpha block?
41. Define Frank-Starling law.
42. What is Monroe Kellie Doctrine law?
43. What is stereognosis? Where is its center?
44. What are the functions of frontal lobe?
45. What are mechanoreceptors? Give example.
46. What is summation? Mention its types
47. What are cholinergic and adrenergic receptors?
48. Draw the structure of rods and cones.
49. What is the difference between the spasticity and rigidity?
50. Define histotoxic hypoxia.

I. ESSAY QUESTIONS

1. **Write in detail the electron microscopic structure of skeletal muscle and the Molecular mechanism of muscular contraction.**

Structure of Skeletal Muscle

Refer to 2006 paper.

Molecular Mechanism of Muscle Contraction

- Muscle, on excitation by action potential results in contraction
- So the electrical phenomenon has lead to a mechanical response
- The linking of the electrical event to a mechanical response is given as Excitation-Contraction coupling.

Excitation-contraction Coupling

When the motor nerve to the skeletal muscle is excited, the neurotransmitter acetylcholine (ACh) is released at the neuromuscular junction.

↓

The ACh binds to **Nicotinic ACh receptors** in the muscle membrane below the nerve—*the motor end plate*.

↓

On binding of ACh with receptor (which by itself is a channel) results in opening of the Non-specific cation channels followed by influx of sodium ions and there is a local depolariztion of motor end plate—***End plate potential (EPP).***

The EPP excites the neighboring muscle membrane and action potential is generated in the muscle membrane.

↓

The AP spreads to the T-Tubule and activates Dihydropyridine recptors (DHP) which in turn triggers the calcium release channels called the Ryanodine receptors in SR and calcium ions are released.

↓

Calcium diffuses into the cytoplasm and gets attached to the Troponin C. Binding of Calcium with Troponin C triggers many events resulting in muscle contraction.

Muscle Contraction

- Sliding theory or Ratchet theory had been put forward to explain muscle contraction by AF Huxley and HE Huxley in 1954
- This theory postulates that the actin filament slide over the myosin filament following the formation of actin-myosin complexes and crossbridge cycling
- At rest, the myosin binding site on actin is covered by tropomyosin and inhibits binding of actin and myosin
- On binding of calcium with Troponin C, tropomyosin molecule changes its configuration and moves out, exposing myosin binding sites on actin
- For each tropomyosin molecule moving out, 7 actin molecules are exposed.

Cross-bridge Cycling

- Each myosin head has two binding sites
- One for binding with actin and other one is an ATPase which hydrolyzes ATP
- On attaching with one ATP, the ATPase hydrolyses the ATP molecule and the energy is stored in the head and thereby it is energized
- ADP and Pi are also attached to the head
- The energized head is 90°perpendicular to thin filament (refer Fig. 1)
- **Power stroke:** When troponin C binds with Ca^{2+}, actin binding sites for myosin are exposed and the perpendicular energized head binds to actin
- Immediately after binding, the head flexes from 90° to 45° and ADP and Pi are released. This is said to be the power stroke or cross bridge cycling
- The bent head is detatched from actin molecule when another ATP molecule binds to the myosin head
- This ATP is again hydrolyzed and the head is re-energized and ready to undergo the next cycle
- As a result of repeated cross bridge cycling, the actin filament from either side is moved towards the center of A band and there is muscle contraction.

Muscle Relaxation

- After the excitation process, Ca^{2+} in the cytosol is pumped back into the SR by cacium ATPase pump on SR membrane
- On removal of Ca^{2+}, Troponin C realigns Tropomyosin back to the position of covering of myosin binding sites in actin and the muscle relaxes.

Changes happening in the sarcomere following muscle contraction:

- H zone disappears
- Sarcomere shortens
- A band width remains same
- I band width decreases
- Z lines are brought closer.

2. **Discuss the composition, mechanism and regulation of gastric secretion.**

Refer answers to 2005 paper.

3. **Define Cardiac output. Discuss the factors regulating the cardiac output. Add a note on Fick's principle.**

- Cardiac output (CO) is defined as the amount of blood ejected by each ventricle per minute
- CO = Stroke volume (SV) × Hear rate (HR)
- NV = 70 mL/beat × 70/min = 4900 mL/min.

Determinants of Cardiac Output

- CO = Stroke volume (SV) × Heart rate (HR)
- So factors affecting either of them will alter CO (refer Fig. 2).

Factors Affecting SV

i. Preload

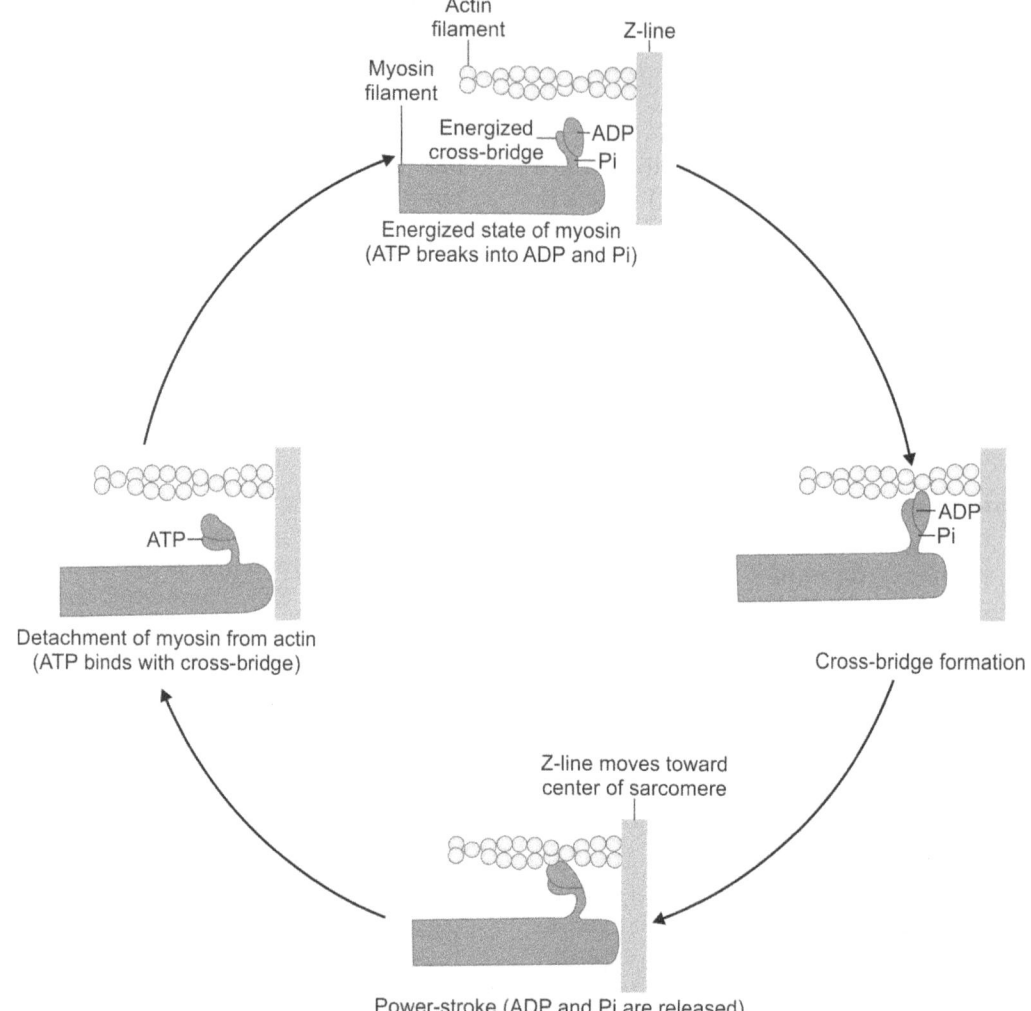

Fig. 1: Cross-bridge cycling in skeletal muscle contraction.
(*Source:* GK Pal)

ii. Afterload
iii. Contractility.

Factors Affecting HR

HR is affected by nerves supplying heart (sympathetic and parasympathetic nerves) and cardiac centers.

Preload

- The initial muscle length is the **preload** (the extent to which the muscle is stretched before contraction)
- Preload is decided by the **end diastolic volume (EDV)**
- EDV is decided by the **venous return (VR)**
- Preload affecting stroke volume is based on the Frank-starling's law
- It states that within physiological limits, the force of contraction is directly proportional to the initial length of the muscle.

Cause for Application of Frank-Starling's Law

Increase in EDV →↑ stretch of muscle fiber → Optimum interaction of thick and thin filament increases →↑ force of contraction

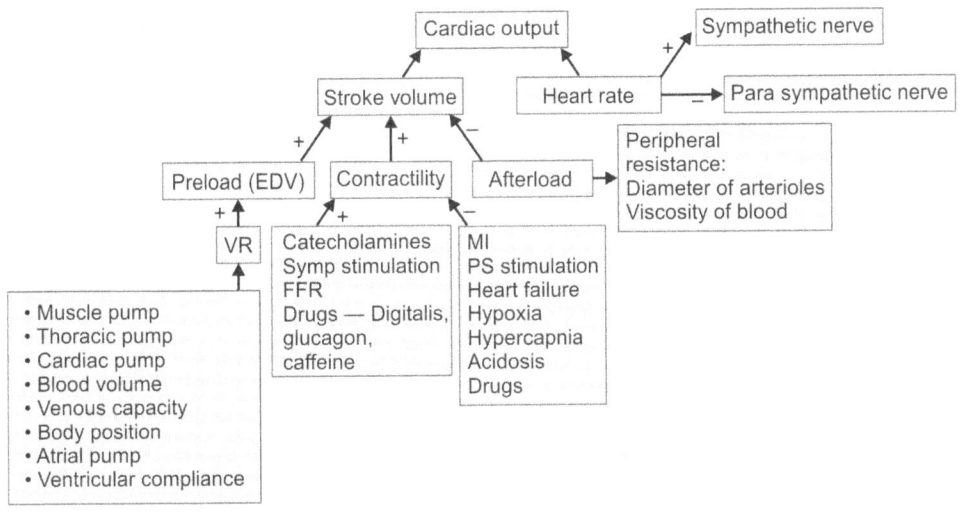

Fig. 2: Regulation of cardiac output.
(VR: venous return; FFR: force frequency relation; MI: myocardial infarction;
PS: parasympathetic; EDV: end-diastolic volume)

EDV is dependent on

I. **Venous return, Which is dependent on:**
   a. Skeletal muscle pump: Contraction of limb muscles press on the veins and increases forward movement of blood in the veins
   b. Thoracic pump: Increase in respiration depresses the diaphragm and decreases intrathoracic pressure and thereby it acts like a suction force to increase VR
   c. Abdominal pump: During respiration compression of abdominal muscles press on the veins and favors venous emptying
   d. Cardiac pump: Vis A Tergo (Force from behind), Vis A Fronte (Force from front)
   e. Total blood volume: As the blood volume increases VR increases and vice versa
   f. Capacity of venous system: Sympathetic stimulation to the veins causes venoconstriction and thereby increases venous emptying
   g. Body position: On standing there is venous pooling due to gravity and it may decrease the VR.

II. **Ventricular compliance**
   - Affected by damage to myocardium as in MI, pericardial effusion, cardiac tamponade.
   This type of regulation of stroke volume in relation to change in initial length of muscle fiber is said to be **heterometric regulation**.

Contractility

Contractility is increase in force of contraction and therby increase in stroke volume without increase in initial muscle length.
- Ventricles are able to do more work per stroke at a given EDV
- Factors which affect contractility— inotropic agents
- There are positive and negative inotropic agents.

Contractility is increased by:
i. Autonomic activity (sympathetics are positively inotropic)
ii. Muscle mass: Increase in myocardial mass increases contractility as after regular exercise
iii. Concentration of hormones and chemicals
iv. Heart rate: Force frequency relationship— there is increase in myocardial contractility

as the heart rate increases within a limit. It could be due to increased availability of intracellular Ca^{++}.

Factors increasing contractility, Positive inotropic agents:

- Sympathetic stimulation
- Circulating catecholamines
- Force frequency relationship
- Digitalis
- Glucagon
- Insulin
- Thyroxine
- Chemicals like xanthine, theophylline.

Factors decreasing contractility, negative inotropic agents:

- Loss of myocardium as in myocardial infarction
- Hypoxia
- Hypercapnia
- Acidosis
- Acetylcholine.

Regulation of stroke volume by affecting contractility of myocardium is **homometric regulation**. Here the force of contraction is affected without much change in muscle length.

Afterload

- It is the force against which the heart muscle shortens
- Cardiac output is inversely proportional to Afterload
- **Cardiac output = 1/Afterload (Anrep effect)**
- Afterload is decided by peripheral resistance
- **Peripheral resistance is decided by:**
  1. Vessel diameter
  2. Viscosity of blood.
- **This is also included in homometric regulation.**

Regulation of Heart Rate

- Heart rate (HR) is also a factor affecting CO
- HR is in turn regulated by autonomic nerves
- Sympathetic stimulation—increases heart rate
- Parasympathetic stimulation—decreases heart rate
- Normally decrease in HR decreases CO
- But in severe tachycardia →↓ duration of diastole →↓ ventricular filling →↓ CO.

Measurement of Cardiac Output

Fick's Principle

- Fick's principle is defined as the amount of substance taken up by an organ or the whole body per unit of time and is equal to the arteriovenous difference of the substance times the blood flow
- Substance taken by an organ = A-V difference × Blood flow
- Blood flow = Substance taken by the organ/A-V difference
- Here the substance taken up is oxygen consumed by the whole organ divided by arteriovenous oxygen difference $A_{(O2)} - V_{(O2)}$ across the lungs
- Output of left ventricle = O_2 consumption by the whole body (mL/min)/$A_{(O2)} - V_{(O2)}$
- O_2 consumed is derived with spirometry
- Arterial blood sample is taken from peripheral artery
- Venous sample is collected from pulmonary artery
  = 250 mL/min/200 mL/L - 150 mL/L
  = 250 mL/min/50 mL/L
  = 5 L/min.
- **Advantage:** Accurate and no chemical is injected
- **Disadvantage:** Needs hospitalization, catheterization etc.

---

4. **Trace the visual pathway and the effects of lesion at various points in the pathway.**

Refer answers for 2004 paper.

---

5. **Define GFR. Explain briefly about mechanism of factors regulating GFR.**

Refer answers for 2005 paper.

---

6. **Define hemostasis. Describe briefly about the mechanism of clotting. Add a note on hemophilia.**

Refer answers to 2007 paper.

7. **Name the functional Division of Cerebellum. Describe the structure, connections and functions of cerebellum. Mention any two signs of cerebellar lesion.**

- Also called as small brain
- It is located posterior and inferior to the cerebral hemispheres
- Cerebellum is connected to the brainstem by superior, middle and inferior cerebellar peduncles
- Cortex is extremely folded and has a surface area 75% as that of cerebral cortex
- It has a central body called vermis and 2 lateral hemispheres
- Vermis is so called as it resembles a worm. It is bent on itself. It has a superior and inferior surface
- The vermis consists of the following divisions from above downwards—lingula, central lobule, culmen, declive, folium, tuber, pyramis, uvula and nodule
- In the hemisphere each part is related to the vermis.

Anatomical Divisions

- Each hemisphere is divided by two transverse furrows into lobes—anterior, posterior and flocculonodular lobes.

Phylogenetical Divisions

- **Archicerebellum:** Flocculonodular lobe
- **Paleocerebellum:** Consists of vermis and paravermal portions
- **Neocerebellum:** Consists of cerebellar hemispheres.

Functional Divisions

1. **Vestibulocerebellum:** It includes the Flocculonodular lobe
2. **Spinocerebellum:** Includes the Paleocerebellum
3. **Cerebrocerebellum:** Includes the Neocerebellum.

Refer answers 2006 and 2009 paper.

8. **Describe the structure and function of the conducting system of the Heart. List the properties of cardiac muscle.**

Properties of cardiac muscle are:
i. Automaticity
ii. Rhythmicity (chronotropism)
iii. Conductivity (dromotropism)
iv. Excitability (bathmatropism)
v. Contractility (inotropism).

Conducting system of the heart:
Refer answers to 2004 paper.

II. SHORT NOTES

1. **Neuromuscular junction.**
Refer answers to 2008 paper.

2. **Regulation of salivary secretion.**
Refer answers to 2008 paper.

3. **Functions of pancreatic juice.**
Refer answers to 2005 paper.

4. **Erythropoiesis.**
Refer answers to 2006 paper.

5. **Micturition reflex.**
Refer answers to 2006 paper.

6. **Spermatogenesis.**
Refer answers to 2006 paper.

7. **Glucagon.**

- It is a polypeptide hormone secreted by the α cells of islets of Langerhans of endocrine pancreas
- It circulates in plasm unbound and its half-life is 6 minutes
- Normal fasting level is 100–150 pg/mL
- Mechanism of action: Since it is a protein hormone it has a membrane receptor and on binding, it activates the second messenger cascade and its actions are mediated through cAMP. It has metabolic effects on various substrates.

Effects on Carbohydrate Metabolism

a. It increases blood glucose levels by various mechanisms like glycogenolysis and gluconeogenesis
b. In liver, it activates the enzyme phosphorylase and breaks down glycogen
c. Glycogenolysis is favoured by activating phospholipase C and increasing cytoplasmic Ca^{2+} in the hepatocytes

d. It has no glycogenolytic action on muscles
e. It increases gluconeogenesis with the help of pyruvate, lactate, glycerol and amino acids.

Effect on Lipid Metabolism

a. It is lipolytic and ketogenic in nature
b. It stimulates lipolysis in adipose tissue and release of fatty acids and glycerol. It also has lipolytic actions in the liver
c. In the liver fatty acids are oxidised resulting in energy production and ketone body formation. It induces ketogenesis in liver by decreasing Malonyl-CoA.

Other Actions

a. It increases amino acid uptake by liver and increases gluconeogenesis
b. It has calorigenic effects
c. It is positively inotropic as it increases myocardial cAMP
d. Stimulates secretion of insulin, growth hormone and pancreatic somatostatin

Insulin-Glucagon Ratio

- Insulin is glycogenic, anti-gluconeogenic, anti-lipolytic and anti-ketogenic
- It is a hormone of storage/abundance and stores the absorbed nutrients
- Glucagon has the opposite actions of insulin and is the hormone of energy release. So the levels of both the hormones must be kept in consideration
- It is given as molar ratio of Insulin and glucagon (I:G)
- I:G ratio in balanced diet is 2.3
- On fasting, the ratio drops to 0.5
- This helps in mobilization of substrates and supply of glucose to vital organs
- In conditions after carbohydrate load or after a meal the I:G ratio reaches 10.

Regulation of Glucagon Secretion

Factors which stimulate glucagon secretion

- Amino acids (amino acids which are gluconeogenic like arginine, alanine, serine, cysteine etc)
- Hormones like CCK, gastrin and cortisol
- Exercise
- Infections
- Stress
- β adrenergic stimulators
- Theophylline
- Acetylcholine.

Factors which inhibit glucagon secretion

- Glucose
- Somatostatin
- Secretin
- FFA
- Ketones
- Insulin
- α adrenergic stimulators
- GABA.

8. **Fetoplacental unit.**

Refer answers to 2010 paper.

9. **Secondary active transport.**

- Active transport across cell membrane involves use of energy and is an uphill transport
- The substances move against the concentration and electrical gradient
- Primary active transport derives the energy directly from hydrolysis of ATP. Therefore the carrier molecules are ATPases like Na^+-K^+ ATPase
- Secondary active transporter uses energy from ATP hydrolysis indirectly. The Na^+-K^+ ATPase which is present in all cells, carries 3 molecules of Na^+ from ICF to ECF and 2 K^+ from ECF to ICF. By the action of this pump there is a concentration gradient established for Na^+ to move into the cell. This inward Na^+ gradient is coupled to transport other ions like glucose; the Na-Glucose transporter (SGLT) in epithelial cells in intestines and kidneys
- Secondary active transporters can be symports or antiports
- Low sodium concentration in the cell favours Na^+ influx and the symport will move glucose into the cell only when both Na^+ and glucose binds to it. So the Na^+ gradient is used to transport glucose across the membrane
- In cardiac myocytes the Na^+ gradient is used to transport Ca^{2+} to the ECF. So Na^+-

Ca^{2+} exchanger is an antiport moving Na$^+$ into the cell and Ca^{2+} out of the cells
- There are also Na$^+$-Amino acid symport, Na$^+$-I$^-$ symport, Na$^+$, K$^+$, 2Cl$^-$ symport, etc.

10. Fibrinolytic system.
Refer answers to 2010 paper.

11. Normal ECG in Lead II.
Refer answers to 2005 paper.

12. Regulation of corornary blood flow.
Refer answers to 2005 paper.

13. Compliance of lung.
Refer answers to 2003 paper.

14. Carbon dioxide transport.
Refer answers to 2010 paper.

15. Dysbarism.
Refer answers to 2005 paper.

16. Functions of Thalamus.
Refer answers to 2008 paper.

17. REM sleep.
Refer answers to 2009 papers.

18. Decerebrate rigidity.
Refer answers to 2006 paper.

19. Taste pathway.
Refer answers to 2005 paper.

20. Theories of hearing.
Refer answers to 2010 paper.

21. Resting membrane potential.
- There is a potential difference across the membrane of all cells and the inside of the cell is more negative than the outside of the cell. This is said to be the membrane potential. The membrane potential at rest in a cell is said to be the resting membrane potential (RMP)
- The RMP in excitable cells like the nerve and muscle cells are important as the change in the potential makes the cell to become more excited or inhibited
- RMP is due to unequal distribution of ions on either side of the membrane and various forces acting on the membrane.

They are:
- Unequal distribution of ions across the cell membrane
- Differences in the permeability of the membrane to various ions
- Na$^+$ - K$^+$ pump or Na$^+$ - K$^+$ ATPase.

The RMP of Various Cells
- RMP of the nerve is –70 mV
- RMP of skeletal membrane is –90 mV
- RMP of cardiac muscle is –90 mV
- RMP of smooth muscles is variable.

Unequal distribution of ions across the cell membrane: Presence of an impermeable ion on one side of the membrane affects the movement of permeable ions. To maintain neutrality on either side of the membrane the permeable ions rearrange. It is given by the 'Gibbs-Donnan Equilibrium'.

Selective Permeability of the Membrane to Ions

The membrane allows certain molecules to move freely across and restrict movements of certain ions. It is highly permeable to K$^+$ and Chloride at rest and only moderately permeable to Na$^+$. It is totally impermeable to intracellular proteins and phosphates which are anions. The high permeability for K$^+$ allows it to move out of the cells and the anions are impermeable and they line up along the interior of the membrane to create the negative membrane potential.

Efflux of K$^+$ continue till the negativity inside the movement opposes the K$^+$ efflux. This is the point where the chemical gradient for K$^+$ is opposed by the electrical gradient. The membrane potential now is said to be the equilibrium potential. At this point net movement of K$^+$ seizes.

RMP of a cell is thereby decided by the equilibrium potential of the ion for which the membrane is permeable. It can be calculated if the ionic concentrations on either side of the membrane is known for each ion and if the permeability of membrane for the ions is known, by using the Nernst equation.

Neuronal cell membrane is highly permeable to K⁺ at rest and therefore the MP is equal to K⁺ equilibrium potential. But there is a small amount of sodium influx also happening at rest and therefore the membrane potential reaches -70mV.

Concentration of Ions in ICF and ECF

- Cations: Na⁺ are high in the ECF (140 mEq/L) and K⁺ are high in the ICF (150 mEq/L)
- Anions: Cl⁻ and HCO_3^- are high in ECF and in ICF proteins and PO_4^- are high.

Na⁺–K⁺ Pump

This pump, by creating a gradient for Na⁺ helps to maintain the RMP. It also contributes minimally for genesis of RMP as the pump extrudes 3 Na⁺ ions out of the cell and 2 K⁺ ions into the cell. So a loss of a single positive ion creates a net negativity inside the membrane.

Factors Responsible for Genesis of RMP

- High permeability of cell membrane to K⁺ at rest
- An inward gradient for Na⁺ and less permeability of membrane for Na⁺ (which does not balance K⁺ efflux)
- Total impermeability of membrane to anions like proteins and phosphate

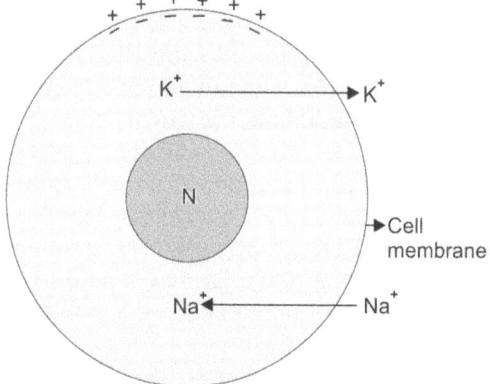

Fig. 3: Genesis of RMP. At rest, an electrical potential difference exists across the membrane of a cell with the inside being negative than the outside of a cell. This is because the cell membrane is more permeable to K⁺ at rest than to Na⁺. So K⁺ efflux is more than Na⁺ influx. This is responsible for the RMP.
(*Source:* GK Pal)

leading to lining up of negative charges on the interior of cell membrane
- Na⁺-K⁺ pump: They offer minimum role in generating RMP but they help in maintaining RMP.

22. Negative feedback mechanism with example.
Refer answers to 2005 paper.

23. Pathophysiology of diabetes mellitus.
Refer answers to 2007 paper.

24. Small intestinal movements.
Refer answers to 2006 paper.

25. Neuro endocrinal reflex.
Refer answers to 2004 paper.

26. Functions of placenta.
Refer answers to 2010 paper.

27. Describe the phases of gastric juice secretion.
Refer answers to August 2005 paper.

28. Hormonal regulation of menstrual cycle.
Refer answers to 2007 paper.

29. Dwarf.

Dwarfism is due to deficiency of growth hormone or growth hormone releasing hormone (GHRH), deficiency of Insulin like growth factor 1 (IGF -1), Growth hormone (GH) receptor insensitivity and thyroid hormone deficiency.

Causes for Dwarfism

- Isolated growth hormone deficiency may be due to GRH deficiency or due to abnormalities of GH secreting cells
- Sometimes the GH levels may be normal or even elevated, but the GH receptors are insensitive to GH due to loss-of function mutation of the genes for GH receptors – This is Laron dwarfism
- African pygmies are a type of dwarfism and are due to reduction of plasma level of growth-hormone binding protein and there is also absence of rise in IGF-1 at the time of puberty

- Cretinism is hypothyroidism in children and it results in stunted growth and mental retardation
- Dwarfism is also seen in conditions of Precocious puberty
- Gonadal dysgenesis is also a cause of dwarfism
- Various bone and metabolic disorders also result in dwarfism.
- **Psycho-social dwarfism:** This type of dwarfism is seen in children who are subjected to chronic abuse and neglect. It is also called as Kaspar Hauser syndrome.
- **Achondroplasia:** It is the most common type of dwarfism. Here the trunk is normal and limbs are short. It is an autosomal dominant condition caused by mutation in the gene that code for fibroblast growth factor receptor 3.

Symptoms

- In a hypothyroid dwarf there is short stature, pot belly, enlarged tongue and delayed sexual maturity. There is definite mental retardation, idiotic facies.
- In pituitary dwarfism: There is short stature, proportionated growth retardation, normal mental development, sexual maturation may or may not be delayed and immature facies is seen.

30. Composition and functions of saliva.

Refer answers to 2003 paper.

31. Non-respiratory functions of lung.

Refer answers to 2007 paper.

32. What is FRC? How will you measure FRC and its clinical Importance?

Refer answers to 2005 paper.

33. Artificial respiration.

Refer answers to 2004 paper.

34. Referred pain and its theories.

Refer answers to 2006 paper.

35. Special features of coronary circulation.

- There are 2 coronary arteries—right and left. Right artery supplies the right atrium and right ventricle and left coronary artery supplies left atrium and ventricles
- There are no anastomoses between the two arteries and therefore they are end arteries. Therefore blockage of vessels results in ischemia or infarction in the areas supplied by those arteries
- There are phasic changes in blood flow through coronaries. In systole, as the myocardium contracts, the blood vessels are compressed and there is no blood flow through the coronaries. In diastole as the myocardium relaxes the vessels dilate and blood flow increases through the vessels
- The endocardial vessels show the maximum phasic variation in blood flow. Therefore these areas suffer from hypoxia and are prone for ischemia in compromised states
- Metabolic regulation is well-developed in coronary vessels. The blood flow increase in coronaries is based on the need of the myocardium
- Coronary circulation is adjusted based on the activites of the myocardium as in exercise, the coronary blood flow can be increased by 4–5 times to meet the body's demand. So it has adequate blood flow reserve
- The myocardium extracts nearly 80% of O_2 from arterial blood and therefore the AV difference of O_2 is high. So to increase further O_2 supply, the blood flow should increase
- The rate of blood flow through the coronary vessels is the second highest next to the renal blood flow. It is 250 mL/min
- The rate of O_2 consumption is the highest of all the organs in the body. It is about 9.7 mL/100g of tissue/min.

36. Color vision.

Refer answers to 2005 paper.

37. Taste pathway.

Refer answers to 2005 paper.

38. Explain dark adaptation.

Refer answers to 2005 paper.

39. What is myasthenia gravis? Explain the biological basis of its treatment.

Refer answers to 2005 paper.

40. Brown-Sequared syndrome.

Refer answers to 2008 paper.

III. SHORT ANSWERS

1. Milieu interior.

- Milieu interior was the term coined by Claude Bernarde
- It denotes the internal environment of the body
- Cells can perform their functions properly only when the internal sea/internal environment of the body is kept a constant
- Internal sea is the extracellular fluid (ECF)
- Homeostasis was the term coined by WB Cannon and it denotes the maintanence of a constant internal environment.

Following factors should be regulated for homeostasis:

- Regulation of plasma pH
- Regulation of body temperature
- Regulation of water and electrolyte balance
- Supply of nutrients, O_2, enzymes and hormones
- Removal of metabolites and waste products.

It is regulated by negative and positive feedback mechanisms.

Example of negative feedback: Regulation of blood pressure is an example of negative feedback regulation:

Increase in blood pressure
↓
Sensed by baroreceptors
↓
Stimulation of cardiac vagal center and inhibition of vasomotor center
↓
Decrease in heart rate and stroke volume
↓
Decrease in cardiac output
↓
Decrease in blood pressure

Example of positive feedback: Parturition reflex is an example of positive feedback regulation:

At the end of term
↓
Increase in sensitivity of oxytocin receptors
↓
Oxytocin binds to its receptor and induces contraction of uterine muscles
↓
Contraction of uterus and descent of fetal head
↓
Stretch of cervix
↓
Stimulation of stretch receptors in cervix
↓
Impulse travels through afferent sensory nerves
↓
Impulses reach hypothalamus
↓
Secretion of oxytocin from hypothalamus
↓
More contraction of uterus

Further descent of head and the cycle continues till the fetus is born.

2. Functions of large intestine.
Refer to 2008 paper.

3. Steatorrhea.
Refer answers to 2007 paper.

4. Dietary fiber.
Refer answers to 2009 paper.

5. Multiunit smooth muscle.

- There are two types of smooth muscles—single-unit and multi-unit muscles
- Multi-unit smooth muscle: These type of muscles are present in ciliary body of eye, iris, precapillary sphincters, piloerector muscles, large airways of lungs etc.
- There are no gap junctions between these muscle fibers, whereas gap junctions are present in single-unit muscles
- Single-unit muscle with the gap junctions act as a syncytium, but the multi unit muscles do not act as syncytium
- Multi-unit muscles like the skeletal muscles are dependent on neural control but are not under voluntary control as it is supplied by autonomic nerves.

6. Sarcomere.

- It is the structural and functional unit of a myofibril. In the myofibril, thick and thin filaments are arranged in repeating pattern; **the sarcomere**
- It is the portion of muscle fiber between two Z lines (refer Fig. 4)
- The average length is 2 μm.

7. Cytokines.

- These are hormone-like substances that regulate immune response
- They are secreted by lymphocytes, macrophages, endothelial cells, neurons, glial cells and other cells
- Cytokines are named after their actions, like B cell-differentiating factors, B cell-stimulating factor. Once the amino acid sequence of cytokine is identified it is named as **interleukins**
- B cell-differentiating factor is now named as interleukin-4
- There are interleukins-1, 2, 4, 5, 6, 8, 11, 12, Tumor necrosis factor α, Lymphotoxin (Tumor necrosis factor β), Transforming growth factor β, Granulocyte-macrophage CSF, Interferons α, β and γ
- The cytokines have both systemic and paracrine actions. IL-1, 6 and TNF-α cause fever and IL-1 increases slow wave sleep and reduces appetite
- Chemokines, which attract WBCs towards site of inflammation, are also belonging to the cytokine family.

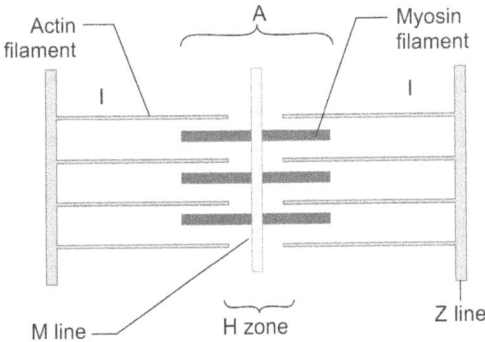

Fig. 4: Sarcomere.
(*Source:* Sembulingam)

Some of the actions of cytokines are:
a. IL-1 and 2: Activation of T cells and macrophages, promotes inflammation
b. IL-4: Activation of lymphocytes, monocytes and IgE
c. IL-5: Differentiation of eosinophils
d. IL-6: Differentiation of B cells, stimulates production of acute phase proteins
e. IL-8: Chemotaxis.

8. Autoimmune disease.

- During the process of development of immunity, the lymphocytes are presented with self and non-self antigens and the cells and antibodies responding to self antigens are eliminated – Tolerance
- Sometimes antibodies against self antigens are not eliminated and it results in Autoimmune diseases
- It can be B cell or T cell mediated, it can be organ-specific or systemic in nature.

Examples are:
a. Type 1 diabetes mellitus: Antibodies against beta cells in Islet of pancreas
b. Myasthenia gravis: Antibodies for Nicotinic acetylcholine receptors in NMJ
c. Multiple sclerosis: Antibodies against myelin basic protein and several other components of myelin
d. Grave's disease: Antibodies for TSH receptors and the receptors are activated resulting in hyperthyroidism
e. Molecular mimicry: Antibodies against certain bacteria will cross-react with body constituents, as in rheumatic fever where antibodies against Streptococcus attacks the cardiac myosin induces damage to heart.

9. Na$^+$- K$^+$ pump.

- It is present in all cells of the body
- It is an electrogenic pump as it pumps 3 Na$^+$ out of the cell and 2 K$^+$ into the cell. It catalyzes hydrolysis of ATP and uses the energy to move the ions
- Its activity is inhibited by Ouabain and digitalis used for heart failure
- It has α and β subunits. Na$^+$ and K$^+$ are transported through α subunit. α subunit

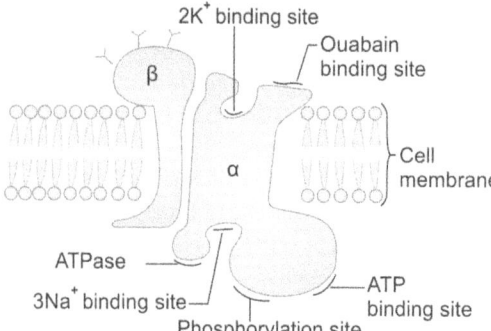

Fig. 5: Sodium-potassium pump. The pump has 2 subunits—α and β subunits. α-subunit has the binding sites for Na⁺ (intracellularly) and extracellular binding sites for K⁺ and Ouabain. Intracellularly there are phosphorylation and ATP binding sites.
(Source: GK Pal)

is larger and has intracellular Na⁺ and ATP binding sites and a phosphorylation site
- When Na⁺ binds to α subunit, ATP also binds and is converted to ADP and the P is added to phosphorylation site (refer Fig. 5)
- This changes the configuration of the pump and extrudes Na⁺ into ECF. K⁺ then binds extracellularly, dephosphorylating α subunit and comes back to original configuration and releases K⁺ intracellularly
- β-subunit is a glycoprotein and has no transport action but its presence is needed for pump activity
- Extracellularly there are binding sites for K⁺ and Ouabain
- Pump activity is regulated by 2nd messengers and hormones
- Thyroid hormone, aldosterone and insulin increase the pump activity, whereas dopamine decreases the pump activity.

10. EMG.

- The process of studying the electrical activity of the muscles on a cathode ray oscilloscope is called as electromyography
- It gives an idea about the activation of motor units
- It can be recorded in humans by placing small metal disks on the skin over the muscle to be examined as the recording electrode or by using a hypodermic needle electrode
- The record obtained with these electrodes is the electromyogram.

Activities Normally Seen in a Muscle
At rest:
- There is no spontaneous activity at rest
- Insertion activity: It may be prolonged in denervated muscle and absent when it is not in a muscle.

On voluntary action:
- During activation of one motor unit, the electrical potential recorded is the motor unit potential (MUP). It lasts for 5 msec and amplitude is 1 millivolt
- Minimal stimulation: Only few motor units close to needle give off electrical discharge
- On increasing stimulation: Firing rate of small units increase till larger units start firing
- During maximal stimulation: Many motor units are contracting and MUPs are superimposed on each other and it is not possible to identify individual components.

Abnormal Activites in a Muscle
- Fasciculation potentials are abnormal involuntary contractions in muscle fibers of single motor unit and they resemble MUPs. This happens when a motor neuron is irritated in certain diseases
- Fibrillation potentials are of short duration and low amplitude
- These potentials are recorded when the nerve is cut and has undergone degeneration for few weeks
- These are due to electrical activity in individual muscle fibers. These potentials disappear when the nerve grows and makes contact with the muscle
- They are seen only in lower motor neuron lesions
- Uses of electromyogram: Used to diagnose neuromuscular diseases, myopathies and peripheral nerve lesions.

11. State Frank-Starling law of the heart.

It states that within the physiological limits, the force of contraction is directly proportional to the initial length of the muscle.

Cause for Frank-starling Law

- Increase in EDV →↑ stretch of muscle fiber → Optimum interaction of thick and thin filament increases →↑ force of contraction.

12. List short-term regulation of blood pressure.

Refer answers to 2010 paper.

13. Intrapleural pressure.

- It is the pressure in the space between the two pleurae: Visceral and parietal pleura
- It is negative or subatmosperic
- At rest, when the respiratory muscles are relaxed and airways are kept open it is around –2.5 mm Hg (refer Fig. 6)
- The negative pressure is due to two opposing forces acting on each other.

They are:

a. The recoiling tendency of the lung towards inwards due to the presence of elastic tissue in the lungs and surface tension of the fluid which cause collapse of lungs
b. The recoiling tendency of the muscle of the thoracic cage towards outward results in expansion of thorax
- These two forces act opposite to each other pulling apart the two layers of the pleurae and thereby creating a negative pressure in the space
- During inspiration, as the chest wall expands, the negative pressure becomes more (–6 mm Hg) negative and thereby pulls on the lungs to create a negative intrathoracic pressure
- During expiration, the inspiratory muscle activity is cut off and the chest wall begins to recoil back to expiratory position and the lungs recoil inwards and the intrapleural pressure is back to –2.5 mm Hg.

14. State dead space and its normal value.

- Dead space volume is the part of the pulmonary ventilation that does not take part in gaseous exchange.

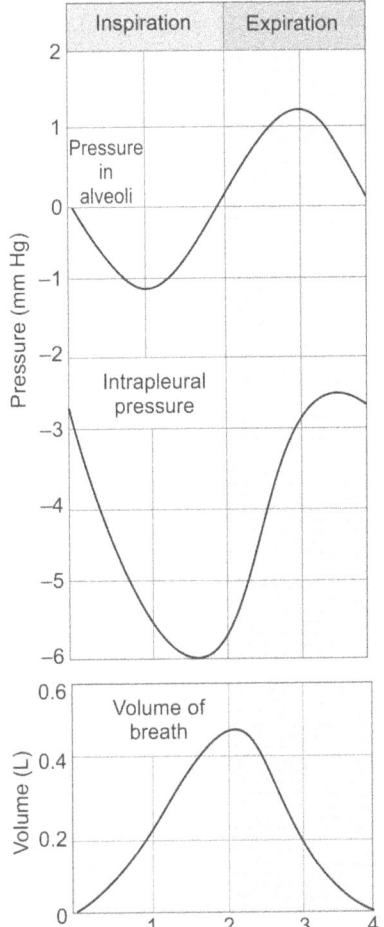

Fig. 6: Intrapleural pressure, intra-alveolar pressure and lung volume in inspiration and expiration.
(Source: GK Pal)

They are of three types:

a. **Anatomical dead space:** It is the volume of air present in the conducting zone of airways where no gaseous exchange takes place. It is from the nose to terminal bronchioles. Normal volume is 150 mL
b. **Alveolar dead space:** It is the volume of air in the alveoli which do not take part in gas exchange as in lung disorders. But in normal condition this volume is zero
c. **Physiological dead space or total dead space** = Anatomical dead space + Alveolar dead space.
= 150 + 0 = 150 mL.

15. Define histotoxic hypoxia with an example.

- Hypoxia is O_2 defeciency at the tissue level
- Histotoxic hypoxia is a condition in which the amount of O_2 delivered to the tissue is adequate but the tissue is unable to utilise O_2 due to toxic poisoning as in cyanide poisoning
- Here tissue oxidative process is affected by inhibition of cytochrome oxidases and other oxidative enzymes
- It is treated with Methylene blue or nitrites which form methemoglobin and this reacts with cyanide to form cyanmethemoglobin which is a less toxic compound.

16. What is Bell–Magendie law?

- Bell-Magendie law states that in the spinal cord the dorsal nerve roots are sensory and ventral nerve roots are motor.

17. Four functions of reticular activating system.

- RAS plays a role in sleep-wakefulness. It also induces alertness
- It plays a role in development of EEG waves, learning and memory
- Controls muscle tone—mainly through the descending reticular formation
- Since many visceral areas are located here it regulates visceral functions.

18. Functions of prefrontal lobe.

- In animals it is considered to be the seat of intelligence but in humans it is the seat of mind
- It controls the mood and feelings of the subject
- It is involved in higher functions like emotions, learning and memory
- It controls various intellectual activities like planning of future, concentration on actions, solving mathematical problems etc.
- It helps in appreciation and discrimination of odors
- It initiates movements in relation to emotions
- It plans the sequence of movements for an action along with motor cortex for actions.

19. What is endochochlear potential?

- The fluids in the cochlear compartments are responsible for the endocochlear potentials
- Endolymph in the scala media contains high K^+ concentration than the perilymph in the scala vestibuli and scala tympani
- There is a potential difference of +80 mV between the compartments with perilymph and endolymph due to this difference in ionic concentration. Positive inside scala media and negative outside it
- This potential is the endocochlear potential
- It is produced by the continuous K^+ secretory activity of stria vascularis lining the lateral wall of scala media.

Significance of this potential:

- The lower parts of the hair cells in organ of Corti are bathed in perilymph and the hairs are bathed in endolymph. There is difference in potentials of the hair cells in relation to perilymph (-70 mV) and endolymph (-150 mV)
- This potential difference sensitizes the hair cells to even minute bending of stereocilia and thereby responds to even minute sounds.

20. Delta waves in EEG.

- Frequency of these waves is 1–5 Hz
- Amplitude is 20–200 µV
- Delta waves occur in sleep in adults but present in infants during wakefulness
- When present in an awake adult it indicates brain damage.

21. Four functions of plasma protein.

Refer answers to 2004 paper.

22. Helper cells.

- There are 4 types of T lymphocytes—Helper T cells, Cytotoxic T cells, Suppressor T cells and Memory T cells.

Helper T cells
- These are the major types of T cells
- As the name implies they help the immune system; both cell-mediated and humoral immunity
- They secrete many interleukins and thereby help the immunity
- They are also called as CD 4 cells.

Helper T cells are activated in the following mechanisms
- Antigen which has entered the body is phagocytosed, digested and processed inside the macrophages and the peptide fragment of the antigen in the phagosome combines with the vesicle containing MHC II
- After fusion of the vesicles, the antigen binds with MHC II and both are incorporated in the cell membrane of Antigen presenting cell (Macrophage)
- The APC with the antigen and MHC II circulate in blood or in lymphatic tissues and the T cells with the receptor for the antigen recognize the antigenic fragment
- The T cell gets activated and undergoes differentiation and proliferation to form Helper T cells
- Helper T cells secrete Interleukin-2 which by autocrine and para crine influence activate other Helper T cells and also activate B cells and Cytotoxic T cells
- As the Helper T cells activate cytotoxic T cells and B cells it has an important role in cellular immunity and humoral immunity.

23. Kernicterus.
- It is seen in hemolytic disease of the newborn
- In this condition there is Rh incompatability between the Rh negative mother and Rh postive fetus
- The RBCs with Rh antigen from fetal blood enters mother's circulation at the time of delivery of first fetus
- Mother's immune system produces Anti D antibodies against D antigen and if the mother conceives for the second time with a Rh fetus, antibodies cross the placenta and affects Rh positive fetus
- It results in massive hemolysis and the bilirubin level increases and results in jaundice
- In fetus, the blood-brain barrier (BBB) is immature and the bilirubin crosses the BBB and affects the basal ganglia since it has affinity for bilirubin
- There are symptoms of motor dysfunctions.

24. Secondary active transport.
Refer answers to 2011 paper.

25. Rigor mortis.
- Rigor mortis is stiffening of muscles after the death of an individual
- Stiffness is due to sustained attachment of myosin heads to the actin filament due to loss of ATP
- After myosin cross-bridge attachment to actin filament, removal of the cross-bridge needs attachment of an ATP molecule
- After death there is no more ATP synthesized therefore the myosin heads stay attached to actin filament resulting in stiffness of muscle
- Rigidity disappears after some hours due to release of enzymes from lysosomes which will digest the muscle proteins
- The appearance and disappearence of rigor mortis is used to identify the time of death.

26. Name the second messengers.
Refer answers to 2008 paper.

27. Name the hormones involved for the growth.
- Thyroid hormone, growth hormone, androgen and estrogen are essential for growth
- Insulin is also essential for growth.

28. What is Turner's syndrome—three features?
- Turner's syndrome is a defect due to nondisjunction

- It is a condition in which a pair of chromosomes fails to separate so both go to one daughter cell during meiosis
- In individuals with XO chromosomal pattern, the gonads are rudimentary or absent so that the female external genitalia develops
- There is short stature, no sexual maturity at puberty and congenital abnormalities are present
- It is also called as Gonadal dysgenesis or ovarian agenesis.

29. APUD cells of its secretion.

- APUD (amine precursor uptake and decarboxylation) cells are present in the GIT and they secrete amines and polypeptides
- These cells are present in other organs like the lungs
- They are also neuroendocrine cells and carcinoid tumor originates from these cells.

30. Law of intestine.

Peristaltic waves are stimulated by distension of intestines. The wave created by distension spreads on either directions but the wave towards the oral side dies out. Therefore the peristaltic waves proceed only from oral to aboral direction and moves chyme only in the aboral direction.

31. Double Bhor effect.

- The fetal blood coming back to placenta carries more CO_2 and the CO_2 is released into the maternal blood
- The maternal blood pH drops because of the mixing of CO_2 and the maternal blood is more acidic than fetal blood
- So in this situation, the hemoglobin-oxygen dissociation curve shifts to left in fetal blood and in maternal blood to right side—Double Bohr's effect
- This helps fetus to receive sufficient oxygen.

32. Aldosterone escape.

- Aldosterone acts on the renal tubules in the DCT and Collecting duct
- It increases Na⁺ and water reabsorption in the renal tubules
- Therefore aldosterone increases water reabsortion and increases ECF volume
- However in hyperaldosteronism the increased retention of salt and water does not result in edema
- The absence of edema in hyperaldosteronism is due to release of Atrial natriuretic peptide (ANP) from right atrium following volume expansion
- ANP acts on the kidneys and induces natriuresis. This is said to be aldosterone escape phenomenon.

33. What are different types of water absorption?

There are two types of water reabsrption in the kidneys—obligatory and facultative reabsorption.

Obligatory reabsorption: 85% of the filtered water is reabsorbed by osmosis along with the solute reabsorption and this happens irrespective of body water balance. 67% of this is reabsorbed from PCT and 15 – 18% from Loop of Henle.

Facultative reabsorption: 15% of water reabsorption may or may not happen and is based on the body water balance. It happens in the collecting duct by action of ADH.

34. What is Houssay animal?

- It is an animal that has been pancreatectomized and hypophysectomized
- It is named after the discoverer of the principle that animals are more sensitive to insulin after removal of the pituitary, and that after this operation the intensity of diabetes in de-pancreatized animals is diminished
- This is because of decreased effect of growth hormone on blood glucose levels due to hypophysectomy.

35. Name the hormones involved in calcium homeostasis, and the main organs that will act.

The hormones involved in calcium homeostasis are:

Parathormone: It acts on the bones and stimulates bone resorption and thereby increases blood calcium levels. It also acts on the kidneys and increases calcium reabsorption. PTH stimulates synthesis of 1, 25 Dihydroxy cholecalciferol and thereby indirectly stimulates calcium absorption from the GIT.

1, 25 Dihydroxycholecalciferol: Acts on the GIT and stimulates absorption of calcium from the GIT. It also acts on the kidneys to increase calcium reabsorption.

PTH and 1, 25 Dihydroxycholecalciferol increase blood calcium levels.

Calcitonin: It is the only hormone which decreases blood calcium levels. It acts on the bones and kidneys. On the bones it decreases bone resorption and in kidneys it increases calcium excretion in urine.

36. Draw the diagram of alveocapillary membrane and write the thickness of it.

- The alveolocapillary membrane is also called as the respiratory membrane
- It seperates the blood in the capillaries and the air in the alveoli
- The gases which have to move from alveoli to capillary or in the opposite direction they have to diffuse across this membrane
- It is made up of alveolar epithelial lining, basement membrane and the capillary endothelial lining
- The thickness of the membrane is 0.2 to 0.5 µm (refer Fig. 7).

37. What is scuba?

Refer answers to 2010 paper.

38. Who discovered J receptors? What is its Physiological significance?

- 'J' receptors are Juxtapulmonary capillary receptors located adjacent to alveoli and can be stimulated by substances in pulmonary capillary blood
- They are the endings of unmyelinated C fibers in the alveoli
- It was discovered by an Indian Physiologist Dr AS Paintal
- They are stimulated by hyperinflation of lungs and also by intravenous or intracardiac injection of chemicals like capsaicin
- The immediate responses are apnea followed by rapid breathing, bradycardia and hypotension: These responses are called as **Pulmonary chemoreflex**
- Similar responses are seen in pulmonary edema, congestion and embolism due to chemicals released in these states.

39. What are otolith organs?

- There are two sac like structures in the vestibular apparatus, the utricle and saccule
- These are called as the otolithic organs
- Their receptor cells, hair cells are located in the receptor organs maculae
- The hairs of these cells are embedded in a gelatinous mass containing crystals of calcium carbonate – the Otoliths or Otoconia
- So these organs are called as otolithic organs (refer Fig. 8).

40. What is alpha block?

Refer answers to 2008 paper.

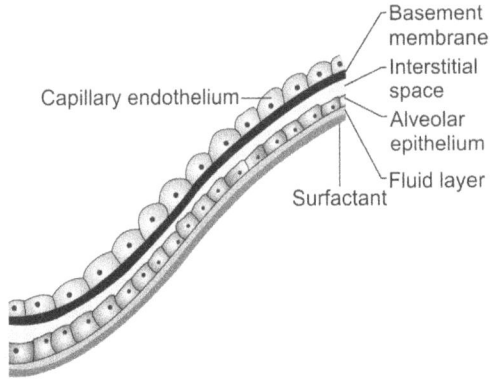

Fig. 7: Respiratory membrane.
(*Source:* Sembulingam)

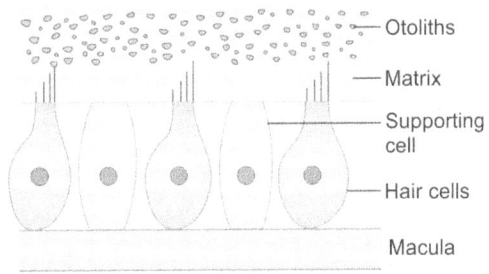

Fig. 8: Otolithic organ.
(*Source:* GK Pal)

41. Define Frank-Starling law.
Refer answers to question number 11, same section.

42. What is Monro-Kellie Doctrine law?
- Monro-Kellie doctrine: According to this phenomenon at any given time the contents within the cranial cavity is a constant
- The contents includes the brain, blood and CSF. So if any one component increases it is at the expense of the other two
- For example if there is an increase in cerebral venous pressure there is a similar increase in intracranial pressure (ICP) and these two decrease the blood flowing through the arteries.

43. What is stereognosis? Where is its center?
- The ability to identify familiar objects by handling them and without seeing them is called stereognosis
- The center is in the cerebral cortex, parietal lobe posterior to postcentral gyrus.

44. What are the functions of frontal lobe?
- Frontal lobe is divided into two main areas—precentral cortex and prefrontal lobe.

Precentral Cortex

This consists of the areas: Primary motor area (Area 4), Premotor area (Area 6), Supplementary motor area and Frontal eyefield (Area 8).

Functions
i. Primary motor area is responsible for initiation of voluntary movements in opposite half of the body and for speech. It aslo contributes 30% fibers for the corticospinal tract
ii. Premotor area also contributes 30% fibers for CST. It programs the skilled motor activity and thereby directs area 4 for its execution. It gives rise to certain extrapyramidal fibers like corticorubral, corticothalamic, fibers etc.
iii. Supplementary area coordinates movements on both sides of the body
iv. Frontal eye field controls voluntary conjugate movements of the eye.

Prefrontal Lobe

Refer answer for question number 18 in this same paper.

45. What are the mechanoreceptor? Give example.
- These are receptors which provide information about touch, pressure and vibration stimuli from the skin
- They are nerve endings of unmyelinated axon surrounded by lamellated connective tissue
- For example: Pacinian corpuscle (Receptor for vibration), Meissner's corpuscle (Receptor for touch).

46. What is summation? Mention its types.
- Summation means adding up of impulses
- In the synapse, following release of neurotransmitters there could be depolarisation or hyperpolarisation of the membrane
- These are called as postsynaptic potentials and they belong to the category of graded potentials
- So these individual potentials from many synapses can summate and excite the membrane and take it to the firing level
- There are two types of summations - Spatial and Temporal summation
- Temporal summation: The same input stimulates the postsynaptic neuron repeatedly and thereby excites it
- Spatial summation: Here many inputs stimulate the postsynaptic neuron simultaneously to excite it.

47. What are cholinergic and adrenergic receptors?

Cholinergic Receptors

- The receptors for acetylcholine are called as cholinergic receptors
- They are present on the postsynaptic neurons or the muscle membrane or on the secretory glands
- They are of two types—nicotinic and muscarinic receptors.

Adrenergic Receptors

- The receptors for adrenaline and noradrenaline are called as adrenergic receptors
- They are of two main types—α and β receptors
- There are subtypes for each one
- They are α1, α2, β1, β2, and β3 receptors.

48. Draw the structure of rods and cones.

See Figure 9.

49. What is the difference between the spasticity and rigidity?

Spasticity	Rigidity
Seen in pyramidal tract lesion	Seen in extrapyramidal lesion
Increased tone in only antagonistic muscles	Increased tone in both agonists and antagonists
Resistance to stretch is seen in initial phase and disappears later	Resistance is seen throughout the passive movement
Clasp-knife type	Cogwheel type and lead pipe rigidity

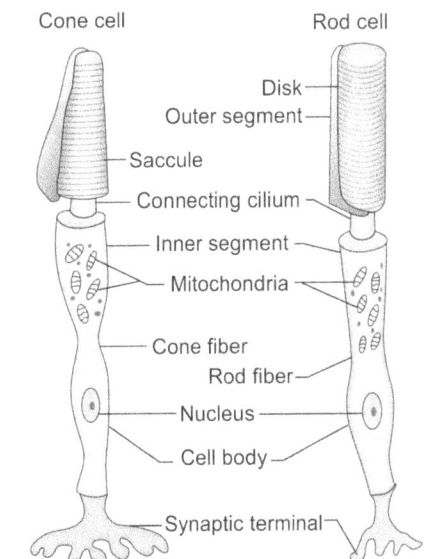

Fig. 9: Structure of rods and cones.
(*Source:* Sembulingam)

50. Define histotoxic hypoxia.

Refer answers to question 15, same section.

MBBS Examination 2012

ANSWER ALL QUESTIONS

I. Essay Questions (5/10/15 Marks each)

1. Explain the sliding filament hypothesis and outline the main events in the cross-bridge cycle. (10 marks)
2. Draw an oxygen dissociation curve and describe how oxygen is transported in the blood. Depict the Bohr's effect. (10 marks)
3. What are the components of gastric secretion? Explain the regulation of gastric secretion. (5 marks)
4. Classify pain. What are the receptors for pain? Describe the dual pathways for pain. What is analgesic system in the brain? (5 marks)
5. What are the normal blood sugar levels? Which hormones regulate the blood sugar level and how? Add a note on diabetes mellitus. (15 marks)
6. Discuss stages of erythropoiesis and the factors affecting it. Add a note on sickle cell anemia. (15 marks)
7. Define cardiac output. Discuss the factors affecting cardiac output and any one method of determination. What is the significance of ejection fraction in ventricular functioning? (15 marks)
8. List the ascending tracts in the spinal cord and discuss the tracts of posterior column with diagram. (15 marks)

II. Short Notes (2/5 Marks each)

1. Anticoagulants. (2 marks)
2. G protein. (2 marks)
3. Calcitriol. (2 marks)
4. Thyroid function tests. (2 marks)
5. Describe the Reflex Arcs involved in micturition. (2 marks)
6. Explain the renal contribution to pH control. (2 marks)
7. Tubuloglomerular feedback mechanism. (2 marks)
8. Functions of plasma proteins. (2 marks)
9. Hemophilia. (2 marks)
10. Countercurrent blood flow in the villi. (2 marks)
11. Frank-Starling law of the heart. (2 marks)
12. Cardiac pacemaker potential. (2 marks)
13. Draw a labelled diagram of a normal ECG in lead II. Write a brief note on PR interval. (2 marks)
14. Non-progressive shock. (2 marks)
15. Travelling waves in the ear. (2 marks)
16. Ventilation-perfusion ratio. (2 marks)
17. Caisson disease. (2 marks)
18. Brown-Sequard syndrome. (2 marks)
19. Functions of ascending reticular activating system. (2 marks)
20. Role of Purkinje cells of cerebellum. (2 marks)
21. Functions of platelets. (5 marks)
22. Composition and functions of gastric juice. (5 marks)
23. Molecular basis of skeletal muscle contraction. (5 marks)
24. Sertoli cells. (5 marks)
25. Rh blood group. (5 marks)
26. Movements of small intestine. (5 marks)
27. Functions of placenta. (5 marks)

28. Functions of mitochondria. (5 marks)
29. Puberty. (5 marks)
30. Functions of glucocorticoids. (5 marks)
31. Chemical regulation of respiration. (5 marks)
32. Functions of middle ear. (5 marks)
33. Hypovolemic shock. (5 marks)
34. Ventilation-Perfusion ratio. (5 marks)
35. Parkinson's disease with treatment. (5 marks)
36. Classification of nerve fibers. (5 marks)
37. Heart sounds. (5 marks)
38. Errors of refraction with correction. (5 marks)
39. Transport of oxygen in blood. (5 marks)
40. Waves of EEG. (5 marks)

III. Short Answers (1/2 Marks each)

1. Functions of Na^+-K^+ pump. (1 mark)
2. Saltatory conduction. (1 mark)
3. Conn's syndrome. (1 mark)
4. Laron dwarfism. (1 mark)
5. Aquaporins. (1 mark)
6. Anion gap. (1 mark)
7. Macula densa. (1 mark)
8. Opsonization. (1 mark)
9. Immunological memory. (1 mark)
10. Cholelithiasis. (1 mark)
11. Enterogastric reflex. (1 mark)
12. Peristaltic rush. (1 mark)
13. Progeria. (1 mark)
14. Pills. (1 mark)
15. Permissive action. (1 mark)
16. Astigmatism. (1 mark)
17. Ocular dominance columns. (1 mark)
18. Dicrotic notch. (1 mark)
19. Cardiac reserve. (1 mark)
20. Reynold's number. (1 mark)
21. J point. (1 mark)
22. Extrasystole. (1 mark)
23. Bell-Magendie law. (1 mark)
24. Cogwheel rigidity. (1 mark)
25. Betz cells. (1 mark)
26. Homunculus. (1 mark)
27. Anomic aphasia. (1 mark)
28. Timed vital capacity. (1 mark)
29. Pneumotaxic center. (1 mark)
30. Asphyxia. (1 mark)
31. Inulin clearance. (2 marks)
32. Oxytocin. (2 marks)
33. Fever. (2 marks)
34. Second messengers. (2 marks)
35. Functions of bile salts. (2 marks)
36. ESR. (2 marks)
37. Hypocalcemic tetany. (2 marks)
38. Placental hormones. (2 marks)
39. Myasthenia gravis. (2 marks)
40. Immunoglobulins. (2 marks)
41. Reynold's number. (2 marks)
42. Summation. (2 marks)
43. Herring-Breuer inflation reflex. (2 marks)
44. Taste receptor. (2 marks)
45. PR interval in ECG. (2 marks)
46. Chronaxie. (2 marks)
47. CSF formation. (2 marks)
48. Phasic changes in coronary circulation. (2 marks)
49. FEV1. (2 marks)
50. Dopamine. (2 marks)

I. ESSAY QUESTIONS

1. **Explain the sliding filament hypothesis and outline the main events in the cross-bridge cycle.**

Refer answer to 2011 paper.

2. **Draw an oxygen dissociation curve and describe how oxygen is transported in the blood. Depict the Bohr's effect.**

Refer answer to 2004 paper.

3. **What are the components of gastric secretion? Explain the regulation of gastric secretion.**

Refer answer to 2005 paper.

4. **Classify pain. What are the receptors for pain? Describe the dual pathways for pain. What is analgesic system in the brain?**

- Pain is an physical adjunct of an imperative protective reflex
- Pain can be induced by—mechanical, thermal or chemical stimuli
- **Two types of pain**—fast pain and slow pain

- **Receptors**—free nerve endings of Aδ and unmyelinated C fibers.

Pain Pathway

Refer answers to 2009 paper.

Analgesic System in the Brain

Pain modulation takes place in 2 places:
1. At the peripheral nerve endings
2. At the spinal cord level.

Peripheral Nerve Endings

Endorphins and Enkephalins combine with Nociceptors and decrease the response to stimuli.

At the Spinal cord

- **Peripheral mechanism: By gate control theory** – large Aβ fibers (when stimulated by touching or rubbing the painful area) ↓ Nociception in C fibers
- **Central pain suppressing mechanism:** Opioids secreted from areas in brain stem inhibit pain transmission in the spinal cord.

Gate control mechanism:

- Pain sensation is carried by Aδ and unmyelinated C fibers and they ascend up as spinothalamic tract
- Touch and pressure senstaions are carried by large myelinated Aβ fibers and they ascend up as dorsal column tract in spinal cord
- Dorsal column fibers in the spinal cord give a branch to inhibitory interneurons which secrete enkephalins and which in turn end on the second order neurons in pain pathway
- So, when there is pain in an area, touching or pressing that region stimulates the large Aβ fibers which in turn inhibit pain pathway and thereby there is decreased pain perception
- So the large Aβ fibers gate the pain pathway.

Central pain suppressing mechanism:

- Pain pathway, as it ascends up gives branches to periaqueductal grey (PAG) in midbrain
- There is a pain suppressing descending pathway from PAG to medulla and to spinal cord
- Axons of the neurons in PAG terminate on serotonergic neurons in Raphe magnus nuclei in Medulla
- They secrete Enkephalin here
- Axons of serotonergic neurons in raphe magnus nuclei descend and terminate on the inhibitiory interneurons in spinal cord
- They secrete serotonin and stimulate internuncial neurons which in turn inhibit second order neurons in the pain pathway by secreting enkephalin (refer Fig. 1).

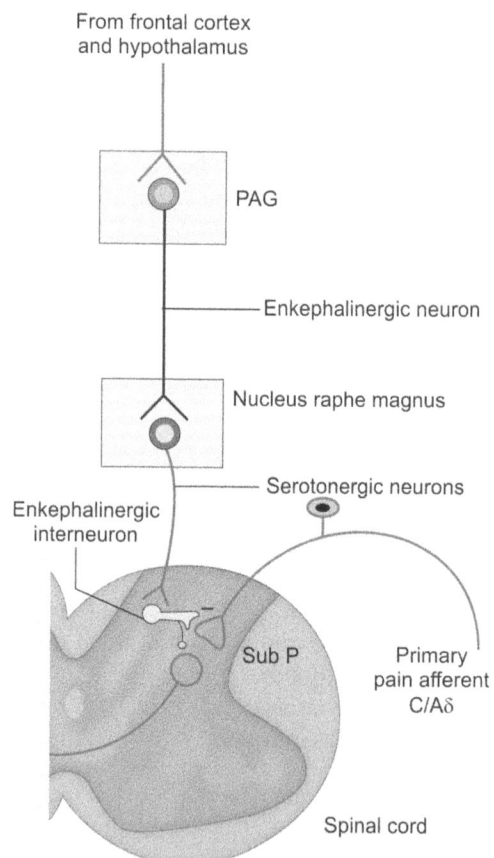

Fig. 1: Endogenous pain inhibition by spinal cord and brainstem structures. PAG: Periaqueductal grey. It has enkephalonergic neurons which end on serotonergic neurons of raphe magnus nucleus in medulla. They send out axons which end on Enkephalonergic neurons in spinal cord and decreases pain.
(*Source:* GK Pal)

5. **What are the normal blood sugar levels? Which hormones regulate the blood sugar level and how? Add a note on diabetes mellitus.**

Refer answer to 2007 paper.

6. **Discuss stages of erythropoiesis and the factors affecting it. Add a note on sickle cell anemia.**

Refer answer to 2006 paper.

Sickle Cell Anemia

- It is a hereditary disorder and the individuals affected have hemoglobin S (HbS)
- In hemoglobin S, the glutamic acid is replaced by Valine at the 6th position in beta chain of globulin portion of hemoglobin
- In conditions of hypoxia, the hemoglobin S crytalises and normal RBC changes its shape to become sickle shaped and the mebrane is rigid and undergoes rapid hemolysis and results in hemolytic anemia.

7. **Define cardiac output. Discuss the factors affecting cardiac output and any one method of determination. What is the significance of ejection fraction in ventricular functioning?**

Refer answers to 2011 paper.

Ejection Fraction

- It is the percentage of end diastolic volume which is ejected per beat
- Stroke volume is given as the percentage of EDV
- EF = SV/EDV × 100
- Normal value is about 65%
- It is a good indicator of left ventricular functioning.

8. **List the ascending tracts in the spinal cord and discuss the tracts of posterior column with diagram.**

Ascending Tracts in the Spinal Cord

I. Dorsal column—fasciculus gracilis and fasciculus cuneatus
II. Spinothalamic tracts—lateral and anterior spinothalamic tracts
III. Spinocerebellar tracts—dorsal and ventral spinocerebellar tracts
IV. Spinotectal tract
V. Spino-olivary tract
VI. Spinovestibular tract
VII. Spinoreticular tract.

Tracts of Posterior/Dorsal Column

- The posterior or dorsal column consists of the Tracts of Goll and Burdach
- They ascend up in two fasiculi—fasciculus gracilis and fasciculus cuneatus
- They are made up of large myelinated fibers which carry sensations like touch, pressure, vibration, stereognosis, tactile localisation, tactile discrimination and proprioception
- Gracile fasciculus lies medially and carries these sensations from the hind limb and trunk, the cuneate fasciculus lies laterally and carries impulses from the upper half of the body and upper limbs
- It is also called as the lemniscal system
- First order neurons have their cell bodies in the dorsal root ganglia
- The peripheral axons of these neurons are nerve fibers from the receptors
- The central axons from the dorsal root ganglia enter the spinal cord and ascend up in the dorsal column as the dorsal column tract
- Gracile and cuneate fasciculi reach medulla and synapse with ipsilateral nucleus gracilis and nucleus cuneatus respectively
- From these nuclei, the second order neurons arise and cross to the opposite side and ascend up as the medial lemniscus
- Medial lemniscus terminate on the venteroposterolateral nucleus (VPLN) of the opposite side thalamus
- Third order neuron arises from the thalamus and terminates in the somatosensory area 1 (Broadmann area 3, 1, 2) in postcentral gyrus (refer Fig. 2).

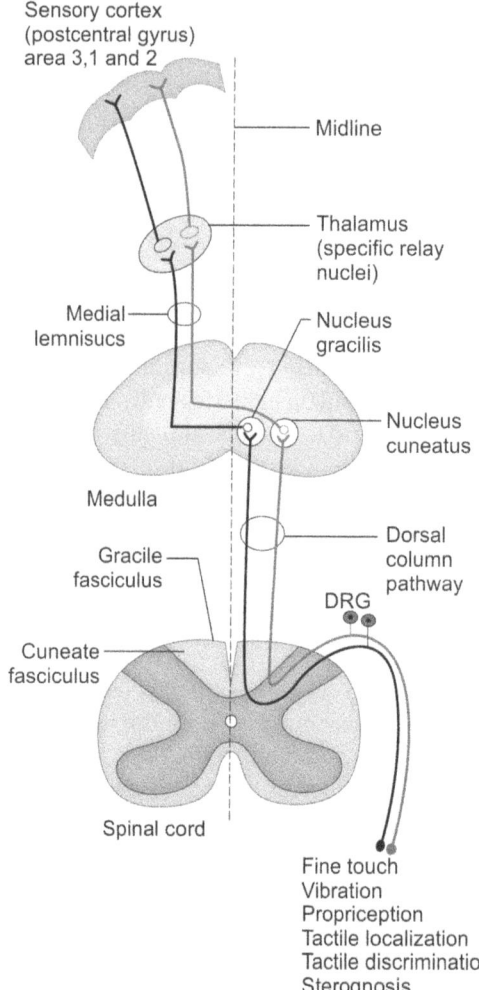

Fig. 2: Pathway of dorsal column tract.
(*Source:* GK Pal)

II. SHORT NOTES

1. Anticoagulants.
Refer answers to 2007 paper.

2. G protein.
- G proteins are nucleotide regulatory proteins that bind to GTP
- GTP is the guanosine analog of ATP
- There are two types of G proteins—Small G proteins and Large G proteins
- When signal reaches a G protein, the protein exchanges GDP for GTP and brings about the response. On completion of action, the intrinsic GTP ase activity of the protein converts GTP to GDP.

***Small G proteins:* These are involved in various cellular functions.**
- They are members of **Rab family:** Regulate vesicle traffic within a cell
- The **Rho/Rac family**, which mediates interaction between cytoskeleton and cell membrane
- The **Ras family** which regulates growth by transmitting signals from cell membrane to nucleus.

Larger Heterotrimeric G Proteins
- They couple cell surface receptors to catalytic units on the membrane that catalyzes formation of intracellular second messengers or couple receptors to ion channels
- There are 3 subunits for the G Protein - α, β and γ
- Only α Subunit is bound to GDP
- On binding of the ligand to G-protein coupled receptor, GDP is exchanged for GTP and α subunit is seperated from β and γ subunits (refer Fig. 3)
- The intrinsic GTPase activity of the α subunit converts GTP to GDP and the action is terminated.

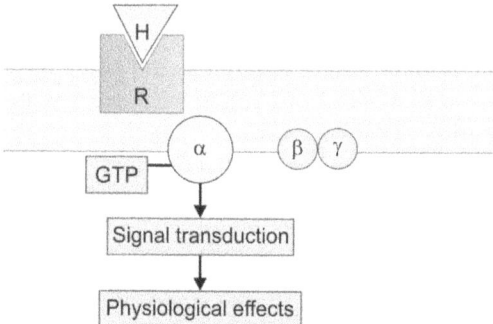

Fig. 3: On binding of hormone to G-Protein bound receptor activates G-protein. α Subunit seperates and G protein exchanges GDP for GTP. This induces series of actions and is responsible for hormone action.
(*Source:* GK Pal)

- There are 5 families of G protein—G_s, G_i, G_t, G_q and G_{13}.

Mechanism of Action through G Protein-Coupled Receptors

- Ligand (hormone) binds to the G_s protein coupled receptor
- On binding of ligand and receptor, α subunit of G protein seperates from β and γ subunits
- On seperation of α subunit, the catalytic enzyme—adenylyl cyclase (enzyme) attached to G protein is activated
- Adenylyl cyclase converts ATP to cAMP
- cAMP activates the enzyme protein kinase A which phosphorylates proteins and brings about changes (refer Fig. 4).

3. Calcitriol.

Calcitriol is the active form of vitamin D3 and is also called as 1, 25 Dihydroxycholecalciferol.

Synthesis of Calcitriol

Vitamin D3 is the precursor for synthesis of Calcitriol. Vitamin D3 is got from 2 sources:

Dietary intake: Fish and egg yolk are rich sources of vitamin D3. The daily requirement in India with good sunlight is 200 IU or 5 µg.

From the skin: Keratinocytes in the skin synthesize Vitamin D3 from 7-dehydrocholesterol, which is an intermediate in synthesis of cholesterol, by the action of sunlight. Pre Vitamin D3 is formed and is converted to Vitamin D3.

- Vitamin D3 is released into blood where it is bound to vitamin D binding protein and reaches the liver

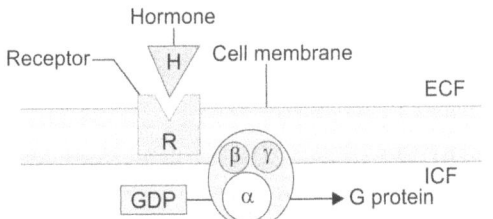

Fig. 4: G-Protein. Hormone binds to G-Protein bound receptor on the cell membrane; G Protein in inactive form is bound to GDP. There are 3 subunits for G-Protein-α, β, and γ. (*Source:* GK Pal)

- In liver, the next step in synthesis happens. Vitamin D3 is converted to 25 hydroxycholecalciferol by the enzyme 25 hydroxylase. This next reaches the kidneys in bound form
- The last step in synthesis happens in the kidneys. The enzyme 1α hydroxylase converts 25 hydroxycholecalciferol to 1, 25 dihydroxycholecalciferol or calcitriol. 24, 25-dihydroxycholecalciferol, a less active metabolite is also formed.

Regulation of Synthesis of Calcitriol

- **Plasma calcium levels:** Increase in plasma calcium levels decreases parathormone secretion which in turn decreases synthesis of calcitriol. Decrease in blood calcium levels increases PTH levels and calcitriol synthesis increases
- **Plasma phosphate levels:** Phosphate levels regulate synthesis of calcitriol by negatively inhibiting the enzyme 1, α hydroxylase
- **Levels of calcitriol:** The calcitriol has a direct negative feedback effect on its synthesis. It also acts on the parathyroid gland and inhibits synthesis of PTH
- **Other factors** like prolactin, estrogen, growth hormone, human chorionic somatomammotrophin and calcitonin stimulate synthesis and thyroid hormone excess and acidosis decrease synthesis.

Actions of Calcitriol

- **Action on GIT:** It increases absorption of calcium from the GIT by increasing its permeability of brush border of the enterocytes. It also increases synthesis of Calbindin, a calcium binding protein in enterocytes
- **Actions on bones:** It induces bone resorption and mineralization. In presence of PTH, calcitriol induces bone resorption
- **Action on kidneys:** It increases reabsorption of calcium and phosphates from the renal tubules
- **Other actions:** Increases calcium transport into skeletal muscles and bones, stimulation and differentiation of immune

cells, it regulates growth and induces formation of growth factors.

Applied Aspects

a. **Rickets:** It is a metabolic bone disease occurring due to deficiency of Vitamin D and there is defective calcification of bone matrix. It is seen in growing children.

Types of rickets:
- Nutritional rickets: Due to dietary deficiency of Vitamin D, either due to poor intake or poor absorption
- Due to inadequate exposure to sunlight: This happens in cities with less sunlight and children show symptoms by 6 months to 2 years of age
- Vitamin D resistant rickets: Vitamin D deficiency is not there but there is inactivating genetic mutation for renal hydroxylase and calcitriol is not formed
- Type II Vitamin D-resistance rickets—There is inactivation mutation of the gene for 1,25 dihydroxychloecalciferol receptor.

Symptoms of rickets:
- Weakness and bowing of weight-bearing bones, dental defects, hypocalcemia
- There could be widening of wrist, collapse of chest wall, kyphosis, pelvic deformities, frontal bossing and rickety rosary—beading of costochondral junction of ribs.

b. **Osteomalacia:** This is the adult counterpart of rickets.
Symptoms are vague like muscle pain and weakness, bony tenderness and Tetany in few cases.

4. Thyroid function tests.
Refer answers to 2003 paper.

5. Describe the Reflex Arcs involved in micturition.
Refer answers to 2009 paper.

6. Explain the renal contribution to pH control.

- Acids are produced by the body as byproducts of metabolism
- **They are of two types:**
  i. Volatile acids - Carbonic acid formed from CO_2
  ii. Non-volatile acids

Non-volatile acids are produced by the body as:
- Products of metabolism
- From diets like protein
- Strenuous exercise
- Starvation
- Renal tubular generation

Regulation of Acid-base Balance of Kidneys

It is by 3 processes:
i. H^+ secretion in PCT, Loop of Henle (LOH) and Collecting duct (CD) as Free H^+ (Very minimal), as Titrable acid and as Ammonium
ii. HCO_3^- reabsorption
iii. Generation of new HCO_3^- in Distal convoluted tubule (DCT) and collecting duct (CD)

- In most of the segments, H^+ secretion is coupled to HCO_3^- reabsorption as in proximal convoluted tubule (PCT)
- In PCT and Thick ascending limb of Loop of Henle (TAL of LOH) it is by Na^+ - H^+ exchanger and in I cells of CD it is by ATP driven proton pumps
- The renal epithelium secretes nearly 4300 mEq of H^+ daily, of which 85% is from PCT, 10% from DCT and 5% from CD.

H^+ Secretion in PCT

- The filtrate that reaches PCT contains Na^+, HCO_3^-, Cl^-, Glucose, amino acids etc.
- Epithelial cells lining the PCT secretes H^+ through the secondary active transporter Na^+ - H^+ exchanger
- The epithelial cells lining PCT has the enzyme carbonic anhydrase (CA). It also has many mitochondria
- In the cells, CO_2 released following metabolism, combines with water in the presence of CA to form H_2CO_3
- H_2CO_3 splits into H^+ and HCO_3^-
- On the luminal membrane, the Na^+-H^+ exchanger secretes H^+ into the lumen in exchange for reabsorption of Na^+

- As H^+ is being secreted, HCO_3^- is reabsorbed into the interstitium on the basolateral side through an anion exchanger in exchange for Cl^-
- Cl^-, on entering the cell diffuses into the lumen
- So for every H^+ being secreted into the lumen one bicarbonate is reabsorbed
- The H^+ which has entered the lumen does not stay as free H^+ and is buffered by the filtered HCO_3^-
- $H^+ + HCO_3^- \rightarrow CO_2 + H_2O$
- CO_2 enters into the epithelial cells and is recycled to form H^+ and HCO_3^-
- So the HCO_3^- which is reabsorbed is not the same HCO_3^- which was filtered
- The H^+ which was added to the tubular fluid does not decrease the pH of the fluid as it is buffered completely by the HCO_3^-
- So the pH of tubular fluid is not altered much in PCT (refer Fig. 5)
- Mechanism of H^+ secretion in LOH is similar to that of PCT secretion and it happens in the thick ascending limb of LOH.

Secretion of H^+ in DCT and Collecting Duct (Fig. 6)

- Epithelial cells lining DCT and 'I' cells of CD secrete H^+ through the primary active transporter – H^+ pump or H^+-K^+ pump
- These cells also contain CA and it catalyses:
  - $CO_2 + H_2O \rightarrow H_2CO_3$
  - $H_2CO_3 \rightarrow H^+ + HCO_3^-$
- H^+ is secreted into the lumen through the pumps
- HCO_3^- is reabsorbed into the interstitium
- The H^+ secreted binds to the monobasic phosphate (HPO_4^-) the major buffer present in the tubular fluid in DCT and CD. (By the time the fluid reaches DCT and CD, HCO_3^- is reabsorbed completely and therefore the buffering is done only by HPO_4^- and NH_3)
- The H^+ secreted is buffered and results in formation of:
  - $HPO_4^- + H^+ \rightarrow H_2PO_4$ (Titrable acid) (refer Fig. 6)
  - $NH_3 + H^+ \rightarrow NH_4$ (Ammonium)
- Since the H^+ is buffered and stays back in the fluid, pH drops in the tubule and reaches the value 6
- So this is the site in the renal tubule where maximal acidification of urine happens
- Here new bicarbonate is also generated.

Generation of New Bicarbonate

It is by two mechanisms:

i. Non-bicarbonate buffering:

- The H^+ secreted in excess of HCO_3^- reabsorption is buffered in the DCT by HPO_4^{2-} to form the **Titrable acid – H_2PO_4**
- The amount of H_2PO_4 formed is equal to new HCO_3^- formed and re-absorbed.

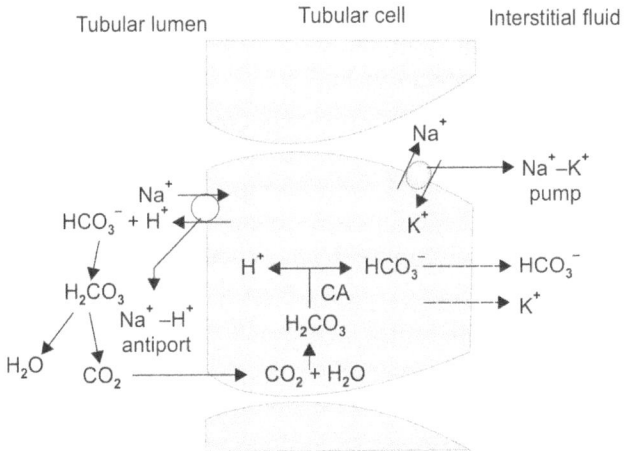

Fig. 5: Secretion of H^+ and reabsorption of HCO_3^- in PCT.
(*Source:* GK Pal)

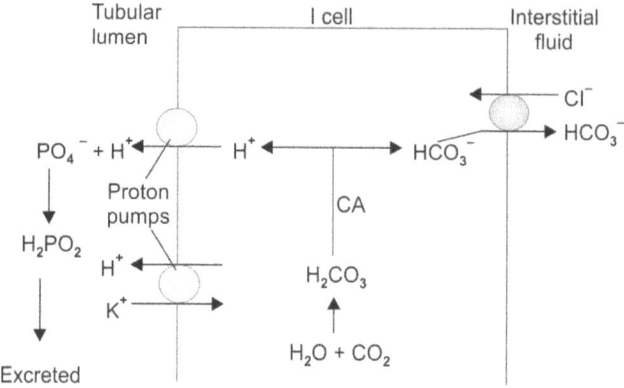

Fig. 6: H+ Secretion in DCT and Collecting duct.
(*Source:* GK Pal)

ii. By glutamine catabolism:
- Glutamine → Glutamate + NH_4
- Glutamate → α-Ketoglutarate + NH_4 + 2 HCO_3
- $NH_4 \leftrightarrow NH_3 + H^+$
- Glutamine metabolism happens in the PCT and it generates 2 HCO_3 and NH_3 for buffering H+ (refer Fig. 7)
- NH_3 is easily diffusible across cell membranes whereas NH_4 is not permeable through membranes
- In TAL of LOH, NH_4 is reabsorbed through Na^+-K^+-$2Cl^-$ where NH_4 occupies the transporter instead of K^+ and is taken into the interstitium. Here it stays in equilibrium with NH_3. NH_3 diffuses into cells of CD and is secreted into the CD lumen where it binds to H+ form NH_4. NH_4 cannot diffuse across the cell membrane and therefore stays in the urine to be excreted
- In metabolic acidosis, the amount of excretion of NH_4 is increased and decreases urinary pH accordingly.

7. Tubuloglomerular feedback mechanism.
Refer answers to 2008 paper.

8. Functions of plasma proteins.
Refer answers to 2009 paper.

9. Hemophilia.
Refer answers to 2008 paper.

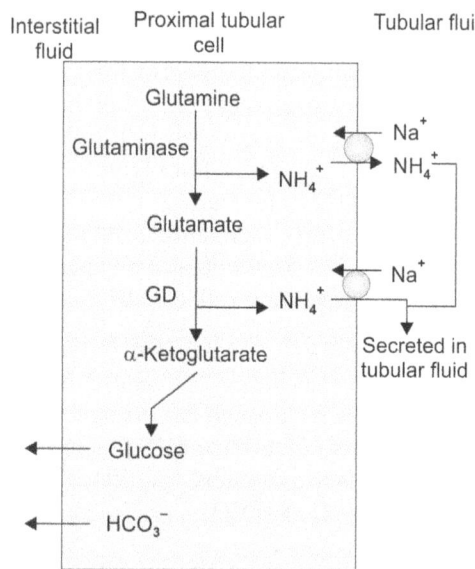

Fig. 7: Formation of ammonium and its excretion.
(*Source:* GK Pal)

10. Countercurrent blood flow in the villi.
- Countercurrent flow means flow of fluids, in two closely placed parallel tubes, in opposite directions and there is exchange of substances between the fluids in the tubes
- This mechanism is present in the kidneys, villi of intestines and in the cutaneous vessels
- In the intestinal villi it is between the capillaries and venules and the main arterioles

- The blood flow in these two vessels is in opposite directions
- The substance getting exchanged here is oxygen
- The countercurrent mechanism favors diffusion of oxygen from ascending arterial limb into the descending venous limb (without going through capillaries)
- So in conditions of slow flow rates, O_2 diffuses out of arterioles and enters the venules at the base of the villus.
- So the cells of the tips of villi suffer from hypoxia and they are prone for necrosis.

11. Frank-Starling law of the heart.

Refer answers to 2011 paper.

12. Cardiac pacemaker potential.

Refer answers to 2005 paper.

13. Draw a labelled diagram of a normal ECG in lead II. Write a brief note on PR interval.

Refer answers to 2005 and 2011 papers.

14. Non-progressive shock.

- It is a stage in shock where the amount of blood lost is less than 1 L. Various body mechanisms try to compensate the decrease in circulatory volume and try to correct the blood loss and cause full recovery without any treatment
- It is also called as compensated stage.

The following are the compensatory mechanisms:

- Immediate **tachycardia** and increase in pulse rate: Due to dcerease in blood volume, baroreceptors are inhibited which results in sympathetic nerve stimulation
- Sympathetic stimulation causes **vasoconstriction** in all the vessels except cerebral and coronary vasculature
- Sympathetic nerves also cause **venoconstriction** which results in increased venous return and thereby increased cardiac output and blood pressure
- Due to loss of RBC and stagnant blood flow, chemoreceptors are stimulated → **Tachypnea** → Thoracic pumping → Increases venous return (VR) and thereby Cardiac output and BP increase
- **Restlessness,** due to release of adrenaline → skeletal muscle activity → increase in VR
- Movement of interstitial fluid into capillaries → **Increases blood volume**
- Increased **secretion of Renin, Angiotensin II and aldosterone** → Reabsorption of electrolytes and water from tubules → Increase in blood volume
- Increased secretion of ADH
- Long-term compensations are increase in **erythropoiesis and plasma protein synthesis.**

15. Travelling waves in the ear.

- When sound waves travel in the middle ear and hit on foot plate of stapes and as a result it vibrates
- This creates pressure waves in the perilymph of scala vestibuli like ripples in water
- The waves displace the basilar membrane and make the hairs of the hair cells to tilt and thereby stimulate the nerves in the bases of the hair cells
- Wave of displacement of basilar membrane starts at the base of cochlea near the oval window and gradullay moves towards the apex
- These pressure waves are called as **Travelling waves**
- The site of maximum displacement of the basilar membrane is dependant on the frequency of sound waves
- Higher frequency sounds create maximum amplitude of pressure waves and thereby maximum displacement of basilar membrane at the base of cochlea and lower frequency waves induce a wave close to the apex of cochlea
- So based on place of stimulation of hair cells, the frequency or pitch discrimination of sound is possible.

16. Ventilation-perfusion ratio.

Refer answer 34 in this paper.

17. Caisson disease.

Refer answers to 2005 paper.

18. Brown-Sequard syndrome.

Refer answers to 2008 paper.

19. Functions of ascending reticular activating system.

- Reticular formation (RF) is located in the core of brainstem starting from the upper part of spinal cord to the lower part of diencephalon
- It is like a mesh with many neurons interspersed among bundles of axons
- Neurons in RF have both sensory and motor functions
- Ascending reticular activating system (ARAS) is a part of RF consisting of sensory fibers projecting to cerebral cortex (refer Fig. 8)
- It is an ascending column of fibers.

Functions of ARAS

- It helps to maintain consciousness and also arousal from sleep
- Controls sleep and wakefulness
- It helps in learning and memory
- Involved in genesis of EEG waves.

20. Role of Purkinje cells of cerebellum.

- Purkinje cells are present in the middle layer (Purkinje cell layer) in the cerebellar cortex
- It is the largest neuron with large amount of dendritic branches
- The dendrites of Purkinje cells project to the outermost layer of the cortex (Molecular layer) where they synapse with axons of the neurons in this layer
- The climbing fiber which is one of the afferents coming into the cerebellum ends on the Purkinje cells. Climbing fiber consists of Olivocerebellar tract which arises from Inferior olivary nucleus in Medulla
- Purkinje cells are the only output from the cerebellar cortex which project to the deep cerebellar nuclei
- The efferents leave the cerebellum from the deep nuclei (refer Fig. 9)
- Purkinje cells are involved in learning of motor tasks
- It has been experimentally proved by increased activity in climbing fibers when a motor task is being learnt

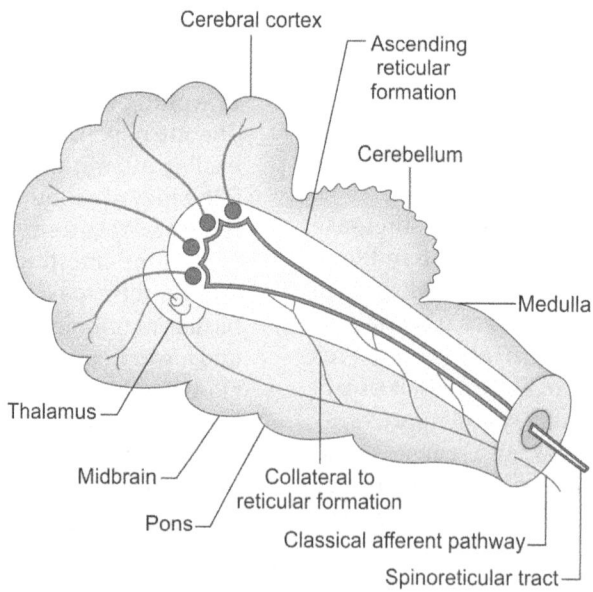

Fig. 8: Ascending reticular activating system.
(*Source:* Sembulingam)

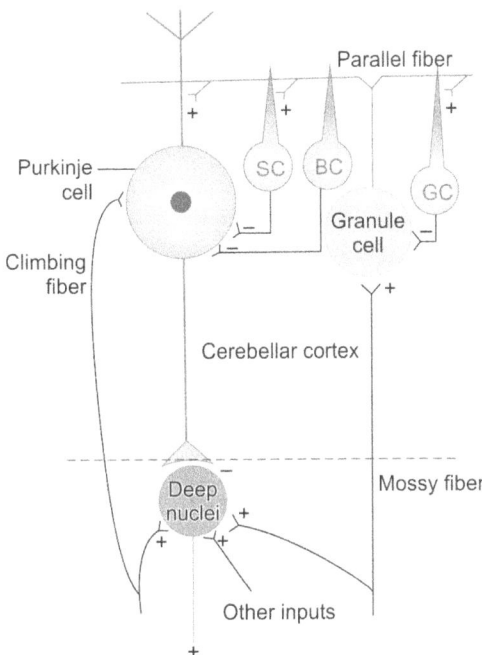

Fig. 9: Purkinje cells in cerebellar cortex. Afferents to cerebellum through climbing fibers end on Deep nuclei and Purkinje cell. Mossy fibers end on Granule cells. Output of cerebellar cortex is only through Purkinje cell.
(SC: Stellate cell; BC: Basket cell; GC: Golgi cell)
(*Source:* GK Pal)

21. Functions of platelets.
Refer answers to 2008 paper.

22. Composition and functions of gastric Juice.
Answers to 2005 and 2009 papers.

23. Molecular basis of skeletal muscle contraction.
Refer answers to 2011 paper.

24. Sertoli cells.
Refer answers to 2008 paper.

25. Rh blood group.
Refer answers to 2007 and 2009 papers.

26. Movements of small intestine.
Refer answers to 2006 paper.

27. Functions of placenta.
Refer answer to 2010 paper.

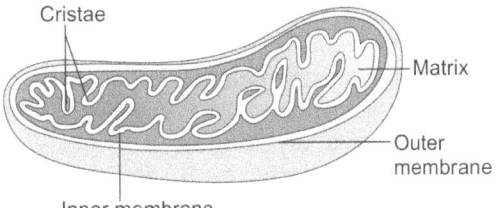

Fig. 10: Structure of Mitochondria.
(*Source:* Sembulingam)

28. Functions of mitochondria.
- Mitochondria is a sausage shaped organelle present in almost all the cells
- It has an outer and an inner membrane. The inner membrane is folded to form the cristae
- The space between two layers—intracristal space
- The space inside the inner membrane—the matrix (refer Fig. 10)
- Mitochondria are the power generating units of the cell and they are present more in cells involved in energy-requiring processes
- They produce energy rich ATP which is essential for many metabolic activities of the cell
- The outer membrane is studded with oxidative enzymes and they provide the raw materials for the reactions inside the matrix
- In the interior, there are enzymes which break down the substrates like carbohydrates, fats and proteins into CO_2 and H_2O
- The enzymes in the inner membrane are NADH dehydrogenase, Succinic dehydrogenase, Cytochrome C and Cytochrome oxidase
- During these reactions H^+ are pumped out and a proton gradient is created which will drive the enzyme, ATP synthase to form ATP
- Mitochondrion has its own genome but the DNA is less when compared to nuclear DNA
- It is helpful for synthesis of many components of oxidative phosphorylation
- It has a role in initiation of apoptosis of the cell.

29. Puberty.
- Puberty is defined as the period when the endocrine and gametogenic functions of

the gonads have developed to the level of reproduction
- The age of puberty in females is between 8-13 years and in boys it is between 9-14 years of age
- In males, testosterone is secreted in the fetus before birth and another time in the neonatal period. After that the Leydig cells (which secrete testosterone) remain quiescent
- Gonads of both sexes reach final maturation at puberty and start secreting sex hormones.

Control of Puberty

a. **Control by GnRH:**
   - Final maturation of the gonads and their hormone secretion are under the control of gonadotrophins
   - Gonadotrophins from anterior pituitary are under the control of GnRH from hypothalamus
   - At the time of puberty, GnRH starts to secrete in a pulsatile fashion. This pulsatility of GnRH secretion is kept under control by a neural mechanism till the time of puberty.

b. **Control by Leptin:**
   - The other control mechanism is thought to be the body weight of the individual. A critical body weight has to be reached to attain puberty
   - It is now understood that Leptin, a hormone secreted from adipose tissue is the link between body weight and onset of puberty.

Components of Puberty

- There are two components of puberty—a sudden growth spurt and development of secondary sexual characteristics
- The changes happening in puberty at various stages are given below in males and females:

Pubertal Changes in Females

Stages of puberty	Age in years	Changes in females
Stage 1	Upto 7½	Pre-adolescent
Stage 2	10½	Thelarche (appearance of breast bud)
Stage 3	11½	• Pubarche (appearance of axillary and pubic hair) • Breast enlargement (elevation) • Growth spurt
Stage 4	13	• Menarche (start of menstrual cycle) • Breast areola elevate and projects
Stage 5	14	• Adult genitalia • Secondary sexual characteristics

Pubertal Changes in Males

Stages	Age in years	Characteristics
Stage 1	7½	Pre-adolescent
Stage 2	12	Enlargement of testis
Stage 3	14	• Enlargement of penis • Appearance of axillary and pubic hair
Satge 4	15	• Further growth of testis, penis and genitalia • Growth spurt
Stage 5	16½	Adult genitalia and secondary sexual characteristics

Hormonal Changes during Puberty

- **FSH and LH** levels are low from birth to childhood. But at the time of puberty their levels increase following the pulsatile secretion of GnRH
- **Adrenal androgen** increases towards puberty, 8-10 years in girls and 10-12 years in boys. This called as Adrenarche. It is essential for the growth of axillary and pubic hair in both males and females
- **Growth hormone** levels are intermittent with peaks every day. At the time of puberty, the frequency and amplitude of these peaks are increased and it induces growth spurt in boys and girls
- **Thyroid hormone** levels also increase at the time of puberty and is needed for the growth hormone to promote growth
- **Sex hormone** levels increase after puberty.

Applied Aspects of Puberty

Precocious puberty: Early onset of puberty below 8 years of age.
It can be:
- True precocious puberty
- Pseudoprecocious puberty

True Precocious Puberty

It is usually due to decreased inhibition of pulsatile secretion of GnRH. Therefore there is an early otherwise normal puberty. It is more common in girls.

Causes:
a. Constitutional (without any cause)
b. Cerebral—disorders of posterior hypothalamus, tumors, infections
c. Gonadotrophin independent precocity.

Pseudoprecocious Puberty

This is due to early devlopment of secondary sexual characteristics without gametogenesis due to abnormal exposure of males to androgens and females to estrogens.

Causes:
a. Adrenal: Congenital virilizing hyperplasia, Androgen secreting tumors in males and estrogen secreting tumors in females
b. Gonadal: Leydig cell tumors of testis and Granulosa cell tumors of ovaries.

Delayed Onset of Puberty or Absent Puberty

Puberty is considered to be delayed if in females the menarche does not appear till 17 years of age and no testicular development till age of 20 in males.

Causes:
- Failure of hypothalamus or anterior pituitary to secrete gonadotrophins as in Panhypopituitarism
- Primary gonadal failure as in Klinefelter syndrome or Turner's syndrome.

Symptoms:
- Short stature
- Features of other endocrinal abnormalities
- Delay in puberty.

30. Functions of glucocorticoids.
Refer answers to 2006 paper.

31. Chemical regulation of respiration.
Refer answers to 2005 paper.

32. Functions of middle ear.
Refer answers to 2003 paper.

33. Hypovolemic shock.

It is a syndrome in which there is inadequate tissue perfusion related with absolute or relative decrease in cardiac output. It is also called as 'cold shock'.

Types of Shock
i. Hypovolemic shock
ii. Distributive shock
iii. Cardiogenic shock
iv. Obstructive shock.

Causes for Hypovolemic Shock
- Trauma
- Hemorrhage
- Surgery
- Burns
- Fluid loss due to vomiting or diarrhea.

Stages of Shock
Reversible and irreversible shock.

Hypovolemic Shock

Symptoms are:
a. Hypotension
b. Rapid thready pulse
c. Skin is cold and clammy with greyish tinge
d. Intense thirst
e. Rapid breathing
f. Restlesness
g. Increased lactic acid production.

Stages of Shock
Reversible and irreversible shock.

1. Reversible or Non-progressive Shock

It is a stage in shock where the amount of blood lost is less than 1 L and various body mechanisms try to compensate the decrease in circulatory volume and to correct and cause full recovery without any treatment.

It is also called as compensated stage.

The following are the compensatory mechanisms: Refer "Compensatory mechanisms" in answer 14 of the same paper.

Refractory Shock
- Depending upon the amount of blood lost many patients die soon after the blood loss

- Some recover with the compensatory mechanisms and with appropriate treatment
- But in some patients the shock persists for hours and it progresses to refractory shock. There is no improvement with treatment and cardiac output stays decreased
- This happens because of operation of various positive feedback mechanisms
- Severe blood loss → Depression of vasomotor center → Vasodilatation and decrease in heart rate → Further drop in BP → Further drop in cerebral blood flow → further depression of VMC and cardiac areas
- Severe shock → Coronary blood flow is decreased due to hypotension and tachcardia → Decreased myocardial contractility → Further decrease in cardiac output → Further decrease in coronary blood flow
- Acidosis makes the situation worse.

If no treatment is advocated refractory shock leads to:
- Depletion of ATP
- Tissue damage and necrosis
- Acute tubular necrosis in kidneys
- Respiratory distress: Shock lung syndrome.

Treatment

Treatment should aim at correcting the cause and restoring the circulatory volume.

General Treatment
- Patient should be kept at room temperature
- Raise the foot end of patient's bed to increase venous return.

Treating the Cause
- In hemorrhagic, traumatic and surgical shock the cause is blood loss, so immediately compatible whole blood should be transfused
- IV fluids can be given temporarily
- In burn shock, plasma is lost and there is hemoconcentration. So plasma should be infused. Plasma expanders which hold the fluid in the capillary can also be given.

34. Ventilation-perfusion ratio.

- It is the ratio of ventilation to the lungs to the blood flow through pulmonary circulation
- Alveolar ventilation (V_a) is 4000 L/min and perfusion (Q) is equal to cardiac output, 5 L/min
- So V_a/Q ratio = 4/5 = 0.8
- Ventilation as well as perfusion increases from the apex to the base of the lungs due to the effect of gravity
- But rate of increase of perfusion is more than the increase in ventilation
- So V_a/Q ratio is more in the apex (3.3) than the base (0.63)
- The high O_2 content in the apex favors the growth of TB bacilli there
- The V_a/Q ratio can get altered in conditions of uneven ventilation and non-uniform blood flow to alveoli as in certain disease conditions.

Decreased V_a/Q Ratio

- In conditions where there is inadequate ventilation to the alveoli and normal perfusion, the oxygenation of blood and removal of CO_2 are not normal
- So alveolar PO_2 falls and PCO_2 rises (refer Fig. 11A)
- So it is like the deoxygenated blood empties directly into the left atrium
- So it is like a physiological shunt.

Causes

Bronchial asthma, pneumothorax, emphysema, pulmonary fibrosis.

Increased V_a/Q Ratio

- When perfusion through pulmonary capillary is decreased in relation to alveolar ventilation the ratio increases
- Alveolar PCO_2 falls and PO_2 increases (refer Fig. 11B)
- As the alveolus is under-perfused it is like wasted ventilation and is like increased physiological dead space.

Causes

- Anatomical shunts in the heart like Fallot's tetralogy

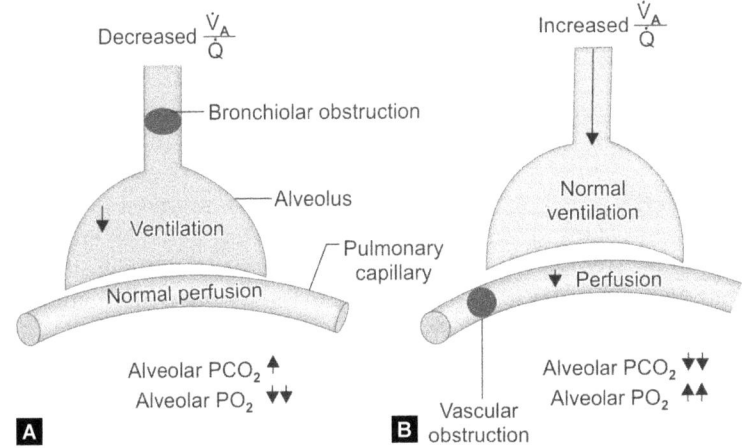

Figs. 11A and B: V_a/Q ratio in complete airway obstruction and complete circulatory obstruction conditions.
(*Source:* GK Pal)

- Decrease in vascular bed as in emphysema
- Pulmonary embolism.

35. Parkinson's disease with treatment.

Refer answers to 2005 paper.

36. Classification of nerve fibres.

- Nerve fibers are classified based on their functions—sensory and motor nerves
- Based on myelination—myelinated and unmyelinated nerves
- But the most accepted classification is the Erlanger-Gasser classification
- It is based on the myelination, thickness of the nerve and its conduction velocity.

I. Erlanger-Gasser Classification

Fiber type	Functions	Fiber diameter (μm)	Conduction velocity (m/s)	Myelination
Aα	Proprioception, Somatic motor	12–20	70–120	Myelinated
Aβ	Touch, Pressure	5–12	30–70	"
Aγ	Motor to muscle spindle	3–6	15–30	"
Aδ	Pain, cold, touch	2–5	12–30	"
B	Preganglionic autonomic	<3	3–15	"
C Dorsal root	Pain, temperature, mechano reception, some reflex response	0.4–1.2	0.5–2	Unmyelinated
Sympathetic	Postganglionic sympathetics	0.3–1.3	0.7–2.3	"

I. Numerical classification:

Sensory nerves are classified as Ia, Ib, II, III and IV

Number	Origin	Fiber type
Ia	Muscle spindle, Annulospiral ending	Aα
Ib	Golgi tendon organ	Aα
II	Muscle spindle, Flower spray ending Touch, pressure	Aβ
III	Pain and cold receptor Some touch receptor	Aδ
IV	Pain, temperature and other receptor	Dorsal root C

II. Classification based on sensitivity of nerves to agents like hypoxia, pressure and local anesthetics:

Susceptibility to	Most susceptible	Intermediate	Least susceptible
Hypoxia	B	A	C
Pressure	A	B	C
Local anaesthetics	C	B	A

37. Heart sounds.

Refer answers to 2006 paper.

38. Errors of refraction with correction.

Refer answers to 2004 paper.

39. Transport of oxygen in blood.
Refer answers to 2004 paper.

40. Waves of EEG.
Refer answers to 2006 paper.

III. SHORT ANSWERS

1. Functions of Na⁺-K⁺ pump.
- It pumps out 3 Na⁺ molecules from ICF to ECF and takes in 2 molecules of K⁺. When Na⁺ is pumped out water also move along with it. Thereby it maintains cell volume and prevents rupture of cell
- It maintains the resting membrane potential of the cell. This is essential for transmission of impulses in nerves and muscles
- It is the major energy-using process of the cells in the body and therefore it is responsible for the basal metabolic rate
- It maintains a high intracellular K⁺ levels and a high Na⁺ concentration in the ECF.

2. Saltatory conduction.
Refer answers to 2005 paper.

3. Conn's syndrome.
Refer answers to 2009 paper.

4. Laron dwarfism.
- Laron dwarfism is a type of dwarfism in which the plasma growth hormone levels are normal or even elevated but the growth hormone receptors are insensitive to the hormones
- The insensitivity is due to a loss-of-mutation of the gene for the receptors
- The plasma level of IGF-1 is also reduced.

5. Aquaporins.
- Water diffusion across the cell membrane in human beings depends on water channels made of proteins—aquaporins
- There are 12 aquaporins identified and classified as two groups—AQP 0, 1, 2, 4, 5, 6 and 8 are permeable only to water and AQP3, 7, 9, 5 and 10 are permeable to water and small solutes like glycerol.
- Aquaporins 1, 2 and 3 are found in the kidneys, aquaporin-4 in the brain, 5 in the salivary glands, lacrimal glands and in respiratory tract
- Aquaporins responding to ADH in the kidneys belong to aquaporin-2. AQP 1 is present in apical and basolateral membranes of cells in PCT
- They are stored in the collecting duct epithelial cells in endosomes and on activation by ADH, the vesicles translocate to the luminal cell membrane and causes water reabsorption
- Aquaporin-9 is found in the human leucocytes, liver, lungs and spleen.

6. Anion gap.
- Anion gap refers to the difference in plasma concentration of cations (other than Na⁺) and concentration of anions (other than Cl⁻ and HCO_3^-) and consists mostly of proteins which are anionic, HPO_4^-, SO_4^{2-} and organic acids
- The normal value is 12 mEq/L. It is used to differentiate between types of metabolic acidosis.

Factors which Increase Anion Gap
- Decrease in plasma concentration of Ca^{2+}, K⁺ or Mg^{2+}
- Increase in concentration of plasma proteins
- Increase in plasma levels of organic anions like lactate or foreign anions.

Factors which Decrease Anion Gap
- When the above cation levels are increased in the plasma
- When the plasma albumin levels are decreased.

Anion Gap is Increased in
- Diabetic ketoacidosis
- Lactic acidosis
- All forms of acidosis.

7. Macula densa.
- It is a component of juxtaglomerular apparatus
- It is a specialized renal tubular epithelial cell at the junction of thick ascending limb of loop of henle with distal convoluted tubule

- They are in close contact with Juxtaglomerular cells and lacis cells, the mesangial cells
- It is also close to afferent and efferent arterioles
- They act as chemoreceptors
- They sense the NaCl content in the tubular fluid
- By sensing this they are responsible for the tubuloglomerular feedback and regulation of renal blood flow and thereby the GFR.

8. Opsonization.

- Opsonization is a process of coating the bacteria, after it enters the circulation, to make them tasty for the phagocytes to engulf them and favors phagocytosis
- Opsonins are—IgG, complement proteins; C5a, C3b.

9. Immunological memory.

The antibody response to an antigen is of 2 types:
- *Primary response:* It is the first response when the body encounters the antigen for the first time. The immunological response happens after 4 to 30 days
- *Secondary immune response:* This is the body's response to an antigen entering for the second time into the host's system. The response is swift, rapid and abundant. This is because the immune system retains the memory of an antigen exposed previously and responds immediately due to the presence of memory cells (Both T and B cells). This memory is retained for long periods—immunological memory.

  It is seen in both humoral and cell-mediated immunities.

10. Cholelithiasis.

Presence of stones in gallbladder and bile duct is cholelithiasis.

There are two types of stones:
a. **Cholesterol stones**—85% of biliary stones are cholesterol stones. Bile salts and lecithin solubilizes cholesterol and keeps it in solution.
   - But if levels of cholesterol increases or levels of bile salts decrease, cholesterol stones are formed
   - The factors which favour gall-stone formation are: Bile stasis, supersaturation of bile with cholesterol and nucleation factors like glycoproteins in the mucus favors gall stone formation.

b. **Calcium bilirubinate stones**—15% of stones belong to this type.

Symptoms:
- Bile stones by themselves do not produce any symptoms but when they are in the bile duct and cause obstruction, they induce severe colicky pain
- There may be obstructive jaundice also.

It is diagnosed by ultrasound or cholecystography.

11. Enterogastric reflex.

- Entry of acidic chyme into the duodenum inhibits gastric secretion
- Presence of digested proteins and acid in duodenum inhibits gastric emptying—by enterogastric reflex
  - *Inhibition of gastric secretion:* Presence of food in the intestine initiates a reflex through enteric nervous system and extrinsic sympathetic and vagus nerves and thereby inhibits gastric acid secretion. The presence of acids and protein break down products in upper intestine and its distension inhibits gastric secretion
  - *Inhibition of gastric emptying:* The food when it enters the duodenum initiates a nervous reflex and inhibits gastric emptying through—enteric nerves, extrinsic inhibitory sympathetic nerves and through inhibition of vagus nerve to stomach.

The factors in duodenum which intiates enterogastric reflex and inhibit gastric emptying are:
a. Distension of duodenum
b. Irritation of duodenal mucosa
c. Degree of acidity of chyme in duodenum
d. Hyper and hypo-osmolality of chyme in duodenum
e. Presence of protein break down products in the duodenal chyme.

12. Peristaltic rush.

- Normally peristaltic waves are weak
- But in conditions of severe intestinal irritation as in intestinal infections there is intense rapid, powerful peristalsis—*peristaltic rushes*
- It is mediated through autonomic nerves and brainstem and also by intrinsic enhancement of myentric plexuses
- The strong peristaltic waves move the chyme for longer distances within minutes and thereby sweep the contents of intestine into the colon and thereby relieve the intestine of its irritating chyme and distension.

13. Progeria.

- Progeria is called as Hutchinson-Gilford Progeria syndrome
- It is an extremely rare, progressive genetic disorder that causes children to age rapidly, beginning in their first two years of life
- Children with progeria appear normal at birth
- During the first year, signs and symptoms, such as slow growth and hair loss, begin to appear.

Signs and Symptoms

- Slow somatic growth, with below-average height and weight
- Narrowed face, small lower jaw, thin lips and beaked nose
- Head disproportionately large for face
- Prominent eyes and incomplete closure of the eyelids
- Hair loss, including eyelashes and eyebrows
- Thinning, spotty, wrinkled skin
- Visible veins
- High-pitched voice
- Heart problems or stroke are the eventual cause of death in most children with progeria
- The average life expectancy for a child with progeria is about 13 years, but some with the disease die younger and some live 20 years or longer.

Cause of Progeria

- Researchers have discovered a single gene mutation responsible for progeria
- The gene, known as lamin A (LMNA), makes a protein, necessary for holding the center (nucleus) of a cell together
- When this gene has a defect, researchers believe the genetic mutation makes cells unstable, which appears to lead to progeria's aging process.

14. Pills.

By pills we mean the oral contraceptive pills used for contraception. In females, they are usually synthetic preparation of estrogen, progesterone or combination of both.

The pills can be of different types:

a. Combined pill or classical pill
b. Sequential pill
c. Minipill
d. Post-coital pill.

Combined pill: It is a combination of estrogen and progesterone. It contains a strip of 21 tablets and is consumed for 21 days from 5th day of menstrual cycle. After 21 days, on stopping the tablets, withdrawal bleeding happens. Again from 5th day the next cycle is started.

It acts by:

- Prevents ovulation, as the high estrogen levels disorganize the LH and FSH secretions
- Prevents implantation of fertilized ovum as the endometrial changes are disorganized
- Progesterone makes the cervical mucus thick and prevents sperm penetration.

Sequential pill: It has high dose of estrogen and minimal amounts of progesterone. It is not used nowadays as the high estrogen levels may induce endometrial cancer or breast cancer.

Minipill: It is progesterone only pill. It does not affect ovulation but makes the cervical mucus thick and prevents sperm penetration.

Post-coital pill: It is used within 72 hours of unprotected intercourse. It has high doses of estrogen and is given for 4–6 days. In this condition the high estrogen prevents implantation of the fertilized ovum rather than inducing changes in gonadotrophin secretion.

Depot preparation: These are implants of progesterone and they are subdermally implanted and prevent pregnancy for 5 years. The only problem is, it can cause amenorrhea.

There are also male contarceptive pills:

Gossypol: A phenolic derivative of cottonseed oil. It induces azoospermia.

Testosterone: High testosterone levels induce azoospermia.

15. Permissive action.

The presence of glucocorticoids is essential for the physiological actions of other hormones—permissive action of glucocorticoids.

The permissive actions of cortisol are:

- Vasoconstrictive action of catecholamines require the presence of glucocorticoids
- Lipolytic actions of catecholamines need the presence of glucocorticoids
- For bronchodilator action of catecholamines
- For calorigenic action of glucagon and catecholamines
- Synthesis of surfactant by fetal lung and for the lung maturation.

16. Astigmatism.

Refer answers to 2009 paper.

17. Ocular dominance columns.

- Ocular dominance columns are a feature of the visual cortex
- The cells in Lateral geniculate body (In thalamus) and the layer 4 cells of visual cortex receive inputs only from one eye
- Layers of cells receiving inputs from one eye alternate with cells receiving input from the other eye
- If radioactive amino acids are injected in one eye they are incorporated into proteins and by way of axoplasmic flow go out of the eye through axons of ganglion cells, to geniculate body and via geniculocalcarine fibers to visual cortex
- So in layer 4 of visual cortex, the radioactive labelled endings from the injected eye alternate with unlabelled endings from uninjected eye
- As a result when viewed from above a vivid pattern of alternating dark and light stripes are seen
- These are said to be the Ocular dominance columns.

18. Dicrotic notch.

Refer answers to 2009 paper.

19. Cardiac reserve.

- It is the amount of blood that can be pumped out of each ventricle in excess of the normal cardiac output (as in during exercise)
- Normal value is 15–25 L/Min.

20. Reynold's number.

Refer answers to 2010 paper.

21. J point.

- It is the point in ECG where the S wave meets the isoelectric line
- This is an indicator of end of ventricular depolarisation and start of ventricular repolarisation (refer Fig. 12).

22. Extrasystole.

- Extrasystole is a premature beat originating from an ectopic focus either in the atrium or the ventricle
- If it is from atria it is atrial extrasystole and if it is from ventricle it is a ventricular extrasystole
- The electrical activity from the ectopic focus in an ECG is called as an ectopic wave

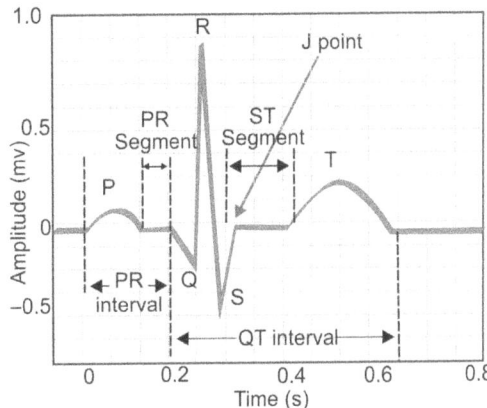

Fig. 12: Normal ECG in Lead II. J point is marked with arrow.
(Source: GK Pal)

- Configurations of the ectopic waves are abnormal (P wave or QRS complex)
- Atrial extrasystole can be benign and are seen in conditions like anxiety, excess consumption of coffee, tea
- QRS complex of the ventricular ectopics are bizarred in shape and appears earlier than expected
- There is a compensatory pause following the extrasystole
- Ventricular extrasystole is also seen in both normal and abnormal conditions.

23. Bell-Magendie law.

Refer answers to 2011 paper.

24. Cogwheel rigidity.

- It is a type of rigidity seen muscles in Parkinson's disease
- Here resistance to passive movement disappears intermittently during the stretch of the muscle.
- It is like series of catches during passive movement.

25. Betz cells.

- The cerebral cortex is histologically divided into 6 layers
- Layer 1: Molecular layer or plexiform layer
- Layer 2: External granular layer
- Layer 3: External pyramidal layer
- Layer 4: Internal granular layer
- Layer 5: Internal pyramidal layer
- Layer 6: Fusiform layer
- Layer 5 contains the large pyramidal cells called as the Giant cells of Betz
- These are usually seen in the primary motor area (area 4)
- Their dendrites reach the outer layer and their axons project to the brainstem and spinal cord and terminate there.
- They give rise to 3% of fibers to corticospinal tract

26. Homunculus.

- Representation of the whole body in the somatosensory area 1 and primary motor cortex are called as sensory homunculus and motor homonculus respectively
- The whole body is represented upside down in the homunculus (refer Fig. 13)

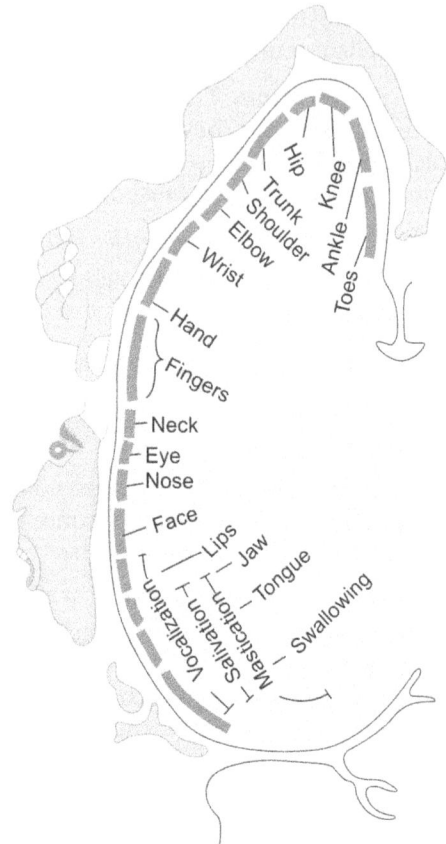

Fig. 13: Homunculus.
(Source: Sembulingam)

- In sensory homunculus the body parts with more number of receptors have a larger representation. For example the lips, fingers which have more numbers of receptors have a larger area of representation than the trunk and lower limbs
- In motor homunculus the parts with fine, skilled movements have larger areas of representation, for example, hand, thumb etc.

27. Anomic aphasia.

- It is a type of difficulty in speech due to lesion in the angular gyrus (area 39)
- The person has no difficulty in speech or understanding of auditory information
- But there is trouble in understanding written language and pictures because the visual information is not processed and transmitted to Wernicke's area
- It is also called as word blindness.

28. Timed vital capacity.
Refer answers to 2007 paper.

29. Pneumotaxic center.
- It is the respiratory center in the pons
- Located in nucleus parabrachialis and Kolliker-Fuse nucleus in the rostral medulla
- It is active during both inspiration and expiration
- It co-ordinates switching between inspiration and expiration
- Normally it inhibits apneustic center.

30. Asphyxia.
Refer answers to 2005 paper.

31. Inulin clearance.
Refer answers to 2005 paper.

32. Oxytocin.
- Oxytocin is an oligopeptide with 9 amino acids and is secreted from posterior pituitary
- It is synthesized from magnocellular neurons of paraventricular nucleus of hypothalamus and is secreted into circulation from posterior pituitary.

Functions of Oxytocin
- It stimulates milk ejection reflex (Refer answers for August 2008 question paper)
- It induces parturition reflex (Refer answers for august 2008 question paper)
- It also acts on non-pregnant uterus to facilitate sperm transport
- In males, it is secreted during ejaculation and causes contraction of smooth muscles of vas deferens to propel the sperm towards urethra.

33. Fever.
- Fever is the increase in body temperature above normal range. It is a symptom of infection
- Fever can be induced by infections like bacterial or viral infections
- It can be non-infectious as in inflammations like rheumatoid arthritis, injuries, malignancies etc.
- It is induced by chemical called as pyrogens. They can be exogenous or endogenous pyrogens
- *Exogenous pyrogens* enter the body from outside through micro-organisms. For example, endotoxin of gram-negative bacteria is an exogenous pyrogen.

Endogenous Pyrogen
Refer answers to 2010 paper.

Fever is a defense mechanism against the disease. It eliminates the disease by:
- The high temperature kills the micro-organisms
- Fever stimulates enzymatic activity and kills the pathogen
- Fever stimulates production of antibodies.

34. Second messengers.
- Second messengers are intracellular signalling molecules formed as a result of series of reactions following the binding of peptide/protein hormones with their cell membrane receptors
- Hormone binding with the receptor is the first messenger.

The major second messengers are:
- Cyclic AMP (cAMP)
- Diacyl glycerol (DAG)
- Inositol triphosphate (IP3)
- Cyclic GMP (cGMP)
- Ca^{2+}.

Second messengers formed depends on the hormone signaling of the effector cells.

The signal transduction pathways activated are depending on G protein activation of membrane enzymes.

35. Functions of bile salts.
a. *Digestion and absorption of fats:* Bile salts have detergent action and emulsifies fats into smaller molecules on which the pancreatic lipase acts and aids in digestion of fats
b. *Absorption of fats:* The bile salts along with lecithin forms micelles because of their amphipathic nature. The lipids are kept in the core of the micelles and are made water-soluble and carried to the enterocytes. The micelle move to the brush border of the enterocytes and the lipids diffuse out of the micelle and is absorbed into the brush border

c. **Choleretic action:** Bile salts are present in the bile and they stimulate further secretion of bile from the liver
d. Bile salts on entering the intestine are converted into bile acids and are added to the bile acid pool of the body
e. Bile salts also help in *absorption of fat-soluble vitamins*
f. Bile salts along with lecithin solubilize cholesterol and *prevent formation of gallstones*
g. Bile salts are synthesized from cholesterol and when its excretion is increased more *cholesterol is lost* from the circulation.

36. ESR.

- Erythrocyte sedimentation rate is the rate at which the RBCs get settled down when anti-coagulated blood is allowed to stand in a narrow tube
- This happens because the RBCs have the property of piling on each other – Rouleaux formation
- The piled up RBCs get heavy and they settle down.

The stages of ESR are:
- Stage of aggregation
- Stage of falling
- Stage of settling down.

The normal value is 3–7 mm/hr in males and 5–9 mm/hr in females.

Factors Affecting ESR

It depends on the shape and number of RBCs and Plasma factors like fibrinogen and Globulin.

RBC

Biconcave shape favors rouleaux formation, spherical and sickle cells inhibit Rouleaux formation.

Anemia increases ESR and Polycythemia decreases ESR.

Plasma Factors

- Fibrinogen and globulin neutralize the negative charges on RBC and attract them and favours rouleaux formation
- Acute phase reactive proteins secreted during acute infections and inflammations will also neutralize the negative charges on RBC and increase ESR.

Other factors are body temperature and plasma viscosity.

Significance of ESR

- ESR is increased in many diseases and therefore does not have any diagnostic value
- It is elevated in chronic inflammatory conditions like rheumatoid arthritis
- It is used to assess the prognosis of a disease when the patient is getting treated.

Variations in ESR

Physiological variations:

Increased in pregnancy, is more in females and newborns.

Pathological variations:

- Increased in:
  a. Acute and chronic inflammations
  b. Tuberculosis
  c. Malignancies
  d. All anemias except hereditary spherocytosis and sickle cell anemia.
- Decreased in:
  a. Polycythemia
  b. Sickle cell anemia
  c. Hereditary spherocytosis.

37. Hypocalcemic tetany.

Refer answers to 2008 paper.

38. Placental hormones.

Refer answers to 2010 paper.

39. Myasthenia gravis.

Refer answers to 2005 paper.

40. Immunoglobulins.

- Immunoglobulins (Ig) or antibodies are of 5 types
- The structure of IgG forms the basic structure of all other types of Igs
- IgG is "Y" shaped and made of 4 polypeptide chains—2 heavy chains and 2 light chains
- The chains are held together by disulfide bonds (refer Fig. 14)
- The two heavy chains are long and light chains are short

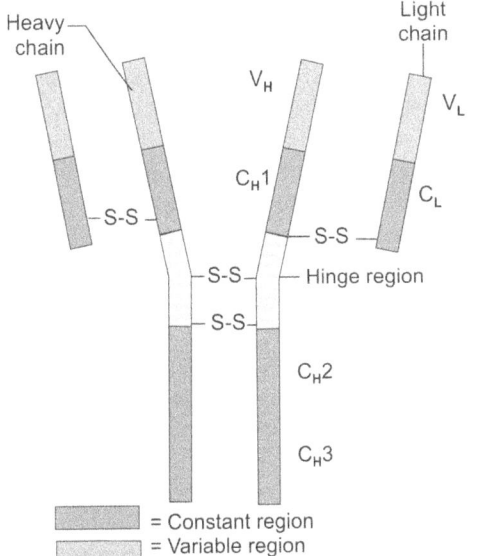

Fig. 14: Structure of immunoglobulin.
VL - Variable region of light chain, VH - Variable region of heavy chain, CL - Constant region of light chain CH1, CH2 & CH3 - Constant regions of heavy chain.
(*Source*: Sembulingam)

- There are 2 types of light chains κ (kappa) and λ (lambda) and there are 8 types of heavy chains
- Each light chain is in parallel with a part of heavy chain and the rest of heavy chain is a separate limb on each side.
- The adjoining region is the hinge or joining segment (J) and the amino acids are moderately variable
- The remaining region is said to be the constant region (C) and is common to all the Igs of the particular type of immunoglobulin
- Each light chain also has a V, and a C segment
- The V segment of both the chains (Fab portion) is the antigen binding sites and the Fragment crystallizable (Fc) portion of the molecule is the effector portion which mediates the reactions of antibodies.

Types of Immunoglobin

- IgG: It is a monomer and it has the function of complement activation and is an opsonin. It can cross the placenta. Rh antibodies belong to this category
- IgA: It is a monomer or dimer. It is present in the secretions of the body like the tears, breast milk etc, therefore it is called as 'secretory immunoglobulin'
- IgM: Complement fixation, ABO antibodies belong to this category
- IgD: Antigen recognition by B cells
- IgE: Reagin activation, releases histamine from basophils and mast cells.

Refer answers for 2009 paper for formation and functions of immunoglobulins.

41. Reynold's number.

Refer answers to 2010 paper.

42. Summation.

Refer answers to 2011 paper.

43. Herring - Breuer inflation reflex.

- Hering and Breuer found that over inflation of the lungs results in decreased output through the phrenic nerves to the diaphragm and thereby stimulates expiration
- This reflex is a protective reflex to prevent over inflation of the lungs
- The receptors are slowly adapting nerve endings of the myelinated vagus nerves in the airways of the lungs
- This reflex is stimulated by steady increase in lung volume resulting in immediate and prolonged expiration
- It is more useful in infants than adults and it regulates the tidal volume in infants.

44. Taste receptor.

- Taste receptors are epithelial cells and are located in the taste buds
- Cells in taste receptor are of three types:
  - Type 1 and 2—are supporting cells
  - Type 3 cells—receptor epithelial cells which have microvilli projecting into the taste pore on the dorsum of the tongue and they respond to the tastants.
- They extend to full length of the taste buds
- They are replaced constantly in 10 days
- Each taste bud has 50–150 taste receptor cells
- Each bud is innervated by 50 nerves at bases of receptor cells
- Each nerve innervates 5 taste buds

- On sectioning the nerve taste bud degenerates
- Taste buds are located in—fungiform, filiform and vallate papillae.

45. PR interval in ECG.
Refer answers to 2011 paper.

46. Chronaxie.
Refer answers to 2009 paper.

47. CSF formation.
Refer answers to 2009 paper.

48. Phasic changes in coronary circulation.
Refer answers to 2011 paper.

49. FEV1.
Refer answers to 2012 paper.

50. Dopamine.
- It is secreted by small intensely fluorescent cells (SIF) in the autonomic ganglia and in the brain. It is also secreted by the adrenal medulla
- In basal ganglia, it is secreted by the nigrostriatal pathway and is very important clinically as the defeciency of dopamine in this pathway results in Parkinson's disease
- Dopamine in circulation causes renal and mesentric vessel vasodilatation. It can also indirectly through release of norepinephrine can cause vasoconstriction. The net effect is increase in systolic BP and no change in diastolic BP. Therefore it is used in treatment of traumatic and cardiogenic shock
- It is synthesized from the amino acid tyrosine
- It is metabolised to inactive compounds by Monoamine oxidase (MAO) and Catechol-O-Methyltransferase (COMT) pathways
- There are 5 different types of receptors for dopamine—D1, D2, D3, D4, and D5
- Most of the receptors act through G proteins
- D2 and D4 receptors are increased in Schizophrenia and blockers of these receptors help to treat schizophrenia
- It is the neurotransmitter responsible for addiction behavior. The part of brain associated with addiction is Nucleus accumbens in the base of striatum.

MBBS Examination 2013

ANSWER ALL QUESTIONS

I. Essay Questions (7.5 Marks each)

1. Define hemostasis. Describe in detail about extrinsic and intrinsic mechanism of clotting?
2. Give an account of composition and functions of pancreatic juice. How is the secretion regulated?
3. Define cardiac cycle. Describe in detail the pressure volume changes that occur during a cardiac cycle with suitable diagram.
4. Describe the connections and functions of hypothalamus.
5. What are blood groups? Discuss their importance.
6. Describe the hormonal regulation of human menstrual cycle.
7. Describe the process of transport of carbon dioxide from tissues to lungs.
8. Describe in detail the photochemical mechanism of vision and mechanism of dark adaptation.
9. Describe digestion and absorption of fat in the digestive tract. Write a note on steatorrhea.
10. What do you understand by the terms innate and acquired immunity? Describe the phenomenon of cell-mediated immunity.
11. Define the term blood pressure. Discuss the determinants and regulation of blood pressure.
12. Trace the pathway for perception of pain. Discuss the descending pain modulatory pathways. Discuss the terms 'Gating of pain' and 'Referred pain'.

II. Short Notes (2.5 Marks each)

1. Erythroblastosis fetalis.
2. Isotonic and isometric contraction.
3. Facilitated diffusion.
4. Enterohepatic circulation.
5. Juxtaglomerular apparatus.
6. Countercurrent exchanger.
7. Transport maximum (Tm).
8. Acromegaly.
9. Steps in thyroxine synthesis.
10. Stages of spermatogenesis.
11. Functional residual capacity and its significance.
12. Types of hypoxia and its cause.
13. Respiratory membrane.
14. Neural centers for regulation of respiration.
15. Dead space.
16. Pacemaker potential.
17. Cardiac index.
18. Dark adaptation.
19. Functions of basal ganglia.
20. Vestibulocerebellum.
21. Tests for ovulation.
22. Contraceptives.
23. Thyroxine synthesis.
24. Tetany.
25. Dialysis.
26. Gastric emptying.
27. Enterohepatic circulation.
28. Functions of saliva.
29. Autoimmune disease.
30. Decompression sickness.
31. Middle ear functions.
32. Define cardiac output. What are the methods to measure the cardiac output?

33. Heart sounds.
34. Define synapse and describe its properties.
35. Describe the functions of thalamus.
36. What are the functions of basal ganglia?
37. Describe the physiology of speech.
38. Decerebrate rigidity.
39. Functions of prefrontal lobe.
40. G-Protein coupled receptors.
41. Primary active transport.
42. Autoregulation of GFR.
43. Renal glycosuria.
44. Mechanism of bicarbonate generation in distal tubule.
45. Stimuli for secretion of aldosterone and actions of aldosterone.
46. Pancreatic C-peptide and its significance as a laboratory test.
47. Cretinism—its cause, features and strategy to prevent it.
48. What is the function of corpus luteum of pregnancy? How is it supported?
49. Parturition.
50. Ionic basis of the pacemaker potential.
51. Windkessel effect of aorta.
52. Illustrate with a diagram, the left ventricular volume and pressure changes during a cardiac cycle.
53. Role of myelin sheath in conduction of nerve impulse.
54. Functions of hypothalamus.
55. Clinical features of cerebellar lesions.
56. Physiological roles of muscle spindle.
57. Chemical regulation of respiration.
58. Hamburger's chloride shift.
59. Role of surfactant in pulmonary function.

III. Short Answers   (1 Mark each)

1. Chronaxie.
2. Motor unit.
3. Apoptosis.
4. Osmotic diuresis.
5. LH surge.
6. Somatomedins.
7. Hormones of adrenal cortex.
8. Types of diabetes.
9. Action of paratharmone on bone.
10. Menarche.
11. Muscles of inspiration.
12. P50.
13. End diastolic volume.
14. Attenuation Reflex.
15. Perimetry.
16. Summation.
17. Referred pain.
18. Types of memory.
19. Thalamic syndrome.
20. Kluver Bucy syndrome.
21. Functions of sodium potassium ATPase pump.
22. Mention the normal value of GFR and substance used to measure GFR.
23. Enumerate heat loss mechanism.
24. Peristalsis.
25. What is the role of vitamin K in the body?
26. What is the normal blood calcium level?
27. Name the hormones of adrenal cortex.
28. Name the hormones of placenta.
29. Cryptorchidism.
30. Why are ovarian cycles suppressed during lactation?
31. What is P50?
32. What are the types of hypoxia?
33. Mention common refractory errors of the eye.
34. SA node as pacemaker.
35. PR interval.
36. Reflex arc.
37. Functions of cerebrospinal fluid.
38. What is righting reflex?
39. Name the nuclei responsible for hunger and satiety in human being.
40. What is referred pain?
41. Extracellular fluid volume and blood volume in an adult male weighing 70 kg.
42. Calcium transporters on the membrane of sarcoplasmic reticulum.
43. Mechanism of edema in congestive cardiac failure.

44. State a manifestation of hypocalcemic tetany. Give one cause leading to this condition.
45. List the vitamin K-dependent coagulation factors.
46. Rh status of mother, father and child for occurrence of Rh incompatibility.
47. Role of tropomyosin in muscle contraction.
48. Type of acetylcholine receptor on skeletal muscle and its function.
49. Hormones secreted by hypothalamus.
50. Hormonal defect in: (a) Addison's disease (b) Conn's syndrome.
51. List the calcium transporters on the sarcoplasmic reticular membrane in the ventricular muscle.
52. State Starling's law of the heart.
53. What is the effect of 2, 3 diphosphoglycerate on the oxygen-hemoglobin dissociation curve? Does it help in loading or unloading of oxygen?
54. What are the types of hypoxia?
55. Region of the cochlea which vibrates most for the highest sound frequency in the audible range.
56. Visual field defect when the optic chiasma is cut in the center.
57. State the refractive error in astigmatism. How is it corrected?
58. What is 'Blind spot'?
59. Receptors for vestibular sensation.
60. Name of tracts made up by second order neurons in the pathway for: (a) Fine touch (b) Pain.

I. ESSAY QUESTIONS

1. **Define hemostasis. Describe in detail about extrinsic and intrinsic mechanism of clotting?**

Refer answers for 2003 and 2007 papers.

2. **Give an account of composition and functions of pancreatic juice. How is the secretion regulated?**

Refer answers for 2006 paper.

3. **Define cardiac cycle. Describe in detail the pressure volume changes that occur during a cardiac cycle with suitable diagram.**

Refer answers for 2005 paper.

4. **Describe the connections and functions of hypothalamus.**

Refer answers to 2008 paper.

5. **What are blood groups? Discuss their importance.**

Refer answers to 2007 paper.

6. **Describe the hormonal regulation of human menstrual cycle.**

Refer answers to 2007 paper.

7. **Describe the process of transport of carbon dioxide from tissues to lungs.**

Refer answers to 2010 paper.

8. **Describe in detail the photochemical mechanism of vision and mechanism of dark adaptation.**

Structure of Rods and Cones

- Rods are named because of their structure
- They have 4 parts—outer segment, inner segment, nucleus and synaptic terminal
- The cones also have similar parts but the outer segment differs
- In the rods, outer segments contain membranous disks arranged in stacks (refer Fig. 1)
- The disks contain the photopigment (Rhodopsin)
- They are constantly renewed
- In cones the outer segment is broader at the base and tapers above and there are no stacks of disks, but there are infoldings of membrane
- Cone pigments are present in the membrane of infoldings.

Photopigments

- The photopigments are made up of two parts—opsin and retinal
- Opsin is a glycoprotein and there are 4 types in the eye, one for rods and 3 for three different cones
- Retinal is derived from vitamin A and exists as *cis*-retinal form

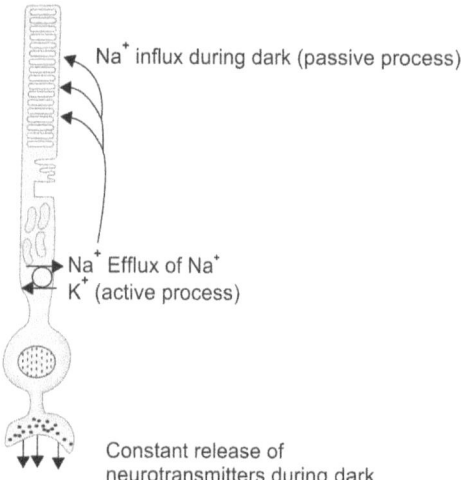

Fig. 1: Structure of rod and the flow of Na⁺ current from inner segment to outer segment in darkness results in depolarisation and release of neurotransmitters.
(Source: GK Pal)

- Photo sensitive pigments are present in the rods and cones
- In the rods it is: Rhodopsin—Retinene1 + Scotopsin
- In cones also, there is Retinene 1 but 3 different types of Opsins in the 3 types of cones
- The 3 cone pigments are: Red-sensitive pigment (560 nm), Green-sensitive pigment (530 nm) and Blue-sensitive pigment (420 nm). (Numbers denote the absorption of light by the pigments at various wavelengths of light)

Phototransduction

- When light strikes the eye there are potential changes which results in generation of action potential in ganglion cells and is transmitted via Optic nerves
- This conversion of light energy to electrical action potential is called as phototransduction
- Before seeing what happens when light strikes the eye, we should know what happens in the eye in dark.

In Darkness

- There are Na⁺ channels in the outer segments of the rods and cones. And they are open in dark. There is a gradient for Na⁺ movement from inner to outer segment and also to the terminals of the rod
- These Na⁺ channels are cGMP dependent and in darkness, guanylyl cyclase hydrolyses GTP to cGMP and cGMP keeps the channel open
- This results in decrease in potential in the synaptic terminal which results in opening of voltage-gated Ca^{2+} channels
- There is Ca^{2+} influx followed by exocytosis of neurotransmitter vesicles (glutamate)
- So the photoreceptor is depolarised in dark or rest.

In Presence of Light

- In the dark, the retineine$_1$ in rhodopsin is in 11-*cis* configuration
- When light strikes the eye the only action of eye is to change the shape of retineine to all-*trans* configuration (refer Fig. 2)
- After the conversion, retineine seperates from Opsin which is called as "Bleaching" effect
- This in turn activates the configuration of Opsin and the changed Opsin will activate the associated G protein, transducin

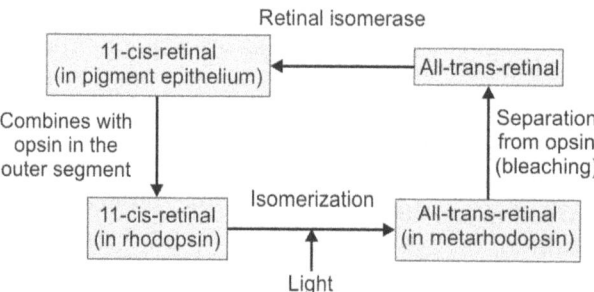

Fig. 2: Effect of light on conversion of Reteneine$_1$.
(Source: GK Pal)

- The G protein exchanges GDP for GTP and the α subunit seperates and remains active till the intrisic activity of GTPase hydrolyzes the GTP
- The activated α subunit activates cGMP phosphodiesterase which converts cGMP to 5'GMP
- Decline in cytoplasmic levels of cGMP causes closure of Na^+ channels and there is hyperpolarisation of the rods
- On activation of the receptors, there is hyperpolarization of rods, which finally results in depolarisation of ganglion cells and propagation of action potentials in Optic nerves
- After this, some of the all-*trans* retinal gets converted back to 11-*cis* retineine by the enzyme retinal isomerase then reassociates with opsin, to replenish Rhodopsin
- Some 11-*cis* retineine is also synthesized from Vitamin A.

Light strikes the eye
↓
Change in configuration of retineine1 of Rhodopsin
↓
Change in confirmation of photopigment
↓
Activation of transducin
↓
Activation of Phosphodiesterase
↓
Decrease in level of cytoplasmic cGMP levels
↓
Closure of cGMP dependent Na^+ channels
↓
Hyperpolarisation of rods
↓
Decreased release of neurotransmitter
↓
Response in bipolar and other cells
↓
Action potential in ganglion cells and impulse transmission in optic nerve

9. **Describe digestion and absorption of fat in the digestive tract. Write a note on steatorrhea.**

Dietary fat consists of neutral fats—triglycerides and also phospholipids, cholesterol, free fatty acids and lecithin. It also has fat-soluble vitamins.

Digestion of Fats

- There are fat-digesting enzymes in the mouth, stomach and pancreatic juice
- Lingual lipase is secreted by the Ebner's gland on the dorsal surface of tongue
- Lingual lipase starts its action while in the stomach and digests 30% of triglycerides. Gastric lipase is of little importance in digestion of fats except in conditions of pancreatic insufficiency
- Most of the digestion of fats begin in the duodenum by the action of pancreatic lipase
- It acts on the fats emulsified by bile salts
- Action of lipase is potentiated by the action of colipase, an enzyme which is also present in the pancreatic juice.

Emulsification of Fats by Bile Salts

- Emulsification means breaking down of large fat molecules into smaller molecules by the detergent action (lowering of surface tension) of bile salts
- The bile salts are amphipathic and their hydrophobic tails face the center (where fat droplets are placed) and the heads are hydrophilic and they face the water in the lumen
- This property along with the intestinal movements break the fat droplets to smaller molecules
- The breaking down of fats into smaller molecules is essential as it increases the surface area on which the pancreatic lipase can act
- Pancreatic lipase is water-soluble and it can act only on lipid-water interface of the fats.

Digestion of Fats by Lipolytic Enzymes

- Fat digestion begins mostly in duodenum by the action of pancreatic lipase
- Pancreatic juice is rich in enzymes and HCO_3^- and thereby it changes the pH of chyme from 6 to 7. This is the optimal pH for the action of lipases

- Colipase is an enzyme secreted by pancreas which opens up a lid like structure in the amphipathic helix so that Lipase can act on triglycerides
- Lipase acts on 1- and 3- bonds of triglycerides and on 2-bond at a low rate and the products of digestion are free fatty acids and 2-monoglycerides
- The other lipase present in pancreatic juice is bile salt- activated lipase and it hydrolyzes the cholesterol esters, esters of fat-soluble vitamins, phospholipids and triglycerides
- Cholesteryl ester hydrolase in pancreatic juice hydrolyzes cholesterol esters
- Phospholipase A2 hydrolyzes Phospholipids and seperates fatty acids from them
- There are similar brush border lipases which act on the lipids in a similar way.

Absorption of Fats and Steatorrhea

Refer answers to 2007 paper.

10. What do you understand by the terms innate and acquired immunity? Describe the phenomenon of cell-mediated immunity.

Refer answers to 2006 paper.

11. Define the term blood pressure. Discuss the determinants and regulation of blood pressure.

Refer answers to 2006 paper.

12. Trace the pathway for perception of pain. Discuss the descending pain modulatory pathways. Discuss the terms 'Gating of pain' and 'Referred pain'.

Refer answers to 2009 and 2012 papers.

II. SHORT NOTES

1. Erythroblastosis fetalis.

Refer answers for 2010 paper.

2. Isotonic and isometric contraction.

- Muscle contains both elastic and viscous elements
- Elastic elements are the connective tissue in the muscle fibers and there are series and parallel elastic elements
- The parallel ones are in between the muscle fibers and the series are at the ends of the muscles connecting the muscle to the bones
- The viscous elements are the contractile component of the muscle
- So when a muscle contracts there can be differences in the response of the elastic and viscous elements
- Based on that the muscle contraction is classified as—isometric and isotonic contractions.

Isometric Contraction

- As the name implies, in this type of contraction length of the muscle remains same but tension developed in the muscle is increased
- The muscle length remains the same because as the contractile components are shortening the series elastic elements are stretched and thereby the tension increases but length remains the same (refer Fig. 3)
- There is no shortening and therefore no movement is happening here
- Work done = Force × Distance and since no distance is changed here, there is no actual work done in isometric contraction.

Examples of Isometric Contraction

- Contraction of arm muscle while pushing against the wall
- Contraction of anti-gravity muscles of the body.

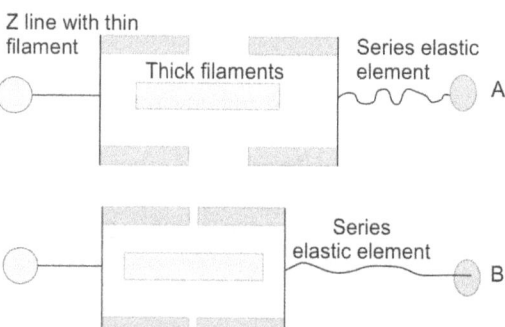

Fig. 3: Isometric contraction. A—Relaxed state of muscle, B—Contracted state of muscle.

Isotonic Contraction

- In this type of contraction the muscle length shortens but the tension developed in the muscle remains the same
- Here the contractile component and parallel elastic elements shorten and series elastic components are not stretched
- Since the muscle shortens there is work being done in this type of contractions.

Examples

- Contraction of upper limb muscles while lifting an object
- Walking
- Swimming.

3. Facilitated diffusion.
Refer answers for 2009 paper.

4. Enterohepatic circulation.
Refer answers for 2009 paper.

5. Juxtaglomerular exchanger (apparatus?)
Refer answers to 2009 paper.

6. Countercurrent exchanger.
Refer answers to 2003 paper.

7. Transport maximum (Tm).
Refer answers to 2008 paper.

8. Acromegaly.
Refer answers to 2008 paper.

9. Steps in thyroxine synthesis.
Refer answers for 2009 paper.

10. Stages of spermatogenesis.
Refer answers to 2006 paper.

11. Functional residual capacity and its significance.
Refer answers to 2011 paper.

12. Types of hypoxia and its cause.
Refer answers to 2006 paper.

13. Respiratory membrane.
Refer answers to 2011 paper.

14. Neural centers for regulation of respiration.
Refer answers to 2007 paper.

15. Dead space.
Refer answers to 2010 paper.

16. Pacemaker potential.
Refer answers to 2005 paper.

17. Cardiac index.
Refer answers to 2010 paper.

18. Dark adaptation.
Refer answers to 2005 paper.

19. Functions of basal ganglia.
Refer answers to 2007 paper.

20. Vestibulocerebellum.

Functional Divisions of Cerebellum

1. **Vestibulocerebellum:** It includes the flocculonodular lobe (refer Fig. 4)
2. **Spinocerebellum:** Includes the paleocerebellum
3. **Cerebrocerebellum:** Includes the neocerebellum.

Vestibulocerebellum

Connections

- **Afferents**: Receive input from vestibular nuclei and primary vestibular apparatus
- **Efferents**: Projects to the vestibular nucleus → vestibulospinal tract and medial longitudinal fasciculus → motor neurons of anterior horn
- **Functions**:
  1. Modulate muscular activity to achieve postural equilibrium or posture
  2. Coordinate movements of eye with movements of head
  3. Involved in eye movements and maintain balance.

21. Tests for ovulation.
Refer answers to 2009 paper.

22. Contraceptives.
Refer answers to 2004 paper.

23. Thyroxine synthesis.
Refer answers to 2009 paper.

24. Tetany.
Refer answers to 2008 paper.

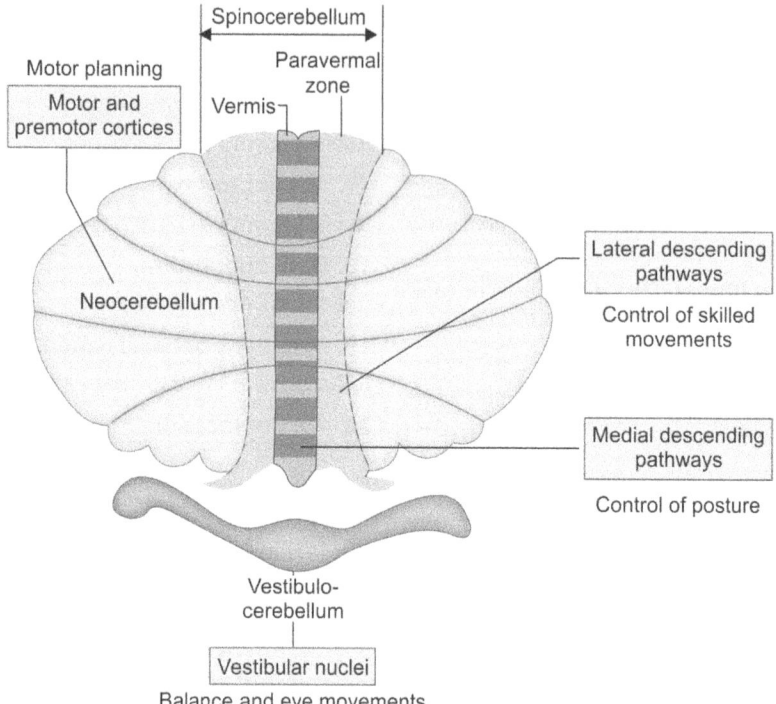

Fig. 4: Functional divisions of cerebellum with their connections and functions.
(*Source:* GK Pal)

25. Dialysis.
Refer answers to 2007 paper.

26. Gastric emptying.
Refer answers to 2009 paper.

27. Enterohepatic circulation.
Refer answers to 2009 paper.

28. Functions of saliva.
Refer answers to 2003 paper.

29. Autoimmune disease.
Refer answers to 2011 paper.

30. Decompression sickness.
Refer answers to 2005 paper.

31. Middle ear functions.
Refer answers to 2003 paper.

32. Define cardiac output. What are the methods to measure the cardiac output?
Refer answers to 2011 paper.

33. Heart sounds.
Refer answers to 2006 paper.

34. Define synapse and describe its properties.

- Junction between two neurons is said to be the synapse
- Neurons communicate with each other through **synapse**.

Properties of Synapse

a. Summation—spatial or temporal
b. Convergence and divergence
c. One way conduction of impulses
d. Synaptic delay
e. Facilitation
f. Subliminal fringe
g. Occlusion
h. Synaptic plasticity and learning
i. Synaptic fatigue.

a. Summation

- Summation means adding up of impulses. In the synapse, following release of neurotransmitters there could be depolarisation or hyperpolarisation of the membrane. These are called as

postsynaptic potentials and they belong to the category of graded potentials
- So these individual potentials from many synapses can summate and excite the membrane and take it to the firing level
- There are two types of summations—spatial and temporal summation
- Temporal summation: The same input stimulates the postsynaptic neuron repeatedly and thereby excites it
- Spatial summation: Here many inputs stimulate simultaneously to excite it.

b. Convergence and Divergence

When many presynaptic neurons end one postsynaptic neuron it is convergence and when one presynaptic terminal divides and ends on many postsynaptic neurons—divergence.

c. One Way Conduction

Impulse transmission always happen from presynaptic to postsynaptic neurons as the receptors for the neurotransmitter released from presynaptic terminal is present on the postsynaptic membrane.

d. Synaptic Delay

There are many steps involved in the impulse transmission from the presynaptic neuron to postsynaptic neuron so there is a delay of 0.5 msec in each synapse.

e. Facilitation

- When a single stimulus is applied to the neuron some response is obtained but if repeated stimuli are given the response is better than the single stimulus response
- So the previous stimulus has been facilitatory for the second and third one.

f. Subliminal Fringe

- It is a partially excited stage of the neuron.
- Let us say presynaptic neuron A ends on postsynaptic neurons X and Y
- Another presynaptic neuron B ends on postsynaptic neurons Y and Z
- When A and B fire simultaneously, the postsynaptic neuron Y is excited fully and starts firing an action potential
- But the postsynaptic neurons X and Z are in partially excited state or in a subliminal fringe of Y.

g. Occlusion

- The response obtained by stimulating two presynaptic neurons together is less than the response obtained by stimulating each one individually
- This is because of common postsynaptic neurons in both the groups.

h. Synaptic Plasticity

The changes that occur in a synpase after repeated stimulation is called as synaptic plasticity

i. Synaptic Fatigue

On repeated stimulation the synapse goes in for fatigue due to exhaustion of neurotransmitters.

35. Describe the functions of thalamus.

Refer answers to 2011 paper.

36. What are the functions of basal ganglia?

Refer answers to 2007 paper.

37. Describe the physiology of speech.

- Understanding spoken and written words and to express ideas in speech and writing is language
- It is a role of the dominant or categorical hemisphere
- It is one of the higher functions of cerebral cortex
- Speech is thought to be a mode of communication between human beings
- There are two forms of speech—written words and spoken words
- Speech involves coordinated activities of central and peripheral speech apparatus.

Areas Involved in Language

All areas for language are around the Sylvian fissure. They are:
a. **Wernicke's area (Area 22):** Comprehension of auditory and visual information
b. **Broca's area (Area 44):** Processes the information comprehended by Wernicke's area into a coordinated pattern for vocalization

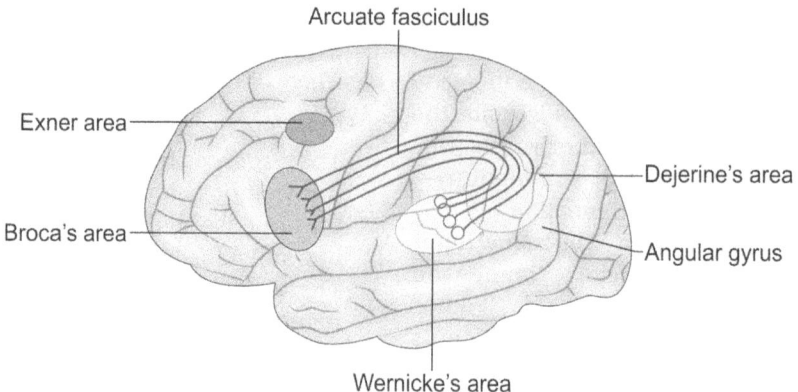

Fig. 5: Speech areas in cerebral cortex.
(*Source:* GK Pal)

c. **Arcuate fasiculus:** Transmits information from Area 22 to 44
d. **Angular gyrus (Area 39):** Processes information from that are read and converted to auditory form of words in Area 22
e. **Motor area (refer Fig. 5).**

Mechanism of Speech

- Speaking and understanding are complex behavior handled by various areas
- Two important areas are: Broca's area and Wernicke's area
- Broca's area is said to be the motor speech area
- Wernicke's area is responsible to recognize and understand spoken words and is the sensory speech area.

Example: When a person asks a question orally how do you answer?

The question is received in area 41 (primary auditory area).
↓
Wernicke's area (interprets and understands the question)
↓
Sends information to Broca's area and it fires
↓
Broca's area sends information to area 4 and muscles for speech contract and the answer is given.

- The same thing happens when a person starts reading a book
- The impulse is received in area 17 → area 18 → angular gyrus → Wernicke's area → Broca's area (if he wants to read it aloud).

Mechanism of Written Speech

- Perception of written words is due to the presence of an intact visual cortex
- Area 17 receives impulses from both retinae through optic nerves. And perceives visual impulses
- From here impulses reach the visual association area (area 18 and 19) – Interpretation happens here
- Generation of new ideas/thought in response to written words—angular gyrus (area 39—visual speech center)
- Impulses reach Broca's area for coordination and to form a pattern for vocalization or writing
- Finally reaches Exner's area in middle frontal gyrus
- Along with motor cortex initiates appropriate movement of hand and fingers to form written speech.

38. Decerebrate rigidity.

Refer answers to 2011 paper.

39. Functions of prefrontal lobe.

Refer answers to 2011 paper.

40. G-Protein coupled receptors.

- Many hormones (Peptide hormones), neuromodulators and other regulatory molecules act through receptors which are involved in signal transduction pathways that involve heteromeric GTP binding proteins called G - proteins
- G-protein exists in two states—active and inactive states
- In active state, G protein has higher affinity for GTP and in inactive state it prefers GDP
- When agonist molecules (hormones) bind to their G protein-coupled receptors, the receptors interact with G proteins and convert it to active state and G protein binds to GTP (refer Fig. 6)
- The activated G protein in turn interacts with many membrane-bound proteins and enzymes or ion channels to alter their activities
- The activated G protein has intrinsic GTPase activity, thereby GTP is hydrolysed to GDP and the activity is terminated
- Activated G proteins acts on enzymes to increase the intracellular concentrations of second messengers cyclic AMP, cyclic GMP, IP3, Ca^{2+} and diacylglycerol
- G protein mediated cAMP mechanisms are powerful modulators of adenylyl cyclase and cGMP of Phophodiesterase, the enzymes responsible for the synthesis of cAMP and break down of cGMP respectively
- Ca^{2+} channel activities may be modulated directly by G proteins or indirectly by second messengers

- G proteins also regulate K^+ channels, Phospholipase etc.

The G-Protein mediated signal transduction pathways include:

- Peptide hormone binds to membrane receptor
- The ligand bound receptor interacts with G protein and activates it
- Activated G protein binds to GTP
- Activated G protein interacts with one or more of the following—adenylyl cyclase, cGMP phosphodiesterase, Ca^{2+} or K^+ channels or phospholipases
- The cellular levels of the following second messengers may increase or decrease—cAMP, cGMP, Ca^{2+}, IP_3 or diacylglycerol
- The increase or decrease of second messenger changes the activities of one or more second-messenger-dependent protein kinase, cGMP dependent kinase etc.
- The level of phosphorylation of an enzyme or an ion channel is altered or an ion channel activity changes and brings about the final result.

41. Primary active transport.

Active Transport

- It is also carrier mediated
- Moves substances uphill against concentration gradient
- So associated with energy expenditure. Energy is derived from ATP, either directly or indirectly
- Types:
  - Primary active transport
  - Secondary active transport.

Primary Active Transport

Here substances are moved uphill across the cell membrane with the help of energy-driven pumps. It involves energy expenditure which is directly derived from break down of ATP.

Ex.

- Na^+- K^+ Pump
- H^+ -K^+ Pump
- Ca^{2+} ATPase.

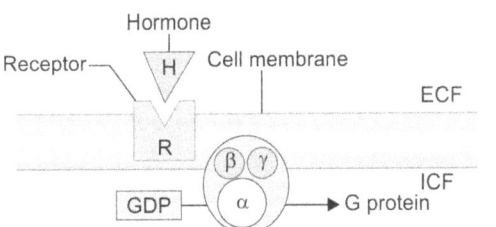

Fig. 6: G-Protein coupled receptor; G protein has 3 subunits—α, β and γ subunits. In inactive state, G Protein is bound to GDP.
(*Source:* GK Pal)

Na⁺- K⁺ Pump
Refer answers to 2011 paper.

Other Primary Active Transportes
a. **Ca^{2+} ATPase:** It is present on the cell membranes, endoplasmic reticulum and sarcoplasmic reticulum of muscles. These pumps help in maintaining a lower concentration of Ca^{2+} in the cytoplasm by pumping it either into ECF or into the SR in muscles
b. **H⁺-K⁺ ATPase:** These pumps are present on the apical membrane of parietal cells in the gastric mucosa and the luminal side of the 'I' cells of the collecting tubule in the nephron. In the stomach the pump is the primary mechanism of secreting H⁺ into the lumen. In nephron, the pump helps in secreting H⁺ into the tubule and thereby acidification of urine
c. **H⁺ ATPase:** It is pesent in the luminal membrane of parietal cells of gastric mucosa and also in the 'I' cells of collecting tubule of nephrons. It is also present in the membrane of lysosomes and endoplasmic reticulum. The acidic nature of the lysosomes is essential for its degenerative actions.

42. Autoregulation of GFR.
The autoregulatory mechanism of GFR is similar to autoregulation of renal blood flow.

Autoregulation of GFR maintains a constant rate of filtration in spite of change in arterial pressure within the range of 80–180 mm Hg.

There are two autoregulatory mechanisms of GFR—myogenic mechanism and Tubuloglomerular feedback.
a. **Myogenic mechanism:** As the renal blood pressure increases the afferent arteriole is stretched and the stretch induces reflex contraction of smooth muscles of the afferent arteriole. This result in vasoconstriction of afferent arteriole and thereby decreases renal blood flow and thereby decreases GFR. This type of regulation happens in the range 80–180 mm Hg mean arterial pressure
b. **Tubuloglomerular feedback:** Refer answers to 2008 paper.

43. Renal glycosuria.
- Renal glycosuria, also known as glucosuria, is the excretion of glucose in urine in detectable amounts at normal blood glucose concentrations in the absence of any signs of generalized proximal renal tubular dysfunction. It happens due to a reduction in the renal tubular reabsorption of glucose
- The inherited form of this disorder is called familial renal glucosuria (FRG)
- FRG is a rare disorder mainly due to mutations in the sodium-glucose co-transporter 2 gene (*SGLT2*)
- Over seventy mutations have been identified
- Glucosuria in these patients can range from <1 to >150 g/1.73 m^2 per day (normal value: range 0.03 to 0.3g/d)
- In general, renal glucosuria is a benign condition and does not require any specific therapy. Glucosuria may also be associated with tubular disorders such as Fanconi-de Toni-Debre syndrome, cystinosis, Wilson disease, hereditary tyrosinemia, or oculocerebrorenal osteodystrophy (Lowe syndrome)
- Renal glucosuria has also been reported in patients with acute pyelonephritis in the presence of a normal blood glucose level. Glucose loss in the urine may vary from a few grams to more than 100 g (556 mmol) per day.

44. Mechanism of bicarbonate generation in distal tubule.

Renal Regulation of Acid-base Balance is by 3 Processes
- Secretion of H⁺ by renal tubules
- Reabsorption of HCO_3^-
- Generation of new HCO_3^-.

H⁺ secretion in the tubules is coupled to reabsorption of HCO_3^-.

Generation of New HCO_3^-

- This happens in the distal convoluted tubule
- It happens during the formation of titrable acid and NH_4
- Formation of titrable acid.

Refer answers to 2012 paper.

45. Stimuli for secretion of aldosterone and actions of aldosterone.

Refer answers to 2005 paper.

46. Pancreatic C-peptide and its significance as a laboratory test.

- Insulin is a peptide hormone and is synthesized in the endoplasmic reticulum (ER) of beta cells and transferred to Golgi apparatus and is packaged to membrane bound vesicles
- Like other polypeptide hormones insulin is synthesized as a large preprohormone
- Preproinsulin has 23 amino acid signal peptide which is removed as it enters the ER
- The rest of the molecule is folded to form the proinsulin and has two polypeptide chains A and B and they are connected by disulfide bonds
- The peptide segment connecting the A and B chains is said to be the C-peptide
- It facilitates the folding and then gets seperated and is stored inside the granules before secretion (refer Fig. 7)
- Proinsulin is processed by two proteases and the C-peptide is cleaved
- C-peptide has no physiological actions.

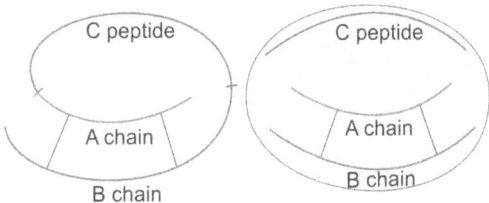

Fig. 7: Structure of insulin with C-peptide. Insulin is a polypeptide hormone with 51 amino acids. It is formed as Preproinsulin and Proinsulin (86 AA). A and B chains of Proinsulin are connected by the C-chain. There are disulphide bridges between C-peptide chain B chain. On cleavage of C-peptide chain, insulin is formed and stored in secretory vesicle along with C-peptide.
(*Source:* GK Pal)

Significance of C-peptide

- Normally 90–97% of the products released from B cells is insulin along with equimolar amounts of C-peptide
- The rest is mostly proinsulin
- C-peptides can be measured by radio-immunoassay and its levels give an index of B cell function in patients receiving exogenous insulin.

47. Cretinism—its cause, features and strategy to prevent it.

Hypothyroid children from birth or from in utero are called cretins and the disease is said to be cretinism.

The main causes for cretinism are:

- Maternal iodine defeciency
- Fetal thyroid dysgenesis
- Inborn error of thyroid hormone synthesis
- Maternal antithyroid antibodies that cross the placenta and damage fetal thyroid
- Fetal hypopituitary hypothyroidism.

If the mother's thyroid status is normal, mother's T4 can cross the placenta and thereby the fetal growth and development are normal till birth.

The child with cretinism has the following symptoms:

- Stunted growth
- Mental retardation
- Potbelly
- Enlarged and protruding tongue
- Hoarse cry
- Poor feeding
- Umbilical hernia
- Retarded bone age
- Deaf mutism and rigidity
- Respiratory distress syndrome.

Prevention of cretinism:

- Worldwide congenital hypothyroidism is the most common cause of preventable mental retardation
- So if thyroid screening is done immediately after birth and thyroid hormone replacement is done early the prognosis for normal growth and development is good and mental retardation can be prevented

- If the mother is hypothyroid as in iodine defeciency the mental development is further affected and response to treatment is less after birth
- This can be prevented by using iodized salts by the mothers.

48. What is the function of corpus luteum of pregnancy? How is it supported?

- Corpus luteum in early pregnancy is "the Source" of progesterone
- Progesterone is essential for the maintanence of pregnancy and survival of fetus
- It also secretes the hormone relaxin
- In pregnancy, relaxin relaxes the pubic symphysis and other pelvic joints and softens the cervix. It also inhibits uterine contractions and aids in development of mammary glands.

Maintanence of Corpus Luteum

- Human chorionic gonadotrophin (hCG) secreted by syncytiotrophoblasts in pregnancy is luteinizing and luteotrophic in nature
- The hCG is detected in maternal blood as early as 6 days after conception and starts increasing and reaches a peak by 3 months after which it starts decreasing
- The major role of hCG is to maintain/support corpus luteum and thereby maintains secretion of progesterone and thereby maintains pregnancy
- After 3 months the hCG levels decline and corpus luteum seizes to function and after that phase the progesterone synthesis is taken over by placenta.

49. Parturition.

- The duration of normal pregnancy is 40 weeks from 1st day of last menstrual cycle
- Delivery of the fetus at term is said to be parturition.

Parturition Reflex

Refer answers to 2004 paper.

50. Ionic basis of the pacemaker potential.

Refer answers to 2012 paper.

51. Windkessel effect of aorta.

Refer answers to 2008 paper.

52. Illustrate with a diagram, the left ventricular volume and pressure changes during a cardiac cycle.

Refer answers to 2009 paper.

53. Role of myelin sheath in conduction of nerve impulse.

Refer answers to 2004 paper (short note 4).

54. Functions of hypothalamus.

Refer answers to 2013 paper.

55. Clinical features of cerebellar lesions.

Refer answers to 2008 paper.

56. Physiological roles of muscle spindle.

Refer answers to 2005 paper.

57. Chemical regulation of respiration.

Refer answers to 2005 paper.

58. Hamburger's chloride shift.

Refer answers to 2005 paper.

59. Role of surfactant in pulmonary function.

Refer answers to 2009 paper.

III. SHORT ANSWERS

1. Chronaxie.

- Chronaxie is the time required for stimulus of double the strength of Rheobase current to excite a tissue. It is an indicator of excitability of tissues
- Rheobase is the minimum strength of current given for a particular duration which is able to excite a tissue
- Chronaxie and excitability are inversely related
- Nerve has a shorter chronaxie and smooth muscles have a longer chronaxie.

2. Motor unit.

- Motor unit is a single motor neuron with all its branches and all the muscle fibers supplied by it (refer Fig. 8)
- The size of the motor unit is decided by the muscle fibers supplied by it

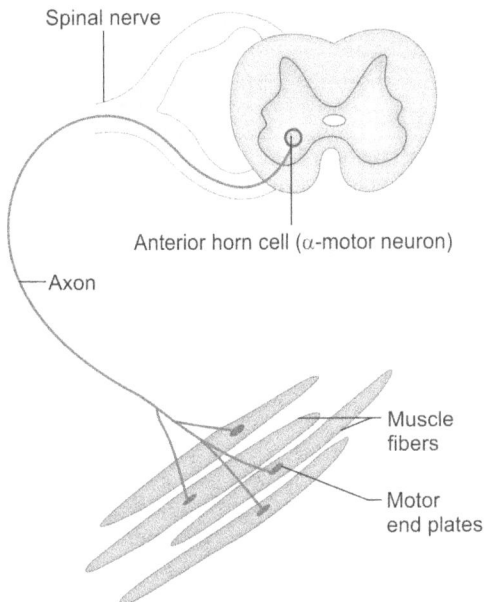

Fig. 8: Motor unit.
(*Source:* GK Pal)

- The ones which supply the intrinsic muscles of the hand have only less than 10 fibers and produce less tension but the ones which supply back muscles are large motor units and have hundreds of fibers
- All the muscle fibers in a single motor unit are of the same type, i.e. either oxidative type or glycolytic type
- Based on this, the motor units may be classified as either Oxidative or slow and glycolytic or fast motor units.

3. **Apoptosis.**

- Apoptosis is "Programmed cell death"
- It is also said to be "cell suicide' as the cell's own genes program the cell death
- It is a common happeneing in the growth and development and also in adulthood.

Examples are:
a. In the nervous system development many neurons are removed by apoptosis while remodelling and formation of synapse
b. In immune system development, apoptosis removes the inappropriate clones of immunocytes and is responsible for the destruction of lymphocytes by glucocorticoids
c. It is responsible for removal of webs between fingers in developmental period of fetal life
d. It is responsible for regression of duct system in development of sexual organs
e. In adults, cyclical breakdown of endometrium and menstruation is also an example of apoptosis

- Apoptosis is triggered by Fas ligand in the membrane of natural killer cells and T lymphocytes and Tumor necrosis factor
- Fas ligand binds with its receptors triggering apoptosis and it activates an important pathway through the mitochondria which releases Cytochrome C and it in turn activates Caspases, a cysteine protease
- It results in DNA fragmentation, cytoplasmic and chromatin condensation and membrane bleb formation and cell break up and removal of debris by phagocytosis.

4. **Osmotic diuresis.**

- The presence of large quantities of unreabsorbed solutes in the tubular fluid results in increased volume of urine— **osmotic diuresis**.
- This usually happens when solutes are not reabsorbed in the PCT. So the solutes exert an osmotic effect as the volume of tubular fluid decreases and concentration of solute increases
- They start holding back water in the tubules
- This decreases the gradient across which Na⁺ has to be reabsorbed. Na$^+$ reabsorption requires a particular gradient and when water stays back in tubule with unreabsorbed solutes this gradient reaches a limiting level—The limiting gradient
- So now, sodium also stays in the tubule and water also stays along with it
- Now this isotonic fluid reaches the loop of Henle. Here the decreased concentration

- of solutes in medullary interstitium prevents further reabsorption of Na⁺ and water
- There is decreased medullary osmolarity because the reabsorption of Na^+, K^+ and Cl^- is decreased in ascending limb as the limiting gradient is reached
- Fluid passes through DCT and Collecting duct and because of absence of medullary gradient for water reabsorption, water stays back in tubule
- This results in marked increase in urine volume and excretion of Na⁺ and other electrolytes
- Solutes which can cause such osmotic diuresis are Mannitol and similar polysaccharides
- In diabetes mellitus, when there is high plasma glucose levels it leads to appearance of glucose in tubular fuid and all the above effects and osmotic diuresis is produced
- In Osmotic diuresis, in contrast to water diuresis, solutes and water are not reabsorbed in PCT and urinary volumes are very high and urine is isotonic in nature.

5. LH surge.

- Just before ovulation there is an LH surge and it triggers the ovulation
- The surge happens 9 hours before the ovulation
- High LH level is necessary for the final maturation and rupture of Graafian follicle
- The estrogen levels are also rising in the preovulatory phase
- It is a unique pattern here, the high estrogen levels positively stimulates further secretion of LH and LH stimulates estrogen secretion and it reaches a peak level (6–10 times baseline value) 9 hours before ovulation
- The FSH levels also increase (2–3 times)
- LH acts on the granuosa and Theca cells and make them secrete progesterone
- Now progesterone levels rise just before ovulation and estrogen levels decrease
- All the above hormonal changes results in Ovulation
- So without the LH surge Ovultion does not happen.

6. Somatomedins.

- Somatomedins are polypeptide growth factors secreted by the liver and other tissues
- They resemble Insulin, except for the C-peptide, they are called as Insulin like growth factors (IGF)
- There are two types; Somatomedin C (IGF-1) and Insulin like growth factor II (IGF-II).

IGF–I

- The secretion of IGF-I is independent of GH in fetal period and is dependent on GH after birth
- It is low during childhood, reaches a peak in puberty and declines thereafter
- Receptors of IGF-I are similar to insulin receptor
- They induce skeletal and cartilage growth and protein metabolism
- They stimulate collagen formation.

IGF–II

- Its secretion is independent of GH levels and is always constant
- Receptors of IGF-II are Mannose 6-Phosphate receptors
- IGF-II plays a major role in fetal growth.

7. Hormones of adrenal cortex.

- The adrenal cortex is in 3 layers and each layer secretes different hormones
- The outermost layer is the zona glomerulosa. It secretes the mineralocorticoid—aldosterone and 11-deoxycorticosterone
- The middle layer is the zona fasiculata. It secretes glucocorticoids—corticosterone and cortisol
- The innermost layer the zona reticularis secretes adrenal androgens—dehydroepi-androsterone (DHEA) and androsternedi-one (refer Fig. 9)
- The middle and inner layer secrete both glucocorticoids and androgens but more

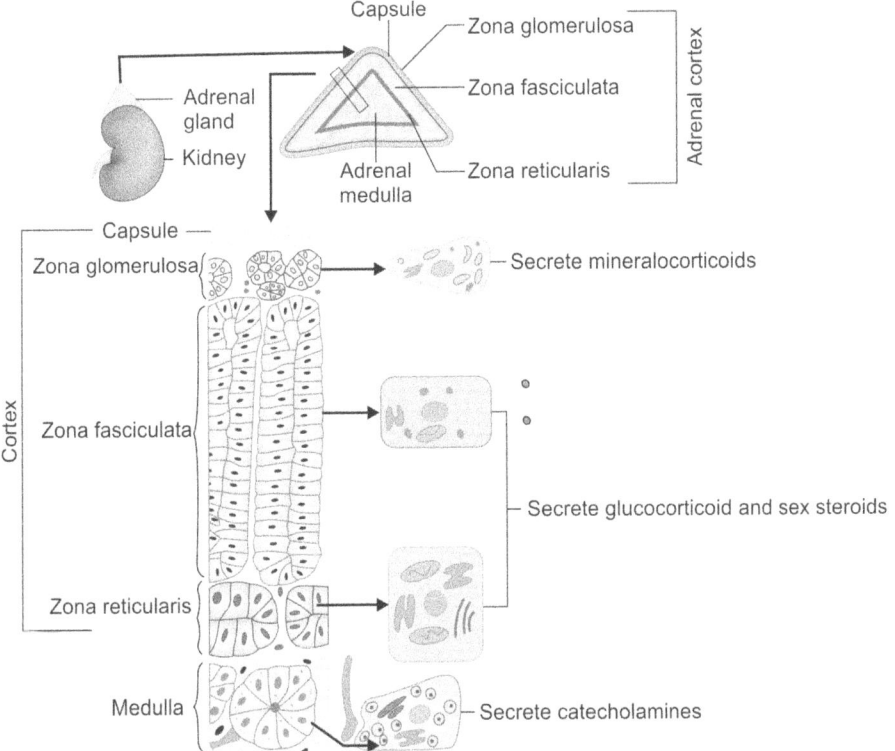

Fig. 9: Layers of adrenal cortex and the hormones they secrete. Zona glomerulosa secretes aldosterone, zona fasciculata secretes glucocorticoids and some amount of androgens, zona reticularis secretes androgens and some amount of glucocorticoids.
(*Source:* GK Pal)

of glucocorticoids from zona fasiculata and more of androgens from zona reticularis.

8. Types of diabetes.

- The term "Diabetes" in Greek and Roman denotes the passing of large volumes of urine
- There are of two types—diabetes mellitus and diabetes insipidus
- In diabetes mellitus urine tastes sweet and in diabetes insipidus it has no taste
- **Diabetes mellitus** is due to deficiency of the hormone insulin and **diabetes insipidus** is due to deficiency of antidiuretic hormone

a. **Diabetes mellitus** is of two types—Type 1 diabetes mellitus or Insulin dependent diabetes and Type 2 diabetes mellitus or Non-insulin dependent diabetes mellitus

- **Type 1 DM:** There is autoimmune destruction of Beta cells in Islets of Langerhans and the insulin secretion is less or even completely absent. The patient is treated with Insulin injections
- **Type 2 DM:** Here the insulin secretion is normal but the insulin receptors are insensitive to insulin. It occurs after the age of 40 years and is treated with anti-hyperglycemic agents.

The symptoms are polyuria, polydipsia, polyphagia, hyperglycemia, weight loss, glycosuria, ketosis, acidosis and coma.

b. **Diabetes insipidus** is of two types—neurogenic or central diabetes insipidus and nephrogenic diabetes insipidus

- **Neurogenic DI:** There is defect in synthesis of ADH from hypothalamus

- **Nephrogenic DI:** Here the synthesis and secretion of ADH is normal but there could be congenital defects of receptors to ADH or mutations of genes for aquaporins and defects in aquaporins, the water channels on the luminal side of principal cells of collecting duct.

Symptoms of DI are polyuria, polydipsia. They pass a large volume (upto 23 L/day) of hypotonic urine (30 mOsm/kg H_2O).

9. Action of paratharmone on bone.

Refer answers to 2008 paper.

10. Menarche.

Menarche is the first menstrual period at the time of puberty. It is the last stage of puberty. It occurs by 11-14 years of age. The initial periods are anovulatory and regular ovulation happens after 1 year.

11. Muscles of inspiration.

- **Primary muscles** of inspiration are diaphragm and external intercostals.
- **Accessory muscles** are—scalene, sternocleidomastoid, neck and back muscles and muscles of upper respiratory tract.

12. P50.

- It is the partial pressure of oxygen in the arterial blood at which 50% of the hemoglobin is saturated with oxygen
- Normal value is 27 mm Hg
- P_{50} is inversely related to hemoglobin affinity for oxygen.

13. End-diastolic volume.

- It is the volume of blood in the ventricle at the end of diastole
- Normal value is 130 mL
- It is decided by the venous return
- It is the preload for the ventricular muscle.

14. Attenuation reflex.

Refer answers to 2005 paper (Short note 7).

15. Perimetry.

- It is an instrumental method to map the peripheral field of vision
- Each eye is mapped seperately
- The instrument used is perimeter
- Lister's perimeter is used
- The chart for recording the field of vision has circles—isopters, drawn at 10° intervals and radial line—meridians, drawn at 10° intervals
- The field of vision of each eye is mapped in the isopters and meridians
- One eye is checked at a time
- One eye is covered and the other eye is fixed on a central point
- A small target is moved towards the central point along selected meridians and along each meridian the site where the object is first visible is plotted in degrees of arc away from the central point
- These points are joined to form the eye's visual field
- Field of vision of each eye is not circular as it is cut off medially by the nose and superiorly by the roof of orbit

16. Summation.

Refer answers to 2012 paper.

17. Referred pain.

Refer answers to 2009 paper.

18. Types of memory.

- **Memory** is the process by which acquired information is stored and can be retrieved
- **Memory is classified based on how long it is stored and retrieved—short-term or long-term memory**
  - Short-term memory: Ability to recall ongoing experiences for a few seconds
  - Long-term memory: If the information is repeatedly used, it results in reinforcement of the synaptic pathway and results in long term memory
- **Another classification is based on how the learned details are retrieved—either with conscious awareness or without conscious awareness:**
  - Explicit or declarative memory: Memory for events, facts and names. Here conscious awareness of the subject is needed

- Implicit memory or procedural memory: Ability to learn and remember motor skills. There is no need of conscious awareness.

19. Thalamic syndrome.

Refer answers to 2010 paper.

20. Kluver-Bucy syndrome.

Lesions of the temporal lobe, especially the amygdala leads to temporal lobe syndrome or **Kluver-Bucy syndrome**. Study has been conducted in monkeys to identify the symptoms following the lesion in temporal lobe.

Features of Kluver-Bucy Syndrome

- Inability to identify objects visually, inspite of normal vision—visual agnosia
- Loss of hearing since the auditory area is in the temporal lobe
- Tends to examine any object orally (oral tendencies)
- Hyperphagia
- Hypersexuality
- Tends to show attention to all peripheral stimuli—hypermetamorphosis
- Change in eating habits, monkeys start eating meat
- Absence of fear, monkeys tend to handle the snakes
- Loss of recent memory.

21. Functions of sodium potassium ATPase pump.

Refer answers to 2011 paper.

22. Mention the normal value of GFR and substance used to measure GFR.

- GFR is defined as the rate at which the filtrate is formed in all the nephrons of both the kidneys per unit of time
- The normal values are: 125 mL/min, 90-140 mL/min or 180L/day.

Measurement of GFR

It is done by measuring renal clearance of inulin and creatinine.

23. Enumerate heat loss mechanism.

a. **Cutaneous vasodilatation:** Warm blood flows to the periphery and heat is lost to the environment

b. **Heat is lost from the body to the environment by:**
   i. Conduction: Heat is exchanged between objects (of different temperatures) in contact with each other
   ii. Radiation: It is transfer of heat by infrared electromagnetic radiations from one object to another object which are not in contact with each other.
c. **Vaporization of sweat**
d. **Increased respiration (panting in animals)**
e. **Urination and defecation.**

24. Peristalsis.

Refer answers to 2004 paper.

25. What is the role of vitamin K in the body?

- Vitamin K is a cofactor for the enzyme which catalyzes the conversion of glutamic acid residues to - γ carboxyglutamic acid residues in the liver
- Six clotting factors, synthesized in the liver, require the conversion of glutamic acid to γ carboxyglutamic acid. They are Factors - II, VII, IX and X, and Protein C and S
- Vitamin K antagonists: Coumarin derivatives like Warfarn, Dicoumarol etc.
- They prevent the action of Vitamin K by competitively binding with Vitamin K receptors.

26. What is the normal blood calcium level?

- The normal plasma calcium level is 10 mg/dL (5 mEq/L, 2.5 mmol/L)
- It is partly protein-bound and partly diffusible.

Diffusible calcium – 6 mg/dL (1.5 mmol/L)

- Ionized calcium (50% of total plasma calcium)—5 mg/dL (1.25 mmol/L)
- Complexed to HCO_3^-, citrate etc—1 mg/dL (0.25 mmol/L).

Non-diffusible calcium—4 mg/dL.

27. Name the hormones of adrenal cortex.

The hormones of adrenal cortex are:
a. Mineralocorticoids—C_{21} steroids
   - Aldosterone
   - Deoxycorticosterone.

b. Glucocorticoids—C_{21} steroids
   - Cortisol
   - Cortisone
   - Corticosterone.
c. Adrenal androgens—C_{19} steroids
   - Dehydroepiandrosterone
   - Androstenedione.

28. Name the hormones of placenta.
a. Human chorionic gonadotrophin (hCG)
b. Human chorionic somatomammotrophin (hCS)
c. Estrogen
d. Progesterone
e. Relaxin
f. Prolactin
g. Corticotrophin releasing hormone (CRH)
h. β-endorphin
i. α-Melanocyte stimulating hormone
j. Gonadotrophin releasing hormone
k. Inhibin.

29. Cryptorchidism.
- The testis develops in the abdomen and descends to the scrotum during fetal development
- The descent of the testis is under the control of Mullerian inhibiting substance and gonadotrophins
- Undescended testis is called as cryptorchidism
- It is seen in 2% in less than 1 year old children and is less than 0.3% after puberty
- It is treated with gonadotrophins
- The treatment has to be started early as the incidence of malignancy in undescended testis is high than when it is present in the scrotum.

30. Why are ovarian cycles suppressed during lactation?
- The nursing mother does not have regular menstrual cycle
- The menstrual cycles are absent for 6 months in women who do not nurse their infants
- Mothers who nurse regularly have amenorrhea for 25 to 30 weeks
- This is because; nursing stimulates prolactin secretion and prolactin—inhibits GnRH secretion, inhibits action of GnRH on the pituitary and antagonizes the action of gonadotrophins on the ovaries
- Ovaries are inactive, ovulation is inhibited and estrogen and progesterone output falls to low levels
- So the chance of a nursing female of becoming pregnant is very low and is a birth control mechanism.

31. What is P50?
Refer short answers Q no. 12.

32. What are the types of hypoxia?
Refer answers to 2006 paper.

33. Mention common refractory errors of the eye.
Refer answers to 2004 paper.

34. SA node as pacemaker.
- SA node is the pacemaker of the heart and it is said to be the pacemaker as it discharges electrical impulses at a rapid rate than the other regions and this depolarisation spreads through the conducting system to other regions before they depolarise on their own
- It is located at the junction of SVC with the right atrium
- SA node contains cells which are round with gap junctions. They are 'P' cells or the pacemaker cells
- They are supplied by sympathetic and parasympathetic nerves
- They fire at a rate of 100/min.

35. PR interval.
Refer answers to 2011 paper.

36. Reflex arc.
Reflex is defined as the involuntary response to a threshold stimulus obtained by stimulating a sensory receptor.
The simplest reflex arc has a single synapse.
Components of a reflex arc: Receptor → afferent nerve → Integrating center → Efferent nerve → Effectors (refer Fig. 10).

37. Functions of cerebrospinal fluid.
- CSF offers mechanical protection by acting as a shock absorber
- CSF offers the optimum chemical environment for accurate neuronal signaling

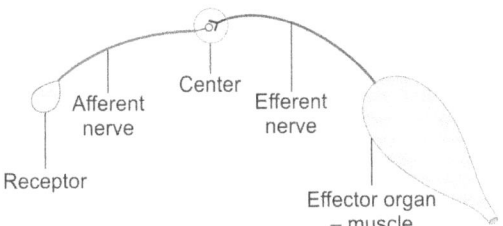

Fig. 10: Reflex arc.
(*Source:* Sembulingam)

- CSF acts as a circulating medium for exchange of nutrients and waste products between the blood and nervous tissue
- Continuous formation and drainage removes metabolic wastes
- Acts as lymph
- Provides nutrition
- Reduces the weight of brain.

38. What is righting reflex?

- Righting reflexes help to maintain the normal standing position and keep the animal's head upright.
- These reflexes are integrated in the nuclei of midbrain.

39. Name the nuclei responsible for hunger and satiety in human being.

Refer answers to 2010 paper.

40. What is referred pain?

Refer answers to 2009 paper

41. Extracellular fluid volume and blood volume in an adult male weighing 70 kg.

- ECF volume in a 70 kg adult (20% of the body weight) – 14 L
- Blood volume is calculated as 100/100-Hematocrit. Plasma volume is 3.5 L and Hct is 38
- So Total blood volume = 3500 × 100/100-38 = 5645 mL.

42. Calcium transporters on the membrane of sarcoplasmic reticulum.

Calcium transporters on SR membrane are Ryanodine receptors, IP3 receptor and Ca^{2+}-Mg^{2+} ATPase.

43. Mechanism of edema in congestive cardiac failure.

In congestive heart failure there is increase in venous pressure which results in increased capillary pressure. This leads to increased filtration pressure and thereby increased interstitial fluid and edema.

44. State a manifestation of hypocalcemic tetany. Give one cause leading to this condition.

Carpopedal spasm is a feature of tetany. The hand takes a peculiar posture—flexion at metacarpophalangeal joints, extension at interphalangeal joints and opposition of thumb. Spasm of feet is rare and if it happens there is plantar flexion of toes and the toes are drawn up.

It is seen in hypoparathyroidism.

45. List the vitamin K-dependent coagulation factors.

In the liver the following clotting factors synthesis depends upon Vitamin K:
Factor II or Prothrombin
Factors VII, IX and X
Protein C.

46. Rh status of mother, father and child for occurrence of Rh incompatibility.

For Rh incompatability to occur the Rh status are:
- Mother is Rh Negative
- Father is Rh Positive
- Fetus is Rh Positive.

47. Role of tropomyosin in muscle contraction.

- Tropomyosin is a regulatory protein
- It is double stranded and is placed in the groove in the Actin filament
- It covers the Myosin binding sites of Actin
- On release of Ca^{2+} from SR, Ca^{2+} binds to Troponin C
- After the binding of Troponin C and Ca^{2+}, Tropomyosin is lifted from the myosin binding sites and the myosin binding sites of actin are exposed and the myosin heads bind to actin
- This brings about cross-bridge cycling and muscle contraction.

48. Type of acetylcholine receptor on skeletal muscle and its function.

- The type of acetylcholine receptor on the muscle fiber is nicotinic acetylcholine receptor
- It is a non-specific cation channel by itself
- When two molecules of acetylcholine binds to the receptor, the channel opens and allows entry of Na^+, as it is the major cation in the ECF
- Na^+ influx results in development of depolarizing end plate potential (EPP) in the motor end plate
- EPP excites the neighboring muscle membrane which in turn generates action potential.

49. Hormones secreted by hypothalamus.

They are:
- Growth hormone releasing hormone (GHRH)
- Growth hormone inhibiting hormone (GHIH) or somatostatin
- Prolactin inhibiting factor (PIF) or dopamine
- Thyrotrophin releasing hormone (TRH)
- Corticotrophin releasing hormone (CRH)
- Gonadotrophin releasing hormone (GnRH).

50. Hormonal defect in: (a) Addison's disease (b) Conn's syndrome.

- Addison's disease: Decreased synthesis of mineralocorticoids and glucocorticoids
- Conn's syndrome: Primary hyperaldosteronism—increased synthesis of aldosterone.

51. List the calcium transporters on the sarcoplasmic reticular membrane in the ventricular muscle.

The calcium transporters on the SR membrane of ventricular muscles are – Ryanodine receptors and IP3 receptors on the SR membrane to release Ca^{2+} and Ca^{2+}- Mg^{2+} ATPase to pump back calcium into the SR.

52. State Starling's law of the heart.

Refer answers to 2011 paper.

53. What is the effect of 2, 3 diphosphoglycerate on the oxygen-hemoglobin dissociation curve? Does it help in loading or unloading of oxygen?

- 2, 3 DPG is a product of glycolysis via Embden-Meyerhof pathway got from 3-phosphoglyceraldehyde
- It is a highly charged anion that binds to deoxyhemoglobin
- HbO_2 + 2, 3 DPG $\leftrightarrow$ Hb - 2, 3 DPG + O_2. So in presence of 2, 3 DPG the affinity hemoglobin to O_2 decreases and it releases O_2. So the Oxy-Hb dissociation curve shifts to the right
- It helps in unloading of O_2.

54. What are the types of hypoxia?

Refer answers to 2006 paper.

55. Region of the cochlea which vibrates most for the highest sound frequency in the audible range.

The basilar membrane at the base of the cochlea vibrtaes the most for the highest sound frequency in the audible range.

56. Visual field defect when the optic chiasma is cut in the center.

In the crossing of optic chiasma the nasal retinal fibers from both the eyes are damaged and the field defect here is bitemporal hemianopia.

57. State the refractive error in astigmatism. How is it corrected?

Refer answers to 2009 paper.

58. What is 'blind spot'?

The optic nerve leaves the eye and the retinal blood vessels enter the eye at a point 3 mm medial to and sligtly above the posterior pole of the eye.

It is called as the optic disk and is viewed through the ophthalmoscope.

There are no receptors of vision (Rods and Cones) in this area, so called as the 'blind spot'.

59. Receptors for vestibular sensation.

- The vestibular apparatus in the inner ear consists of – 3 semicircular canals and 2 sac like structures—utricle and saccule

- The receptors for vestibular sensation are the hair cells and they are located in the cristae in the ampulla of semicircular canals and the macula or otolithic organ of the utricle and saccule

60. Name of tracts made up by second order neurons in the pathway for: (a) Fine touch (b) Pain.

- Fine touch—dorsal column pathway
- Pain—lateral spinothalamic tract.

MBBS Examination 2014

ANSWER ALL QUESTIONS

I. Essay Questions (7.5/10 Marks each)

1. Describe the physiological roles of the different types of granulocytes circulating in blood. (7.5 marks)
2. Define glomerular filtration rate (GFR). What are its determinants? Discuss the phenomenon of autoregulation of GFR. Describe the best test for estimation of GFR. What is the routinely used clinical test to assess renal function? (7.5 marks)
3. Define the terms Cardiac output and Total peripheral resistance and discuss their determinants. (7.5 marks)
4. What are the neural mechanisms involved in spontaneous breathing? Discuss chemical regulation of respiration. Distinguish between the two types of respiratory failure. (7.5 marks)
5. What is the composition of gastric juice? Describe the mechanism of HCl secretion. Give a detailed account on the regulation of gastric secretion. (10 marks)
6. Define blood pressure. Discuss in brief the various factors which influence the pressure. Add a note on hypertension. (10 marks)
7. Define anemia. Classify them. List the important investigations to confirm the various types of anemia. (10 marks)
8. Define cardiac cycle. Describe the sequence of events during cardiac cycle in detail with suitable diagrams. (10 marks)

II. Short Notes (2.5/5 Marks each)

1. cAMP signaling pathway, with an example. (2.5 marks)
2. Colloid oncotic pressure and its importance. (2.5 marks)
3. Excitation-contraction coupling in skeletal muscle. (2.5 marks)
4. Types of polycythemia and complications due to this condition. (2.5 marks)
5. Findings of 'tests of hemostasis' in hemophilia. (2.5 marks)
6. Functions of macrophages. (2.5 marks)
7. Physiological role of corticosteroids. (2.5 marks)
8. Function of any one hormone of posterior pituitary. (2.5 marks)
9. Composition of bile and the physiological role (if any) of the components. (2.5 marks)
10. Pathophysiology of peptic ulcer. (2.5 marks)
11. Describe the 3 bipolar limb leads of ECG. What is the significance of: (a) PR interval (b) ST segment in an ECG? (2.5 marks)
12. Discuss the changes in ventricular volume during different phases of the cardiac cycle with a diagram. (2.5 marks)
13. Discuss any two pulmonary function tests which can detect obstructive lung disease. (2.5 marks)
14. Trace the pathway for perception of fine touch. (2.5 marks)
15. Operant conditioning. (2.5 marks)

16. Clinical features of cerebellar lesions. (2.5 marks)
17. Define muscle tone and discuss the phenomenon responsible for it. What conditions lead to alterations of tone? (2.5 marks)
18. Endogenous opioid peptides. (2.5 marks)
19. Refractory errors of the eye. (2.5 marks)
20. Discuss the phenomena by which sound waves in air induce action potentials in the cochlear nerve. (2.5 marks)
21. Hypersecretion of growth hormone. (5 marks)
22. Tissue macrophage system. (5 marks)
23. Neural regulation of respiration. (5 marks)
24. Functions and tests of cerebellum. (5 marks)
25. Transport across cell membrane. (5 marks)
26. Ovarian and endometrial changes of menstrual cycle. (5 marks)
27. Brown-Sequard syndrome. (5 marks)
28. Oxygen dissociation curve. (5 marks)

III. Short Answers (1/3 Marks each)

1. Membrane transporters involved in clearance of calcium from cytoplasm. (1 mark)
2. Concentrations of sodium and potassium in intra and extracellular fluids. (1 mark)
3. Phenomena involved in the act of swallowing. (1 mark)
4. Role of ATP in relaxation of muscle. (1 mark)
5. Draw a schematic diagram of the sarcomere and label its components. (1 mark)
6. Opsonins. (1 mark)
7. Cells which express major histocompatibility complex II. (1 mark)
8. Significance of glycosylated hemoglobin. (1 mark)
9. Name 4 enzymes in pancreatic secretion. (1 mark)
10. Hormonal imbalance causing: (a) Acromegaly (b) cretinism. (1 mark)
11. List the types of shock. (1 mark)
12. Define preload and state its effect on cardiac function. (1 mark)
13. Baroreceptor reflex. (1 mark)
14. What is myocardial infarction? State one ECG change in this condition. (1 mark)
15. Role of myelin sheath in conduction of nerve impulse. (1 mark)
16. Conditions where plantar response is 'extensor'. (1 mark)
17. Finding in Weber's test in conduction deafness of the left side. (1 mark)
18. Muscle actions responsible for: (a) Normal expiration (b) Forced expiration. (1 mark)
19. Oxygen carrying capacity of blood. (1 mark)
20. Hypoxic vasoconstriction—where does it occur and what are its complications? (1 mark)
21. Permissive action of hormone. (3 marks)
22. Role of vitamin D in calcium homeostasis. (3 marks)
23. Contraception in males. (3 marks)
24. Corpus luteum. (3 marks)
25. Vitamin K dependent clotting factors. (3 marks)
26. Atonic bladder. (3 marks)
27. Functions of skin. (3 marks)
28. Secondary active transport. (3 marks)
29. Motor unit. (3 marks)
30. Refractory period. (3 marks)
31. Heart sounds. (3 marks)
32. Waves of ECG in Lead II. (3 marks)
33. Different types of hypoxia. (3 marks)
34. Aphasia. (3 marks)
35. Stages of sleep. (3 marks)
36. Optic pathway. (3 marks)
37. Functions of ascending reticular activating system. (3 marks)
38. Components of vestibular apparatus. (3 marks)
39. Features of Parkinson's disease. (3 marks)

40. Functions of middle ear. (3 marks)
41. Functions of plasma proteins. (3 marks)
42. Non-excretory functions of kidney. (3 marks)
43. Myasthenia gravis. (3 marks)
44. Stages of spermatogenesis. (3 marks)
45. Cystometrogram and its significance. (3 marks)
46. Hormones regulating calcium homeostasis. (3 marks)
47. Enterohepatic circulation. (3 marks)
48. Enzymes involved in digestion of fat. (3 marks)
49. Structure of platelets. (3 marks)
50. Functions of saliva. (3 marks)
51. Dead space. (3 marks)
52. Hering Breuer reflex. (3 marks)
53. Korotkoff sounds. (3 marks)
54. Draw a diagram of the pathway of crude touch and label it. (3 marks)
55. Functions of CSF. (3 marks)
56. Fluent aphasia. (3 marks)
57. Receptor potential. (3 marks)
58. Motor homunculus. (3 marks)
59. Attenuation reflex. (3 marks)
60. Taste pathway. (3 marks)

I. ESSAY QUESTIONS

1. **Describe the physiological roles of the different types of granulocytes circulating in blood.**

Granulocytes in blood are:

- Neutrophils (refer Fig. 1)
- Eosinophils
- Basophils.

Physiological Roles of Neutrophils

- Neutrophils are the first line of defense

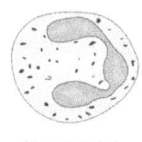 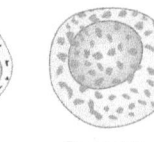 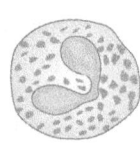

Neutrophil   Basophil   Eosinophil

Fig. 1: Granulocytes.
(Source: GK Pal)

- It does the defense mechanism by phagocytosis.

Phagocytosis

- Neutrophils are the first ones to reach the site of infection followed by macrophages
- They come out of the blood vessels by a process called **Emigration**
- Adhesion molecules like *selectins* and *integrins* help in emigration
- Phagocytes are attracted to sites of infection or inflammation by **Chemotaxis**
- Substances inducing chemotaxis are called **Chemotaxins**
- On reaching the pathogens or tissue debris, phagocytes adhere to them—**Adherence**
- Then they put out processes – Pseudopods and ingest the particles—**Ingestion**
- The ingested particle is enclosed in a vesicle—**Phagosome**
- Phagosome attaches to lysosomes in the neutrophil to form—**Phagolysososme**
- The lysosomes put out hydrolytic enzymes like *lysozymes*
- The phagocytes have oxidative enzymes in them which form lethal oxidative metabolites like—O_2^-, H_2O_2 and hypochlorites
- Antimicrobials – **Defensins** in phagocytes kill the micoorganisms
- By all these killing mechanisms the microbes are killed and degraded or form **residual bodies** (refer Fig. 2).

Other Functions

- Neutrophils release many chemical mediators like leukotrienes, thromboxane A2 which mediate inflammatory reaction
- It mediates febrile response by releasing endogenous pyrogens.

Eosinophils

Structure of Eosinophils

- Size is same as that of neutrophils (10–14 µm)
- Bilobed nucleus and lobes are connected by thick chromatin strand—gives a spectacle shaped appearance

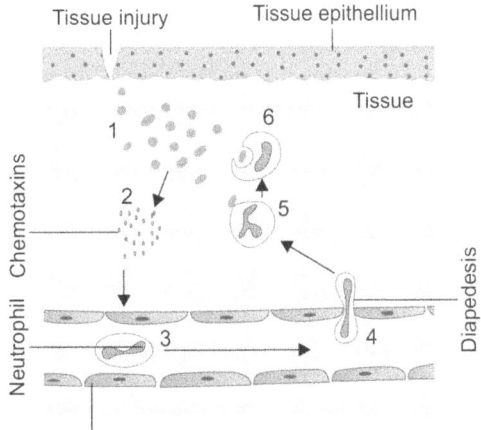

Fig. 2: Phagocytosis; Neutrophils marginate towards the wall of capillary followed by diapedesis, chemotaxis and engulfing the microbes.
(*Source:* GK Pal)

- Cytoplasm has coarse, orange pink granules
- Granules contain—eosinophil peroxidase, eosinophilic cationic protein, major basic protein, histaminase, catalase etc.
- Mostly present in tissues.

Physiological Roles
- Leave the capillaries and enter tissue spaces where allergic reactions occur
- Releases an enzyme, histaminase that combats the effects of histamine released by basophils
- They inhibit mast cell degranulation
- They are weakly phagocytic and phagocytose Ag-Ab complexes
- Eosinophils also release substances (major basic protein) which kill the parasitic worms
- So eosinophil counts increase in allergy and worm infestation.

Basophils
- They are similar to mast cells
- They are mildly phagocytic
- They enter tissues at sites of infection or tissue damage and release histamine, heparin and serotonin
- These chemicals are responsible for the inflammatory reactions
- They also release eosinophilic chemotactic factor which attracts eosinophils to combat the inflammatory reactions by removing Ag-Ab complexes
- Mast cells and basophils release the inflammatory mediators and are responsible for allergic reactions
- Basophils release heparin which is an anticoagulant and thereby removes minute clots and prevents clotting of blood.

2. **Define glomerular filtration rate (GFR). What are its determinants? Discuss the phenomenon of autoregulation of GFR. Describe the best test for estimation of GFR. What is the routinely used clinical test to assess renal function?**

- Glomerular filtration rate is defined as the volume of plasma filtered by all the nephrons of both the kidneys per unit of time
- Normal value is 125 mL/min or 180 L/day.

The determinants of GFR are:
- Filtration co-efficient (K_f): It is the product of permeability of the glomerular membrane and its surface area. As the Kf increases GFR increases and as K_f decreases GFR decreases
- Glomerular capillary hydrostatic pressure (P_{GC}): It is dependent on arterial blood pressure, renal blood flow and afferent and efferent arteriolar resistance. P_{GC} is directly proportional to GFR
- Capillary oncotic pressure (p_{GC}): GFR is inversely proportional to p_{GC}
- Hydrostatic pressure in Bowman's space: It opposes filtration and GFR is inversely related to GFR
- Sympathetic stimulation: Stimulation leads to vasoconstriction and decreased RBF and GFR.

Autoregulation of GFR
Refer answers to 2013 paper.

The best test to estimate GFR
Refer answers to 2005 paper.

Routinely used Clinical Test used to Assess Renal Function
- A fall in GFR is the first and only clinical sign of kidney disease

- So measurement of GFR is used to assess kidney diseases
- Since measurement of GFR by Inulin clearance is cumbersome in clinical setting, plasma creatinine is measured and it is level is inversely proportional to GFR. From the serum creatinine level estimated GFR (eGFR) is calculated
- But the fall in GFR should be substantial for the rise in plasma creatinine.

3. Define the terms cardiac output and total peripheral resistance and discuss their determinants.

Cardiac output is defined as the amount of blood ejected by each ventricle per minute.

Cardiac output = Stroke volume × Heart rate

Normal value = 5–6 L/min.

Total peripheral resistance is defined as the resistance offered to the blood flow in the blood vessels.

Determinants of peripheral resistance are diameter of blood vessels and viscosity of blood.

Determinants of Cardiac Output
Refer answers to 2011 paper.

Determinants of Peripheral Resistance
Refer answers to 2013 paper.

4. What are the neural mechanisms involved in spontaneous breathing? Discuss chemical regulation of respiration. Distinguish between the two types of respiratory failure.

Neural Regulation of Respiration
Refer answers to 2007 paper.

Chemical Regulation of Respiration
Refer answers to 2005 paper.

Two Types of Respiratory Failure

Respiratory failure is due to inadequate gas exchange. There are two types of failures—Type 1 and Type 2 failure.
1. **Type 1 failure:** Here only the PO_2 level in the arterial blood is low and PCO_2 level is either normal or low. It may be due to mismatch in ventilation/perfusion ratio and the defect here is poor oxygenation of blood
2. **Type 2 failure:** Here PO_2 level is below 60 mm Hg and also hypercapnea is present, PCO_2 is >50 mm Hg. Seen in conditions of increased airway resistance like bronchial asthma, decreased breathing effects as in brainstem lesion, skeletal deformity like kyphosis and a decrease in diffusion area as in chronic bronchitis.

5. What is the composition of gastric juice? Describe the mechanism of HCl secretion. Give a detailed account on the regulation of gastric secretion.

Refer answers to 2005 paper.

6. Define blood pressure. Discuss in brief the various factors which influence the pressure. Add a note on hypertension.

Refer answers to 2003 paper.

Factors Influencing BP

Blood pressure = Cardiac output × Peripheral resistance.
- Cardiac output = Stroke volume × Heart rate
- *Stroke volume:* It is decided by:
  - End diastolic volume (Preload): Preload is directly proportional to Stroke volume and cardiac output. It is based on Frank-Starling's law.

    Factors affecting preload are—blood volume, skeletal muscle pump, thoracic pump as in respiration, ventricular compliance and atrial contraction
  - Contractility: Force of contraction of the myocardium without increase in initial length of the muscle fiber. It is said to be the inotropic property of the heart. Sympathetic stimulation, catecholamines, glucagon and digitalis are positively inotropic. Hypoxia, hypercapnia, acidosis are negatively inotropic
  - Afterload: It is the peripheral resistance against which the heart contracts. It is determined by peripheral resistance. Afterload is inversely related to stroke volume and cardiac output.

- *Heart rate (HR):* It is regulated by:
  - Parasympathetic nerves: Decrease HR
  - Sympathetic nerves: Increase HR.

Peripheral resistance
- *Diameter of blood vessels*
  a. Vasomotor tone: Regulated by sympathetic nerve supply (increases the tone). Vasoconstriction increases the PR and thereby the blood pressure is increased.
- *Viscosity of blood*
  a. Plasma proteins
  b. Number of RBCs.

Hypertension
- It is defined as the sustained elevation of systemic arterial pressure
- Blood pressure is determined by cardiac output and peripheral resistance
- Systolic BP is determined by cardiac output and therefore affected by stroke volume and heart rate. These determinants are subjected to daily activities. Therefore elevation in systolic BP is not usually considered as hypertension
- Diastolic BP is determined by peripheral resistance. PR is in turn decided by calibre of blood vessel and viscosity of blood. Sustained elevation of diastolic BP results in hypertension. It is usually associated with elevation of systolic BP also
- 120/80 mm Hg is normal BP
- 120-139/80-89 mm Hg—prehypertension
- Above 140/90 mm Hg—hypertension.

Types of Hypertension (HT)
- Primary or essential hypertension
- Secondary hypertension.

Primary or Essential Hypertension
- In over 90% of the individuals with hypertension, the cause is unknown. This is said to be primary HT. It could be due to sympathetic hyperactivity, increased sodium intake, increase in blood volume etc.
- It can be in the benign form or it can progress to malignant HT.

Benign form:
- There could be moderate or great increase in BP upto 210/110 mm Hg. But there is also fluctuation of systolic BP—so it is called as Labile HT
- In late stages, systolic BP is increased and fixed and does not come back to normal
- Anti-hypertensives are prescribed
- It causes cardiac hypertrophy, arteriosclerosis of the vessels and increased incidence of myocardial infarction. There are renal changes like albuminuria, hematuria etc.

Malignant hypertension:
- BP is very much increased even upto 260/150 mm Hg
- There are arteriolar lesions
- Patients show symptoms of papilledema, cerebral symptoms and renal failure
- If patient is not treated, usually death occurs within 6 months to 2 years.

Secondary Hypertension
- Blood pressure is increased due to some other underlying disease.

It can be due to:

Renal diseases like glomerulonephritis, pyelonephritis, renal tumors, polycystic kidney disease etc.

Goldblatt hypertension: Due to renal artery stenosis. They are of two types:
a. One kidney one clip Goldblatt hypertension: One kidney is removed and the renal artery of the other kidney is stenosed. Here rise in BP is independent of Renin levels
b. Two kidney one clip Goldblatt hypertension: Two kidneys are present and constriction of the renal artery of one kidney. The rise in BP is dependent on increased renin levels.

Cardiovascular diseases like atherosclerosis.

Endocrinal Diseases
- Pheochromocytoma
- Cushing's syndrome
- Primary hyperaldosteronism or Conn's syndrome
- Acromegaly
- Glucocorticoid remediable hyperaldosteronism
- Myxedema.

Neurogenic hypertension (Refer answers to 2010 paper).

Hypertension in pregnancy: Due to pressor peptides secreted from placenta hypertension is present with preeclampsia or eclampsia.

Congenital diseases like Liddle's syndrome where there is excessive retention of salt and water.

Coarctation of aorta: Congenital narrowing of the aorta especially the thoracic aorta results in severe hypertension in upper half of the body.

Chronic treatment with oral contarceptive (OC) pills:
- OC pills contain estrogen and progesterone
- Estrogen increases production of Angiotensinogen resulting in elevated Angiotensin II levels
- Normally this would decrease Renin secretion and that brings Ang II levels to normal
- But in consumption of OC pills this feedback is incomplete resulting in hypertension—Pill hypertension.

Effects of Hypertension

On the Heart
- The consistent increase in peripheral resistance leads to increase in afterload which increases the work of the myocardium resulting in left ventricular hypertrophy
- Myocardial oxygen requirement increases due to increased ventricular muscle mass
- So even minimal narrowing of coronary vessels results in ischemia
- Gradually the ability to compensate for the high peripheral resistance is exceeded and the heart fails.

On the Blood Vessels
- There is increased incidence of atherosclerosis
- High BP also leads to stiffness of vessels and their compliance is lost
- They are prone for cerebral thrombosis and cerebral hemorrhage.

Kidneys
- Atherosclerosis of renal vessels affects renal functions like filtration and tubular functions
- Renal failure is an important complication in HT.

7. Define anemia. Classify them. List the important investigations to confirm the various types of anemia.

- **Anemia is defined as the decrease in red cell count or hemoglobin content in blood**
- Anemia is classified based on the cause of anemia and based on the structure of red cells.

A. Morphological Classification or Wintrobe's Classification

Based on the size and the presence of hemoglobin content inside the cell it is classified as:
i. Normocytic normochromic anemia: The RBC size (MCV) and the hemoglobin content (MCH and MCHC) is normal. It is seen in hemorrhagic anemia, hemolysis and aplastic anemia
ii. Microcytic hypochromic anemia: The cell volume and the hemoglobin content are decreased. Mean corpuscular volume (MCV), mean corpuscular hemoglobin (MCH) and mean corpuscular hemoglobin concentration (MCHC) are below normal. It is seen in iron defeciency anemia
iii. Macrocytic anemia: MCV is above normal range. There is macrocytosis and the hemoglobin concentration is normal. This type is normally seen in Vitamin B12 and Folic acid deficiency.

B. Etiological Classification or Wintrobe's Classification

Anemia is usually due to either decreased production from the bone marrow or increased destruction (refer Fig. 3).

Classification of Anemia
i. Decreased red cell production:
   a. Decreased production due to stem cell failure: Aplastic anemia
   b. Dietary defeciencies:
      - Iron defeciency anemia

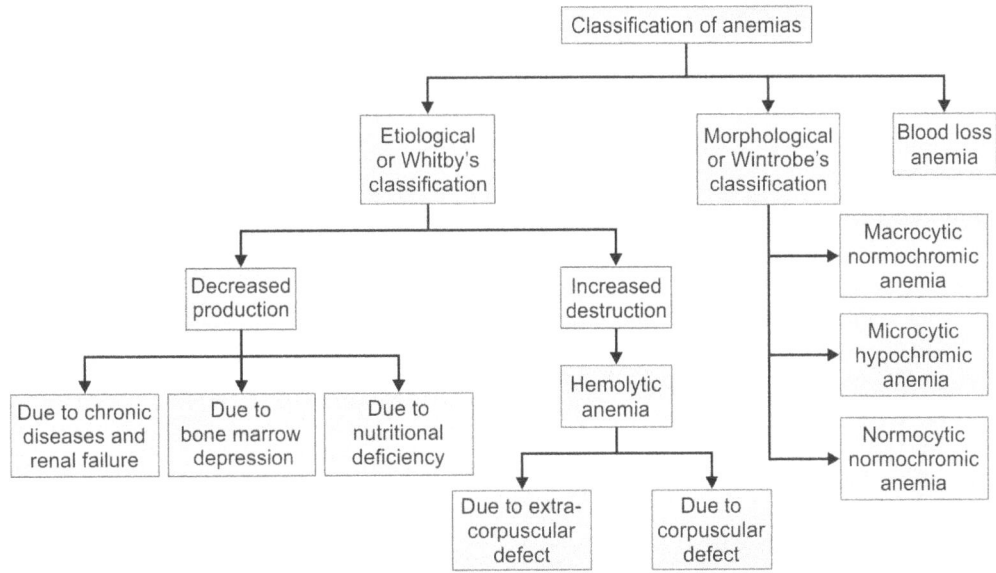

Fig. 3: Classification of anemias.

- Megaloblastic anemia: Due to defeciency of folic acid and vitamin B12 defeciency
- Pernicious anemia: Anemia due to vitamin B12 deficiency due to deficiency of Intrinsic factor
- Protein deficiency

ii. Increased destruction of red cells:
  a. Hemolytic anemias: Congenital and acquired
     Congenital:
     a. Membrane defects: Hereditary spherocytosis and hereditary elliptocytosis
     b. Hemoglobin defects:
        * Hemoglobinopathies (defects in hemoglobin): Sickle cell anemia (HbS, in the beta chain in the 6th position glutamic acid is replaced by Valine), abnormal hemoglobin like HbC, HBE, HbD
        * Thalassemias (deficiencies of hemoglobin: Deficiency of α or β chain)—major and minor.
     c. Enzyme defects: Deficiency of glucose-6-phosphate dehydrogenase and pyruvate kinase.
     Acquired:
     - Due to antigen-antibody reactions
     – Erythroblastosis fetalis, incompatible blood transfusions etc.
  - Infections: Malaria
  - Drug induced: Quinine, asprin etc
  - Snake venom
  - Hypersplenism: Excessive destruction of RBCs
  - Burns.

iii. Blood loss anemia:
  – Acute hemorrhage: Trauma, surgery etc.
  – Chronic blood loss: Menorrhagia, worm infestation.

iv. Anemia due to chronic renal failure: Due to decreased production of erythropoietin

v. Anemia associated with chronic diseases.

Investigations to Detect the Types of Anemia

Most common types of anemias are iron deficiency and Vitamin B12 deficiency anemias. So the investigations done to detect these anemias are discussed below.

Iron Deficiency Anemia

- **Blood picture and red cell indices:**
  – Hb concentration↓
  – RBCs in peripheral smear are microcytic hypochromic
  – Red cell indices like MCV, MCH, MCHC are reduced.
- **Bone marrow findings:**
  – Erythroid hyperplasia
  – Marrow is iron-deficient.

- **Biochemical findings:**
  - Serum iron decreases < 50 µg% (normal 60–160 µg%)
  - Serum ferritin low
  - Total iron binding capacity (TIBC) is increased.

Megaloblastic Anemia
- **Blood changes:**
  - RBCs are macrocytic normochromic.
  - RBC count decreases < 1 million/cumm
  - Hb decreases <12g/dL
  - MCV increases 95–160 fL (Normal 78–94 fL)
  - MCH increases to 50 pg
  - MCHC normal as both MCV and MCH has increased
  - In peripheral smear there are nucleated RBCs
  - Reticulocyte count increases >5%
  - WBC and platelet counts decrease.
- **Biochemical findings:**
  - Plasma concentration of vitamin B12 decreases in pernicious anemia.
  - Serum folate level decreases in anemia due to folic acid deficiency.

8. **Define cardiac cycle. Describe the sequence of events during cardiac cycle in detail with suitable diagrams.**

Refer answers to 2005 paper.

II. SHORT NOTES

1. **cAMP signaling pathway, with an example**

- Cyclic adenosine monophosphate (cAMP) is an important second messenger for peptide hormones
- Many chemicals like norepinephrine, adrenocorticotrophic hormone (ACTH), antidiuretic hormone (ADH), angiotensin II, calcitonin, corticotropin-releasing hormone (CRH), follicle-stimulating hormone (FSH), luteinizing hormone (LH) etc act via cAMP
- It is said to be the cAMP-adenylyl cyclase pathway.

The following is the signaling pathway:
- Peptide hormone binds to the membrane bound receptor

- The receptor is bound to G-protein
- On binding of hormone to receptor, GDP is released from G-protein and replaced by GTP and G-protein is activated
- Activated G-protein in turn stimulates or inhibits the membrane bound enzyme adenylyl cyclase
- Adenylyl cyclase catalyses the conversion of cytoplasmic ATP to cAMP. When the G-protein is stimulatory (Gs) the cAMP levels increase and when the G-protein is inhibitory (Gi) The cAMP is decreased
- cAMP in turn activates a cascade of enzyme system like protein kinase A
- Protein kinase A catalyzes the phosphorylation of proteins, changing their confirmation and functions
- cAMP is inactivated to 5'AMP by the enzyme phosphodiesterase and activity is terminated (refer Fig. 4).

For example, the activation of phosphorylase kinase enzyme in the liver by epinephrine via cAMP and protein kinase A is given below:

Epinephrine
↓
β2 receptor
↓
Gs
↓
Adenylyl cyclase
↓
ATP → cAMP
↓
Protein kinase A activated
↓
Inactive phosphorylase
β kinase +ATP → Activated phosphorylase β kinase
↓
Phosphorylase β +ATP → Phophorylase A
↓
Glycogen → Glucose-1-phosphate

2. **Colloid oncotic pressure and its importance.**

- Colloidal oncotic pressure is the osmotic pressure generated by larger molecules, especially proteins in plasma

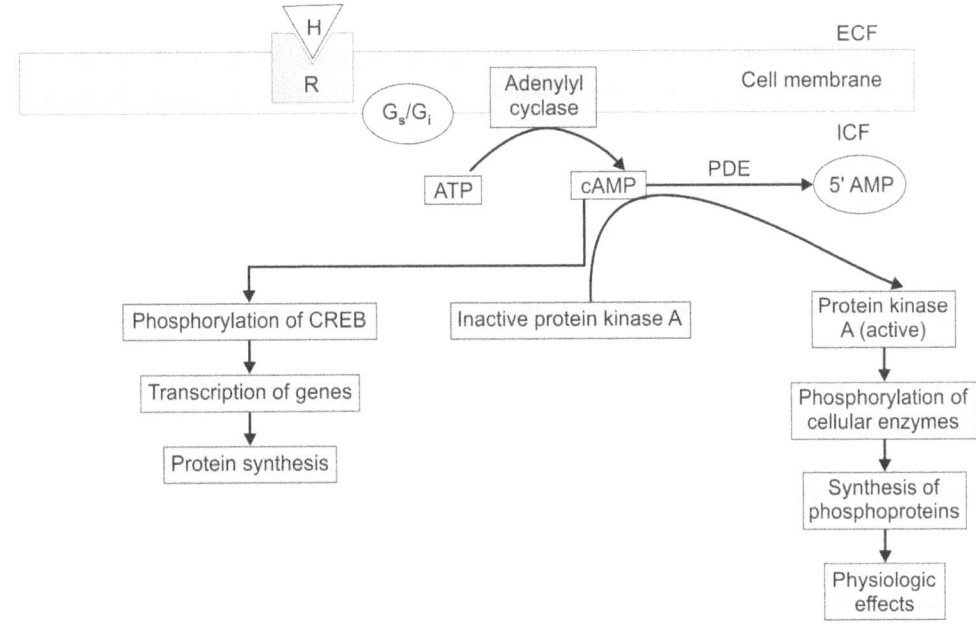

Fig. 4: Activation Gs—adenylyl cyclase—cAMP signaling pathway.
(H: Peptide hormone; R: Receptor; Gs/Gi: Stimulatory G protein/Inhibitory G protein; cAMP: Cyclic adenosine monophosphate; PDE: Phosphodiesterase; CREB:cAMP responsive element-binding protein)
(*Source:* GK Pal)

- The oncotic pressure exerted by plasma proteins is 26–28 mm Hg
- It is the important force involved in fluid movement across the capillaries
- Among the plasma proteins, albumin is the major protein to exert the oncotic pressure
- The pores in between the endothelial cells are smaller in size and therefore do not allow the movement of proteins and other colloids across them
- The colloids have a high molecular weight and are present in large amounts
- Therefore the capillary membrane is like an impermeable membrane to colloids and they exert an osmotic pressure of an average of 25 mm Hg
- The rate of filtration of fluid across the capillary wall at any time is dependent upon the balance of Starling's forces
- One of the starling's forces is the plasma oncotic pressure and other forces are— capillary hydrostatic pressure, interstitial hydrostatic pressure and osmotic pressure in the interstitium
- So the hydrostatic pressure gradient (hydrostatic pressure in capillary—hydrostatic pressure in interstitium) and the osmotic pressure gradients (colloidal oncotic pressure in capillary—colloidal osmotic pressure in interstitium) decide filtration across capillaries
- In the arteriolar end of the capillaries, the hydrostatic pressure is 36 mm Hg and the interstitial hydrostatic pressure varies in different tissues, it is subatmospheric in subcutaneous tissues, positive in liver and 6 mm Hg in the brain
- The oncotic pressure in capillary is 25 mm Hg and in the interstitium it is negligible
  - So fluid movement = $K[(Pc + \pi i) - (Pi + \pi c)]$
  - K = Filtration co-efficient
  - Pc = Hydrostatic pressure in capillary (37 mm Hg in arteriolar end and 17 mm Hg in venous end)
  - Pi = Hydrostatic pressure in interstitium (1 mm Hg)
  - πc = Colloidal oncotic pressure in plasma (25 mm Hg)
  - πi = Colloidal osmotic pressure in interstitium (0 mm Hg)

- Pc and πi favors filtration and Pi and πc opposes filtration.
- In the arteriolar end of capillaries the hydrostatic pressure in capillaries exceeds the oncotic pressure and therefore filtration of fluid happens here
- Along with the fluid filtered, nutrients also enter the tissues
- As fluid moves out of the capillaries, in the venous end, the hydrostatic pressure in capillaries drops to 17 mm Hg and the colloid oncotic pressure is 25 mm Hg and this favors reabsorption in the venous end of capillaries along with the metabolic wastes
- In the glomerulus, throughout length of the capillary, the hydrostatic pressure exceeds the oncotic pressure and therefore fluid moves out of the capillaries throughout the length of the capillary.

Applied Aspects

In hypoproteinemia due to malnutrition, liver diseases (synthesis of protein is less) and in nephrosis (albumin is lost in urine), the plasma colloidal oncotic pressure decreases resulting in edema.

3. **Excitation-contraction coupling in skeletal muscle.**

Refer answers to 2003 paper.

4. **Types of polycythemia and complications due to this condition.**

Polycythemia is increase in RBC count above the normal value. It can be physiological or pathological.

Physiological Polycythemia

- Age: At birth the count is high (6–7 million cells/cumm) and after birth it starts decreasing due to destruction of RBCs
- High altitude: Hypoxia in high altitude stimulates production of erythropoietin which in turn stimulates RBC production
- Excessive exercise.

Pathological Polycythemia—2 Types

a. *Primary polycythemia or polycythemia vera:* It is a type of myeloproliferative syndrome and is due to a cancerous condition of the bone marrow. The counts increase more than 10 million cells/cu mm. A high WBC count may also be seen. In this condition erythropoietin levels may be very low

b. *Secondary polycythemia:* It happens due to hypoxic conditions in the body as in lung (emphysema, COPD) and cardiovascular diseases (cyanotic heart diseases). The hypoxia stimulates synthesis of eryhtropoietin and thereby increased production of RBCs.

Complications of Polycythemia

Increase in RBC count, increases the viscosity of blood and thereby increases the peripheral resistance leading to hypertension and left heart failure.

5. **Findings of 'tests of hemostasis' in hemophilia.**

Hemophilia is a bleeding disorder due to the absence of clotting factor VIII, IX and XI. It is a genetic disorder and is x-linked recessive diesease. The males are always affected and the females are carriers.

The Laboratory Tests in Hemophilia

a. **Bleeding time** is normal as the platelet count and the capillary integrity is normal
b. **Capillary fragility test** is normal
c. **Platelet count** is also normal
d. **Coagulation time:** It is the time taken for the blood to clot in a capillary tube by formation of fibrin thread. It is prolonged in hemophilia
e. **Prothrombin time:** It is done by Quick's one stage method. Here the anticoagulated plasma of the patient is mixed with commercially available tissue thromboplastin and calcium chloride solution and is incubated at 37°C. The time at which a gel is formed is taken to be the PT. Normally it is around 11–16 seconds. Only extrinsic pathway is assessed by this method and therefore it is normal in hemophilia
f. **Partial thromboplastin time (PTT):** Here to the anticoagulated plasma, Kaolin (surface agent), calcium chloride and cephalin are added and incubated at 37°C.

The time taken to form the gel is the PTT. It gives an idea about the intrinsic pathway. Normal PTT is 40 seconds. It is prolonged in hemophilia

g. **Thromboplastin generation test:** This test assesses the intrinsic pathway of coagulation and the normal value is 12 seconds. It is prolonged in hemophilia.

6. Functions of macrophages.

The macrophages have the following functions:

a. **Phagocytosis:** As a phagocyte it is very powerful and it emigrats into the tissues following the bacterial invasion. But this happens 24 hours after the neutrophil action and therefore it is said to be the **second line of defense**. It engulfs the bacteria and digests it; the process of digestion of bacteria is similar to that of the neutrophils—by producing free radicals - H_2O_2 and lowering the pH. It can also engulf other substances like the cell debris, dead RBCs, Foreign bodies etc.

b. **Secretory function:** Monocytes and macrophages secrete many chemicals like—interleukins, IL-1, TNF-α, binding proteins like transferrin, lysozyme, proteases, acid hydrolase etc.

IL-1 has many important functions—it acts as a WBC growth factor in red bone marrow, it is an endogenous pyrogen etc.

TNF α: It induces shock in septicemia due to gram negative bacterial infections, destroys invading bacteria, etc.

Transferrin is an iron binding protein in plasma to carry iron and also makes it unavailable for bacteria and thereby prevents its multiplication

c. **Role in lymphocyte-mediated immunity:** Macrophages act as Antigen presenting cells in immune reactions. It engulfs the microorganism and digests it and attaches the antigenic component to the MHC II molecule in the macrophage. The antigen-MHCII complex now moves towards the membrane of the macrophage and is inserted there. This macrophage moves towards the lymphnodes and the antigen is presented to the Lymphocytes.

The Lymphocytes with the receptor for the antigen binds to the APC and is activated for further differentiation and division

d. Monocyte-Macrophage seceretory products also play a *key role in healing and repair.*

7. Physiological role of corticosteroids.

Refer answers to 2009 paper.

8. Function of any one hormone of posterior pituitary.

- Oxytocin is an oligopeptide with 9 amino acids and is secreted from the posterior pituitary
- It is synthesized from magnocellular neurons of paraventricular nucleus of hypothalamus and is secreted into circulation from posterior pituitary.

Functions of Oxytocin in:

i. It stimulates milk ejection reflex (Refer answers for August 2008 question paper)
ii. It induces parturition reflex (Refer answers for August 2008 question paper)
iii. It also acts on non-pregnant uterus to facilitate sperm transport
iv. In males it is secreted during ejaculation and causes contraction of smooth muscles of vas deferens to propel the sperm towards urethra.

9. Composition of bile and the physiological role (if any) of the components.

Composition of Bile

Bile is formed from hepatocytes in liver. Some substances are added to bile from blood (e.g. Bile pigments).

The composition of bile is:

- It contains water and solids
- Water – 97.5%
- Solids – 2.5%
- Solids includes organic and inorganic substances
- Organic substances: Bile salts, bile pigments, cholesterol, fats, fatty acids, lecithin, mucin
- Inorganic substances—Na^+, K^+, Cl^-, HCO_3^- and Ca^{++}.

Functions of Bile Salts
Refer answers to 2009 paper.

10. Pathophysiology of peptic ulcer.
There are two types of ulcers:
1. **Duodenal ulcer**
2. **Gastric ulcer**
- Ulcer is due to disruption of the mucosal barrier or excess secretion of gastric juice
- Acid or pepsin in gastric juice digests the mucosa leading to ulcer.

Mucosal barrier is formed by:
- Mucus secreted by the neck cells and surface mucosal cells in the mucosal lining. It also contains mucin, phospholipid, HCO_3^- and water
- Prostaglandins secreted by epithelial cells have antisecretory activity (HCl) and increases HCO_3^- and mucus secretion
- Epithelium of mucosa has low permeability, rapid turnover and HCO_3^-, mucus secretions from there
- Bicarbonate secretion from gastric mucosal cells increases the pH.

Factors which impair mucosal defense
a. Defective mucus secretion
b. Drugs like NSAIDs, cortisol etc: They inhibit secretion of mucus and bicarbonate
c. Alcohol
d. Type of Food
e. Smoking: ↓mucus and pancreatic secretions. Causes reflux of duodenal contents
f. Stress
g. Reflux of gastric contents
h. Delayed gastric emptying
i. H.pylori infection: Causes local inflammation in antral mucosa and disrupts the barrier.

Factors which increase HCl secretion:
- Genetic factors: Increased parietal cell mass, increased post-prandial gastrin response
- Psychosomatic factors: Anxiety increases secretion
- Food: Alcohol, tea, coffee, spicy food
- Rapid gastric emptying
- Zollinger-Ellison syndrome: It is a gastrin secreting tumor of pancreas.

11. Describe the 3 bipolar limb leads of ECG. What is the significance of (a) PR interval (b) ST segment in an ECG?
- In bipolar leads both the elctrodes are active and one electrode is connected to the negative terminal and the other electrode is connected to the positive terminal of the electrocardiogram
- The placements of three bipolar limb leads are based on the Einthoven's triangle
- It is an equilateral triangle with each side of the triangle as the axis of each lead and heart as source of current in the center
- The 3 corners of the triangle are formed by the two shoulders and the pubic region. Since the body fluid acts as a good conducting media the leads can be placed in the two arms and left foot
- The two electrodes have to be placed in the corners of the triangle
- Bipolar limb leads: Lead I, II and III
  - **Lead I:** The two active electrodes are placed in the right and left arms. Left arm is connected to positive terminal and right arm is connected to negative terminal
  - **Lead II:** It is between the right arm and left foot. Right arm is connected to negative terminal and left foot to positive terminal
  - **Lead III:** It is between left arm and left foot. Left foot is connected to positive terminal and left arm is connected to negative terminal (refer Fig. 5).

As the electrical activity of the heart moves toward the positive lead an upward deflection is recorded in that lead.

P-R Interval
- It is between the onset of P wave to the onset of QRS complex (refer Fig. 6)
- The normal duration is 0.12–0.2 seconds
- It is the time taken for impulse conduction from SA Node to the AV node
- Prolonged PR interval signifies AV conduction block.

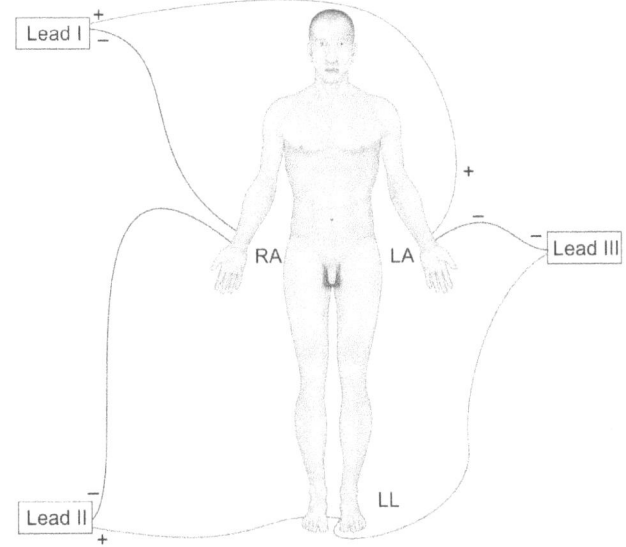

Fig. 5: Placement of bipolar limb leads.
(*Source:* Sembulingam)

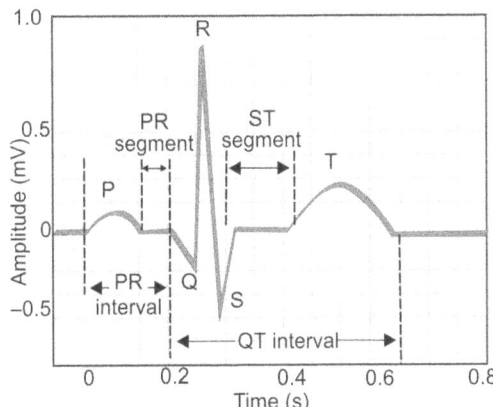

Fig. 6: Waves, segments and intervals in a normal ECG recorded in Lead II.
(*Source:* GK Pal)

ST Segment

- It is an isoelectric line between the end of QRS complex and beginning of T wave
- Normal duration is 0.04–0.08 sec
- It is in relation to ventricular repolarisation
- ST segment is clinically significant as it is 'the indicator' of myocardial infarction.
- In myocardial infarction ST segment is elevated. Based on the elevation of ST segment in particular leads overlying the walls of the heart the area of infarct can be identified.

12. Discuss the changes in ventricular volume during different phases of the cardiac cycle with a diagram.

Volume changes in the ventricles during various phases of cardiac cycle:

Ventricular Systole

Isovolumetric contraction phase:
- There is no change in the volume of the ventricle in this phase.

Ventricular ejection phase:
- During this phase blood is ejected out of both the ventricles—stroke volume. It is about 80 mL
- The end-diastolic volume is about 130 mL and therefore after ejection 50 mL remains in the ventricle—end-systolic volume
- Ejection fraction is the ratio of EDV ejected per systole.

Ventricular Diastole

- Protodiastole is the phase just before closure of semilunar valves. There is continuous drop in ventricular pressure and no blood flowing into the ventricles. So volume doesn't change (refer Fig. 7)
- Isovolumetric relaxation phase: As the name implies no change in ventricular

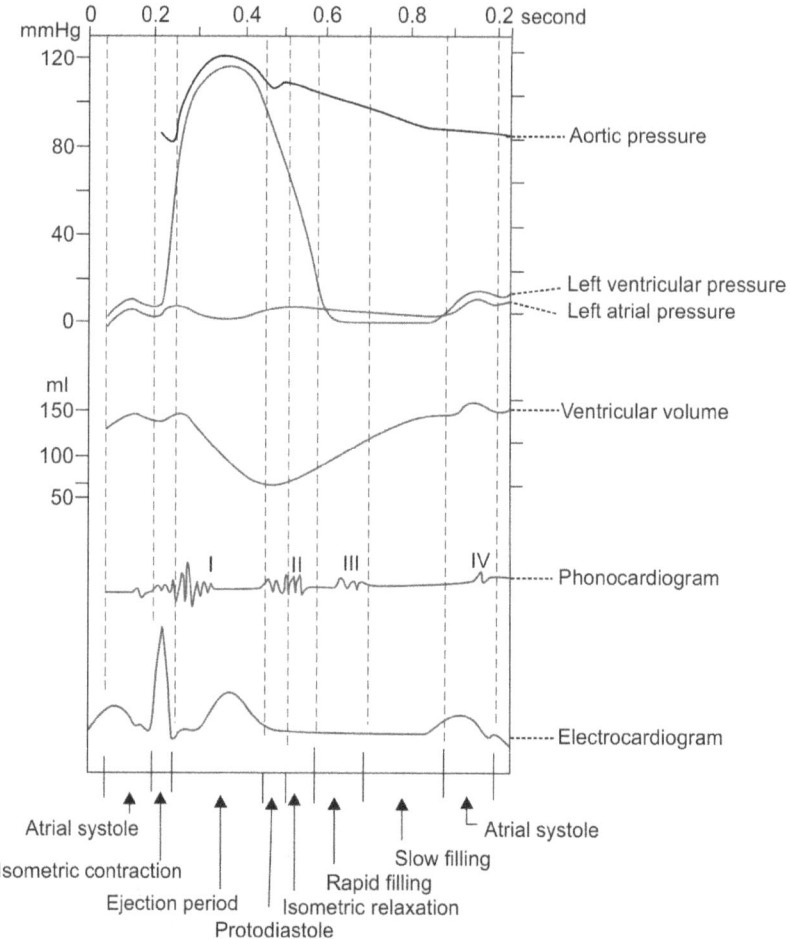

Fig. 7: Changes in ventricular volume in various phases of cardiac cycle.
(*Source:* Sembulingam)

volume as the AV valves and semilunar valves are closed and therefore no blood flows in or flows out
- First rapid filling phase and diastasis: This phase starts with opening of AV valves. The ventricular pressure is very low, almost zero and there is pressure gradient allowing rapid inrush of blood into the ventricles. Almost 75% of the ventricular filling happens in this phase (105 mL of EDV) (refer Fig. 8)
- Atrial systole or second rapid filling phase
  - The last 25% of ventricular filling happens due to atrial contraction or systole
  - The EDV of 130 mL is reached in both the ventricles.

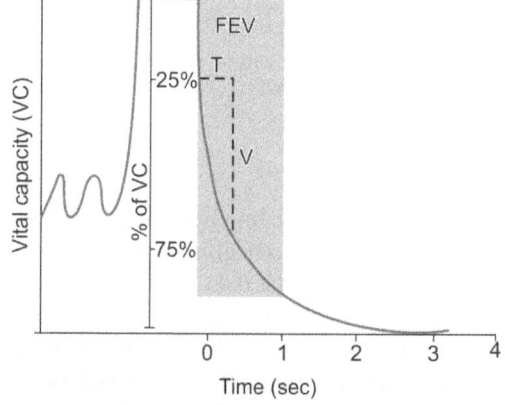

Fig. 8: Timed Vital capacity in normal individuals. FEV1 is around 80% of FVC. The same recording can be used to calculate forced expiratory flow rate between 25% - 75% of expiratory flow with T as time and V as Volume in the curve.
(*Source:* GK Pal)

13. Discuss any two pulmonary function tests which can detect obstructive lung disease.

- The major problem in obstructive lung disease is during expiration. The major feature is decrease in expiratory flow rate
- The most important tests done to detect the obstructive airway diseases are—maximum mid-expiratory flow rate (MMEFR) and FEV_1/FVC ratio.

MMEFR

- It is the flow rate in the middle 50% of FVC
- It is given as forced expiratory flow rate at 25-75% of the lung volume ($FEF_{25-75\%}$) (refer Fig. 8)
- Normally it is around 300 L/min
- This parameter indicates the patency of the smaller airways and therefore is affected in chronic obstructive lung disorders like bronchial asthma.

Timed Vital Capacity

Timed vital capacity (TVC) or forced vital capacity (FVC) is the maximum volume of air which has been breathed out as maximally, forcefully and rapidly as possible following a maximum inspiration. As it includes the words rapidly, time factor is included here. So it is a dynamic lung volume and is divided into the following components:

- FEV_1: It is the volume of FVC forcefully breathed out in the first second of expiration and the normal value is 80% of FVC
- FEV_2: It is the volume of FVC forcefully breathed out in the first two seconds of expiration. Normal value is 95% of FVC
- FEV_3: It is the volume of FVC forcefully breathed out in the first 3 seconds of exhalation. Normal value is 98–100% of FVC
- In obstructive lung disorders the vital capacity is normal but the FEV_1 is decreased
- FEV_1 less than 72% is a definite indicator of obstructive lung disorder.

14. Trace the pathway for perception of fine touch.

Refer answers to 2012 paper.

15. Operant conditioning.

- It is a reflex response to a stimulus, that previously elicited little or no response, aquired by repeatedly pairing the stimulus with another stimulus which normally produces a response
- The stimulus that normally produces a response is the unconditioned stimulus (UCS) and the stimulus which elicits a response after pairing with UCS is the conditioned stimulus (CS)
- There are two types of conditioned reflexes—Classical conditioning and Operant conditioning.

Operant Conditioning

- It is a form of conditioning in which the animal is taught to do a task in order to obtain a reward or to avoid a punishment
- UCS is the pleasant or unpleasant event and CS is light or an event which alerts the animal to do the task
- For example, the animal kept in a Skinner box where there is a lever and when the animal presses the lever it can escape an electric shock to its feet
- The animal learns to avoid pressing the lever
- This is called as conditioned avoidance reflex or negative reinforcement
- Similarly in another experiment when the animal presses the lever it is provided with food pellet
- Initially it presses the lever accidentally and then it continues to do learning that it receives the food pellet
- This is positive reinforcement of learning.

16. Clinical features of cerebellar lesions.

Refer answers to 2008 paper.

17. Define muscle tone and discuss the phenomenon responsible for it. What conditions lead to alterations of tone?

Refer answers to 2010 paper.

- Muscle tone is altered in UMN and LMN lesions
- In UMN lesions, the inhibitory control of higher centers over the stretch reflex is

removed and therefore there is hypertonia in the muscles
- In LMN lesion, the final common pathway to the muscles is affected which results in hypotonia in the muscles
- In cerebellar lesion there is hypotonia.

18. Endogenous opioid peptides.
Refer answers to 2005 paper.

19. Refractory errors of the eye.
Refer answers to 2004 paper.

20. Discuss the phenomena by which sound waves in air induce action potentials in the cochlear nerve.
Refer answers to 2010 paper.

21. Hypersecretion of growth hormone.

Acromegaly
- It is a clinical condition due to excess secretion of growth hormone (GH) in adults (after the fusion of the epiphyseal plates in the long bones)
- It is usually due to a tumor of growth hormone producing cells (somatotrophs) in the anterior pituitary gland
- Rarely, it can also be due to hypothalamic tumors secreting GH releasing hormone
- There is no increase in height of the individual
- But because of excess levels of GH, there is thickening of bones and proliferation of soft tissues like connective tissue and skin
- This leads to coarse disfigured appearance. "Acro" means extremity and "megaly" is large.

Clinical Features of Acromegaly
a. The tumor in the anterior pituitary compresses the optic chiasma resulting in visual disturbances
b. Enlargement of sella turcica and headache
c. Enlarging tumor may destroy other pituitary cells and decrease in levels of other hormones secreted from anterior pituitary may happen
- *Clinical features due to excess GH levels:*
   a. Acromegalic face: Jaw and cheek bones become more prominent, lips are thickened, nose is broad and thick, enlarged brows and coarse skin
   b. Prognathism: Protrusion of the lower jaw due to elongation and thickening of mandible
   c. Enlarged spade like hands, broad fingers and large feet
   d. Body hair is increased
   e. Kyphosis: Since the vertebral bones continue to grow the person has kyphosis
   f. They develop osteoarthritis
   g. Organomegaly: Internal organs like heart, liver, spleen and kidneys are enlarged
   h. High levels of GH decreases insulin sensitivity in the tissues and the patient has hyperglycemia and are prone to develop diabetes mellitus.

Gigantism
It is due to hypersecrteion of GH in children before the closure of epiphysis.

Symptoms
- Abnormal height (7-8 ft tall)
- Enlarged hands and feet
- Gynecomastia
- Loss of libido
- Hyperglycemia which may result in diabetes mellitus
- They also have symptoms similar to acromegaly due to the compression of tumor on neighboring neural structure.

22. Tissue macrophage system.
- Monocytes are formed in the bone marrow. They circulate in blood for 10-20 hours
- They are the largest blood cells, 12-20 μm in size (2-2.5 times the size of RBCs)
- Nucleus occupies almost 50% of the cell volume and the rest is the cytoplasm. The granules in cytoplasm do not take the regular staining and therefore not visible. So is an agranulocyte
- Monocytes after circulation, enter various tissues through the capillary membrane and swell up to become the macrophage

- They live for months to years as a tissue macrophage
- They exist as either fixed macrophages or mobile macrophage
- The monocytes, macrophages and specialized endothelial cells in bone marrow, spleen and lymph nodes are grouped as reticulo-endothelial system
- They are destroyed once their phagocytic action is over
- Tissue macrophages are named according to the sites where they are present.

Following are the Tissue Macrophages

a. ***Pulmonary alveolar macrophage (PAM):*** The PAMs are present in the walls of the alveolus. It is one of the routes of entry of microbes from the environment. Macrophages phagocytose the microorganisms and if possible digests them and release them into the lymph

b. ***Kupffer cells in the liver sinusoids:*** The other route of entry for micro-organisms is through GIT. Bacteria absorbed from ingested food enters the portal circulation and reaches the liver and are phagocytosed and destroyed by kupffer cells lining the sinusoids

c. ***Macrophages in the spleen and bone marrow:*** Trabeculae of red pulp and sinuses of the spleen are lined by macrophages and they are very narrow passages and when blood squeezes through this path, unwanted debris and older cells like senile RBCs are phagocytosed and removed by the macrophages.
   In the bone marrow also there are macrophages to take care of microorganisms that enter through other routes of entry into the body

d. ***Tissue macrophages in skin and subcutaneous tissues (histiocytes):*** Normally skin forms a protective barrier to prevent entry of micro-organisms, but in case of breakage of the protective skin barrier infections may enter and they are taken care by the skin macrophages

e. ***Macrophages in lymph nodes:*** There are macrophages in lymph nodes also

f. ***Osteoclasts:*** Osteoclasts also belong to the family of monocytes and when they come in contact with stromal cells of bone marrow, they get converted to osteoclasts and they erode the bone and help in its remodelling

g. ***Microglia:*** Microglia is a type of neuroglial cell and it belongs to the monocyte family and they have the property of scavenging foreign particles in the nervous system.

Functions of Monocyte-macrophage system:

a. Active phagocytosis, they are the second line of defence
b. They enter tissues to become macrophages. They are given different names in various tissues – Kupffer cells in liver, PAM in lungs etc.
c. They also take part in immune response (As APCs)
d. They synthesize many substances like IL-1, TNF-α, Lysozyme, proteases etc.
e. They also help in healing and repair of tissue.

23. Neural regulation of respiration.

Refer answers to 2007 paper.

24. Functions and tests of cerebellum.

Functions of Cerebellum

Refer answers to February 2009 question paper (Essay 3).

Tests of Cerebellum

- **Finger nose test:** The patient is asked to extend the hand and to bring the tip of his index finger and touch the tip of nose. He is asked to repeat it alternately with both the hands rapidly
- **Adiadochokinesis:** Rapid and alternate pronation and supination of the forearm
- **Finger to finger test:** The patient is asked to bring his arms to the sides and then asked to bring the tips of index fingers together in front as an arc and to touch the tips
- **Drawing a circle in air** with finger tip
- **Buttoning** and unbuttoning the shirt
- **Heel knee test:** The subject is asked to place the heel of one leg on the knee of

another leg and to move the heel along the medial side of the tibia
- Walking in straight line.

25. Transport across cell membrane.
Refer answers to 2009 paper.

26. Ovarian and endometrial changes of menstrual cycle.
Refer answers to 2008 question paper.

Changes in the Uterine Endometrium

The uterine changes are given in 3 phases:
- Proliferative phase
- Secretory phase
- Menstrual phase.

Proliferative Phase

This phase correlates with follicular phase of ovarian cycle. Estrogen secreted from the follicle stimulates growth of uterine endometrium and therefore it thickens. Glands in the endometrium and the blood vessels grow. This phase is from day 5 till the day of ovulation.

Secretory Phase

This phase is from day of ovulation to 25th day. It correlates with the luteal phase of the ovarian cycle. Progesterone levels are high and they make the endometrium secretory by acting on the glands. Maximum action is 5 - 7 days after ovulation. The secretion is rich in glycogen and can nourish the fertilized ovum. Secretory endometrium is favorable for implantation of fertilized ovum.

If fertilization does not happen the corpus luteum starts to regress and the progesterone and estrogen levels drop. Withdrawal of hormonal support of the endometrium and release of prostaglandins result in vasoconstriction of the spiral arteries, uterine ischemia happens and endometrial necrosis and shedding of endometrium happens.

Menstrual Phase

It starts with the menstrual bleeding with the shedding of outer 2/3rd of endometrium, unfertilized ovum and contnues for 5 days.

27. Brown-Sequard syndrome.
Refer answers to 2008 paper.

28. Oxygen dissociation curve.
Refer answers to 2004 paper.

III. SHORT ANSWERS

1. Membrane transporters involved in clearance of calcium from cytoplasm.

a. Ca^{2+} transporters to clear Ca^{2+} from cytoplasm of a cell is by the following transporters in the cell membrane – Ca^{2+}-H^+ ATPase and Na^+ - Ca^{2+} exchanger

b. Ca^{2+} ATPase is the transporter on the sarcoplasmic reticulum membrane in skeletal muscles to pump back Ca^{2+} into SR resulting in muscle relaxation.

2. Concentrations of sodium and potassium in intra and extracellular fluids.

	Intracellular concentration (mmol/L of H_2O)	Extracellular concentration (mmol/L of H_2O)
Na^+	15	150
K^+	150	5.5

3. Phenomena involved in the act of swallowing.
Refer answers to 2003 paper.

4. Role of ATP in relaxation of muscle.
- After the cross-bridge cycling of the energized head of myosin, the head stays attached to actin molecule
- For the head to get detached another molecule of ATP has to get attached to the myosin head so that the head is removed from the attachment site
- The final relaxation happens after the cytoplasmic Ca^{2+} is decreased by pumping the Ca^{2+} into the sarcoplasmic reticulum
- This is done by the primary active transporter Ca^{2+}-ATPase
- A single molecule of ATP is broken to provide energy for the pumping of Ca^{2+} into SR.

5. **Draw a schematic diagram of the sarcomere and label its components.**

See Figure 9.

6. **Opsonins.**
- Opsonins are chemical substances which coat the microorganisms and make it tastier for phagocytosis by the neutrophils or macrophages
- Complementary protein C3b and the immunoglobulin IgG are opsonins.

7. **Cells which express major histocompatibility complex II.**

MHC II proteins are present in the antigen presenting cells like macrophages, dendritic cells and B cells and activated T cells.

8. **Significance of glycosylated hemoglobin.**
- There are small amounts of hemoglobin A that are represented as glycated hemoglobin
- One of these is Hemoglobin A_{1c} (HbA_{1c}). It has a glucose attached to the terminal valine in each β chain and is of special interest because its quantity increases in poorly controlled diabetes mellitus
- It gives an idea about the average blood glucose levels for the past 3 months.

9. **Name 4 enzymes in pancreatic secretion.**
- Trypsin, chymotrypsin, carboxypeptidase—proteolytic enzymes
- Pancreatic amylase—enzyme for digesting carbohydrates.

10. **Hormonal imbalance causing: (a) Acromegaly (b) Cretinism.**

Acromegaly: Hypersecretion of growth hormone in adults after the fusion of epiphysis.

Cretinism: Hypothyroidism in children.

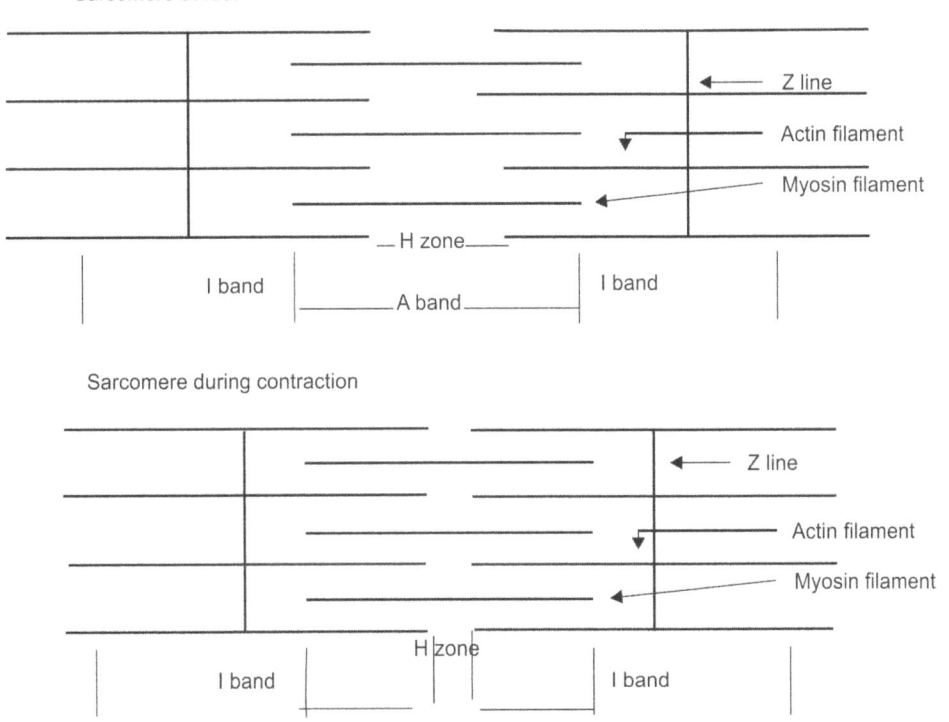

Fig. 9: Structure of sarcomere.
(*Source: Sembulingam*)

11. List the types of shock.

Types of Shock
i. Hypovolemic shock
ii. Distributive shock
iii. Cardiogenic shock
iv. Obstructive shock.

12. Define preload and state its effect on cardiac function.

- Preload is the tension developed in the muscle before the muscle sarts contracting. In cardiac muscle, the initial muscle length is the **preload** (the extent to which the muscle is stretched before contraction)
- Preload is decided by the **end-diastolic volume (EDV)**
- EDV is decided by the **venous return**
- According to Frank-Starling's law "**Within physiological limits, the force of contraction is directly proportional to the initial length of the muscle**"
- Therefore preload is directly proportional to stroke volume and to cardiac output.

13. Baroreceptor reflex.

Refer answers to 2003 paper.

14. What is myocardial infarction? State one ECG change in this condition.

Myocardial infarction (MI) is myocardial cell death due to ischemia. It happens when the ischemia is prolonged and the obstruction of coronary vessels is more than 75%.

ECG Change in MI

The most significant ECG change in MI is elevation of the ST segment in the leads overlying the infarct.

15. Role of myelin sheath in conduction of nerve impulse.

Refer answers to 2013 paper.

16. Conditions where Plantar response is 'extensor'.

- Normal response to plantar reflex is plantar flexion of big toe and flexion and adduction of other toes.

Babinski's Sign

- It is an extensor plantar response. There is dorsiflexion of big toe and abduction and dorsiflexion of other toes
- It is seen infants in physiological conditions and in upper motor neuron lesion, especially corticospinal tract lesion in pathological conditions.

17. Finding in Weber's test in conduction deafness of the left side.

- Weber's test is a tunning fork test
- Here the base of the vibrating tunning fork is placed on the vertex or in the forehead
- In normal conditions the subject hears equally in both the ears through bone conduction
- In conduction deafness, on placing the tunning fork sounds are heard better in the deaf ear due to the absence of masking sounds.

18. Muscle actions responsible for (a) Normal expiration (b) Forced expiration.

- Muscles involved in normal expiration: Normal expiration happens by passive recoil of the lungs. There is no muscle action during normal expiration
- Muscles involved in forced expiration: Anterior abdominal wall muscles and the internal intercostal muscles.

19. Oxygen carrying capacity of blood.

- Oxygen is carried in blood in two forms: Dissolved form and as Oxyhemoglobin
- The maximum amount of oxygen that can be carried by hemoglobin is called as the Oxygen carrying capacity of blood
- O_2 **transported as Oxyhemoglobin:** 1.34 mL of O_2 is carried by each gram of hemoglobin. In an average adult, 15g of hemoglobin is present in each decilitre of blood
- Therefore 1.34 × 15 = 20.1 mL of blood is carried in 100 mL of arterial blood. So 20.1 mL/100 mL of O_2 is the O_2 carrying capacity of blood.

20. Hypoxic vasoconstriction—where does it occur and what are its complications?

- Hypoxic vasoconstriction is seen in the pulmonary arteries
- In systemic arteries hypoxia induces vasodilatation and thereby increases blood flow to remove the hypoxic stimulus
- Hypoxic vasoconstriction diverts the blood flow from underventilated airways towards normal alveoli. Hypoxia directly causes contraction of vascular smooth muscles.

21. Permissive action of hormone.

Cortisol amplifies effects of certain processes of other hormones where it does not act directly.

Examples:
- It does not induce glycogenolysis by itself but augments glycogenolysis by glucagon
- It also augments vaso responsiveness of blood vessels to catecholamines
- Lipolytic actions of catecholamine is possible only in the presence of cortisol
- Thyroid hormone is essential for inducing the growth promoting effects of growth hormone.

22. Role of vitamin D in calcium homeostasis.

- Vitamin D has a potent effect in increasing the blood calcium levels. Vitamin D by itself does not increase blood calcium levels
- It gets converted to 1, 25 Dihydroxy-cholecalciferol in the skin, liver and kidneys
- 1, 25 Dihydroxycholecalciferol or calcitriol is the active form of Vitamin D.

Actions of Calcitriol

- It acts in the intestines to increase absorption of calcium from ingested food. It acts by inducing the calcium binding protein on the intestinal cells and therby transports calcium from intestinal lumen to the cell cytoplasm. It also increases activity of Ca^{2+} stimulated ATPase in the brush border of cell membrane
- It decreases Ca^{2+} excretion through the kidneys by stimulating reabsorption of Ca^{2+} from the renal tubules
- It also plays an important role in both bone resorption and deposition of calcium.

23. Contraception in males.

Refer answers to 2004 paper.

24. Corpus luteum.

Refer answers to 2008 paper.

25. Vitamin K dependent clotting factors.

- Vitamin K is a cofactor for the enzyme which catalyzes conversion of glutamic acid residues to γ-carboxyglutamic acid residues in the liver
- Six clotting factors, synthesized in the liver, require the conversion of glutamic acid to γ-carboxyglutamic acid.
- They are factors—II, VII, IX and X, and protein C and S.

26. Atonic bladder.

- Atonic bladder is due to deafferentation of the bladder
- Destruction of the afferent nerves to bladder results in inhibition of impulses from the bladder due to stretching of the bladder while it is getting filled
- Loss of afferent impulses results in absence of micturition reflex
- All bladder reflexes are lost in spite of intact efferent control to bladder
- Instead of emptying of bladder it gets filled to its capacity and there is overflow dribbling of urine
- It happens in Tabes dorsalis and crush injury to spinal cord.

27. Functions of skin.

Refer answers to 2006 paper.

28. Secondary active transport.

- In secondary active transport, substances are moved against the concentration gradient with the help of energy derived indirectly from ATP. Na^+- K^+ Pump, when it pumps out 3 Na^+ from the cell, creates a concentration gradient for Na^+ influx into the cell
- This inward gradient of Na^+ is utilised for movement of other ions across the cell membrane

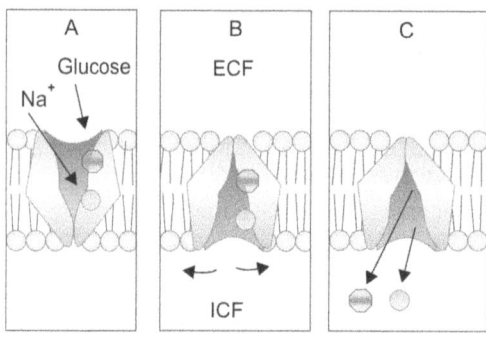

Fig. 10: Na⁺- Glucose symport, a secondary active transporter
(*Source:* Sembulingam)

- So the transporters of secondary active transport moves Na⁺ in exchange (Sodium counter-transporter) or along (Sodium cotransporter) with another molecule (both organic and inorganic substances) (refer Fig. 10).

Examples:

- Na⁺—Glucose symport
- Na⁺—Amino acid symport
- Na⁺—H⁺ exchanger
- Na⁺—Ca⁺⁺ exchanger.

29. Motor unit.
Refer answers to 2013 paper.

30. Refractory period.
Refer answers to 2004 paper (Short note: Nerve action potential).

31. Heart sounds.
Refer answers to 2006 paper.

32. Waves of ECG in Lead II.
Refer answers to 2005 paper.

33. Different types of hypoxia.
Refer answers to 2006 paper.

34. Aphasia.

Fluent Aphasia or Wernicke's Aphasia

- Lesion in the sensory speech area – Wernicke's area (Area 22). It can happen due to blockage of vessels supplying the area or injury
- Also called as fluent aphasia
- Here the person is able to hear spoken words or identifying written words
- But cannot comprehend spoken or written words
- Motor speech is intact. So speech is not disturbed. Person speaks excessively
- Impairment of written words as they are not able to comprehend written words also.

Non-fluent Aphasia or Broca's Aphasia

- In lesion of Broca's area there is normal comprehension of speech but there is poverty of speech
- This type of aphasia is called as Non-fluent aphasia
- Broca's area is the motor speech area (Area 44) and is located in the foot of the Primary motor cortex (Area 4)
- In spoken speech, impulses from the ear are transmitted to the primary auditory area (Area 42) in the temporal lobe
- From area 42, the impulse reaches the auditory association areas and then to the sensory speech area – Wernicke's area (Area 22). Here comprehension of speech happens
- From the Wernicke's area impulses are transmitted to the Broca's area
- It regulates the functions of the muscles of the lips, tongue, pharynx and larynx and it helps in vocalisation of the reply.

Global Aphasia

- Lesion in both the Wernicke's area and Broca's area results in Global aphasia
- All aspects of speech are impaired
- The patient is not able to comprehend or repeat words.

Anomic Aphasia

- It is a type of difficulty in speech due to lesion in the Angular gyrus (Area 39)
- The person has no difficulty in speech or understanding of auditory information
- But there is trouble in understanding written language and pictures because the visual information is not processed and transmitted to Wernicke's area
- It is also called as word blindness.

35. Stages of sleep.
Refer answers to 2006 paper.

36. Optic pathway.
Refer answers to 2004 paper.

37. Functions of ascending reticular activating system.
Refer answers to 2011 and 2012 papers.

38. Components of vestibular apparatus.
- It is the sensory organ which detects the sensation of equilibrium
- It is made of membranous tubes and chambers in the petrous part of temporal bone.
- It consists of 3 Semicircular canals and 2 sac like structures—utricle and saccule and the membranous labyrinth within (refer Fig. 11)
- Semicircular canals detect angular acceleration and thereby help in regulation of body posture and visual fixation
- Utricle and saccule detect linear acceleration and position of head in relation to gravity.

39. Features of Parkinson's disease.
Refer answers to 2005 paper.

40. Functions of middle ear.
Refer answers to 2005 paper.

41. Functions of plasma proteins.
Refer answers to 2004 paper.

42. Non-excretory functions of kidney.
a. *Endocrine functions of kidneys:* Kidneys help in synthesis of 1, 25 Dihydrocholecalciferol, Erythropoietin, Renin, Prostaglandins and Thromboxane A2
b. *Regulation of acid-base balance:* Kidneys excretes H^+, titrable acid, NH_4 and reabsorbs HCO_3^- and thereby regulates plasma pH
c. *Regulation of ECF volume:* Kidneys are capable of excretion and reabsorption of water as per the requirements of the body. Hormones like ADH, aldosterone and ANP act on the kidneys to regulate ECF volume
d. *Regulation of blood pressure:* Kidneys play a major role in long-term regulation

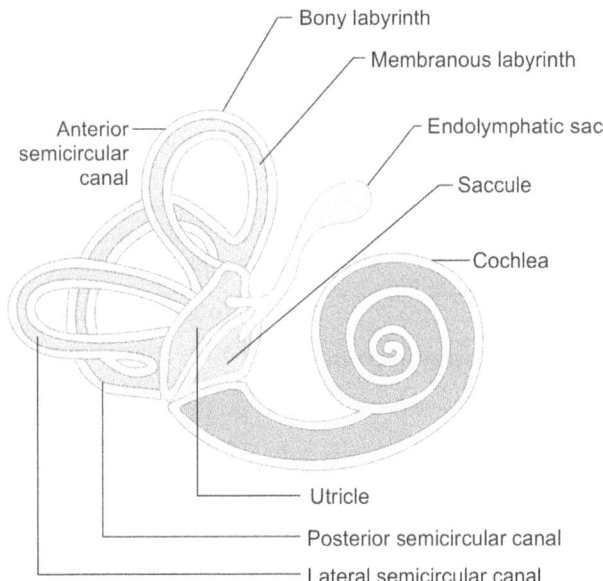

Fig. 11: Components of inner ear. It contains the vestibular apparatus—saccule, utricle and three semicircular canals. Inner ear also contains cochlea, the organ of hearing
(*Source:* Sembulingam)

of blood pressure. Renin-angiotensin-aldosterone mechanism acts through the kidneys to regulate BP

e. **Regulation of ECF osmolality:** Kidneys reabsorbs Na, Cl and water and thereby regulates EFC osmolality
f. Kidneys also help in **gluconeogenesis** in conditions of starvation.

43. Myasthenis gravis.
Refer answers to 2005 paper.

44. Stages of spermatogenesis.
Refer answers to 2006 paper.

45. Cystometrogram and its significance.
Refer answers to 2005 paper.

46. Hormones regulating calcium homeostasis.
Refer answers to 2008 paper.

47. Enterohepatic circulation.
Refer answers to 2009 paper.

48. Enzymes involved in digestion of fat.
Refer answers to 2013 paper.

49. Structure of platelets.
Refer answers to 2004 paper.

50. Functions of saliva.
Refer answers to 2003 paper.

51. Dead space.
Refer answers to 2010 paper.

52. Hering-Breuer reflex.
Refer answers to 2007 paper (Short note: Neural regulation of respiration).

53. Korotkoff sounds.
Refer answers to 2007 paper.

54. Draw a diagram of the pathway of crude touch and label it.
Refer answers to 2010 paper.

55. Functions of CSF.
Refer answers to 2009 paper.

56. Fluent aphasia.
Refer answers to 2009 paper.

57. Receptor potential.
Receptor potential is a graded potential developed in the receptors.

Pacinian corpuscle, the receptor for touch and vibration was used to study the site of generation of receptor potential.

The corpuscle has concentric lamella surrounding the unmyelinated end of the nerve fiber.

Myelination of nerve starts within the corpuscle and the first node of Ranvier is also within the corpuscle, second node is at the point of the nerve leaving the corpuscle.

On placing recording electrodes over the nerve leaving the corpuscle and while applying graded pressure, a non-propagated depolarizing potential was generated. It is said to be the generator or receptor potential. Its amplitude is dependent on the amount of pressure applied.

It was identified that the degeneration of unmyelinated nerve terminal resulted in absence of this generator potential. So it is the site of generation of receptor potential.

This potential excites the first node of Ranvier and if the potential reaches threshold fires an action potential.

Properties of receptor potential:
- It is a non-propagated potential
- It resembles EPSP in a synapse
- It is a graded response
- It can be summated
- Amplitude depends on stimulus intensity.

58. Motor homunculus.
- Parts of the whole body are represented in the primary motor area (Area 4) and this is said to be the Motor homunculus
- Face is represented bilaterally whereas, other body parts have unilateral representation

- The whole body is represented upside down with the feet above and the face and hands in the lower part of Area 4
- The area of representation for each part of the body is based on the level of skilled activities performed
- So the fingers and hand have larger area of representation than the trunk and lower limbs
- The area of representation for lips and tongue are also larger since they are involved in speech.

59. Attenuation reflex.

Refer answers to 2003 paper (Short note 7).

60. Taste pathway.

Refer answers to 2005 paper.

MBBS Examination 2015

ANSWER ALL QUESTIONS

I. Essay Questions (10 Marks each)

1. Describe the synthesis, storage, release, functions and regulation of secretion of thyroid hormone. Add a note on hypothyroidism.
2. Define cardiac output. Explain the factors regulating cardiac output. Add a note on ejection fraction.
3. Describe the mechanism of coagulation of blood.
4. Describe in detail the pyramidal tract. List out the differences between UMN and LMN lesions.
5. Discuss in detail the gastric secretions with experimental evidences. Add a note on peptic ulcer.
6. Explain the chemical regulation of respiration. Add a note on oxygen toxicity.

II. Short Notes (5 Marks each)

1. Give an account on micturition.
2. Classify the blood groups and indications and complications of blood transfusion.
3. Auditory pathway with suitable diagram.
4. Adjustment in respiratory physiology at high altitudes.
5. Cushing's syndrome.
6. Succus entericus.
7. Functions of hypothalamus.
8. Baroreceptor reflex.
9. Factors necessary for erythropoiesis.
10. Explain the actions of glucocorticoids.
11. Effects of lesions in optic pathway.
12. Determinants of Blood pressure.

III. Short Answers (3 Marks each)

1. Fetoplacental unit.
2. Importance of dietary fibers.
3. Neuromuscular transmission.
4. ESR-clinical significance.
5. Movements of small intestine.
6. Diabetes insipidus.
7. Red cell indices.
8. Extracellular edema.
9. Functions of Sertoli cells.
10. Tests for ovulation.
11. Accommodation reflex.
12. Conducting system of the heart.
13. Artificial respiration.
14. Conditioned reflexes.
15. Surfactant.
16. Central analgesic system.
17. VO_2 max.
18. Functions of CSF.
19. Decompression sickness.
20. Babinski's sign and its clinical significance.
21. Resting membrane potential.
22. Define all-or-none law. How is this law applicable in the skeletal and cardiac muscle.
23. Name the muscle proteins. What is the role of troponin C in muscle contraction?
24. Inulin clearance.
25. Countercurrent exchanger mechanism in kidney.
26. Somatomedin.
27. Action of thyroxine on CVS.
28. Positive feedback mechanism.
29. How does temperature influence spermatogenesis?

30. Effects of estrogen on the uterine endometrium.
31. Dark adaptation.
32. Periodic breathing.
33. Pacemaker potential.
34. Cardiac reserve.
35. Referred pain theories.
36. Features of shock.
37. Peak expiratory flow rate.
38. Oxygen debt.
39. Mass reflex.
40. Impedance matching.
41. Dwarfism.
42. Functions of lymphocytes.
43. Proximal tubular events.
44. Acromegaly.
45. Hormones produced by placenta.
46. Stages of deglutition.
47. Renin-angiotensin system.
48. Oral contraceptives.
49. Chronaxie and rheobase.
50. Significance of glycosylated hemoglobin.
51. Phasic changes in coronary blood flow.
52. AV nodal delay.
53. Properties of reflex.
54. Splanchnic circulation.
55. Functions of middle ear.
56. Nitrogen narcosis.
57. Effects of positive 'g'.
58. Papez circuit.
59. Heart sounds.
60. Differentiate REM and NREM sleep.

I. ESSAY QUESTIONS

1. **Describe the synthesis, storage, release, functions and regulation of secretion of thyroid hormone. Add a note on hypothyroidism.**

Refer answers to 2009 paper.

2. **Define cardiac output. Explain the factors regulating cardiac output. Add a note on ejection fraction.**

Refer answers to 2011 paper.

3. **Describe the mechanism of coagulation of blood.**

Refer answers to 2007 paper.

4. **Describe in detail the Pyramidal tract. List out the differences between UMN and LMN lesions.**

Refer answers to 2008 paper.

Differences between UMN and LMN Lesions

S.No	Upper motor neuron lesion	Lower motor neuron lesion
1.	Damage to motor tracts above anterior horn cell	Damage to the anterior horn cells and below
2.	Muscles affected in groups	Individual muscles affected
3.	Spastic type of paralysis	Flaccid type of paralysis
4.	Deep reflexes are exaggerated	Deep reflexes are lost
5.	There is no muscle atrophy	Paralysed muscles are atrophied
6.	Babinski's sign is positive	Plantar reflex is normal
7.	Muscle tone is increased (hypertonia)	Muscle tone is decreased (hypotonia)
8.	Common site of lesion is at the Internal capsule	Injury to peripheral nerves, poliomyelitis
9.	No involuntary movements	Fasiculations are present
10.	Nerve conduction study is normal	Nerve conduction velocity is decreased

5. **Discuss in detail the gastric secretions with experimental evidences. Add a note on peptic ulcer.**

Refer answers to 2005 paper – Gastric secretion.
Refer answers to 2014 paper – Pathophysiology of peptic ulcer.

Experimental Evidences

Phasic regulation of gastric secretion is studied by many experimental procedures conducted in animals.

a. Experimental Evidence for Cephalic Phase of Gastric Secretion

- It is demonstrated by sham feeding experiment in dogs
- The esophagus of the dog is divided in the middle and both the cut ends are brought and fixed to the abdominal surface
- Now the dog is made to swallow food, but the food comes out of the cut end

- The gastric secretion in this phase is due to the cephalic phase as this is due to the smell, sight and taste of food
- The secretion from the stomach is collected through a tube connected to the lower cut end of esophagus.

b. Experiment to Demonstrate that Vagus Stimulates Gastric Secretion by Pavlov's Pouch

- Under anesthesia, a pouch of the stomach is created with intact nerve and blood supply and is seperated from the stomach. The mucosa is incised and muscle layer is kept intact. The main section of stomach is restored by applying sutures
- An outlet is made from the pouch and is sutured with abdominal wall to drain the secretions from stomach
- The vagus nerve is identified in the neck and divided. After some days the peripheral cut end is stimulated in the unanaesthetised dog. There is secretion of gastric juice rich in HCl and pepsin which indicates that vagus is secretomotor to stomach.

c. Heidenhain's Pouch to Demonstrate Gastrin-mediated Regulation of Gastric Secertion

- Heidenhain's pouch is a modified Pavlov's pouch in which the denervated antral part of stomach is seperated with intact blood supply
- When this pouch is distended there is gastric secretion. Since it is denervated, there is a blood-borne mechanism which mediates the secretion, which could be due to gastrin
- It is confirmed by injecting Gastrin and following which there is similar gastric secretion from the Heidenham's pouch.

6. Explain the chemical regulation of respiration. Add a note on oxygen toxicity.

Refer answers to 2005 paper – Chemical regulation of respiration.

O_2 Toxicity

O_2 toxicity may appear when 100% O_2 is given at a pressure of 4 atm.

- It is due to formation of Free radicals (like O_2^-, H_2O_2)
- They oxidize Polyunsaturated fatty acids (PUFA) and destroy the cellular enzymes.

Symptoms

- Nausea
- Irritability
- Dizziness, tinnitus
- Disorientation
- Muscle twitching
- Convulsions and in severe cases coma
- Congestion and irritation of airways → tracheo-bronchial secretions →↓ Surfactant → Pulmonary edema
- Blurring of vision
- In newborns it results in Retrolental fibroplasia (formation of opaque vacular tissue in eyes) that in turn results in premature retinopathy
- When given for longer periods results in Bronchopulmonary dysplasia and bronchial cysts in newborns when they are treated with 100% O_2 for Respiratory distress syndrome.

II. SHORT NOTES

1. Give an account on micturition.

Refer answers to 2006 paper.

2. Classify the blood groups and indications and complications of blood transfusion.

Classification of Blood Groups

- The blood groups are divided based on the presence of antigens or agglutinogens on the membranes of RBCs
- An individual with a particular antigen will not possess the corresponding antibody or agglutinin in his plasma
- This forms the basis of blood grouping
- There are more than 30 blood group systems based on the presence of nearly 400 antigens
- The blood group systems are: ABO system, Rh system, MNS, Lutheran, P, Kell, Kidd, Duffy, Lewis etc.

- Most of the antigens are cold antigens and therefore they do not react in body temperature
- The ABO and Rh systems are the major blood group systems as they react in body temperature and when they react with their corresponding agglutinins they produce major reactions.

Indications of Blood Transfusion

- Acute blood loss
- Chronic anemia
- Bone marrow failure
- Preparation for surgery or during surgery
- Burns—only plasma is given
- Clotting diseases—fresh frozen plasma given.

Complications of Blood Transfusion

I. Due to Mismatched Transfusion

Happens immediately → Agglutination of RBCs → Hemolysis - Acute hemolytic transfusion reactions. Usually happens in ABO incompatibility.

Complications are:
i. Shivering and fever
ii. Hemoglobinemia and hemoglobinuria
iii. Jaundice
iv. Acute renal failure
v. Clumped RBCs block vessels of vital organs.

II. Due to Faulty Techniques of Giving Blood

- Thrombophlebitis
- Air embolism.

III. Febrile Reactions

- Due to pyrogens in the blood.

IV. Allergic Reactions

- Itching, erythema, nausea, vomiting and anaphylaxis.

V. Transmission of Diseases

- Hepatitis, Malaria, AIDS, Syphilis, etc.

Due to storage of blood

- Increased K^+ content of plasma → On infusion leads to arrhythmias and cardiac arrest.

3. **Auditory pathway with suitable diagram.**
Refer answers to 2010 paper.

4. **Adjustment in respiratory physiology at high altitudes.**
Refer answers to 2003 paper.

5. **Cushing's syndrome.**
Refer answers to 2006 paper.

6. **Succus entericus.**
Refer answers to 2005 paper.

7. **Functions of hypothalamus.**
Refer answers to 2013 paper.

8. **Baroreceptor reflex.**
Refer answers to 2003 paper.

9. **Factors necessary for erythropoiesis.**
Refer answers to 2006 paper.

10. **Explain the actions of glucocorticoids.**
Refer answers to 2004 paper.

11. **Effects of lesions in optic pathway.**
Refer answers to 2004 paper.

12. **Determinants of blood pressure.**
Refer answers to 2013 paper.

III. SHORT ANSWERS

1. **Fetoplacental unit.**
Refer answers to 2010 paper.

2. **Importance of dietary fibers.**
Refer answers to 2009 paper.

3. **Neuromuscular transmission.**
Refer answers to 2011 paper.

4. **ESR—clinical significance.**
Refer answers to 2010 paper.

5. **Movements of small intestine.**
Refer answers to 2004 paper.

6. **Diabetes Insipidus.**

Lack of ADH action – Diabetes Insipidus (DI)

1. **Central or Neurogenic DI:** ADH is not synthesized and secreted from posterior pituitary. It can be treated with

DDVAP (Desmopressin), Clofibrate, Chlorpropamide

2. **Nephrogenic DI:** The synthesis of ADH is normal. But the receptors for ADH in the kidneys do not respond to ADH due to genetic mutations. It is treated with diuretics like hydrochlorthiazide.

Features of DI

1. Polyuria: Urine output is 3 – 20 L/day
2. Polydipsia: Increase in thirst sensation
3. Osmolality of urine is very low (<300 mOsm/L)
4. Dehydration happens if water intake is decreased.

7. Red cell indices.

Mean Corpuscular Volume (MCV)

It refers to the average volume of a single RBC. It is calculated by dividing PCV by the red cell count.

MCV $= PCV \times 10/RBC$ count/µL
$= 45 \times 10/5 = 90$ µm^3

Normal value of MCV is 78-94 µm^3
Decrease in MCV = Microcytosis
Increase in MCV = Macrocytosis.

Mean Corpuscular Hemoglobin (MCH)

MCH is average weight of hemoglobin contained in each RBC. It is calculated by dividing the amount of Hb in 1L of blood by RBC count in 1 L of blood.

MCH $=$ Hb g in L /RBC in L
$=$ Hb g% $\times$ 10/RBC in µL $\times 10^{12}$
$= 15 \times 10/5 \times 10^{12} = 30 \times 10^{-12}$g
$= 30$ pg

Normal value of MHC is 27-30 pg.

Mean Corpuscular Hemoglobin Concentration (MCHC)

It is the amount of hemoglobin expressed as a percentage of RBC volume.

MCHC $=$ Hb g%/PCV $\times$ 100 mL $\times$ 100
$= 15/45 \times 100 = 33.3$%

Normal value = 30-38%
In iron defeciency anemia the RBCs are hypochromic and MCHC is less.

Color Index (CI)

It is the ratio of Hb to RBC.
CI $=$ Percentage of normal Hb/Percentage of normal RBC count
$= 100/100 = 1$

Normal value of CI = 0.85 to 1.15.

8. Extracellular edema.
Refer answers to 2010 paper.

9. Functions of sertoli cells.
Refer answers to 2008 paper.

10. Tests for ovulation.
Refer answers to 2013 paper.

11. Accommodation reflex.
Refer answers to 2003 paper.

12. Conducting system of the heart.
Refer answers to 2004 paper.

13. Artificial respiration.
Refer answers to 2004 paper.

14. Conditioned reflexes.
Refer answers to 2014 paper.

15. Surfactant.
Refer answers to 2008 paper.

16. Central analgesic system.
Refer answers to 2012 paper.

17. VO$_2$ max.
Refer answers to 2010 paper.

18. Functions of CSF.
Refer answers to 2009 paper.

19. Decompression sickness.
Refer answers to 2005 paper.

20. Babinski's sign and its clinical significance.
Refer answers to 2008 paper.

21. Resting membrane potential.
Refer answers to 2011 paper.

22. Define all-or-none law. How is this law applicable in the skeletal and cardiac muscle.

- Only a stimulus of threshold intensity can excite the excitable tissues like a nerve or

a muscle. On excitation they can generate an action potential
- If the stimulus is of subthreshold intensity it does not induce an action potential
- If a suprathreshold stimulus is given, action potentials are produced of the same amplitude as that of the threshold stimulus response
- In skeletal and cardiac muscles when the action potentials are generated it produces maximum response (Contraction)
- In skeletal muscle fiber, when a threshold stimulus is given, it induces an action potential followed by contraction of the individual muscle fiber and results in force generation by the single fiber
- But in a cardiac muscle, since there are gap junctions in between ventricular myocytes and atrial myocytes, when a threshold stimulus is given whole of the atria and ventricles get excited at the same time and each of them contract as individual syncitia. This is needed for the efficient pumping of blood by the myocardium.

23. Name the muscle proteins. What is the role of troponin c in muscle contraction?

There are 3 types of proteins in the muscles—structural proteins, contractile proteins and regulatory proteins.

Structural Proteins

- **Actinin:** Binds actin to Z lines
- **Titin:** Connects Z line to M line, provides scaffolding to sarcomere
- **Desmin:** Binds Z lines to plasma membrane.

Contractile Proteins

- **Actin and Myosin:** Myosin heads bind to attaching sites on actin and bring about cross-bridge cycling and thereby contraction (refer Fig. 2).

Regulatory Proteins

- **Troponin:** There are 3 subunits—Troponin I, T and C. Troponin I inhibits the interaction of myosin with actin, troponin T binds other troponins to tropomyosin

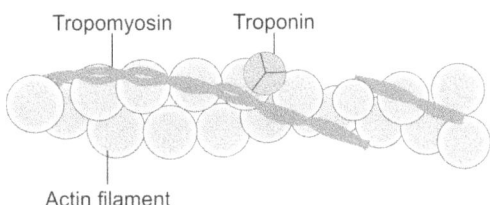

Fig. 1: Muscle proteins in thin filament. It consists of actin, tropomyosin and troponin. Troponin is made of 3 subunits – I, T and C.
(*Source:* GK Pal)

and troponin C binds to calcium ions. Binding of Ca^{2+} to troponin C results in movement of tropomyosin away from the myosin binding sites of Actin, exposing the binding sites which results in cross-bridge cycling and it results in muscle contraction (refer Fig. 1)

- **Tropomyosin:** Covers the myosin binding site of actin. On binding of troponin C to Ca^{2+} tropomyosin is lifted and exposes the myosin binding sites on actin molecules.

24. Inulin clearance.
Refer answers to 2012 paper.

25. Countercurrent exchanger mechanism in kidney.
Refer answers to 2003 paper.

26. Somatomedin.
Refer answers to 2013 paper.

27. Action of thyroxine on CVS.

- Thyroxine increases metabolic rate and therefore, main action of CVS is to increase blood supply to tissues to deliver more O_2.

In Hyperthyroidism

- Heart rate and stroke volume ↑→↑ Cardiac output
- Systolic BP↑ and diastolic BP ↓→ Widened pulse pressure
- Diastolic BP is decreased due to decreased peripheral resistance. Decrease in PR is due to vasodilatation which in turn is due to increased heat production due to increase in metabolism.

In Hypothyroidism

- Heart rate and stroke volume decrease

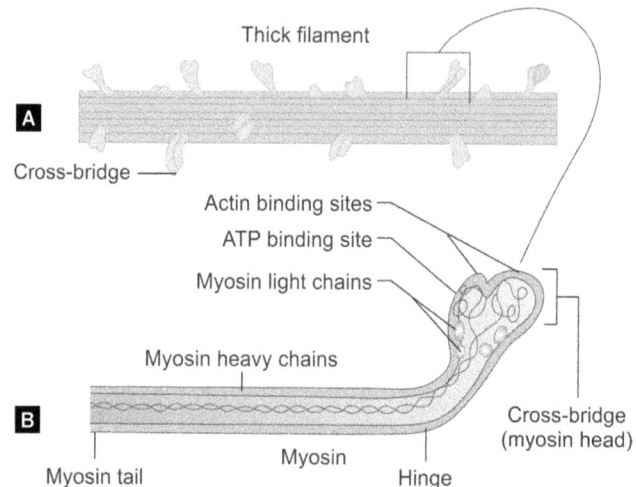

Figs. 2A and B: (A) Arrangement of myosin molecule in thick filament; (B) Structure of myosin molecule.

- Peripheral resistance is usually increased
- The cutaneous vasoconstriction is responsible for the cold skin in hypothyroids.

28. Positive feedback mechanism.
Refer answers to 2007 paper.

29. How does temperature influence spermatogenesis?
Body temperature: Spermatogenesis takes place in a temperature less than the inner body temperature. The testis are kept at a temperature of 32°C. If the testis is exposed to higher temperatures the tubular walls degenerate, inhibits spermatogenesis and sterility results.

30. Effects of estrogen on the uterine endometrium.

Proliferative Phase

- This phase correlates with follicular phase of ovarian cycle
- Estrogen secreted from the follicle stimulates growth of the uterine endometrium and therefore it proliferates
- The glands in the endometrium and the blood vessels also grow. This phase is from day 5 till the day of ovulation.

Secretory Phase

- This phase is from day of ovulation to 25th day
- It correlates with the luteal phase in the ovarian cycle
- Progesterone levels are high and they make the estrogen primed endometrium to become secretory by acting on the glands
- Maximum action is 5–7 days after ovulation
- The secretion is rich in glycogen and can nourish the fertilized ovum
- The secretory endometrium is favorable for implantation of fertilized ovum.

Menstrual Phase

- If fertilization does not happen, corpus luteum starts to regress and progesterone and estrogen levels drop
- Withdrawal of hormonal support of the endometrium and release of prostaglandins result in vasoconstriction of the spiral arteries → uterine ischemia happens and endometrial necrosis and shedding of endometrium happens
- It starts with menstrual bleeding with the shedding of outer 2/3rd of endometrium, unfertilized ovum and continues for 5 days.

31. Dark adaptation.
Refer answers to 2005 paper.

32. Periodic breathing.
Refer answers to 2009 paper.

33. Pacemaker potential.
Refer answers to 2005 paper.

34. Cardiac reserve.
Refer answers to 2012 paper.

35. Referred pain theories.
Refer answers to 2009 paper.

36. Features of shock.
Refer answers to 2012 paper.

37. Peak expiratory flow rate.
- Peak expiratory flow rate is the maximum velocity of flow in liters per minute with which air is breathed out of the lungs
- It is a good indicator of patency of airways
- Normal value is 400–600 L/min or 6 to 10 L/sec
- It can be recorded by using Wright's Peak flow meter
- The other more sensitive test to measure airway patency is maximum mid expiratory flow rate (MMEFR).

38. Oxygen debt.
Refer answers to 2009 paper.

39. Mass reflex.
- This type of reflex is seen in spinal cord lesions
- In lesions of spinal cord, a single afferent impulse can irradiate from one center to another center of spinal cord
- Therefore when a noxious stimulus is applied to the skin, the impulse may radiate to autonomic centers in the spinal cord and produce a **mass reflex** resulting in evacuation of bladder and rectum, sweating, pallor and swings in BP along with withdrawal reflex
- This reflex may be used to train the paraplegic patients to evacuate bladder and bowels by pinching or stroking the skin on the inner aspect of the thigh.

40. Impedance matching.
Refer answers to 2003 paper (Short note 7).

41. Dwarfism.
Refer answers to 2011 paper.

42. Functions of lymphocytes.
Based on the functions the lymphocytes are classified as B Lymphocytes, T Lymphocytes and Natural Killer cells.

A. B Lymphocytes
These cells are formed in the bone marrow and processed there and are transported to the lymph nodes where they are present till their activation. There are two types of B cells. They are Plasma cells and Memory B cells.

Plasma cells: Plasma cells are formed from B cells on antigenic stimulation. Each B cell has a specific receptor for a particular antigen on its membrane. When the antigen is recognized by the specific B cell it undergoes division and differentiation to the specific clone of B cells and transforms into plasma cells. The plasma cells produce the immunoglobulins to destroy that specific antigen. It produces a large quantity of antibodies and release them into circulation.

Memory B cells: A small proportion of the stimulated B cells stay in the lymph node so that on subsequent exposure to the same antigen they produce a rapid, swift and hightened response.

B. T Lymphocytes
T cells are formed from the bone marrow and are processessed in the Thymus gland and are transported to the lymph nodes and stored there till they are activated by the antigen. There are 3 types of T cells – Helper T cells, Cytotoxic T cells and Memory T cells.

Helper T cells: They are also called as CD4 cells as they express CD4 antigen on their cell membrane. They are needed for activation of both cell-mediated and humoral immunity. There are two types – T_H1 and T_H2 cells.

T_H1 cells secrete IL-2 and γ Interferon and are needed for cell-mediated immunity.

T_H2 cells secrete IL-4 and 5 and are needed for humoral immunity.

Cytotoxic T cells: These cells are also called as CD8 cells as they express CD8 antigen on their cell membrane. On activation by T_H1 cells they bind to the antigen and kill it by inserting pores called Perforins on its membrane and it can induce killing by stimulating apoptosis. These cells are responsible for rejection of transplanted tissue, destruction of cancer cells and for delayed allergic reactions.

Memory T cells: Similar to memory B cells the memory T cells also are a small number of stimulated T cells which do not take part in immune attack and remain in the lymph node. On subsequent exposure to the same antigen they get activated immediately to divide and differentiate to a clone of similar cells and they produce a rapid, swift and enormous response to destroy the antigen. They can even live for ever in the lymph node if there is no second exposure.

C. Natural Killer Cells

These cells do not belong to the T or B cell category. They form 10–15% of circulating total lymphocytes.

They are mostly involved in innate defense mechanism. They kill a wide range of micro-organisms without any specificity. They do not need the MHC proteins. They kill viruses and antibody-coated viruses. They are the natural first line of defense against viruses. They also destroy the tumor cells.

43. Proximal tubular events.

- The proximal convoluted tubule (PCT) is an important part of the nephron were 67% of Na^+, Cl^-, K^+ and water are reabsorbed from the tubular fluid
- Na^+ reabsorption in the early part of PCT is along with glucose and amino acid reabsorption and in later part is with Cl^- reabsorption
- Almost most of the HCO_3^-, K^+ and amino acids are reabsorbed in PCT
- Glucose is also reabsorbed completely (SGLT1)
- H^+ is also secreted in exchange for Na^+ (Na^+-H^+ exchanger)
- For every H^+ secreted one HCO_3^- and one Na^+ is reabsorbed
- Na^+ reabsorption here is an energy consuming process due to action of Na^+- K^+ ATPase in the basolateral membrane which creates a gradient for Na^+ to move into the cells from the tubule
- Solute reabsorption is active and water is reabsorbed passively by the osmotic gradient created by solute reabsorption. So the tubular fluid osmolality in PCT is similar to plasma
- Water reabsorption through epithelial cells is via aquaporin 1 present in cell membrane and also through paracellular routes.

44. Acromegaly.
Refer answers to 2008 paper.

45. Hormones produced by placenta.
Refer answers to 2010 paper.

46. Stages of deglutition.
Refer answers to 2003 paper.

47. Renin-angiotensin system.

- Renin is an acid protease and is a glycoprotein hormone secreted from the juxtaglomerular cells of kidneys
- Renin acts on angiotensinogen in plasma and converts it to angiotensin 1
- Angiotensin I is converted to angiotensin II by the angiotensin converting enzyme (ACE)
- ACE is produced by endothelial cells of all blood vessels, especially by the vessels in lungs
- Angiotensin II is in turn converted to Angiotensin III and IV
- The most active form is angiotensin II
- The major actions of angiotensin II are to regulate blood volume and pressure (refer Fig. 3).

Actions of Angiotensin II

a. It is a potent vasoconstrictor
b. It acts on the proximal convoluted tubule to increase reabsorption of Na^+ and water
c. It acts on the adrenal cortex to stimulate the secretion of aldosterone and aldosterone in turn increases salt and water reabsorption from the collecting duct
d. It increases release of norepinephrine from sympathetic nerve terminals

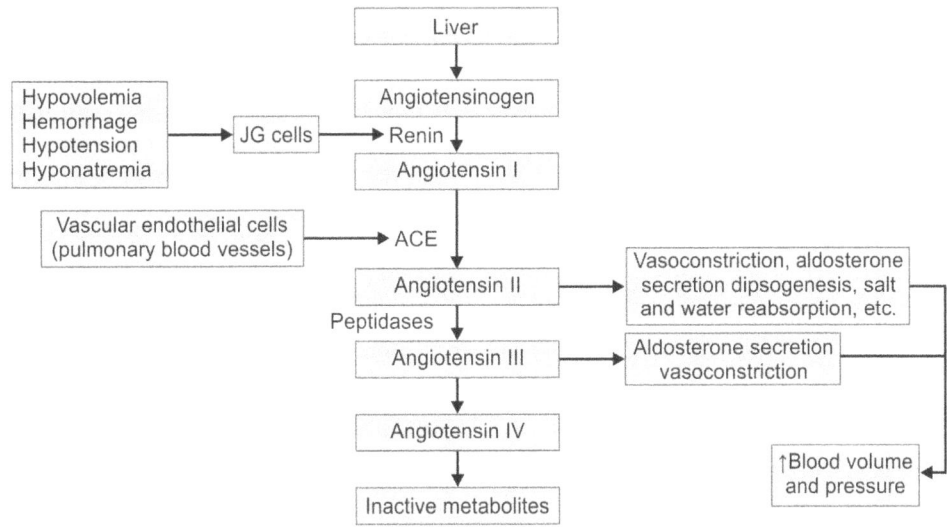

Fig. 3: Renin-angiotensin-aldosterone pathway.
(*Source:* G K Pal)

e. It also acts on the circumventricular organs in the brain—subfornical organ (SFO) and organum vasculosum of lamina terminalis (OVLT) and increase thirst sensation and thereby increases water intake
f. Increases ADH secretion from posterior pituitary
g. It increases secretion of ACTH from anterior pituitary
h. It acts as neurotransmitters in the brain.

Factors Regulating Renin Secretion

Factors that increase secretion:
- Decreased blood volume
- Decreased blood pressure
- Sympathetic nerve stimulation.

Factors that decrease renin secretion:
- Increased blood volume and pressure
- ADH
- Increased plasma Na⁺ concentration
- Angiotensin II.

48. Oral contraceptives.
Refer answers to 2004 paper.

49. Chronaxie and rheobase.
- Minimal intensity of stimulus acting for a given duration that can produce an action potential is the threshold stimulus
- Rheobase: The weakest strength of current that can excite a tissue when given for an adequate time—rheobase. The time for which it is given as utilization time.
- Chronaxiae: The duration of time for which twice the rheobase strength of current is given to produce a response
- Chronaxie gives an idea about the excitability of excitable tissues. Excitability and chronaxie are inversely related. The smooth muscles are least excitable and their chronaxie is longer in duration.

50. Significance of glycosylated hemoglobin.
Refer answers to 2014 paper.

51. Phasic changes in coronary blood flow.
Refer answers to 2005 paper.

52. AV nodal delay.
Refer answers to 2011 paper.

53. Properties of reflex.
a. **Adequate stimulus:** A reflex response can be obtained only when a precise stimulus is applied. The precise stimulus which can initiate the response is the adequate stimulus
b. **Delay:** There is always a delay between application of stimulus and the response due to the presence of synapses in the pathway. More the number of synapses, more will be the delay

c. **One way conduction:** The impulses are always transmitted from the receptor → center → effector
d. **Summation:** Spatial and temporal summation of impulses facilitates responses
e. **Irradiation:** When the stimulus is very strong as that of the noxious stimuli the impulses spread to neighboring neurons and centers and produces a wider response, as in crossed extensor reflex. Mass reflex is an example for irradiation
f. **Final common pathway:** The alpha motor neurons in the spinal cord which supply the extrafusal muscle fibers, is the final pathway through which the excitatory or inhibitory impulses reach the muscles for reflexes
g. **Facilitation:** When repeated stimuli are given there is increased responses in the initial few occasions due to facilitation in the synapse
h. **Inhibition:** During a reflex response, when the agonists are contracting there are inhibitory impulses reaching the antagonists to make them relax. This is because of firing of inhibitory interneurons from the spinal cord which end on the antagonists
i. **After discharge:** When a reflex response is elicited by a stong stimuli, even after cessation of stimulus the response is present. This is said to be After-discharge. It happens due to reverberatory circuits
j. **Rebound phenomenon:** When the reflex activity is inhibited due to some reason and after the inhibition is lifted, the response which we get is a stronger one
k. **Susceptibility to hypoxia:** Reflexes are susceptible to hypoxia
l. **Fatigue:** When a reflex is elicited repeatitively, gradually the response diminishes and finally disappears due to fatigue. The site of fatigue is usually at the synapse
m. **Occlusion:** The muscles contract forcefully when stimulated directly through motor nerve stimulation rather than the reflex stimulation through the sensory nerve. This is due to property of occlusion when stimulated through sensory nerve
n. **Sensitization:** When a noxious stimulus is applied repeatedly the response gets intensified, this is due to presynaptic facilitation. This is said to be sensitization.

54. Splanchnic circulation.

Means Circulation through Abdominal Viscera

- Circulation through GIT
- Circulation through liver
- Circulation through spleen.

Intestinal Circulation

- Resting blood flow to intestine is 20% of cardiac output
- Increases to 50% after a meal
- Supplied by 3 main arteries—celiac trunk, superior and inferior mesentric arteries
- Intestinal mucosa receives 60–70% of the total intestinal blood flow
- Arterioles supply the tips of villi
- Direction of blood flow in arterioles and venules in villi is opposite to each other and form a counter-current system.
- Regulation is by neural and auto-regulation (Metabolic- Adenosine, K^+ and Osmolality)

Hepatic Circulation

- Liver is a vital organ performing metabolic activity
- Hepatic blood flow—28% of cardiac output
- Blood flow to liver is through—hepatic artery (25%) and portal vein (75%)
- Normal blood flow—1500 mL/min (58 mL/100 g/min)
- Hepatic arterial and portal vein blood flow are reciprocal
- Regulation is by neural (sympathetic nerve) and metabolic factors.

Splenic Circulation

- Main blood flow to spleen is through splenic artery
- Nerve supply is by sympathetic vasoconstrictor fibers
- Spleen functions as reservoir for blood especially in animals

- During circulatory shock, splenic contraction releases blood into circulation.

55. Functions of middle ear.
Refer answers to 2003 paper.

56. Nitrogen narcosis.

N₂ Toxicity or N₂ Narcosis
- At high atmospheric pressure environments, as in deep sea, breathing air under high pressure leads to increased pN_2 and high partial pressure of N_2 dissolves it in body fluids and more easily in fats
- N_2 dissolves easily in neuronal membrane, altering their ionic conductance and decreases their excitability—results in N_2 narcosis
- It starts at a depth of 120 feet below sea level and becomes severe at 250 feet.

Symptoms
- N_2 narcosis symptoms are similar to alcohol intoxication
- Causes euphoria: Person becomes jovial, carefree, impairment of mental functions, intelligence and poor muscular coordination
- This problem can be overcome by breathing mixtures of O_2 and helium, but this also leads to disorders like high pressure nervous syndrome.

57. Effects of positive 'g'.
- Force acting on the body due to acceleration is expressed as 'g' units
- 1 'g' is the force of gravity acting on earth's surface
- "Positive g" is force due to acceleration acting in the long axis from head to foot
- During positive 'g' blood is thrown to the lower parts of the body and therefore arterial pressure is high in lower parts and low in the head
- But as the venous pressure and also intracranial pressures are also reduced there is not much decrease in blood flow to brain
- The major problem here is decrease in venous return and thereby decrease in cardiac output
- Cardiac output is maintained for some time due to blood being drawn from venous reservoirs
- At accelerations above 5 'g' there is failure of vision, "Black out" in 5 seconds and unconsciousness immediately after that
- These effects of positive 'g' can be reduced by wearing 'g suits'
- These are double-walled pressure suits containing water or air and they compress the abdomen or legs with force equal to the positive g
- The suit prevents venous pooling and enhances venous return.

58. Papez circuit.
- Hypothalamus along with limbic system participates in the expression of emotions
- This relation is given as the Papez circuit which is responsible for emotions
- Papez circuit is also responsible for memory and learning.

Papez Circuit
- Hippocampus is connected to mamillary bodies through the fornix
- Mammillary body is connected to the anterior thalamic nucleus through mammillothalamic tract
- Anterior thalamic nucleus is connected to cingulate gyrus and it is in turn connected to hippocampus (refer Fig. 4).

59. Heart sounds.
Refer answers to 2006 paper.

60. Differentiate REM and NREM sleep.
Refer answers to 2009 paper.

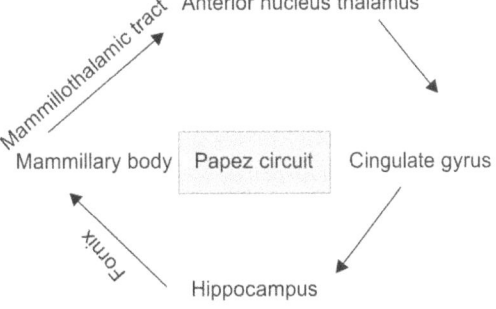

Fig. 4: Papez circuit.

MBBS Examination 2016

ANSWER ALL QUESTIONS

I. Essay Questions   (10 Marks each)
1. What is glomerular filtration rate (GFR)? Enumerate the factors affecting GFR.
2. What is cardiac cycle? Describe the various events in the cardiac cycle.
3. Discuss in detail the stages of erythropoiesis and the factors affecting it. Add a note on polycythemia.
4. Describe the oxygen transport in blood. Add note on fetal hemoglobin.

II. Short Notes   (5 Marks each)
1. Facilitated diffusion.
2. Control of insulin secretion.
3. Golgi tendon reflex.
4. Oxygen-hemoglobin dissociation curve.
5. Neuromuscular junction.
6. Regulation of hydrochloric acid secretion in the gastric parietal cells.
7. Autorhythmicity of heart.
8. Describe the connections and functions of temporal lobe.

III. Short Answers   (3 Marks each)
1. Hemophilia.
2. Differentiate between isotonic and isometric contraction.
3. Erythropoietin.
4. Compound action potential.
5. Gastrin.
6. Addisonian crisis.
7. Law of gut.
8. Intestinal phase of pancreatic secretion.
9. Inhibin.
10. Functions of prostate gland.
11. Putamen circuit of basal ganglia.
12. Caisson disease.
13. Hering-Breuer inflation reflex.
14. Einthoven's law.
15. Endocochlear potential.
16. Describe the normal waves in electroencephalogram (EEG).
17. Presbyopia.
18. Bainbridge reflex.
19. Transpulmonary pressure.
20. Wernicke's and global aphasia.
21. Functions of saliva.
22. Diuretics and their sites of action.
23. Steps in synthesis of thyroid hormones.
24. Enterohepatic circulation.
25. Phagocytosis.
26. Endoplasmic reticulum.
27. Anticoagulants.
28. Functions of estrogen.
29. Importance of Rh typing.
30. Fat absorption.
31. Taste receptors.
32. Functions of utricle and saccule.
33. Sleep-wake theory.
34. Mechanism of accommodation.
35. P-R interval.
36. Trichromatic theory of color vision.
37. Mean arterial pressure.
38. Reward and punishment centers.
39. Changes in cardiac output during exercise.
40. Surfactant.

I. ESSAY QUESTIONS

1. What is glomerular filtration rate (GFR)? Enumerate the factors affecting GFR.

Refer answers to 2005 paper.

2. **What is cardiac cycle? Describe the various events in the cardiac cycle.**

Refer answers to 2005 paper.

3. **Discuss in detail the stages of erythropoiesis and the factors affecting it. Add a note on polycythemia.**

Refer answers to 2006 paper and 2014 papers.

4. **Describe the oxygen transport in blood. Add note on fetal hemoglobin.**

Refer answers to 2004 paper.

- *Fetal hemoglobin (HbF)* has 2 alpha chains and 2 gamma chains making up the globin part of Hb
- 80% of Hb in the fetus at the time of birth is HbF
- Disappears by 5th month of age
- It has greater affinity for oxygen and it shifts the O_2-Hb dissociation curve to the left
- High affinity is due to its poor binding capacity with 2, 3, DPG
- It is also resistant to action of alkalis. Life span is 1–2 weeks.

II. SHORT NOTES

1. **Facilitated diffusion.**

Refer answers to 2013 paper.

2. **Control of insulin secretion.**

There are factors which stimulate and inhibit insulin secretion (refer Fig. 1):

Factors Stimulating Insulin Secretion

a. Glucose
b. Amino acids (leucine, arginine)
c. Intestinal hormones (GIP, GLP, gastrin, secretin, CCK)
d. β-ketoacids
e. Acetylcholine
f. Glucagon
g. cAMP
h. β-adrenergic stimulation
i. Sulfonylureas
j. Theophylline.

Factors Inhibiting Insulin Secretion

a. Somatostatin
b. 2-Deoxyglucose
c. α-adrenergic stimulation
d. β-adrenergic blockers
e. Galanin
f. Diazoxide
g. Thiazide diuretics
h. K^+ depletion
i. Phenytoin
j. Alloxan
k. Insulin.

Effect of Plasma Glucose on Insulin Secretion

- Blood glucose levels have a direct action on β cells to increase insulin secretion
- There is an initial rapid increase in secretion followed by a slow rise
- Glucose enters B cells via GLUT 2 transporters. It is phosphorylated by glucokinase and metabolized to pyruvate in cytoplasm
- Pyruvate then enters mitochondria and is metabolized to CO_2 and H_2O via citric acid cycle

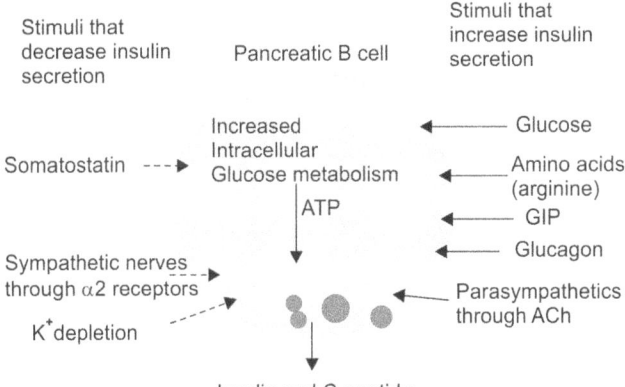

Fig. 1: Regulation of insulin secretion.
(GIP: gastrin inhibitory peptide; ACh: acetylcholine)

- ATP is produced and it enters cytoplasm and inhibits ATP-sensitive K⁺ channels and thereby reduces K⁺ efflux
- This results in depolarisation of B cells and causes opening of voltage-gated Ca^{2+} channels. Calcium influx causes exocytosis of secretory vesicles containing insulin
- Pyruvate metabolism also produces glutamate which in turn causes release of the second pool of secretory granules of insulin.

Effect of Protein and Fat Derivatives on Insulin Secretion

- Insulin stimulates protein synthesis by incorporating amino acids like leucine, arginine into proteins
- It also inhibits fat catabolism
- Secretion of insulin is stimulated by β-keto acids like acetoacetate
- Like glucose, these substrates also induce formation of ATP and close the ATP-sensitive K⁺ channels.

Effect of cAMP on Insulin Secretion

- Stimuli that increase intracellular cAMP increases insulin secretion by increasing intracellular Ca^{2+}
- Factors that increase cAMP levels are β-adrenergic agonists, glucagon and phosphodiesterase inhibitors like theophylline
- Catecholamines while acting through $α_2$-adrenergic stimulation inhibits insulin secretion and while acting on β-adrenergic receptors stimulate insulin secretion. Net efffect is inhibition of secretion.

Effect of Autonomic Stimulation on Insulin Secretion

- Stimulation of vagus nerve to pancreatic islets results in secretion of insulin. The neurotransmitter released is acetylcholine which acts on M4 receptors. It stimulates secretion by increasing intracellular calcium
- Sympathetic nerve stimulation acts through $α_2$-adrenergic receptors and inhibit secretion of insulin.

Effect of Intestinal Hormones on Insulin Secretion

- Elevated plasma glucose levels increase insulin secretion. But it was found that orally adminstered glucose had a greater effect of increasing insulin secretion
- This has been identified due to GI hormone effect on insulin secretion like – Glucagon, Secretin, CCK, Gastrin, Gastric inhibitory peptide (GIP) and Glucagon-like polypeptide (GLP).

Effect of Plasma K⁺ Levels on Insulin Secretion

- Increase in K⁺ levels increase insulin secretion. Insulin decreases plasma K⁺ levels
- Insulin is a major hormone which decreases plasma K⁺ levels following food intake
- Thiazide diuretics causes loss of K⁺ and Na⁺ in urine and thereby decreases K⁺ levels and decreases insulin secretion.

3. Golgi tendon reflex.

- When the skeletal muscle is stretched, muscle spindle is stimulated by the stretch and results in muscle contraction
- This happens only upto a particular level of stretch
- If the tension in the muscle is increased beyond a level, the muscle relaxes
- Relaxation of muscle in relation to strong stretch is called the Inverse stretch reflex or Autogenic inhibition
- The receptor for this reflex is Golgi tendon organ (GTO). Therefore the reflex is also called as Golgi tendon reflex (refer Fig. 2)
- Golgi tendon organ, the receptor for this reflex is present in the tendons of the muscles
- It is stimulated when the extrafusal fibers contract and thereby it induces a stretch to the GTO in the tendon
- The afferents from GTO are carried by the Ib fibers
- Ib fibers end on spinal interneurons and through them they inhibit the motor neurons supplying the same muscles and produces IPSP in them. This causes relaxation of the same muscle

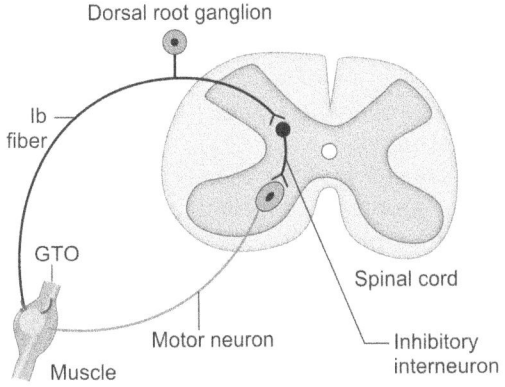

Fig. 2: Golgi tendon reflex or inverse stretch reflex.
(*Source:* G K Pal)

- This reflex helps in regulation of tension developed in the muscle.

4. Oxygen-hemoglobin dissociation curve.
Refer answers to 2004 paper.

5. Neuromuscular junction.
Refer answers to 2011 paper.

6. Regulation of hydrochloric acid secretion in the gastric parietal cells.
Refer answers to 2005 paper.

7. Autorhythmicity of heart.
- Heart has the capacity to beat even after the nerves supplying the heart are removed. This is because of the presence of the pacemaker tissue in the heart
- It is called as the pacemaker as it can generate action potentials repeatedly in a rhythmic manner without any neural stimulation
- The tissues in the heart capable of producing such impulses are; the SA node, AV node, His Bundle, Purkinje fibers and the ventricles
- Even though all the above tissues can function as the pacemaker, SA node is said to be the Primary pacemaker of the heart as it generates impulses at a faster rate (60–100/min) than other tissues
- In case of disease of SA node other pacemakers take up the activity of pacemaking in a hierarchal manner; the AV node, His bundle-Purkinje system and then the ventricle
- Rhythmicity means the heart beats rhythmically with the intervals between each beat remaining a constant
- The impulses from SA node are in a rhythmic manner. It contributes to the autorhythmic property of heart
- The electrical impulses generated in the pacemaker is discussed under the topic of pacemaker potential.

Pacemaker Potential
Refer answers to 2005 paper.

8. Describe the connections and functions of temporal lobe.
Temporal lobe is located inferior to the lateral sulcus.

It has three regions—superior temporal gyrus, inferior temporal gyrus and mediobasal gyrus.

It has the following areas:
- ***Broadman's area 41 and 42:*** This is the primary auditory area located in the superior temporal gyrus. Area 42 is below area 41. It receives afferents from medial geniculate body and is concerned with perception of frequency, intensity and location of sound. It projects to area 22 which helps in understanding speech
- ***Area 22:*** It is located below area 42. It also receives inputs from visual areas and projects to frontal lobe, parietal lobe and cingulate gyrus. It is involved in interpretation of meaning of sound and comprehension of spoken and written words
- ***Wernicke's area:*** Posterior part of area 22 is the Wernicke's area. It is the sensory speech area. It is concerned with understanding of spoken and written words and in meaningful word formation for replying back in form of spoken speech or written words (refer Fig. 3)
- ***Area 20, 21 and 37:*** Present in inferior and middle gyri. It receives inputs from visual areas, thalamus and parietal lobes. It projects to visual areas, amygdala and entorhinal cortex. Area 20 and 21 are concerned with speech and facial recognition. Area 37 is concerned with perception of colors

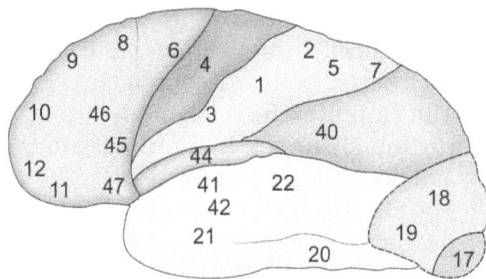

Fig. 3: Lobes of cerebral cortex and Broadman's areas.
(*Source:* GK Pal)

- **Areas 28 and 38:** They are located in the medial parts of temporal lobe. They are concerned with speech, limbic functions and olfaction.

Functions of Temporal Lobe

- It perceives sound and has the capacity to discriminate pitch, intensity and localization of sound
- Wernicke's area has a role in comprehension of spoken and written language
- It has a role in interpretation of sounds
- Since the areas of limbic system, like hippocampus are located here it has a role in memory and emotions
- Areas 20 and 21 are needed for facial recognition
- Has a role in color vision
- It has a role in olfaction.

III. SHORT ANSWERS

1. Hemophilia.

Refer answers to 2008 paper.

2. Differentiate between isotonic and isometric contraction.

Refer answers to 2013 paper.

3. Erythropoietin.

- Erythropoietin is a glycoprotein hormone synthesized and secreted from kidneys and liver
- It is secreted by the interstitial cells in peritubular capillary bed of the kidneys (85%) and by perivenous hepatocytes (15%) in the liver
- It acts on the bone marrow and increases the number of erythropoietin-sensitive committed stem cells in the bone marrow and converts them into mature RBCs
- Level of erythropoietin (EPO) is increased in anemia
- Gene for EPO has been cloned and it can be produced by recombinant technology in animal cells and can be used for treatment of anemia in renal failure
- It can also be used to stimulate RBC production in people who undergo autologous blood transfusion as in elective surgeries.

Regulation of Secretion

- Hypoxia stimulates EPO secretion. There are O_2 sensors which are heme proteins in the kidneys and liver which are stimulated in its deoxy form and inhibited in their oxy form
- It is also stimulated by cobalt salts and androgens
- High altitude alkalosis also stimultes secretion of EPO
- It is also stimulated by β adrenergic stimulation.

4. Compound action potential.

- When a single axon is stimulated, a single peak action potential can be recorded
- But if a mixed nerve is stimulated there is a multipeaked action potential recorded
- This is said to be compound action potential
- This type of multipeaked action potential is recorded in a mixed nerve due to the differences in the speed of conduction of individual fibers
- When such a nerve is stimulated, activity in the fast-conducting fibers arrives at the recording electrode sooner than the slower conducting fibers, this creates multiple peaks
- The number and size of the peaks vary with the type of fibers in the particular nerve being studied.

5. Gastrin.

- Secreted by G cells in stomach in the antrum
- It is a polypeptide hormone
- Three types of gastrin—G34, G17 and G14
- In stomach G 17 is secreted.

Factors Influencing Gastrin Release

- *Stimuli that increase release:*
  1. Gastric distension
  2. Products of protein digestion in stomach
  3. Increased vagal discharge
  4. Calcium and epinephrine.
- *Stimuli that decrease release:*
  1. Low pH in stomach
  2. Somatostatin
  3. Secretin,
  4. Vasoactive intestinal peptide
  5. Calcitonin
  6. Glucagon.

Functions of Gastrin

a. Stimulates secretion of HCl and pepsinogen in stomach
b. Stimulates gastric motility and emptying
c. Contracts lower esophageal sphincter and prevents reflux gastritis
d. Has a trophic action on gastric and intestinal mucosa
e. Stimulates secretion of pancreatic juice
f. Stimulates insulin and glucagon secretion from endocrine pancreas
g. Responsible for gastro-colic reflex
h. Stimulates histamine from Enterochromaffin like cells in GI mucosa and thereby stimulates HCl secretion.

6. Addisonian crisis.

- Primary adrenal insufficiency is due to diseases affecting adrenal cortex and is called as Addison's disease
- It is usually seen as a complication of tuberculosis, due to an autoimmune inflammation of adrenal or malignancy of adrenal cortex
- Here there is deficiency of mineralocorticoids, glucocorticoids and androgens
- Absence of glucocorticoids—patients are tired, lose weight, nausea, vomiting etc. Fasting results in fatal hypoglycemia and any stress leads to collapse of the patient
- Mineralocorticoid deficiency—hypotension, hyponatremia, hyperkalemia and acidosis. They have a small heart due to hypotension which results in decrease workload of the heart
- Adrenal androgen deficiency—loss of hair in females
- Water excretion is decreased and a water load may lead to water intoxication
- Low glucocorticoid levels lead to increase in ACTH levels which results in hyperpigmentation. This is because of melanocyte stimulating hormone (MSH) like action of ACTH.

Addisonian Crisis

- Acute adrenal insufficiency leads to addisonian crisis
- It can happen due to major surgery, trauma and sudden withdrawal of glucocorticoid therapy
- With all the symptoms above they eventually develop severe hypotension and shock which may be fatal
- It can be treated with fluids, electrolytes, glucocorticoid and mineralocorticoid supplements.

7. Law of gut.

Movement of chyme in intestines by peristalsis is always from oral to aboral direction and never in the opposite direction. Peristalsis is stimulated by distension of the gut which induces a contraction ring in the segment of intestine behind the chyme and a relaxing segment ahead of the chyme. This pushes the food towards the anus.

8. Intestinal phase of pancreatic secretion.

Refer answers to 2013 paper.

9. Inhibin.

Refer answers to 2010 paper.

10. Functions of prostate gland.

- It is an accessory gland of male reproductive system
- It is present below the urinary bladder and urethra passes through the prostate gland. This part of the male urethra is said to be the prostatic urethra
- It secretes a milky fluid which forms 20% of semen. It is alkaline in nature.

It contains the following components:
a. Spermine
b. Citric acid
c. Cholesterol
d. Phopholipids
e. Fibrinolysin, finbrinogenase
f. Zinc
g. Acid phosphatase.

Functions of Prostatic Fluid

- Maintains an optimum pH of 6-6.5 in vaginal environment, which is needed for motility of sperm and it favors fertilization
- It converts fibrinogen from seminal fluid into a coagulum which is needed to hold the sperm in uterine cervix
- Later, fibrinolysin in prostatic fluid liquifies the coagulum, facilitating sperm motility and activation.

11. Putamen circuit of basal ganglia.

It is the direct pathway in basal ganglia:
Cerebral Cortex → Striatum (Caudate and Putamen) → Internal segment (IS) of Globus Pallidus (GP) → Thalamus → Motor cortex.

Cortex excites striatum
↓
Striatum inhibits IS of GP
↓
IS of GP inhibits the inhibition of thalamus via thalamic fasciculus (goes to VA and VL nuclei of thalamus)
↓
Impulses from thalamus to prefrontal and premotor cortex and the final effect is disinhibition.

Functions of Putamen Circuit

Putamen circuit in connections with the cerebral cortex controls complex patterns of motor activity—like writing, cutting, hammering nails, vocalisation, controlled movements of eyes and all other skilled movements.

12. Caisson disease.
Refer answers to 2009 paper.

13. Hering-Breuer inflation reflex.
Refer answers to 2012 paper.

14. Einthoven's law.
Refer answers to 2010 paper.

15. Endocochlear potential.
Refer answers to 2011 paper.

16. Describe the normal waves in electro-encephalogram (EEG).
Refer answers to 2012 paper.

17. Presbyopia.
Refer answers to 2004 paper.

18. Bainbridge reflex.

- In a person with low heart rate when rapid infusion of saline is done there is a rapid rise in heart rate
- This reflex was described by Bainbridge in 1915 and therefore called as Bainbridge reflex
- It is a true reflex and the afferents are the vagal afferents. The impulses cause a decrease in vagal tone and thereby increase the heart rate
- This reflex can be blocked by application of atropine or vagotomy
- The receptors are tachycardia-producing atrial receptors.

19. Transpulmonary pressure.

- Transpulmonary pressure (TPP) is the pressure difference across the lung. It is Intrapulmonary pressure minus Intrapleural pressure
- There is a difference in intrapleural pressure in the apex and the base of the lung and therefore transpulmonary pressure is different in the apex and the base
- It is +6 mm Hg in the apex and +1 mm Hg in the base
- It varies with the phases of respiration
- At the end of expiration TPP is 2.5 mm Hg and at end of inspiration it is 6 mm Hg
- Increase in TPP stretches the lungs and therefore it decides the lung volume.

20. Wernicke's and global aphasia.
Refer answers to 2014 paper.

21. Functions of saliva.
Refer answers to 2003 paper.

22. Diuretics and their sites of action.

Diuretics are chemicals which increase excretion of Na⁺ and water and thereby increase urine output.

Site of Action of Diuretics

Drugs acting in PCT:
a. Carbonic anhydrase inhibitors like acetazolamide. They inhibit carbonic anhydrase and thereby increases Na⁺ excretion, decreases H⁺ secretion and bicarbonate reabsorption. Since H⁺ and K⁺ compete with each other (For secretion) along with Reabsorption of Na⁺, there is increased K⁺ secretion and excretion and therefore K⁺ depletion occurs
b. Osmotic diuretics like Mannitol and Isosorbide. They are not reabsorbed in PCT and therefore are retained in the tubule along with water. This in turn alters the gradient for Na⁺ reabsorption and therefore it inhibits Na⁺ reabsorption.

Diuretics acting on Loop of Henle:
a. Loop diuretics like frusemide, bumetamide and ethacrynic acid: They act by inhibiting Na⁺-K⁺-2Cl⁻ transporter. They increase NaCl and K⁺ excretion. K⁺ depletion occurs while treating with these drugs.

Diuretics acting on DCT:
a. Thiazides: They act by inhibiting Nacl symport in DCT. They increase excretion of NaCl and K⁺.

Diuretics acting on Late DCT and Collecting duct:
a. K⁺ sparing diuretics like spiranolactone, triamterene and amiloride act in late DCT and CD by inhibiting actions of aldosterone or epithelium sodium channels (ENaCs). They increase excretion of Na⁺ and retain K⁺ and H⁺.

23. Steps in synthesis of thyroid hormones.
Refer answers to 2009 paper.

24. Enterohepatic circulation.
Refer answers to 2009 paper.

25. Phagocytosis.
Refer answers to 2005 paper.

26. Endoplasmic reticulum.
- Endoplasmic reticulum (ER) are flattened membrane-bound vesicles and tubules. They are continuous with the nuclear membrane (refer Fig. 4)
- There are two types of ER—rough ER and smooth ER.

Rough ER
- They are flattened membrane-bound tubes
- They appear continuous with nuclear membrane of Golgi complex and cell membrane
- The membrane is studded with ribosomes
- It is present in large amounts in cells synthesizing proteins. Their major function is protein synthesis in the cells.

Smooth ER
- It has no ribosomes on the membrane
- It is the site of lipid and steroid synthesis
- It is found abundantly in Leydig and adrenal cortical cells
- In liver it helps in detoxification of toxins
- In skeletal and cardiac muscles it is the site of storage of Ca^{2+}.

27. Anticoagulants.
Refer answers to 2012 paper.

28. Functions of estrogen.
Refer answers to 2009 paper.

29. Importance of Rh typing.
Refer answers to 2009 paper.

30. Fat absorption.
Refer answers to 2013 paper.

31. Taste receptors.
Refer answers to 2010 paper.

32. Functions of utricle and saccule.
Refer answers to 2009 paper.

33. Sleep-wake theory.
Sleep is a state of temporary unconsciuosness from which the individual can be aroused by a sensory stimulus.

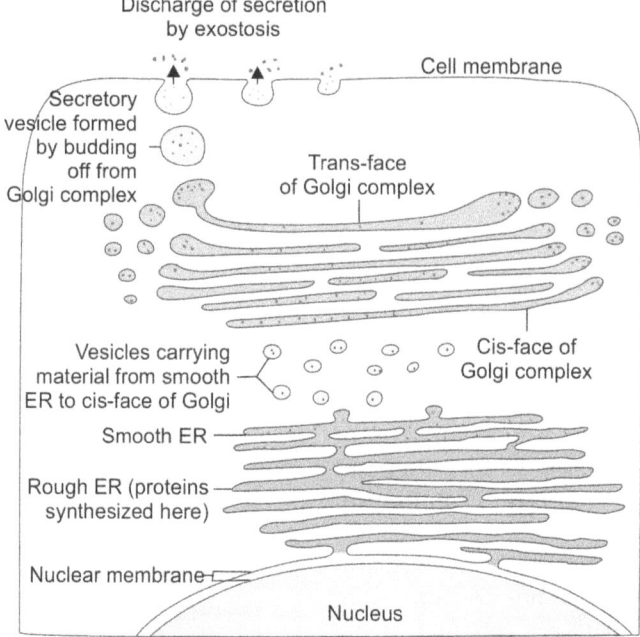

Fig. 4: Structure of endoplasmic reticulum.
(*Source:* GK Pal)

Wakefulness

- Wakefulness is a function of reticular activating system (RAS) in the brain stem
- RAS is a multisynaptic pathway projecting from brainstem to all areas of cerebral cortex. Therefore when stimulated, induces arousal and alertness
- RAS receives inputs from ascending sensory pathways and RAS inturn sends impulses to cerebral cortex and increases responsiveness to the sensory stimuli
- When the firing rate of RAS is decreased it results in sleep. When there is damage to RAS it results in coma.

Sleep

- There are two types of sleep—non-rapid eye movement sleep or NREM sleep or slow wave sleep and rapid eye movement sleep (REM) or paradoxical sleep.

Control of Sleep-wakefulness

- Sleep-wakefulness is regulated by circadian rhythm. The cycle happens in relation to the day-night variations. It is regulated through the retinohypothalamic pathway and suprachiasmatic nucleus in hypothalamus
- Pineal gland also plays a role in sleep-wakefulness. It secretes the hormone melatonin. Melatonin secretion varies with day-night cycle. It is secreted more in the evening and early part of night. Melatonin acts on neurons of RAS to mediate sleep-wake cycle
- There are sleep inducing areas in the brain like:
  - **In diencephalon:** Posterior hypothalamus, intralaminar and anterior thalamic nuclei.
  - **Medullary synchronizing zone:** Medullary reticular formation.
  - **Basal forebrain sleep zone:** Preoptic area and diagonal band of Broca.

  These areas when stimulated induce slow wave sleep
- Neurons in Pons and midbrain induce REM sleep
- There are neurotransmitters in the brain which are responsible for sleep and wakefulness

- **Neurotransmitters for wakefulness:** Serotonin, acetylcholine, histamine, catecholamines and adenosine antagonists like caffeine induce wakefulness
- **Neurotransmitters inducing sleep:** Adenosine, serotonin antagonists, prostaglandin D_2 and sleep peptides in brain.

Theories of Sleep

There are many theories put forward to explain the transition from wakefulness to sleep. They are:
- **Pavlov's theory** says sleep is a conditioned inhibition of brain activity
- **Cerebral ischemia:** Sleep may be due to cerebral ischemia. It can be explained by drowsiness following food intake as there is decreased cerebral blood flow after food intake
- **Biochemical theories:** It is based on action of various chemicals in the brain
  a. Lactic acid accumulation in brain during fatigue can induce sleep
  b. Hypnotoxin from brain can induce sleep
  c. Delta sleep inducing peptide released in the brain may induce sleep.

34. Mechanism of accommodation.
Refer answers to 2003 paper.

35. P-R interval.
Refer answers to 2011 paper.

36. Trichromatic theory of color vision.
- Trichromatic theory of colour vision was put forward by Young and Helmholtz
- According to this theory, it postulates that there are three types of cones with three types of photopigments and each one is maximally sensitive to one primary color (red, green and blue)
- The sensation of a color perceived is based on the frequency of impulses from each cone.

The cone pigments are:
- Red sensitive pigment or erythrolabe or long wavelength pigment. It absorbs light maximally in the yellow portion with a peak at 565 nm. The cones with these pigments are L cones
- Green sensitive pigment or chlorolabe or medium wavelength pigment, and is maximally sensitive in green portion and peaks at 535 nm. The cones with these pigments are M cones
- Blue sensitive pigment or cyanolabe or short wavelength pigment. It absorbs light maximally in the blue-violet portion and peaks at 440 nm. The cones with this pigment are S cones
- Blue, green and red are the primary colors, but cones with maximal sensitivity in yellow portion of the spectrum are sensitive in red portion and responds to red light at a lower threshold than green
- Based on Young-Helmholtz theory, for perceiving a color at least two cone types are needed
- The visual cortex compares the relative frequency of action potentials in the activated cone pathways and finds the wavelength and thereby identifies the color
- Change in intensity is appreciated by change in wavelength
- Gene for Rhodopsin is on chromosome 3 and gene for S cone pigment is on chromosome 7 and for green and red pigment it is on X chromosome.

37. Mean arterial pressure.
- Mean arterial pressure (MAP) is the average pressure in blood vessels throughout the cardiac cycle
- Duration of systole is less than diastolic phase and therefore MAP is not the average of systolic and diastolic pressures
- It is calculated as MAP = Diastolic pressure + 1/3 Pulse pressure
  = 80 + 1/3 × 40 = 93 mm Hg
- Normal MAP is 75 to 100 Hg.

Significance of MAP
- It is the pressure head which is responsible for the tissue perfusion.

38. Reward and punishment centers.
- When we do an act and if we are appreciated/rewarded we tend to repeat the act—motivation
- At the same time when an act has lead to punishment we tend to avoid the act

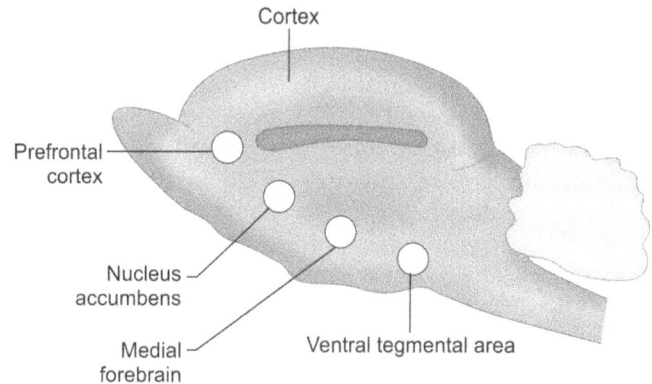

Fig. 5: Reward centers in brain. It extends from ventral tegmentum to nucleus accumbens.
(*Source:* GK Pal)

- There are reward and punishment centers in brain which decides our actions
- There are areas in the brain when electrically stimulated induces a pleasurable feeling and is said to be the **reward center**
- Certain areas when stimulated induce fear or terror—**punishment center**.

Reward Areas

- It consists of the dopaminergic pathway from the ventral tegmentum to nucleus accumbens
- Nucleus accumbens is the major reward center and dopamine is the major neurotransmitter
- This area is also responsible for addiction behaviors
- The other area is the medial band of tissue extending from frontal cortex through the hypothalamus to the midbrain tegmentum (refer Fig. 5).

Punishment/Avoidance Area

It includes the lateral portion of posterior hypothalamus, dorsal midbrain and entorhinal cortex.

39. Changes in cardiac output during exercise.

Refer answers to 2010 paper.

40. Surfactant.

Refer answers to 2008 paper.

MBBS Examination 2017

ANSWER ALL QUESTIONS

I. Essay Questions   (10 Marks each)
1. Define immuninty. How will you classify immunity? Explain in detail cell-mediated immunity.
2. Define blood pressure. Describe in detail short-term regulation of blood pressure. Add a note on hypertension.
3. Enumerate the hormones secreted by anterior pituitary gland. Discuss the actions and regulation of growth hormone.
4. Define hypoxia. Explain in detail the different types of hypoxia. Add a note on hyperbaric oxygen therapy.

II. Short Notes   (5 Marks each)
1. Primary active transport.
2. Excitation-contraction coupling.
3. Stages of deglutition.
4. Micturition reflex.
5. Hyperthyroidism.
6. Compliance.
7. Hypoxic hypoxia.
8. Pacemaker potential.
9. Stages of sleep.
10. Functions of cerebellum.
11. Role of helper T cells.
12. Action potential.
13. Juxtaglomerular apparatus.
14. Achalasia cardia.
15. Fetoplacental unit.
16. Conduction system of heart.
17. Special features of coronary circulation.
18. Vital capacity.
19. Functions of hypothalamus.
20. Properties of synapse.

III. Short Answers   (2 Marks each)
1. Positive feedback mechanism.
2. Rigor mortis.
3. Polycythemia.
4. Bombay blood group.
5. Tubuloglomerular feedback.
6. Functions of large intestine.
7. Migrating motor complex.
8. Diabetes insipidus.
9. Features of Cushing's syndrome.
10. Male contraception.
11. Triple response.
12. Bainbridge reflex.
13. Residual volume.
14. Artificial respiration.
15. Functions of middle ear.
16. Features of Parkinsonism.
17. Papez circuit.
18. Name two facilitatory and inhibitory neurotransmitters and their sites of action.
19. Saltatory conduction.
20. Senstions carried by posterior column.
21. Reticulocyte response.
22. Clot retraction.
23. Sodium potassium pump.
24. Name the muscle proteins. What is the role of Troponin C in muscle contraction?
25. Role of *H.pylori* in peptic ulcer.
26. Gastrocolic reflex.
27. Physiological basis of treatment of diarrhea.
28. Anion gap.
29. Radioimmunoassay.

30. List four differences between dwarfism and cretinism.
31. Reynold's number.
32. Jugular venous pulse.
33. Lead II ECG.
34. Bohr's effect.
35. Dead space.
36. Functions of somatosensory area.
37. Stretch reflex.
38. REM sleep.
39. Features of dark adaptation.
40. Stapedial reflex.

I. ESSAY QUESTIONS

1. **Define imuninty. How will you classify immunity? Explain in detail cell-mediated immunity.**

Immunity is the response the body develops when challenged by an antigen.
Two types of immunity are present:
1. Innate or non-specific immunity
2. Acquired or specific immunity.

Classification of Immunity

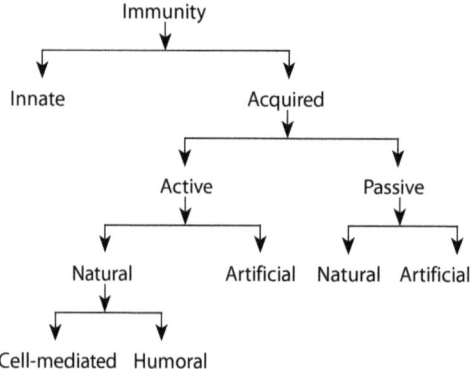

Refer answers to 2006 paper.

2. **Define blood pressure. Describe in detail short-term regulation of blood pressure. Add a note on hypertension.**

Blood Pressure and Regulation

Refer answers to 2010.

Hypertension

Refer answers to 2014 paper.

3. **Enumerate the hormones secreted by anterior pituitary gland. Discuss the actions and regulation of growth hormone.**

Refer answers to 2005 paper.

Regulation of Growth Hormone Secretion

- GH secretion is under the control of hypothalamus. There are two hypothalamic hormones regulating secretion of GH – Growth hormone releasing hormone (GRH) and Somatostatin (SS) which is GH inhibiting hormone (GIH). It undergoes fluctuations in children and young adults
- It is under negative feedback control. GH stimulates secretion of IGF-1 from liver which in turn inhibits secretion of GH and stimulates secretion of SS
- There are various factors which stimulate and inhibit secretion of GH (refer Fig. 1).

Factors Increasing Secretion of GH

1. Hypoglycemia
2. Increase in plasma levels of amino acids
3. Exercise, fasting
4. Stress, emotions
5. Glucagon
6. Puberty
7. Stage IV sleep

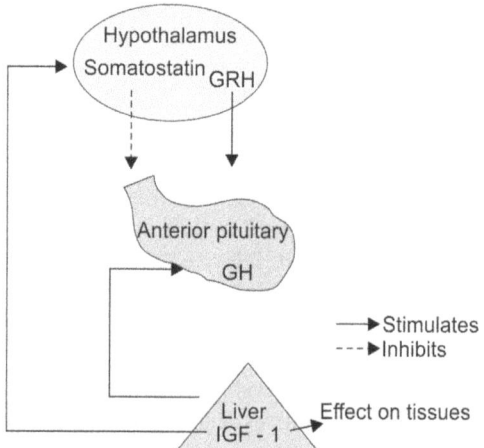

Fig. 1: Regulation of secretion of growth hormone.
(GRH: Growth hormone releasing hormone; GH: Growth hormone; IGF-1: Insulin like growth factor 1)

8. Enkephalins
9. Drugs like, L-Dopa, α receptor agonists
10. Hormones like estrogen, androgen.

Factors Inhibiting Secretion of GH
1. Increase in glucose
2. Increase in FFA
3. Hormones like—cortisol, GH
4. REM sleep
5. Medroxyprogesterone
6. Pregnancy.

4. Define hypoxia. Explain in detail the different types of hypoxia. Add a note on hyperbaric oxygen therapy.

Refer answers to 2006 paper.

Hyperbaric Oxygen
- It is administration of O_2 at high pressure
- Normal O_2 solubility in blood—0.003 mL/100 mL/mm Hg
- It can be increased to 6 mL/100 mL/mm Hg, when inspired PO_2 is 2000 mm Hg. This is possible when 100% O_2 is given at a pressure of 3 atm
- O_2 toxicity may appear when 100% O_2 is given at a pressure of 4 atm.

Indications
- CO poisoning
- Radiation-induced tissue injury
- Gas gangrene
- Very severe blood loss anemia
- Diabetic leg ulcers and other wounds those are slow to heal
- Decompression sickness
- Air embolism.

Symptoms of O_2 Toxicity
It is due to formation of Free radicals (like O_2^-, H_2O_2).
They oxidize PUFA and destroy the cellular enzymes.

Symptoms
- Nausea
- Irritability
- Dizziness
- Disorientation
- Muscle twitching
- Convulsions and in severe cases coma
- Congestion and irritation of airways → tracheo-bronchial secretions →↓ Surfactant → Pulmonary edema.

II. SHORT NOTES

1. Primary active transport.
Refer answers to 2013 paper.

2. Excitation-contraction coupling.
Refer answers to 2003 paper.

3. Stages of deglutition.
Refer answers to 2003 paper.

4. Micturition reflex.
Refer answers to 2006 paper.

5. Hyperthyroidism.

Causes
a. **Thyroid overactivity**
   - Graves' Disease
   - Solitary toxic adenoma
   - Toxic multinodular goiter
   - TSH secreting pituitary tumor
   - Thyroiditis
   - Mutations causing constitutive activation of TSH receptor.
b. **Extrathyroidal causes:**
   - Administration of T_3 and T_4
   - Ectopic thyroid tissue.

Grave's Disease
- Most common cause of hyperthyroidism (60–70%)
- It is an autoimmune disorder with activating antibodies (Ab) to TSH receptor
- More common in women.

Symptoms
Goiter is present.

Symptoms due to action of excess TH on tissues:
- BMR and body temperature ↑
- Heat intolerance
- Nervousness
- Heart rate is increased. Palpitations and fine tremors are present

- Muscle weakness
- Nervousness, irritability and anxiety
- Exaggeration of deep tendon reflexes
- Increased frequency of defecation
- Increased appetite
- Weight loss
- Moist, warm skin
- Bruit over thyroid gland
- Pretibial myxedema
- Fatigue
- Impotence in males
- Oligomenorrhea or amenorrhea in females.

Protrusion of eyeball or Exophthalmos is present only in Grave's disease and not in other types of hyperthyroidism.
- This is due to increase in retro-orbital contents
- Fibroblasts proliferate and develop into adipocytes, which have receptors for circulating TSH Ab → gets activated → release cytokines → inflammation and edema, leading to protrusion of eyeball.

Treatment of Hyperthyroidism

Treated with antithyroid drugs:
- Drugs acting by inhibiting iodide trapping: Monovalent anions like chlorate, pertechnetate, periodate, biiodate, nitrate, perchlorate and thiocyanate
- Drugs acting by inhibiting organification and coupling: Thiourylenes like propylthiouracil and methimazole
- Iodides: Large doses inhibit thyroid function.

6. Compliance.
Refer answers to 2003 paper.

7. Hypoxic hypoxia.
Refer answers to 2005 paper.

8. Pacemaker potential.
Refer answers to 2005 paper.

9. Stages of sleep.
Refer answers to 2014 paper.

10. Functions of cerebellum.
Refer answers to 2006 paper.

11. Role of helper T cells.
Refer answers to 2011 paper.

12. Action potential.
Refer answers to 2004 paper.

13. Juxtaglomerular apparatus.
Refer answers to 2009 paper.

14. Achalasia cardia.
Refer answers to 2008 paper.

15. Fetoplacental unit.
Refer answers to 2010 paper.

16. Conduction system of heart.
Refer answers to 2004 paper.

17. Special features of coronary circulation.
Refer answers to 2011 paper.

18. Vital capacity.
Refer answers to 2006 paper.

19. Functions of hypothalamus.
Refer answers to 2013 paper.

20. Properties of synapse.
Refer answers to 2013 paper.

III. SHORT ANSWERS

1. Positive feedback mechanism.
Refer answers to 2007 paper.

2. Rigor mortis.
Refer answers to 2011 paper.

3. Polycythemia.
Refer answers to 2014 paper.

4. Bombay blood group.
Antigens of ABO blood group systems are glycoproteins and glycolipids. They are attached to H antigen on the RBC membrane. H antigen is a product of H gene. If N-Galactosamine is attached to H antigen, A antigen is derived and the blood group is A. If galactose is attached to H antigen then B antigen is derived and the blood group is B. If both N-galactosamine and galactose are attached the blood group is AB and if only H antigen is present the blood group is O.

In few individuals there is absence of H antigen due to absence of H gene. If routine blood grouping is done, these individuals will be considered as having O blood group. But their serum will contain anti A, anti B and anti H antibodies. So they have to be transfused only with Bombay blood group.

5. Tubuloglomerular feedback.
Refer answers to 2008 paper.

6. Functions of large intestine.
Refer answers to 2008 paper.

7. Migrating motor complex.
Refer answers to 2008 paper.

8. Diabetes insipidus.
It is of two types—neurogenic or central diabetes insipidus (DI) and nephrogenic diabetes insipidus.
- **Neurogenic diabetes insipidus:** There is defect in synthesis of ADH from hypothalamus
- **Nephrogenic diabetic insipidus:** Here the synthesis and secretion of ADH is normal but there could be congenital defects of receptors to ADH or mutations of genes for Aquaporins and defects in aquaporins, the water channels on the luminal side of Principal cells of collecting duct.

Symptoms of DI are polyuria, polydipsia. They pass a large volume (upto 23 L/day) of hypotonic urine (30 mOsm/kg H_2O).

9. Features of Cushing's syndrome.
Refer answers to 2006 paper.

10. Male contraception.
Refer answers to 2004 paper.

11. Triple response.
Refer answers to 2009 paper.

12. Bainbridge reflex.
Refer answers to 2016 paper.

13. Residual volume.
It is the volume of air that remains in the lung after a forceful expiration. Normal value is 1200 mL in males and 1100 mL in females.

14. Artificial respiration.
Refer answers to 2004 paper.

15. Functions of middle ear.
Refer answers to 2003 paper.

16. Features of Parkinsonism.
Refer answers to 2005 paper.

17. Papez circuit.
Refer answers to 2015 paper.

18. Name two facilitatory and inhibitory neurotransmitters and their sites of action.
- **Facilitatory neurotransmitters:** Glutamate and aspartate
- **Inhibitory neurotransmitters:** Glycine and GABA
- Glutamate acts in the cerebral cortex and brainstem. Aspartate acts in the visual cortex
- Glycine is present in the neurons mediating direct inhibition in spinal cord, brainstem, forebrain and retina
- GABA acts in cerebellum, basal ganglia, cerebral cortex and neurons mediating presynaptic inhibition.

19. Saltatory conduction.
Refer answers to 2005 paper.

20. Senstions carried by posterior column.
Refer answers to 2012 paper.

21. Reticulocyte response.
It is the rapid increase and release of newly formed red blood cells and reticulocytes into the circulation following treatment for certain types of anemias like Vitamin B 12 deficiency or Iron deficiency anemias. Reticulocyte response indicates a favorable response to treatment with Vitamin B12 or Iron.

22. Clot retraction.
Refer answers to 2005 paper (Essay).

23. Sodium potassium pump.
Refer answers to 2011 and 12 papers.

24. Name the muscle proteins. What is the role of Troponin C in muscle contraction?
Refer answers to 2015 paper.

25. Role of *H.pylori* in peptic ulcer.
High acid content in the stomach can damage the gastric and duodenal mucosa and cause peptic ulcer. This is prevented by the presence of the 'Mucosal barrier'. This barrier is made up of:
- Mucus secreted by the neck cells and surface mucosal cells
- Prostaglandins secreted by epithelial cells have antisecretory activity (for HCl) and increases HCO_3 and mucus secretion
- Epithelial barrier: Low permeability due to tight juctions between epithelial cells of mucosa, rapid turnover of lining cells and HCO_3 and mucus secretions from there
- Bicarbonate secretion from gastric mucosal cells increases the pH.

When this barrier is disrupted it leads to peptic ulcer. *Helicobacter pylori* disrupts this barrier and thereby is responsible for inducing ulcer. This can be eradicated by giving appropriate antibiotics.

26. Gastrocolic reflex.
Intake of food → Distension of stomach with food → Contraction of rectum → Desire to defecate. This reflex is due to action of the hormone gastrin on colon. Because of this reflex, defecation after a meal is a regular activity for children. In adults, habits, cultural and social factors play a role in defecation.

27. Physiological basis of treatment of diarrhea.
- Diarrhea is treated with ORS (Oral rehydration solution). It helps to replace the salts and water lost. The solution contains a mixture of sodium and glucose
- Physiological basis of using such a combination is due to the presence of the secondary active transporter Sodium-glucose symport (SGLT 1) in the luminal membrane of the epithelial cells in the intestinal mucosa
- The presence of glucose in the intestinal lumen facilitates reabsorption of sodium through SGLT 1. This is the reason the ORS contains sodium and glucose
- Following absorption of sodium, water is also reabsorbed
- Cereals containing carbohydrates can also be used.

28. Anion gap.
Refer answers to 2012 paper.

29. Radioimmunoassay.
- It is a highly sensitive method to measure hormone levels in blood
- First step is to produce an antibody for the hormone to be tested
- Small quantity of antibody is mixed with the sample to be measured
- Some quantity of antibody is mixed with a standard hormone tagged with radioactive isotope
- There should be too little antibody for the tagged hormone and the hormone in the sample to be assayed to compete for binding sites in antibody
- After binding of both have reached equilibrium the antibody-hormone complex is seperated from the solution and the quantity of radioactive hormone bound is measured by radioactive techniques
- If large amount of radioactive hormone was bound it is known that the natural hormone levels are low in the assay sample and vice versa
- To make the test more quantitative, the same procedure is performed for standard solutions of untagged hormone at various concentrations and a standard curve is plotted
- By comparing the radioactive counts recorded from the unknown sample with the standard curve the concentration of hormone in the sample can be determined with an error of 10–15%.

30. List four differences between dwarfism and cretinism.
Refer answers to 2010 paper.

31. Reynold's number.
Refer answers to 2012 paper.

32. Jugular venous pulse.
Refer answers to 2009 paper.

33. Lead II ECG.
Refer answers to 2011 paper.

34. Bohr's effect.
Refer answers to 2009 paper.

35. Dead space.
Refer answers to 2013 paper.

36. Functions of somatosensory area.
Refer answers to 2007 paper.

37. Stretch reflex.
Refer answers to 2005 paper.

38. REM sleep.
Refer answers to 2009 paper.

39. Features of dark adaptation.
Refer answers to 2009 paper.

40. Stapedial reflex.
Refer answers to 2003 paper.

MBBS Examination 2018

ANSWER ALL QUESTIONS

I. Essay Questions (10 Marks each)
1. Expalin in detail synthesis, secretion and functions of thyroid hormone. Add a note on cretinism.
2. Describe the classification, connections and functions of cerebellum.
3. Define hemostasis. Describe the various stages involved in coagulation process.
4. Discuss in detail the neural regulation of respiration.

II. Short Notes (4 Marks each)
1. T lymphocyte.
2. Properties of smooth muscle.
3. Counter-current system in kidney.
4. Composition and functions of pancreatic juice.
5. Female contraception.
6. Triple response.
7. Non-respiratory functions of lungs.
8. Mechanism of receptor potential.
9. Factors regulating cardiac output.
10. Anatomic dead space.
11. Passive transport.
12. Gastric emptying.
13. Peculiarities of renal blood flow.
14. Second messengers.
15. Hypersecretion of growth hormone.
16. Ventricular action potential.
17. Tracts of Goll and Burdach.
18. Venous return.
19. Lung volumes and capacities.
20. Fetal circulation.

III. Short Answers (2 Marks each)
1. Mechanism of action of Botulinum toxin and the basis of Botox injection.
2. What is Steatorrhea?
3. List out four functions of liver.
4. Draw schematically how HCl is formed.
5. What are renal threshold and tubular maximum for glucose?
6. Give an example of neuroendocrine reflex. Briefly outline its pathway.
7. Name four hormones which increase blood glucose levels. What is the mechanism of action of one of this hormone?
8. Compare the actions of adrenaline and noradrenaline on heart and blood vessels.
9. Explain the mechanism of action of contraceptive pills.
10. How does temperature influence spermatogenesis?
11. Neuromuscular blockers.
12. Na^+- K^+ ATPase.
13. Endocytosis.
14. Fibrinolytic agents.
15. Cross matching.
16. Secretin.
17. Enteric nervous system.
18. Mention two substances used for measuring total body water and ECF volume.
19. Loop diuretics.
20. Neuroendocrine reflex.
21. The law of projection.
22. Types of hypoxia.
23. Antegrade amnesia.
24. Draw a normal electrocardiogram. What is Einthoven's triangle?
25. Respiratory exchange ratio.
26. Attenuation reflex.
27. Mean arterial pressure.
28. Reynold's number.

29. Astigmatism.
30. Functions of thalamus.
31. Clinical uses of ECG.
32. P_{50}.
33. Types of deafness.
34. Blood-brain barrier.
35. Anaphylactic shock.
36. Red-green blindness.
37. Reflex arc.
38. Primary taste sensations.
39. Functions of limbic system.
40. Physiological dead space.

I. ESSAY QUESTIONS

1. **Expalin in detail synthesis, secretion and functions of thyroid hormone. Add a note on cretinism.**

Refer answers to 2009 paper.

2. **Describe the classification, connections and functions of cerebellum.**

Refer answers to 2006 & 2009 papers.

3. **Define hemostasis. Describe the various stages involved in coagulation process.**

Refer answers to 2007 & 2008 papers.

4. **Discuss in detail the neural regulation of respiration.**

Refer answers to 2009 paper.

II. SHORT NOTES

1. **T lymphocyte.**

Refer answers to 2008 paper.

2. **Properties of smooth muscle.**

The properties of smooth muscles are classified as electrical and mechanical properties.

There are two types of smooth muscles; Single-unit or Visceral smooth muscles & Multi-unit smooth muscles.

The properties differ in these two types of muscles.

Electrical Properties

- The single-unit smooth muscles do not have a stable resting membrane potential, average potential being –50 mV.
- There are pacemaker cells among the single-unit muscles and are capable of generating action potentials by themselves.
- The pacemaker cells generate slow wave potentials which are slow sine-wave like fluctuations of few millivolts in magnitude and if they reach threshold, action potentials are fired either in the upstroke or downstroke of the waves.
- The smooth muscle action potentials are of either Spike potentials or Plateau potential as in cardiac muscle.
- Depolarisation is due to Ca^{++} influx and repolarisation is due to closure of Ca^{++} channels followed by K^+ efflux.
- The excitation-contraction coupling process is a very slow one in smooth musles as the muscle starts to contract 200msec after the start of the spike and 150 msec after the spike is over.

Mechanical Properties

- *Tone of muscle:* Visceral smooth muscles show slow wave potentials which is followed by continuous and iregualr contractions. This maintained state of contraction said to be the tone of muscles.
- *Length-tension relationship; Plasticity:* Smooth muscles exert variable tension at any given length. When a piece of visceral smooth muscle is stretched, initially the muscle exerts tension and when the stretch is maintained, the tension gradually decreases and may fall below initial tension. Therefore it is not possible to relate muscle length to tension developed and no resting length is assigned to smooth muscles. This property is said to be PLASTICITY of smooth muscles.

It is demonstrated in the muscle wall of urinary bladder. As the bladder gets filled there will be little increase in tension initially in the dertusor muscle then the tension decreases but as it reaches its capacity, the tension rises to a peak and the contracts forcefully and empties the urine.

3. Counter-current system in kidney.
Refer answers to 2003 & 2004 papers.

4. Composition and functions of pancreatic juice.
Refer answers to 2006 paper.

5. Female contraception.
Refer answers to 2004 paper.

6. Triple response.
Refer answers to 2006 paper.

7. Non-respiratory functions of lungs.
Refer answers to 2007 paper.

8. Mechanism of receptor potential.
Refer 2014 paper.
- When a weak stimulus is applied to a receptor, a local non-propagating depolarization potential is produced in the unmyelinated nerve terminal of the receptor (as in pacinian corpuscle). This is the receptor potential.
- If the stimulus intensity is increased, the amplitude of the receptor potential increases to reach a maximum and as it reaches a firing level, current sinks spread to the first node of ranvier and an action potential is fired here.
- In the receptor studied, the Pacinian corpuscle, the receptor or generator potential is produced due to opening of Na^+ channels leading to Na^+ influx.
- In many other receptors various types of stimuli cause opening of Na^+ channels and are responsible for the receptor potential.

9. Factors regulating cardiac output.
Refer answers to 2011 paper.

10. Anatomic dead space.
Refer answers to 2013 paper.

11. Passive transport.
Refer answers to 2009 paper (Short note – Transport across cell membrane).

12. Gastric emptying.
Refer answers to 2009 paper.

13. Peculiarities of renal blood flow.
- Rate of renal blood flow is 1200 mL/min or 400 mL/100 g of tissue per minute
- Renal O_2 consumption is highest next to the heart (6 mL/100 g/min)
- There is a regional difference in blood flow in the cortex and the medulla. Since the glomeruli, where filtration happens, lie in the cortex, cortical blood flow is high (5 mL/g/min) of kidney.
- Medullary interstitial osmolality needs to be maintained and therefore medullary blood flow is low (2.5 mL/g in outer medulla and 0.6 mL/g/min in inner medulla)
- O_2 extraction is less in the cortex (PO_2 is 50 mmHg) and more in the medulla (PO_2 is 15 mmHg). A-V O_2 difference is also less in the cortex and more in medulla.
- The vasculature is also different in the kidneys. The afferent arterioles break down into glomerular capillaries and they in turn reunite to form the efferent arteriole which again breaks down into peritubular capillaries or vasa recta. Renal circulation is therefore a type of portal circulation.
- The pressure in glomerular capillaries is higher than in any other systemic capillaries as the efferent arteriole is partially constricted than the afferent arteriole. Also the renal artery arises directly from the abdominal aorta.
- Autoregulation of renal blood flow is very well developed in the kidneys. This helps in regulating the GFR.

14. Second messengers.
These are intracellular messengers activated by the membrane bound protein/receptors in the target organs on which the peptide hormones act.

The peptide hormones are said to be the 'First messengers'.

These second messengers are activated through G proteins which are attached to the receptors on the cell membrane.

The general principle of second messenger activation is:

Binding of the hormone to its receptor on cell membrane
↓
Activates G Proteins and the membrane-bound enzymes

↓
Formation of second messengers
↓
Activation of Proteinkinase enzymes
↓
Phosphorylation of proteins
↓
Cellular response

The G proteins are - $G_s, G_i, G_q, G_{tl}, G_{13}$

The enzymes activated by G proteins are - Adenylyl cyclase, Guanylyl cyclase, Phospholipase C etc.

The second messengers are – cAMP, cGMP, Ca^{2+}, Inositol triphosphate (IP3), Diacylglycerol (DAG)etc.

Proteinkinases activated by second messengers are:

cAMP dependant kinases
cGMP dependant kinase
Proteinkinase C
Calmodulin dependant kinase
Tyrosine kinases

G proteins:

- G proteins are nucleotide regulatory proteins that bind to GTP.
- GTP is the guanosine analog of ATP.
- There are two types of G proteins – Small G proteins and Large G proteins.
- When signal reaches a G protein, the protein exchanges GDP for GTP and brings about the response. On completion of action, the intrinsic GTP ase activity of the protein converts GTP to GDP
- Large G Proteins couple cell surface receptors to catalytic units on the membrane that catalyzes formation of intracellular second messengers or couple receptors to ion channels.
- There are 3 subunits for the G Protein—α, β and γ (Ref. Fig 1).
- Only α Subunit is bound to GDP.
- On binding of the ligand to G-protein coupled receptor, GDP is exchanged for GTP and α subunit is seperated from β & γ subunits.
- The intrinsic GTPase activity of the α subunit converts GTP to GDP and the action is terminated.

Mechanism of action through G protein-coupled receptors: (Gs-adenylyl cyclase-cAMP pathway)

- Ligand (hormone) binds to the G_s protein coupled receptor
- On binding of ligand and receptor, α subunit of G protein seperates from β and γ subunits (Ref. Fig. 2)
- On seperation of α subunit, the catalytic enzyme – For example, adenylyl cyclase (Enzyme) attached to Gs protein is activated (Ref. Fig. 3).
- Adenylyl cyclase converts ATP to cAMP.
- cAMP activates the enzyme protein kinase A which phosphorylates proteins and brings about changes in the cell.

15. Hypersecretion of growth hormone.

Refer answers to 2014 paper.

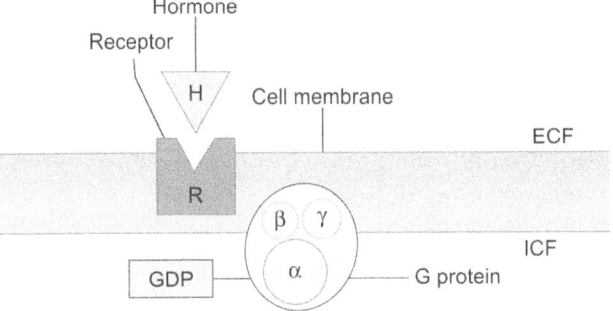

Fig. 1: G-Protein. Hormone binds to G-Protein bound receptor on the cell membrane; G Protein in inactive form is bound to GDP. There are 3 subunits for G-Protein—α, β, & γ.
(H: Hormone; R: Receptor)
(*Source:* GK Pal)

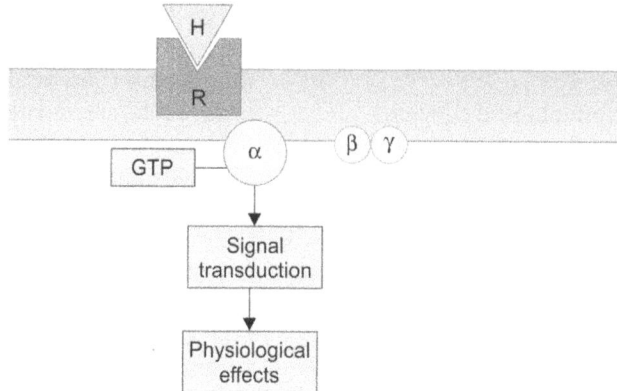

Fig. 2: On binding of hormone to G-Protein bound receptor activates G-Protein. α-Subunit seperates and G protein exchanges GDP for GTP. This induces series of actions and is responsible for hormone action.
(*Source:* GK Pal)

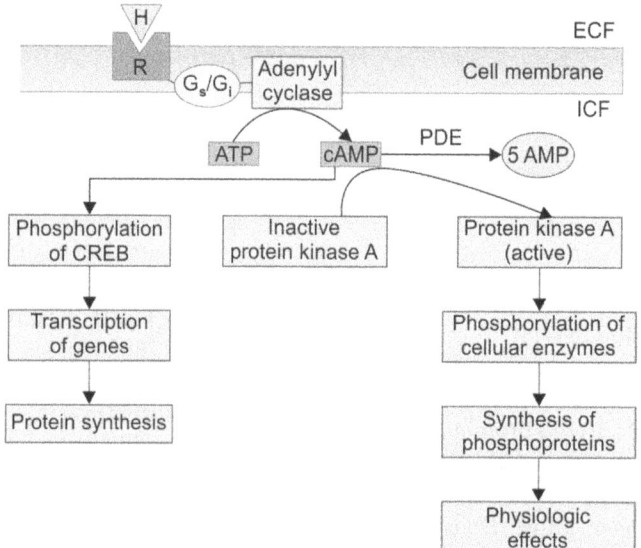

Fig. 3: Mechanism of hormone action through adenylyl cyclase-cAMP pathway.
(H: Hormone; R: Receptor; Gs/Gi: Stimulatory or inhibitory G Protein; PDE: Phosphodiesterase; CREB: cAMP-responsive element-binding protein).
(*Source:* GK Pal)

16. Ventricular action potential.

- The resting membrane potential (RMP) of ventricular muscle is –90 mV
- Following the stimulation from SA Node, through the conducting system, the ventricular myocyte, which is a fast muscle gets excited and it fires an action potential (AP).
- Following the electrical excitation (action potential) the ventricular muscle contracts.
- The ventricular AP has a rapid depolarisation followed by a small rapid repolarisation and a plateau phase (Ref Fig. 4).
- The plateau is followed by replorisation and it reaches the RMP
- The depolarisation is for 2 ms, plateau and repolarisation is for 200 ms or more. By this time the mechanical contraction is half over. So tetanization is not possible in cardiac muscle.

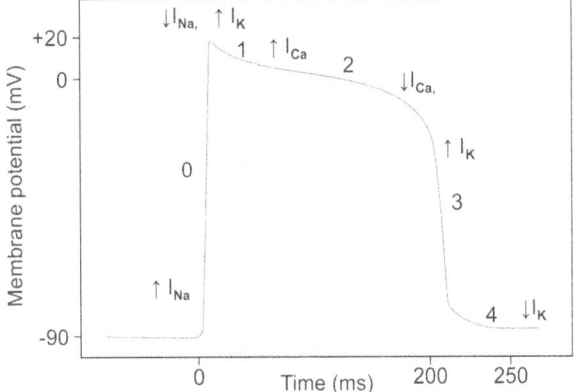

Fig. 4: Ventricular action potential.

Ionic Events Responsible for the AP

- The initial rapid depolarisation (Phase 0) is due to opening of Voltage-gated Na⁺ channels and rapid influx of Na⁺. The spike reaches a potential of +20 mV.
- This is followed by an initial rapid repolarisation (Phase 1) which is due to closure of the Na⁺ channels and opening of K⁺ channels and therefore K⁺ efflux (I_{TO}).
- Initial rapid repolarisation is followed by a plateau phase (Phase 2) due to influx of Ca²⁺ and efflux of K⁺. The calcium channel opening here is a slower Voltage-gated Ca²⁺ channel (L type channels).
- Final repolarisation (Phase 3) is due to closure of Ca²⁺ channels and opening of K⁺ channels (I_{KS}) and K⁺ efflux.
- Phase 4 is the phase of restoration of the RMP.

17. Tracts of Goll and Burdach.

Tracts of Posterior/Dorsal Column

- The posterior or dorsal column consists of the Tracts of Goll and Burdach
- They ascend up in two fasiculi – Fasciculus gracilis and Fasciculus cuneatus
- They are made up of large myelinated fibers which carry sensations like touch, pressure, vibration, stereognosis, Tactile localisation, Tactile discrimination and proprioception.
- Gracile fasciculus lies medially and carries these sensations from the hind limb and trunk, the cuneate fasciculus lies laterally and carries impulses from the upper half of the body and upper limbs.
- It is also called as the Lemniscal system
- First order neurons have their cell bodies in the dorsal root ganglia.
- The peripheral axons of these neurons are nerve fibers from the receptors.
- The central axons from the dorsal root ganglia enter the spinal cord and ascend up in the dorsal column as the dorsal column tract.
- Gracile and cuneate fasciculi reach medulla and synapse with ipsilateral Nucleus gracilus and nucleus cuneatus respectively. (Ref. Fig 5)
- From these nuclei, the second order neurons arise and cross to the opposite side and ascend up as the Medial lemniscus.
- Medial lemniscus terminate on the Venteroposterolateral nucleus (VPLN) of the opposite side thalamus.
- Third order neuron arises from the thalamus and terminates in the opposite Somatosensory area 1 (Broadman's are 3, 1, 2) in postcentral gyrus.

18. Venous return.

- Venous return (VR) is the amount of blood that returns to the right atrium from the periphery through Inferior vena cava and superior vena cava.
- VR decides the End diastolic volume (EDV) which in turn decides the stroke volume (SV).

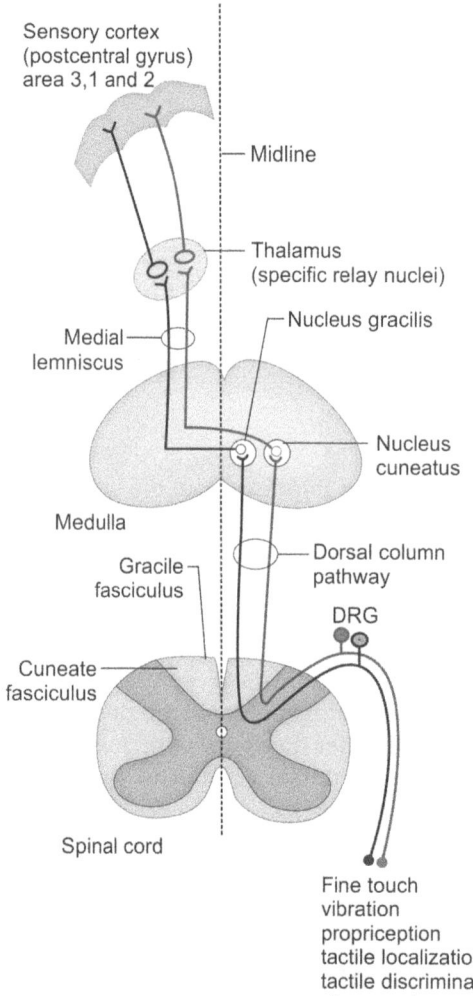

Fig. 5: Pathway of Dorsal column tract.
(DRG: Dorsal root ganglion)
(*Source:* GK Pal)

- SV decides the cardiac output and thereby the systolic blood pressure
- So factors affecting venous return will affect the cardiac output.

Venous return is dependent on:

a. **Skeletal muscle pump**: Contraction of limb muscles press on the veins and increases forward movement of blood in the veins and thereby increases VR.
b. **Thoracic pump**: Increase in respiration depresses the diaphragm and decreases intrathoracic pressure and thereby it acts like a suction force to increase VR.
c. **Abdominal pump**: During respiration compression of abdominal muscles press on the veins and favors venous emptying.
d. **Ventricular compliance**: Decrease in ventricular compliance decreases the ventricualr filling and thereby decreases EDV.
e. **Cardiac pump**: Vis A Tergo (Force from behind), Vis A Fronte (Force from front).
f. **Total blood volume**: As the blood volume increases VR increases and vice versa.
g. **Capacity of venous system**: Sympathetic stimulation to the veins causes venoconstriction and thereby increases venous emptying.
h. **Body position**: On standing there is venous pooling due to gravity and it may decrease the VR.

19. Lung volumes and capacities.

- Respiration is the process in which inspiration of atmospheric air is followed by equal volume of air expired out. The measure of quantities of air at different stages of respiration is given as lung volumes and capacities.
- Lung volumes are individual measures of air in the respiratory system at various stages and capacities are two or more volumes put together.
- Most of the lung volumes and capacities are measured with a Spirometer and the recording is said to be the Spirogram (Ref. Fig. 6). Residual volume and capacities which includes residual volume cannot be measured with spirometer.

Lung Volumes and Capacities

- Lung volumes are – Tidal volume (TV), Inspiratory reserve volume (IRV), Expiratory reserve volume (ERV) and Residual volume (RV)
- Lung capacities are – Inspiratory capacity (IC), Functional residual capacity (FRC), Vital capacity (VC) & Total lung capacity (TLC).

Tidal Volume

- It is the volume of air inspired or expired with each breath during normal breathing.

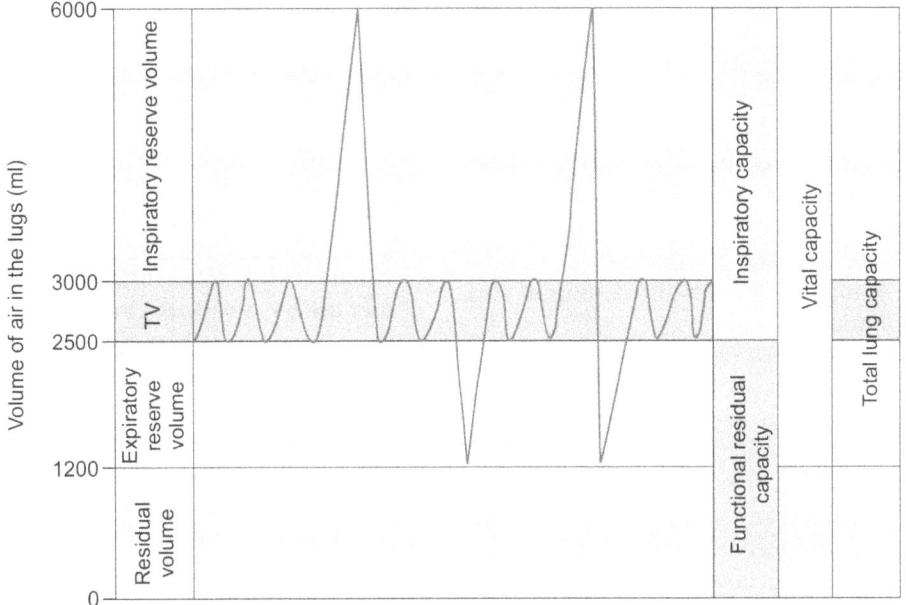

Fig. 6: Spirogram.
(TV: Tidal volume)

- Normal volume is 500 mL in adults.
- It is less in children and increases with age. It increases with exercise and muscular activity.

Inspiratory Reserve Volume

- It is the maximal volume of air inspired by forceful inspiration after a tidal inspiration.
- Normal vlaue is 3.3 L in males and 1.9 L in females.

Expiratory Reserve Volume

- It is the maximal volume of air exhaled from the resting end-expiratory level. (Volume expired by active expiration after passive expiration) 750–1000 mL.
- Normal value is 1 L in men and 700 mL in females.

Residual Volume

- It is the volume of air remaining in the lungs at the end of maximal expiration.
- Normally it is about 1200 mL in males and 1100 mL in females.
- Residual volume is the volume remaining in the lung even after forceful and complete expiration.
- This volume cannot be measured by spirometer.
- It can be measured by subtracting ERV from FRC and FRC is measured by Helium dilution technique.

Lung Capacities

Inspiratory Capacity

- It is the maximal volume of air inspired from resting expiratory level.
- Normal value is 3000–3500 ml IC= IRV + TV.

Functional Residual Capacity

- It is the volume of air remaining in the lungs at the end of resting (normal) expiration.
- Normal value – 2500 mL
- FRC = RV + ERV

Significance of FRC

- This volume of gas in the lungs helps in continuous exchange of gases even in between the breaths.
- It helps maintain a stable O_2 and CO_2 levels in the alveolus.

Measurement of FRC:
- FRC is measured by Helium dilution technique

Helium Dilution Technique
- The subject is made to breathe from a spirometer with a known volume of gas mixture with helium of known concentration.
- He is made to breathe from normal end expiration.
- The remaining volume of air in lungs at end expiration will be equal to FRC.
- If he breathes in after forced expiration RV can be measured.
- Now as the subject breathes through the spirometer many times, the FRC and the gas in spirometer and lung has equilibriated and have equal concentrations of helium. The new concentration of helium is measured and is said to be C2.
- Now the FRC is calculated by using the formula:
    - $C1 \times V1 = C2 \times V2$.
    - V1 - Initial volume of spirometer
    - C1 - Initial concentration of helium
    - V2 - Final volume of spirometer + FRC
    - C2 - Final concentration of helium
    - $V2 = V1 \times C1 / C2$
      $FRC = V2 - V1$
      $= V1 (C1 - C2)/C2$

Vital Capacity
- Maximum volume of gas completely expired from the lungs following a maximal inspiration.
- Normal value - 4800 mL (in males) and = 3200 mL (in females)
- VC = TLC - RV
  or VC = IRV + TV + ERV

Total Lung Capacity (TLC)

It is the total volume of air within the lung after maximum inspiration. It is the maximum volume of air that the lung can contain.
- Normal value - 6000 mL
  TLC = FVC + RV
  OR

TLC = RV + ERV + TV + IRV
- TLC is increased in airway narrowing with air trapping as in bronchial asthma.

20. Fetal circulation.
Refer answers to 2004 paper.

III. SHORT ANSWERS

1. **Mechanism of action of Botulinum toxin and the basis of Botox injection.**
- There are various drugs and toxins acting at the neuromuscular transmission and thereby affect muscle contraction.
- Botulinum toxin is derived from the bacteria *Clostridium botulinum*.
- There are various types in it – toxins A, B, C, D, F and G.
- Toxins B, D, F and G act on the synaptic membrane protein Synaptobrevin.
- Toxin C acts on another protein Syntaxin and toxins A & B act on the protein SNAP- 25.
- By inhibiting these proteins they prevent the release of neurotransmitter vesicle from presynaptic terminal.
- These toxins act at the neuromuscular junction and they inhibit the release of acetylcholine. This induces flaccid paralysis of the muscles.
- Botox produced from botulinum toxin is used to treat conditions involving muscle hyperactivity as in achalasia cardia to relieve the contraction of lower esophageal sphincter.
- It is also injected into facial muscles to relieve facial wrinkles.

2. **What is Steatorrhea?**
Refer answers to 2011 paper.

3. **List out four functions of liver.**
Refer answers to 2008 paper.

4. **Draw schematically how HCl is formed.**
Refer answers to 2005 paper.

5. **What are renal threshold and tubular maximum for glucose?**
- Transport maximum or Tubular maximum (Tm) is the maximum amount of the

solute that can be actively transported (reabsorbed or secreted) per minute by the renal tubules.
- Tm is the level at which the carrier, transporting the substance, gets saturated and beyond this level, the substances are no more reabsorbed or secreted.
- Therefore the amount of substance transported depends on the amount of the solute present in the tubular fluid upto the Tm for the solute.

Tubular Maximum for Glucose (TmG)
- The transporters in the epithelial cells of PCT used for reabsorption of glucose are SGLT2 and GLUT2 on apical and basolateral sides respectively.
- The transporter on reaching its Tm, does not reabsorb glucose anymore and it starts appearing in the urine.
- Tm for glucose in males is 375 mg/min and 300 mg/min in females.

Renal Threshold
- It is the concentration of a solute in plasma at or above which the substance starts appearing in the urine.
- Renal threshold for glucose should have been ideally 300 mg/dL (Threshold = TmG/GFR, so, 375 mg/min/125 mg/min = 300 mg/dL).
- But glucose starts appearing in urine when the plasma concentration reaches 200 mg/dL of arterial plasma and 180 mg/dL of venous plasma.
- This is because the TmG differs in different tubules and there is also difference in removal of glucose by the nephrons when the amount filtered is below TmG.

6. **Give an example of neuroendocrine reflex. Briefly outline its pathway.**

Refer answers to 2003 and 2004 papers.

7. **Name four hormones which increase blood glucose levels. What is the mechanism of action of one of this hormone?**

Hormones which increase blood glucose levels are:
- Glucagon
- Glucocorticoids
- Catecholamines
- Growth hormone
- Throid hormones

Mechanism of Action of Glucagon
- It increases blood glucose levels by various mechanisms like glycogenolysis and gluconeogenesis.
- In the liver it activates the enzyme phosphorylase and breaks down glycogen.
- Glycogenolysis is favoured by activating Phospholipase C and increase in cytoplasmic Ca^{2+} in the hepatocytes. It has no glycogenolytic action on muscles.
- It increases gluconeogenesis with the help of pyruvate, lactate, glycerol and amino acids.

8. **Compare the actions of adrenaline and noradrenaline on heart and blood vessels.**

- Adrenaline and Noradrenaline act on the heart and increase the force and rate of contraction.
- They mediate these actions through $\beta 1$ receptors.
- They also increase the myocardial excitability and therby increase the heart rate.
- They also decrease the AV nodal delay.
- Norepinephrine produces vasoconstriction in almost all blood vessels via $\alpha 1$ receptors.
- Adrenaline causes vasodilatation in blood vessels in skeletal muscles and liver via $\beta 2$ receptors.

9. **Explain the mechanism of action of contraceptive pills.**

Refer answers to 2005 paper.

10. **How does temperature influence spermatogenesis?**

Refer answers to 2015 paper.

11. Neuromuscular blockers.

Blockers of NMJ

Curare: It binds with the ACh receptors and prevents binding of ACh to their receptors. This blocks the neuromuscular transmission.

Bungarotoxin: This is acquired from snake venom. It also prevents impulse transmission by binding the Ach receptors

Succinycholine: They act just like ACh and make the muscle membrane depolarized. But the choline esterase does not have any effect on these substances and therefore the muscle is continuously depolarized and cannot be stimulated again. So it is called as depolarizing blockers.

Botulinum toxin: They are derived from the bacteria *Clostridium tetani* and it prevents release of ACh vesicles from terminal buttons and thereby causes flaccid paralysis.

Neostigmine and Physostigmine : They are reversible Acetylcholine esterase (ACHE) inhibitors. They compete with ACh and prevent the action ACHE and there is continuous action of ACh. It is used to treat diseases like myasthenia gravis.

Pesticides like Organophosphorous: They aslo act by inhibiting ACHE by binding to it and its action is irreversible. It is also present in nerve gases. This type of poisoning leads to respiratory muscle paralysis and death. It can be treated with atropine.

12. Na⁺- K⁺ ATPase.

Refer answers to 2011 paper.

13. Endocytosis.

It is the process by which substances are internalized within the cell. There are 3 types:
- Phagocytosis
- Pinocytosis
- Receptor mediated endocytosis.

Phagocytosis: Engulfing of solid substances (Cell eating) as that of micro-organisms by the neutrophils.

Pinocytosis: Engulfing the liquid components (Cell drinking).

Receptor-mediated endocytosis: Here the substances to be internalized get attached to a receptor protein present on the cell membrane and the whole complex is engulfed.

14. Fibrinolytic agents.

Refer answers to 2010 paper.

15. Cross matching.

- Cross matching is done before blood transfusion along with blood grouping.
- There are two types of cross matching – Major & Minor cross matching.
- *Major cross matching* – Here the donor's RBCs are mixed with the recipient's plasma and assessed for agglutination. The ABO agglutinogens on RBC membranes are highly antigenic and they may cause agglutination when transfused. So this test confirms the safety of transfusion.
- *Minor cross matching* – Here donor's plasma is mixed with recipient's RBCs. This is said to be minor because the plasma of donor will get diluted in recipient's plasma and not much reactions will be produced.

16. Secretin.

Refer answers to 2007 paper (Short note – Gastrointestinal hormones).

17. Enteric nervous system.

- It includes Submucosal and Myentric plexuses.
- Neurons of these plexuses are small interneurons that connect afferent and efferent neurons to smooth muscles, secretory cells and epithelial cells. They are involved in the local GI reflexes.
- Submucosal plexuses are present between the submucosal amd circular muscle layers. They are also called as Meissner's plexus. They regulate the secretory functions of the GIT.
- Myentric or Auerbach's plexus is present between the circular and longitudinal muscle layers in the wall of the gut. It regulates the movements of the GIT.
- They are highly connected to Sympathetic and parasympathetic nerves supplying the GIT and thereby modulate their actions.

- It is also called as the third division of ANS/Mini brain of the gut.
- Neurotransmitters here are – ACh, VIP, Serotonin, enkephalins, substance P, norepinephrine, GABA, ATP, NO and CO.

18. Mention two substances used for measuring total body water and ECF volume.

Substances used to measure total body water – Deutrium oxide and Aminopyrine.

Substances used to measure ECF volume – Inulin and Sucrose.

19. Loop diuretics.
Refer answers to 2016 paper.

20. Neuroendocrine reflex.
Refer answers to 2004 paper.

21. The law of projection.
Law of projection: This law codes the location of stimulus in perception. The law states that, along the pathway anywhere from the receptor to brain, wherever stimulated, the conscious sensation is referred to the location of receptor. This is one of the causes for PHANTOM LIMB phenomenon.

22. Types of hypoxia.
Refer answers to 2006 paper.

23. Antegrade amnesia.
- Amnesia is loss of memory. It could be retrograde or anterograde amnesia.
- Retrograde amnesia: Inability to recall previous events or known facts.
- Anterograde amnesia: Inability to learn new facts or acquire new memories. It is seen in lesion of hippocampus which leads to inability to form new long-term memories. They are able to learn things and retain for a very short period and they cannot convert it to long term memories.

24. Draw a normal electrocardiogram. What is Einthoven's triangle?
Refer answers to 2009 (ECG).
- Einthoven's triangle is an imaginery triangle drawn around the heart (Ref. Fig. 7).
- It is formed by the two arms and the left leg forming the apices of the triangle.
- The two apices at the upper part of the triangle represent the points at which the arms connect electrically with the fluid around the heart.
- The lower part of the apex is formed by the left leg connecting with body fluids.

There are three bipolar limb leads placed in the 3 apices of this triangle.
- **Lead I:** The negative terminal of the electrode is connected to the right arm and the positive terminal is connected to the left arm
- **Lead II:** To record in limb lead II, the negative terminal of the electrocardiograph is connected to the right arm and the positive terminal to left leg.
- **Lead III:** To record in limb lead III, the negative terminal is connected to the left arm and the left leg is connected to the positive terminal.

25. Respiratory exchange ratio.
- Respiratory exchange ratio (R) is the ratio of CO_2/O_2 at any given time whether equilibrium is reached or not.
- Respiratory Quotient (RQ) is the ratio of CO_2 produced to O_2 consumed in a steady state per unit of time.
- 'R' is affected by many factors other than metabolism. For example, during hyperventilation CO_2 is blown out and

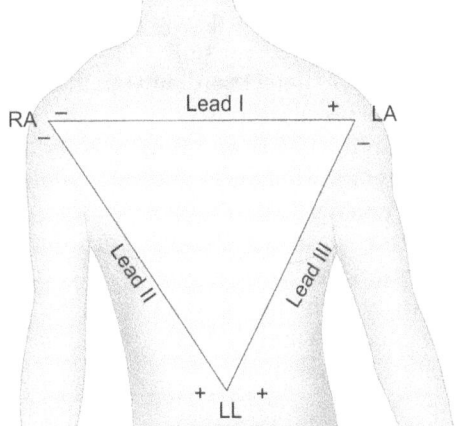

Fig. 7: Einthoven's triangle with placement of bipolar limb leads.
(*Source:* GK Pal)

therefore R rises. In severe exercise 'R' rises even to 2.0 as large amount of CO_2 is blown off, CO_2 is being produced from lactic acid by anerobic glycolysis.
- After exercise, when O_2 debt is being incurred 'R' falls to 0.5
- In metabolic acidosis, 'R' rises because there is a rise in expired CO_2 levels due to respiratory compensation.
- In metabolic alkalosis 'R' is decreased.

26. Attenuation reflex.

Refer answers to 2003 paper (Short note - Functions of middle ear).

27. Mean arterial pressure.

Refer answers to 2016 paper.

28. Reynold's number.

Refer answers to 2008 paper.

29. Astigmatism.

Refer answers to 2004 paper (Short note - Referactory errors of eye).

30. Functions of thalamus.

Refer answers to 2007 paper.

31. Clinical uses of ECG.

- It is used to calculate heart rate by using R-R interval
- It is used to detect conduction defects like arrhythmias and bundle branch blocks
- It is used to detect myocarial infarction and ischemia.
- It is used to analyze the cardiac vector
- It is used to detect electrolyte abnormalities
- It is used to detect cardiomyopathies and chamber hypertrophy
- Continuous ECG monitoring is used in theaters during surgeries and intensive care units.
- Holter monitor is an ambulatory continuous monitoring of electrical activity of the heart for 24 hours and the results are analysed later for abnorml electrical activities.

32. P_{50}.

Refer answers to 2013 paper.

33. Types of deafness.

There are two types of deafness. Conduction deafness and sensorineural deafness.

Conductive deafness: Impaired sound transmission in external or middle ear leading to deafness.
- Causes:
  i. Plugging of external auditory canal by wax or foreign body
  ii. Destruction of ossicles
  iii. Thickening of ear drum
  iv. Rigidity of attachment of stapes
  v. Otitis media
  vi. Blockage of pharyngotympanic tube

Neural deafness: It is due to damage to cochlea, hair cells or neural pathways.
- Causes:
  i. Aminoglycoside antibiotics obstruct mechanosensitive channels in stereocilia.
  ii. Damage to outer hair cells by exposure to prolonged noise.
  iii. Tumor in vestibulocochlear N & cerebellopontine angle.
  iv. Deafness due to mutation of genes.
  v. Degeneration of hair cells in old age
  vi. Meningitis – Viral and bacterial.

Test for deafness: The deafness and types of deafness can be assessed with tests like – Watch test, tuning fork tests and audiometry.

34. Blood-brain barrier.

Refer answers to 2009 paper.

35. Anaphylactic shock.

- Anaphylactic shock is a type of distributive shock. It is a warm shock. It develops due to a rapid and severe allergic reaction especially to an already sensitised antigen and when the person is re-exposed to it.
- The antigen-antibody reaction releases large amounts of histamine. Histamine leads to increased capillary permeability and loss of fluid into interstitial spaces, widespread venodilatation and thereby decrease in venous return and dilatation of arterioles and decrease in arterial pressure.

- All the above features decrease the venous return and cardiac output and may lead to a serious shock which may be fatal.
- This can be treated with sympathomimetic drugs like adrenaline and noradrenaline can be given to cause vasoconstriction and to prevent fluid loss.

36. Red-green blindness.

- Red-green blindness is a sex-linked disease and is the commonest type of colour blindness.
- It is an X-linked recessive disease and therefore males are affected and females act as carriers.
- The father with color blindness passes on this defect to his female children who are carriers and the daughters pass on the defect to half of the male children.
- Therefore this disease skips generations and appears in male children.
- This common occurrence of red-green blindness is due to arrangement of genes for green-sensitive and red-sensitive cone pigments on X chromosome.
- They are located near each other on the q arm of X chromosome and are prone for unequal homologous recombination during development of germ cells.
- This produces hybrid pigments with shifted sensitivities.

37. Reflex arc.

Refer answers to 2013 paper.

38. Primary taste sensations.

Sweet, sour, bitter, salt & Umami.

39. Functions of limbic system.

- It controls autonomic functions and thereby regulate visceral activities
- It has a role in olfaction
- Amygdala and piriform cortex are involved in sexual behavior
- Hippocampus is involved in learning and memory
- Connections with hypothalamus is involved in control of circadian rhythm
- It is the seat of emotions
- Reward and punishment centers are present in limbic system
- Behavioral responses are regulated by amygdaloid nucleus.
- Amygdaloid is responsible for discriminative feeding

40. Physiological dead space.

Refer answers to 2010 paper.

Topic-wise University Questions

1. GENERAL PHYSIOLOGY

Homeostasis

- Feedback mechanisms (2007)
- Milieu interior (2011)
- Negative feedback mechanism with example (2011)
- Positive feedback mechanism (2015, 2017)

Cell Physiology

- Intercellular connections (2004)
- Cytoskeleton (2007)
- GAP junction (2009)
- Endoplasmic reticulum (2016)
- Lipids in cell membrane (2010)
- Functions of mitochondria (2012)
- Apoptosis (2013)

Tissues

- Cells in fibrous tissue, their functions (2010)

Transport Across Cell Membrane

- Carrier-mediated transport (2005)
- A transport across cell membrane (2009, 2014)
- Secondary active transport (2011, 2014)
- Na^+-K^+ pump (2011, 2012, 2013, 2017, 2018)
- Facilitated diffusion (2013, 2016)
- Primary active transport (2013, 2017)
- Passive transport (2018)
- Endocytosis (2018)

Membrane Potentials

- Resting membrane potential (2011, 2015)

Body Fluids

- Determination of plasma volume (2005)
- Classify body fluid compartments, give their normal values, methods to determine ECF volume (2009)
- Measurement of total body water (2010)
- ECF volume and blood volume in a 70 kg adult male (2013)
- Concentration of Na^+ & K^+ in intracellular and extracellular fluids (2014)
- Two substances used to measure total body water and ECF volume (2018)

2. BLOOD

Composition and Functions of Blood

- Functions of blood (2007)

Plasma Proteins

- Types and functions of plasma proteins (2004, 2007, 2009, 2010, 2011, 2012, 2014)
- Albumin:Globulin ratio (2009)
- Functional categorization of plasma proteins (2010)
- Colloid oncotic pressure and its importance (2014)

Red Blood Cells

- Erythropoiesis—stages and regulation (2006, 2009, 2011, 2012, 2015, 2016)
- Significance of ESR (2009, 2010, 2012, 2015)
- Red cell indices (2015)

Hemoglobin

- Fate of hemoglobin (2006)
- Differences between adult hemoglobin and fetal hemoglobin (2008)

Anemia and Polycythemia

- Anemia (2014)

- Sickle cell anemia (2012)
- Types of polycythemia and its complications (2014, 2016, 2017)
- Reticulocyte response (2017)

WBCs

- Phagocytosis (2005, 2009, 2010, 2016)
- Functions of eosinophil (2008)
- Cytokines (2011)
- Opsonization (2012)
- Functions of different granulocytes in circulating blood (2014)
- Functions of macrophages (2014)
- Opsonins (2014)
- Tissue macrophage system (2014)
- Functions of lymphocytes (2015)

Lymph and Edema

- Formation and circulation of lymph (2009)
- Starling forces and edema (2010)
- Mechanism of edema in congestive heart failure (2013)
- Extracellular edema (2015)

Immunity

- Cell mediated immunity (2004, 2017)
- Humoral immunity (2005)
- Essay on immunity (2006, 2013, 2017)
- B Lymphocytes (2007, 2010)
- Physiological principles of tissue transplantation (2008)
- T Lymphocytes (2008, 2018)
- Formation and functions of immunoglobulins (2009, 2012)
- Plasma cells (2009)
- Autoimmune disease (2011, 2013)
- Helper cells (2011, 2017)
- Immunological memory (2012)
- Cells which express MHC II (2014)

Platelets

- Structure and functions of platelets (2004, 2008, 2012, 2014)
- Role of platelets in coagulation (2005))
- Thrombocyte (2006)
- Purpura (2009)

Hemostasis

- Mechanism of clotting by intrinsic pathway (2003, 2007, 2018)
- Extrinsic mechanism of coagulation (2005, 2008)
- Mechanism of coagulation (2011, 2013, 2015)
- Anticoagulants (2007, 2008, 2012, 2016)
- Hemophilia (2007, 2008, 2011, 2012, 2016)
- Heparin (2009)
- Fibrinolysis (2010, 2011, 2018)
- Role of Vitamin K in the body (2013)
- Vitamin K dependant coagulation factors (2013, 2014)
- Finding of tests of hemostasis in hemophilia (2014)
- Clot retraction (2017)

Blood Groups

- Erythroblastosis fetalis (2003, 2006, 2008, 2010, 2013)
- Blood groups (2007, 2010, 2013, 2015)
- Reactions due to incompatible blood transfusion, Autologous transfusion (2008)
- Indications of exchange transfusion (2009)
- Significance of Rh group (2009)
- Landsteiner's laws (2010)
- Kernicterus (2011)
- Rh blood group (2012, 2016)
- Rh status of mother, father and child for occurance of Rh incompatability (2013)
- Indications and complications of blood transfusion (2015)
- Bombay blood group (2017)
- Cross matching (2018)

3. NERVE MUSCLE PHYSIOLOGY

Nerve

- Nerve action potential (2004, 2005, 2007, 2017)
- Compound action potential (2016)
- Saltatory conduction in nerve fibers (2005, 2012, 2017)
- Chronaxie (2009, 2012, 2013, 2015)
- Rheobase (2009, 2015)

- Utilization time (2009)
- Refractory period (2009, 2014)
- Define all or none law, its application in skeletal and cardiac muscle (2015)
- Neuroglia (2004)
- Denervation hypersensitivity (2010)
- Classification of nerve fibers (2012)
- Role of myelin sheath in conduction of nerve impulse (2013, 2014)

Neuromuscular Junction

- Neuromuscular junction (2008, 2009, 2011, 2015, 2016)
- Myasthenia gravis (2005, 2008, 2009, 2011, 2012, 2014)
- Type of acetylcholine receptor on skeletal muscle and its function (2013)
- Neuromuscular blockers (2018)

Muscle Physiology

- Excitation-contraction coupling (2003, 2005, 2007, 2017)
- Structure of skeletal muscle (2006)
- Electron microscopic structure of skeletal muscle and molecular mechanism of muscle contraction (2011, 2012)
- Multiunit smooth muscle (2011)
- Sarcomere (2008, 2011)
- Rigor mortis (2009, 2011, 2017)
- Sliding filament hypothesis and cross-bridge cycling (2012)
- Isotonic and isometric contraction (2013, 2016)
- Motor unit (2013, 2014)
- Calcium transporters in membrane of sarcoplasmic reticulum (2013)
- Role of tropomyosin in muscle contraction (2013)
- Membrane transporters involved in clearance of cytoplasmic calcium (2014)
- Role of ATP in muscle relaxation (2014)
- Draw a schematic diagram of sarcomere and label the parts (2014)
- Name the muscle proteins. What is the role of troponin C in muscle contraction (2015, 2017)
- Plasticity of smooth muscle (2008)
- Properties of smooth muscles (2018)
- Differences between three types of muscles (2008)

4. GASTROINTESTINAL SYSTEM

Salivary Secretion

- Composition, regulation and functions of saliva (2003, 2005, 2008, 2009, 2011, 2013, 2014, 2016)
- Lingual lipase (2010)
- Enteric nervous system (2018)

Deglutition

- Deglutition (2003, 2004, 2006, 2007, 2009, 2010, 2014, 2015, 2016)

Esophagus and Applied Aspects

- Achalasia cardia (2008, 2017)

Stomach: Secretion and Motility

- Composition, mechanism and regulation of gastric secretion (2003, 2005, 2006, 2008, 2009, 2010, 2011, 2012, 2014, 2015, 2016, 2018)
- Experimental evidences for gastric secretion (2015)
- Gastric emptying (2009, 2013, 2018)
- Pathophysiology of peptic ulcer (2014, 2015)
- Role of *H.pylori* in peptic ulcer (2017)

Pancreatic Secretions

- Actions of pancreatic juice (2005)
- Composition, function and regulation of pancreatic secretion (2006, 2011, 2013, 2018)
- Enzymes of exocrine pancreas (2008, 2014)
- Intestinal phase of pancreatic secretion (2015)

Liver, Gallbladder and Bile Secretion

- Functions of liver and jaundice (2008, 2018)
- Components and functions of bile (2009)
- Enterohepatic circulation of bile (2009, 2013, 2014, 2016)

- Hepatic and gallbladder bile (2010)
- Cholelithiasis (2012)
- Functions of bile salts (2012)
- Composition of bile and physiological role of its components (2014)

Small Intestine: Secretion and Motility

- Succus entericus (2005, 2015)
- Movements of small intestine (2006, 2008, 2010, 2011, 2012, 2015)
- Migrating myoelectric complex (2008, 2017)
- APUD cells (2011)
- Law of intestine (2011, 2016)
- Counter-current blood flow in the villi (2012)
- Enterogastric reflex (2012)
- Peristaltic rush (2012)
- Peristalsis (2013)

Large Intestine: Secretions and Motility

- Functions of large intestine (2008, 2011, 2017)
- Dietary fiber (2009, 2011, 2015)
- Colonic movements (2010)
- Defecation (2010)
- Gastrocolic reflex (2017)
- Physiological basis of treatment of diarrhea (2017)

GI Hormones

- Gastrointestinal hormones (2007)
- Gastrin (2016)
- Secretin (2018)

Principles of Digestion and Absorption of Carbohydrates, Fats and Proteins and Applied Aspects

- Fat absorption (2007)
- Digestive proteases (2010)
- Transporters of amino acids in gut and kidneys (2010)
- Micelle formation (2010)
- Steatorrhea (2011, 2013, 2018)
- Digestion and absorption of fat (2013, 2016)
- Enzymes involved in fat digestion (2014)

5. RENAL SYSTEM

Introduction to Renal System and Functional Anatomy of Kidneys

- Functions of Juxtaglomerular apparatus (2009, 2013, 2017)
- Renin-angiotensin system (2015)
- Macula densa (2012)
- Non-excretory functions of kidneys (2014)
- Peculiarities of renal blood flow (2018)

Glomerular Filtration

- Definition, factors affecting and measurement of GFR (2003, 2011, 2013, 2014, 2016)
- Steps involved in formation of urine (2006)
- Glomerular filtration rate (2008, 2009)
- Autoregulation of GFR (2013, 2014)
- Clinical tests to assess GFR (2014)

Tubular Functions

- Tubular maximum for glucose (2008)
- Tubuloglomerular feedback (2008, 2012, 2017)
- Types of water absorption (2011)
- Aquaporins (2012)
- Transport maximum (2013)
- Renal glycosuria (2013)
- Proximal tubular events (2015)
- Tubular maximum and renal threshold for glucose (2018)

Concentration of Urine

- Counter-current excangers in kidney (2003, 2013, 2015)
- Mechanism of concentration of urine (2004)
- Concentration of urine (2007)
- Counter-current mechanism (2009, 2010, 2018)

Acidification of Urine

- Limiting pH of urine (2010)
- Renal contribution of pH regulation (2012)
- Anion gap (2012, 2017)
- Mechanism of generation of HCO_3^- in distal tubule (2013)

Kidney Function Tests

- Kidney function tests (2007)
- PAH clearance (2010)
- Inulin clearance (2012, 2015)

Diuresis and Diuretics

- Diuresis (2009)
- Osmotic diuresis (2013)
- Diuretics and their sites of action (2016)
- Loop diuretics (2018)

Dialysis

- Artificial kidney (2007, 2013)

Nerve Supply of Urinary Bladder, Cystometrogram, Micturition Reflex and Bladder Disorders

- Cystometrogram (2005, 2008, 2010, 2014)
- Nerve supply of urinary bladder and micturition reflex (2006, 2007, 2008, 2009, 2011, 2012, 2015, 2016)
- Abnormalities of micturition (2010)
- Atonic bladder (2014)

Skin

- Functions of skin (2006, 2014)
- Role of sweat glands in thermoregulation (2010)

6. ENDOCRINOLOGY

Introduction to Endocrinology and Second Messengers

- Negative feedback mechanism of hormone regulation (2005)
- Name the second messengers (2008, 2011, 2012)
- G protein (2012)
- G-Protein coupled receptors (2013)
- cAMP signalling pathway with an example (2014)
- Radioimmunoassay (2017)
- Second messengers (2018)

Hypothalamic Hormones

- Name the hormones of hypothalamus (2008, 2013)

Pituitary Hormones: Anterior and Posterior Pituitary Hormones

- Actions of growth hormone (2003, 2009)
- List the hormones of anterior pituitary, Mechanism of action of growth hormone, acromegaly (2005, 2017)
- Regulation of growth hormone secretion (2017)
- Milk ejection reflex (2003)
- Neuroendocrine reflex (2004, 2006, 2008, 2010, 2011, 2018)
- Mechanism of parturition (2005)
- Acromegaly (2008, 2013, 2014, 2015)
- Actions of prolactin (2008)
- List the hormones of pituitary gland (2009)
- Role of oxytocin in female reproduction (2009)
- Differences between cretinism and dwarfism (2010, 2017)
- Dwarf (2011, 2015)
- Name the hormones involved in growth (2011)
- Houssay animal (2011)
- Laron dwarf (2012)
- Progeria (2012)
- Oxytocin (2012)
- Somatomedins (2013, 2015)
- Functions of any one hormone of posterior pituitary (2014)
- Hypersecretion of growth hormone (2014, 2018)
- Diabetes insipidus (2015, 2017)

Thyroid Hormones

- Thyroid function tests (2003, 2012)
- Actions of thyroid hormones (2004)
- Myxedema (2005, 2009)
- Thyrotoxicosis (2006)
- Hypothyroidism (2007, 2009, 2015)
- Synthesis and functions of thyroid hormones (2009, 2013, 2015, 2016, 2018)
- Cretinism (2013, 2014, 2018)
- Regulation of thyroid hormones (2015)
- Action of thyroxine on CVS (2015)
- Hyperthyroidism (2017)

Adrenal Hormones

- Actions, regulation and applied aspects of glucocorticoids (2004, 2006, 2009, 2012, 2014, 2015)
- Metabolic actions of cortisol (2009)
- Cushing's syndrome (2006, 2015, 2017)
- Actions and regulation of secretion of aldosterone (2005, 2013)
- Adrenogenital syndrome (2006)
- Conn's syndrome (2009, 2012, 2013)
- Aldosterone escape (2009, 2011)
- Functions of adrenocortical hormones (2010)
- Permissive action (2012, 2014)
- Hormones of adrenal cortex (2013)
- Addison's disease (2013)
- Addisonian crisis (2016)
- Compare the actions of adrenaline and noradrenaline on heart and blood vessels (2018)

Endocrine Pancreas

- Mechanism of action of insulin (2005)
- Glucose homeostasis, GTT and diabetes mellitus (2007, 2013)
- Actions of insulin (2009)
- Name the hyperglycemic hormones, actions of hypoglycemic hormone, GTT, diabetes mellitus (2010, 2018)
- Glucagon (2011, 2018)
- Pathophysiology of diabetes mellitus (2011, 2012)
- Normal blood sugar levels, hormonal regulation of blood glucose levels (2012)
- Pancreatic C-peptide and its significance as a laboratory test (2013)
- Significance of glycosylated hemoglobin (2014, 2015)
- Control of insulin secretion (2016)

Calcium Regulating Hormones

- Actions and regulation of parathormone (2005, 2008, 2010, 2013)
- Calcitonin (2007)
- Regulation of serum calcium levels, (2008)
- Hormones involved in calcium regulation (2011, 2014)
- Calcitriol (2012)
- Tetany (2008, 2012, 2013)
- Normal blood calcium level (2013)
- Role of Vitamin D in calcium homeostasis (2014)

Bone Physiology

- Remodelling of bone tissue (2010)

Other Hormones

- Erythropoietin (2007, 2016)
- Leptin (2010)
- Atrial natriuretic peptide (2009)

7. REPRODUCTIVE SYSTEM

Sex Determination and Differentiation, Puberty and Menopause

- What is Turner's syndrome, give three features (2011)
- Puberty (2012)
- Menarche (2013)

Male Reproductive System

- Spermatogenesis (2006, 2011, 2013, 2014)
- Functions of Sertoli cells (2008, 2010, 2012, 2015)
- Composition of semen and its use as a diagnostic tool (2009, 2010)
- Blood-testis barrier (2009)
- Mullerian regression factor (2010)
- Cryptorchidism (2013)
- Influence of temperature on spermatogenesis (2015, 2018)
- Functions of prostate gland (2016)
- Testosterone (2003)

Female Reproductive System

Menstrual Cycle

- Ovarian cycle (2006)
- Menstrual cycle, hormonal regulation (2007, 2008, 2010, 2011, 2013, 2014)
- Ovulation (2008)
- Indicators of ovulation (2009, 2013, 2015)

- Corpus luteum (2008, 2009, 2013, 2014)
- LH surge (2013)

Ovarian Hormones
- Functions of estrogen (2009, 2016)
- Actions of relaxin and inhibin (2010, 2016)
- Effect of estrogen on uterine endometrium (2015)

Pregnancy
- Pregnancy tests (2007, 2009)
- Immunological tests for pregnancy (2010)
- Parturition (2013)

Placenta and Lactation
- Functions of placenta (2009, 2010, 2011, 2012)
- Fetoplacental unit (2010, 2011, 2015, 2017)
- Placental hormones (2012, 2013, 2015)
- Lactation
- Describe hormones acting on breast (2006)
- Why are ovarian cycles suppressed during lactation? (2013)

Contraception
- Contraceptives (2004, 2013)
- Female contraceptive methods (2005, 2007, 2018)
- Pills (2012)
- Contraception in males (2014, 2017)
- Oral contraceptives (2015, 2018)

8. CARDIOVASCULAR SYSTEM

Properties of Cardiac Muscle
- Pacemaker potential (2008, 2009, 2012, 2013, 2015, 2017)
- List the properties of cardiac muscle (2011)
- SA node as pacemaker (2013)
- List the calcium transporters on the sarcoplasmic reticulum membrane in ventricular muscle (2013)
- Autorhythmicity of heart (2016)
- Ventricular action potential (2018)

Conducting System of Heart
- Origin and spread of cardiac impulse (2004, 2007, 2015, 2017)
- Excitation-contraction coupling in cardiac muscle (2010)
- Structure and function of conducting system of heart (2011)
- AV nodal delay (2015)

Electrocardiogram
- Draw an ECG, cause for each wave (2005, 2007, 2009, 2018)
- ECG changes in abnormal conditions (2007)
- ECG leads (2007)
- Kirchhoff's law & Einthoven's law (2010, 2016)
- Unipolar limb leads (2010)
- Normal ECG in lead II (2011, 2012, 2014, 2017)
- PR interval (2012, 2013, 2016)
- J Point (2012)
- Extrasystole (2012)
- 3 Bipolar limb leads of ECG, significance of PR segment and ST segment in ECG (2014)
- What is myocardial infarction? State one ECG change in this condition (2014)
- What is Einthoven's triangle? (2018)

Cardiac Cycle and Heart Sounds
- Define cardiac cycle (2005, 2007, 2009, 2013, 2014, 2016)
- Pressure-volume changes in left ventricle, left atrium and aorta in cardiac cycle (2005, 2007, 2009, 2013, 2014)
- Second heart sound (2005)
- Heart sounds (2006, 2007, 2009, 2012, 2013, 2014, 2015)
- Phonocardiogram (2008)
- Events of cardiac cycle (2016)

Cardiac Output
- Preload and afterload in the heart (2010)
- Cardiac index (2010, 2013)
- Define cardiac output, factors regulating cardiac output (2011, 2012, 2013, 2015, 2018)
- Fick's principle (2011)
- State Frank-Starling's law of heart (2011, 2012, 2013)
- Cardiac reserve (2012, 2015)

- Methods of determining cardiac output (2012, 2013)
- Significance of ejection fraction in ventricular function (2012, 2015)
- End diastolic volume (2013)
- Discuss the terms cardiac output and Total peripheral resistance and discuss their determinants (2014)
- Define preload and state its effects on cardiac function (2014)
- Venous return (2018)

Arterial and Venous Pulse

- Labelled diagram of arterial pulse and explain (2009)
- Jugular venous pulse (2009, 2017)
- Tracing of arterial pulse (2010)
- Dicrotic notch (2012)

Vascular System

- Windkessel effect (2008, 2013)
- Endothelins (2010)

Hemodynamics of Circulation

- Total peripheral resistance in vascular system (2003)
- Reynold's number (2008, 2010, 2012, 2017, 2018)

Blood Pressure and Hypertension

- Define blood pressure, give normal values (2003, 2006, 2008, 2013, 2014, 2017)
- Nervous regulation of blood pressure (2008)
- Baroreceptor mechanism of regulation of blood pressure (2003, 2007, 2014, 2015)
- Humoral regulation of BP (2004)
- Regulation of blood pressure (2006, 2013)
- Korotkov's sounds (2007, 2014)
- Short term and long term regulation of blood pressure (2010, 2017)
- Neurogenic hypertension (2010)
- List short term regulation of blood pressure (2011)
- Determinants of blood pressure (2013, 2014, 2015)
- Add a note on hypertension (2014, 2017)
- Bain-bridge reflex (2016, 2017)
- Mean arterial pressure (2016, 2018)

Special Circulation

- Fetal circulation (2004, 2018)
- Regulation of coronary circulation (2005, 2008, 2011)
- Special features of coronary circulation (2011, 2017)
- Triple response (2006, 2009, 2010, 2017, 2018)
- Blood-brain barrier (2009, 2018)
- Phasic changes in coronary circulation (2012, 2015)
- Splanchnic circulation (2015)
- Cerebral circulation (2010)
- Monro-Kellie doctrine law (2011)

Pathophysiology of Shock

- Non-progressive shock (2012)
- Hypovolemic shock (2012)
- List the types of shock (2014)
- Features of shock (2015)
- Anaphylactic shock (2018)

Heart Failure

- Heart failure (2008)

Others

- Anti G suit (2009)
- Effects of positive 'g' (2015)

9. RESPIRATORY SYSTEM

Functional Anatomy of Respiratory System

- Non-respiratory functions of lungs (2007, 2011, 2018)

Mechanics of Breathing

- Compliance of lungs (2003, 2009, 2011, 2017)
- Mechanics of pulmonary ventilation (2007)
- Surfactant (2008, 2009, 2013, 2015, 2016)
- Physiological dead space (2010, 2018)
- Respiratory distress syndrome (2010)
- Intrapleural pressure (2011)
- Dead space and its normal value (2011, 2013, 2014, 2017)
- Anatomic dead space (2018)
- Muscles of inspiration (2013)

- Muscle actions responsible for a) Normal expiration b) Forced expiration (2014)
- Transpulmonary pressure (2016)

Lung Volumes and Capacities

- Definition and measurement of functional residual capacity (2005, 2011, 2013)
- Clinical importance of FRC (2011)
- Maximum breathing capacity (2005)
- Timed vital capacity (2007, 2012)
- FEV1 (2012)
- Peak expiratory flow rate (2015)
- Vital capacity (2017)
- Residual volume (2017)
- Lung volumes and capacities (2018)

Diffusion of Gases

- Diagram of alveolo-capillary membrane and write the thickness of it (2011)
- Respiratory membrane (2013)

Pulmonary Circulation and V/Q Ratio

- Pecularities of pulmonary circulation (2009)
- Ventilation/perfusion ratio (2012)

Transport of Gases

- Oxygen transport (2004, 2012, 2016)
- Fetal hemoglobin (2016)
- Oxygen-dissociation curve (2004, 2007, 2012, 2014, 2016)
- Double Bohr Effect (2011)
- Chloride shift (2005, 2008, 2009, 2013)
- Haldane's effect (2008)
- Bohr's effect and its significance (2009, 2010, 2012, 2017)
- CO_2 transport (2010, 2011, 2013)
- P_{50} (2013, 2018)
- What is the effect of 2,3 DPG on Oxy-Hb dissociation curve? Does it help in loading or unloading of oxygen? (2013)
- Oxygen carrying capacity of blood (2014)
- Respiratory exchange ratio (2018)

Regulation of Respiration

- Chemoreceptors (2005, 2010)
- Chemical regulation of respiration (2005, 2009, 2012, 2013, 2014, 2015)
- Neural regulation of respiration (2007, 2009, 2013, 2014, 2018)
- Who discovered J receptors? What is its physiological significance? (2011)
- Pneumotaxic center (2012)
- Hering-Breuer inflation reflex (2012, 2014, 2016)
- Respiratory failure (2014)
- Hypoxic vasoconstriction - Where does it occur and what are its complications? (2014)

Hypoxia

- Hypoxic hypoxia (2005, 2017)
- Hypoxia (2006, 2007, 2013, 2014)
- Treatment for hypoxia (2007)
- Define histotoxic hypoxia with an example (2011)
- Types of hypoxia (2018)
- Oxygen toxicity (2015)
- Hyperbaric oxygen therapy (2017)

High Altitude Physiology

- Acclimatization to high altitude (2003, 2015)

Deep Sea Physiology

- Decompression sickness/Dysbarism/Caisson's disease (2005, 2006, 2008, 2009, 2010, 2011, 2012, 2013, 2015, 2016)
- SCUBA diving (2010, 2011)
- Nitrogen narcosis (2015)

Abnormal Respirations

- Stages of asphyxia (2005, 2012)
- Cheyne-Stokes respiration (2005)
- Periodic breathing (2009, 2015)

Pulmonary Function Tests

- Spirogram (2006)
- Name two pulmonary function tests to detect obstructive pulmonary disease (2014)

Artificial Respiration

- Artificial respiration (2004, 2008, 2011, 2015, 2017)

10. NERVOUS SYSTEM

Synapse and Neurotransmitters

- Acetylcholine (2009)
- What is summation? Mention its types (2011, 2012, 2013)
- What are cholinergic and adrenergic receptors? (2011)
- Dopamine (2012)
- Define synapse and describe its properties (2013, 2017)
- Name the facilitatory and inhibitory neurotransmitters and their sites of actions (2017)
- Mechanism of action of Botulinum toxin and basis of Botox (2018)

Sensory System: Sensory Modalities, Sensory Cortex

- Sensory cortex (2003)
- Bell-Magendie law (2011, 2012)
- What is stereognosis? Where is its center? (2011)
- Functions of somatosensory area (2017)

Receptors

- Classification of receptors and their properties (2006)
- Phantom limb (2009)
- What are mechanoreceptors? Give an example. (2011)
- Receptor potential (2014)
- Mechanism of receptor potential (2018)
- Law of projection (2018)

Ascending Pathways

- Enumerate the ascending pathways (2009, 2012)
- Anterior spinothalamic tract (2010)
- Discuss the posterior column with a diagram (2012)
- Name of tracts made up by second order neurons in the pathway for—fine touch and pain (2013)
- Trace the pathway for perception of fine touch (2014)
- Tracts of Goll and Burdach (2018)
- Draw the diagram of crude touch pathway and label it (2014)
- Sensations carried by posterior column (2017)

Pain

- Visceral pain (2003)
- Endorphins (2005)
- Referred pain and its theories (2006, 2009, 2011, 2013, 2015)
- Brown-Sequard syndrome (2008, 2009, 2011, 2012, 2014)
- Pathway for pain (2009, 2012, 2013)
- Classify pain (2012)
- Receptors for pain (2012)
- Analgesic system in the pain (2012, 2013, 2015)
- Gating of pain (2013)
- Endogenous opioid peptides (2014)

Motor System: Motor cortex

- Motor homunculus (2014)

Reflexes: Classification, Stretch Reflex

- Stretch reflex (2005, 2017)
- Reciprocal inhibition (2005)
- Clinical classification of receptors with example and its significance (2006)
- Sneezing reflex (2010)
- Reciprocal inhibition (2010)
- Inverse stretch reflex (2010)
- Reflex arc (2013, 2018)
- Mass reflex (2015)
- Properties of reflex (2015)
- Golgi tendon reflex (2016)

Muscle Spindle and Golgi Tendon

- Structure and functions of muscle spindle (2005)
- Causes of muscle tone (2010)
- Physiological roles of muscle spindle (2013)
- Define muscle tone and discuss the phenomenon responsible for it, What conditions lead to alteration of tone (2014)

Descending Tracts: Pyramidal and Extra-pyramidal Tracts

- Name the descending tracts (2006, 2008)
- Describe corticospinal tract and effect of lesions at various levels (2006, 2008, 2015)

- Differences between UMN and LMN lesions (2006, 2015)
- Babinski sign (2008, 2015)
- Differences between spasticity and rigidity (2011)
- Cogwheel rigidity (2012)
- Conditions where plantar reflex is 'extensor' (2014)

Regulation of Posture and Movement
- Righting reflexes (2003, 2013)
- Decerebrate rigidity (2006, 2011, 2013)
- Postural reflexes (2010)
- Spinal animal (2010)

Thalamus
- Functions of thalamus (2007, 2008, 2011, 2013, 2018)
- Thalamic syndrome (2010, 2013)

Basal Ganglia
- Basal ganglia (2005)
- Connections and functions of basal ganglia, clinical disorders and physiological basis of treatment (2007, 2009, 2013)
- Parkinson's disease (2005, 2007, 2009, 2012, 2014, 2017)
- Functions of paleostriatum (2010)
- Putamen circuit of basal ganglia (2016)

Cerebellum
- Connections and functions of cerebellum (2006, 2008, 2011, 2017, 2018)
- Clinical features of cerebellar lesion (2007, 2011, 2013, 2014)
- Climbing, mossy and parallel fibers (2010)
- Functional divisions of cerebellum (2011)
- Role of Purkinje cells of cerebellum (2012)
- Vestibulocerebellum (2013)
- Functions and tests of cerebellum (2014)

Vestibular Apparatus
- Otolith organ: Mechanism of action and functions (2005, 2011)
- Functions of vestibular apparatus (2009)
- Receptors for vestibular sensation (2013)
- Components of vestibular apparatus (2014)
- Functions of utricle and saccule (2016)

Hypothalamus
- Hypothalamic thermostat (2005)
- Nuclei, connections and functions of hypothalamus (2009, 2007, 2008, 2013, 2015, 2017)
- Endogenous pyrogens (2010)
- Brown fat tissue (2010)
- Fever (2012)
- Heat loss mechanisms (2013)
- Control of food intake (2003, 2010)
- Role of hypothalamus in hunger perception (2005)
- Name the nuclei responsible for hunger and satiety in human beings (2013)

Limbic System
- Functions of limbic system (2004, 2018)
- Papez circuit (2015, 2017)
- Reward and punishment centers (2016)

EEG and Sleep
- Berger's rhythm (2006, 2008 (EEG), 2012, 2016)
- EEG changes during sleep (2007)
- Alpha block (2008, 2011)
- Compare REM and NREM sleep (2009, 2015)
- Rapid eye movement sleep (2009, 2011, 2017)
- Clinical significance of EEG (2009)
- Induction of sleep (2010)
- Delta waves in EEG (2011)
- Stages of sleep (2014, 2017)
- Sleep-wake theory (2016)

Reticular Formation
- Four functions of reticular activating system (2011)
- Functions of ascending reticular activating system (2012, 2014)

Learning and Memory
- Associative learning (2003)
- Mechanism of memory (2004)
- Conditioned reflex (2008, 2015)

- Consolidation of memory (2010)
- Types of memory (2013)
- Operant conditioning (2014)
- Anterograde amnesia (2018)

Language and Sleep

- Wernicke's aphasia (2009)
- Broca's area (2010)
- Anomic aphasia (2012)
- Physiology of speech (2013)
- Aphasia (2014)
- Fluent aphasia (2014)
- Wernicke's and global aphasia (2016)

Cerebral Cortex

- Functions of parietal lobe (2007)
- Cerebral circulation (2010)
- Functions of prefrontal lobe (2011, 2013)
- Functions of frontal lobe (2011)
- Betz cells (2012)
- Homunculus (2012)
- Kluver-Bucy syndrome (2013)
- Connections and functions of temporal lobe (2016)

Cerebrospinal Fluid

- Describe formation, circulation and functions of CSF (2009, 2010, 2012, 2013, 2014, 2015)

11. SPECIAL SENSES

Vision

- Accommodation for near vision (2003, 2005, 2015, 2016, 2016)
- Visual pathway and lesions (2004, 2007, 2008, 2009, 2014, 2015)
- Refractory errors of eye (2004, 2006, 2008, 2011, 2012, 2013, 2014)
- Dark adaptation (2005, 2009, 2010, 2011, 2013, 2015, 2017)
- Color vision (2005, 2010, 2011)
- Aqueous humor (2006, 2008, 2010)
- Color blindness (2007)
- Defect in astigmatism and correction (2009, 2010, 2012, 2013, 2018)
- Pupillary light reflex (2009)
- Draw the structure of rods and cones (2011)
- Ocular dominance columns (2012)
- Perimetry (2013)
- Photochemical mechanism of vision (2013)
- Visual field defect when the optic chiasma is cut in the middle (2013)
- What is 'Blind spot'? (2013)
- Presbyopia (2016)
- Trichromatic theory of color vision (2016)
- Red-green blindness (2018)

Hearing

- Functions of middle ear (2003, 2005, 2007, 2007, 2012, 2013, 2014, 2015, 2017)
- Structure of middle ear (2005, 2009)
- Cochlea (2004)
- Cochlear microphonic potentials (2006)
- Travelling wave theory (2008, 2012)
- Rinne's test (2008)
- Organ of Corti (2009)
- Elucidate how pressure vibrations are perceived as sound (2010)
- Explain auditory pathway with neat diagram (2009, 2015)
- Note on conductive deafness (2010)
- Theories of hearing (2010, 2011)
- What is Endocochlear potential? (2011, 2016)
- Attenuation reflex/Stapedial reflex (2013, 2014, 2017, 2018)
- Region of the cochlea which vibrates most for the highest sound frequency in the audible range. (2013)
- Discuss the phenomenon by which sound waves in air induce action potentials in the cochlear nerve (2014)
- Finding in Weber's test in conduction deafness of the left ear (2014)
- Impedence matching (2015)
- Types of deafness (2018)

Taste

- Pathway (2005, 2008, 2010, 2011, 2012, 2014)
- Labelled diagram for taste pathway (2009)

- Gustatory receptors (2010, 2016)
- Primary taste sensations (2018)

12. EXERCISE PHYSIOLOGY

- Respiratory changes during moderate exercise (2004)
- VO_2 max (2008, 2015)
- O_2 debt (2009, 2015)
- Types of muscular exercises. Discuss various physiological changes occurring during and after exercise (2010)
- Changes in cardiac output in exercise (2016)

EU GSPR Authorised Reprsentative
Logos Europe, 9 rue Nicolas Poussin
1700, La Rochelle, France
Phone: +33 (0) 6 67 93 73 78
E-mail: contact@logoseurope.eu

www.ingramcontent.com/pod-product-compliance
Ingram Content Group UK Ltd.
Pitfield, Milton Keynes, MK11 3LW, UK
UKHW051249180426
11947UKWH00020B/1611